Kathn

MW00787876

DOING CBT

Doing CBT

A Comprehensive Guide to Working with Behaviors, Thoughts, and Emotions

DAVID F. TOLIN

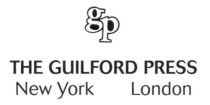

THE GUILFORD PRESS

New York   London

Copyright © 2016 The Guilford Press
A Division of Guilford Publications, Inc.
370 Seventh Avenue, Suite 1200, New York, NY 10001
www.guilford.com

All rights reserved

Except as indicated, no part of this book may be reproduced, translated, stored in a retrieval system, or transmitted, in any form or by any means, electronic, mechanical, photocopying, microfilming, recording, or otherwise, without written permission from the publisher.

Printed in the United States of America

This book is printed on acid-free paper.

Last digit is print number: 9   8   7   6   5

LIMITED DUPLICATION LICENSE

These materials are intended for use only by qualified mental health professionals.

The publisher grants to individual purchasers of this book nonassignable permission to reproduce all materials for which permission is specifically granted in a footnote. This license is limited to you, the individual purchaser, for personal use or use with individual clients. This license does not grant the right to reproduce these materials for resale, redistribution, electronic display, or any other purposes (including but not limited to books, pamphlets, articles, video- or audiotapes, blogs, file-sharing sites, Internet or intranet sites, and handouts or slides for lectures, workshops, or webinars, whether or not a fee is charged). Permission to reproduce these materials for these and any other purposes must be obtained in writing from the Permissions Department of Guilford Publications.

The author has checked with sources believed to be reliable in his efforts to provide information that is complete and generally in accord with the standards of practice that are accepted at the time of publication. However, in view of the possibility of human error or changes in behavioral, mental health, or medical sciences, neither the author, nor the editor and publisher, nor any other party who has been involved in the preparation or publication of this work warrants that the information contained herein is in every respect accurate or complete, and they are not responsible for any errors or omissions or the results obtained from the use of such information. Readers are encouraged to confirm the information contained in this book with other sources.

Library of Congress Cataloging-in-Publication Data

Names: Tolin, David F., author.
Title: Doing CBT : a comprehensive guide to working with behaviors, thoughts, and emotions / David F. Tolin.
Description: New York, NY : The Guilford Press, [2016] | Includes bibliographical references and index.
Identifiers: LCCN 2016023931 | ISBN 9781462527076 (hardback)
Subjects: LCSH: Cognitive therapy. | BISAC: MEDICAL / Psychiatry / General. | SOCIAL SCIENCE / Social Work. | PSYCHOLOGY / Psychotherapy / General. | MEDICAL / Nursing / Psychiatric.
Classification: LCC RC489.C63 T65 2016 | DDC 616.89/1425—dc23
LC record available at https://lccn.loc.gov/2016023931

To Fiona, James, and Katie

Thanks for your support, for your encouragement,
and for putting up with me while I wrote this thing.

About the Author

David F. Tolin, PhD, ABPP, is founder and director of the Anxiety Disorders Center/ Center for Cognitive Behavioral Therapy at The Institute of Living–Hartford Hospital and Adjunct Professor of Psychiatry at the Yale University School of Medicine. The author of over 150 scientific journal articles, Dr. Tolin has served as a principal investigator and scientific reviewer for the National Institutes of Health since 2003. He is a past president of the Society of Clinical Psychology (Division 12) of the American Psychological Association and a recipient of awards for Distinguished Contribution to the Science of Psychology, Distinguished Contribution to the Practice of Psychology, and Distinguished Lifetime Contribution to Psychology from the Connecticut Psychological Association.

Preface

This book is for mental health clinicians of all kinds. You might be a psychologist, a social worker, a psychiatrist, a counselor, or a member of another helping field. You might still be in a training program, or you might be a seasoned practitioner with years or decades of practice under your belt who is looking to sharpen your skills and expand your repertoire.

You also could work in one or more of a diverse array of clinical settings. You might be in an outpatient private practice or clinic. You might work in a community mental health center. You might work on a psychiatric inpatient unit or a residential treatment program. Perhaps you work in a general medical hospital or rehabilitation center. Maybe you're in a school or college setting. Your typical client population could vary as well. Perhaps you treat higher-functioning clients with milder psychiatric problems. Or maybe you treat clients with more severe illness, whether acute or chronic. Maybe you work primarily with children, or with older adults, or with the developmentally disabled.

Regardless of your level of expertise, your professional setting, or the clients you work with, this book is intended to be useful for you. Historically, it's been hard to find good resources that are broad enough to be applicable to all of these practitioners, settings, and clients, yet detailed enough that they can be put to actual use in practice. It's also been hard to find resources that have enough scientific detail to help academically oriented readers grasp the rationale behind the ideas without losing the "how-to's" among the scientific jargon.

This book aims to straddle multiple lines. My hope is that regardless of your clinical title, and whether you are a rookie or an old pro, you will find this material helpful. I am a clinical psychologist, and much of the scientific work described in this book comes from within the discipline of psychology. But I don't assume you have the same background, so I have tried to lay out the concepts in a way that people from all disciplines can use. My principal aim is for this book to show you how to do darn good cognitive-behavioral therapy (CBT) for whatever kinds of clients you work with. But I'm aware that for many readers, this book will also serve as your introduction to this rich and interesting field, and so I want to make sure you get the scientific understanding you need in order to appreciate CBT from all angles: scientific, theoretical, and practical.

We're going to cover a lot of ground in this book. We'll discuss how we understand psychological problems, how we engage our clients, and a wide range of techniques that we use to help our clients improve their lives. In addition, we'll present a number of (fictitious) clinical cases that illustrate what I'm talking about. There are numerous sidebars that describe the science behind what we're doing, arguments and counterarguments, and essential points to remember. I'll give you exercises to try on yourself so you can really embrace key constructs and practice key techniques. I'll introduce and define several terms that might be new to you.

With so many different topics, it's easy to lose sight of the forest for the trees. The "forest" of CBT, as I see it, is this:

• Theory and technique are intertwined. As CBT practitioners, we formulate a theoretical understanding of why a client is suffering, and we introduce therapeutic techniques based on that understanding. In particular, our interventions often target behavioral, emotional, and cognitive mechanisms that are keeping the problem in place or making it worse.

• Behavior, emotion, and thought are all different parts of an interactive process that can function well or not so well. When that interactive process is functioning not so well, maladaptive behaviors, emotions, and thoughts tend to exacerbate each other in a "snowball" effect.

• Conversely, as therapists, we can use the "snowball" effect to our advantage. We can influence the interactive process by intervening at the level of behavior, emotion, or thought—and there is nearly always more than one way to help. The art and science of CBT involve figuring out what kind of intervention will be most helpful for which client.

Whoever you are, wherever you work, and whomever you treat, you want what's best for your clients with psychological problems. I do, too. So how do we know what's best? People have been debating that issue for decades. Here's what we know:

• First, there is no doubt that CBT can be effective for a broad range of mental disorders. CBT, in various forms, has been clearly demonstrated to help clients with anxiety disorders, mood disorders, compulsive disorders, substance use disorders, marital distress, certain personality disorders, somatoform disorders and behavioral medicine concerns, and even psychotic disorders. Furthermore, the scientific evidence tells us that CBT can be just as effective in kids as it is in adults.

• Second, the efficacy of a lot of other forms of psychotherapy is less clear. Note that I don't say they're ineffective; I'm just saying we know much less about how well they work, and for whom they work, than we do about CBT. Certain treatments, such as interpersonal psychotherapy, have been shown to work for certain disorders, such as depression, but they haven't been demonstrated to serve as a solid foundation for a wide range of clients with a wide range of problems the way CBT has.

• Third, we've discovered a lot of helpful things in psychotherapy that have little or nothing to do with theoretical orientation. As just one example, we've learned much from successful psychotherapists of all stripes about how to develop and maintain a successful therapeutic relationship, which is critical for any treatment.

I'm a CBT therapist because, as far as I can tell, CBT is broadly the most effective perspective to take with most clients. And it serves as a general platform for the full range of clients that I might see, such that I don't need to learn one kind of therapy for one kind of client and an entirely different therapy for another kind of client. It's a broadly applicable knowledge base. But at the same time, I appreciate that there are good ideas to be found from many sources, many of which are also backed by solid evidence. For me, the bottom line has never been whether something is CBT or isn't CBT—it's whether any given strategy, technique, or way of talking to the client has been proven to work.

Now, a disclaimer is probably warranted here. Several readers, experts in the CBT field, have reviewed and offered critical comments on various drafts. Nevertheless, this book describes how *I* do CBT. It may or may not resemble how someone else does CBT. My CBT is based on my reading of the available basic and applied research, as well as my own experience treating clients with a range of problems. Throughout the book I don't hesitate to share my opinions with you (I have many), and I let you know when I'm doing so. You might have a different perspective on the research, and your clinical experience may differ from mine. Over time you will probably develop your own CBT. You'll have your own style, things you emphasize or deemphasize, and so on. But I think we can agree on some common ground.

Let's start with a basic commitment to science as a guiding principle. Science isn't a perfect system. Sometimes scientific results are wrong. But over time, science corrects itself, takes a hard look at the available evidence, and helps us separate fact from fantasy. So I propose that we strive to base our case conceptualizations on the best available scientific information about a particular problem and to base our clinical decision making on the best available scientific information about what works. That won't necessarily lead to perfect conceptualizations or slam-dunk treatment plans, but it beats any of the alternatives. That commitment to science also means that we're not going to be theoretically dogmatic. Right now, we know that CBT is the best available treatment for a wide range of problems. But in the future, we might find that something else is better. That's as it should be. So if, 10 years from now, rigorous research determines that the best treatment for social anxiety disorder is bloodletting, then I will be the first to invest in a leech farm.

Let's also recognize that CBT isn't one thing. Rather, it's a collection of conceptual elements and treatments that have come from a variety of sources. The first of these was behavior therapy, which started to gather steam in the 1950s and was based on experimental studies of behavioral change processes and learning principles. The second was cognitive therapy, which started in the 1960s when trained psychoanalysts began to emphasize conscious thought and a focus on the here and now. The behavior therapists and cognitive therapists eventually started realizing that their approaches overlapped a fair amount and created CBT, which was the subject of numerous efficacy trials and became a powerhouse in mental health treatment. Some CBT therapists, starting in the 1980s and 1990s, developed what many have called the "third wave" of CBT, which deemphasizes specific elements of cognitive restructuring and frequently includes elements of mindfulness meditation. This is an ever-evolving field.

Although we could take an approach based on the *Diagnostic and Statistical Manual of Mental Disorders* (DSM) and say "here's how you do CBT for depression," "here's how you do CBT for alcohol abuse," "here's how you do CBT for social phobia," and so on, that's going to leave a lot of our clients out in the cold, since many of them may not have a clear diagnosis or may have more than one problem. So I vote that we deemphasize the DSM in favor of a broad set of principles, based on the best available science, which we can apply to all of our clients, no matter who they are or what problem(s) they have.

Finally, I submit that the distinction often made between psychotherapeutic technique and the psychotherapy relationship is a false one. All psychotherapy, including CBT, is relationship based. Let's just accept that there are a bunch of things a good therapist should do. Some of them are designed to help build a relationship with the client, and some are designed to help the client change his or her thoughts, feelings, and behaviors.

CBT got a bad rap for a while from observers who felt it didn't pay enough attention to people's emotions, focusing exclusively on thoughts and behaviors. Critics charged that we CBTers don't try to understand the reasons problems happen, focusing only on how to treat them; that we don't pay enough attention to the therapeutic relationship and that our therapy is too technique-y; and that we're dogmatic and inflexible, ignoring helpful elements from other theoretical orientations. Some of this criticism has been well deserved, and some of it hasn't. After all, it's possible to deliver any treatment in a dogmatic, inflexible way. But I hope over the course of this book you'll see that it doesn't have to be so. I'll show you how a flexible and open-minded clinician can make the best use of the most evidence-based approach we have. If we start with the idea that CBT is primarily a way of thinking about psychological problems and take a science-informed yet pragmatic approach to case conceptualization, client interaction, treatment selection, and implementation of specific interventions, you'll see that we end up with a compassionate, flexible, and satisfying way of looking at the whole person—feelings, thoughts, behaviors, personal history, environment, interpersonal systems—and coming up with creative, effective ways to help.

Heck, maybe someday we'll stop calling it "CBT" and just call it "therapy."

Acknowledgments

I would like to express my gratitude to the many students and colleagues who helped me formulate and refine the ideas in this book. My postdoctoral fellows Bethany Wootton and Lauren Hallion and my colleagues Kimberli Treadwell and Lizabeth Roemer deserve particular mention for wading through draft after draft and giving me their unvarnished opinions. David Albert, Jennie Bernstein, William Bowe, Brett Deacon, Samantha Moshier, Suzanne Meunier, and Shari Steinman also provided helpful comments and critiques along the way.

Finally, I am grateful to all of the clients who have taught me so much over the years. Thank you, thank you, thank you.

Contents

Purchasers of this book can download and print larger versions
of the Personal Target Worksheets and the clinical tools in Appendix B
at *www.guilford.com/tolin-forms* for personal use or use with individual clients
(see copyright page for details).

CHAPTER 1

Laying Out the Basics

An Overview of This Book

This book is divided into three parts. Part I, "Why Do People Suffer?," is dedicated to using the principles of cognitive-behavioral therapy (CBT) to answer the fundamental question of why our clients are suffering in the first place. Why is this person depressed? Why does that client experience panic attacks? Why does this client engage in self-injury? Why is that client abusing drugs? And so on. Part II, "How Do We Help?," addresses the interventions we use in CBT. As you will see, our "hows" are heavily dependent on our "whys": We select interventions based on our working understanding of why the problem persists. This strategy is at the heart of the **case formulation approach**[1] (Persons, 1989; Persons & Tompkins, 2007), in which information gathered during a thorough assessment is used to develop a formulation about the causes of the problem and the formulation directly informs the selection of interventions. Part III, "Putting It All Together," walks you through several case examples, from the beginning to the end of therapy, so that you can see how these conceptual and interventional elements are woven together in a single case.

Meet Our Clients

Throughout this book, I'll illustrate the concepts and interventions by referring to several fictitious clients, whom you'll get to know over time. Our clients are:

- *Scott* is a 50-year-old socially anxious man seen in private practice. Although he can interact with his wife and children just fine, he becomes paralyzed by fear when talking to his supervisor at work or with people he doesn't know well.

---

[1]Terms in **boldface** type are defined in the "Key Terms and Definitions" sections at the ends of the chapters.

1

- *Suzanne* is a 65-year-old woman, seen in an outpatient counseling clinic, who has symptoms of generalized anxiety disorder (GAD) characterized by excessive worrying and tension. To cope with this anxiety, Suzanne has been abusing her benzodiazepine medication and fears she has become "hooked" on it. She is also highly dependent on others and seems reluctant to make decisions for herself.

- *Melissa* is a 25-year-old lesbian woman who is being treated in a community mental health center. A survivor of chronic sexual abuse during her childhood, Melissa is experiencing complex posttraumatic stress disorder (PTSD) characterized by nightmares, extremely low self-esteem, difficulty sustaining healthy relationships, and difficulty trusting others.

- *Christina* is a 46-year-old African American woman with chronic depression. She feels depressed most of the time and often has difficulty even getting out of bed. Although she is being treated in an outpatient clinic, at times she has had thoughts of suicide, combined with difficulty taking care of herself, that were so severe that she had to be hospitalized.

- *Samantha* is a 10-year-old girl with trichotillomania. She repetitively pulls the hair from her scalp, eyebrows, and eyelashes, resulting in visible and embarrassing bald patches. Her parents brought her to a private specialty clinic.

- *Anna* is a 20-year-old Hispanic college student, seen in her university's counseling center, who suffers from panic disorder and agoraphobia. Ever since moving onto campus, she has been experiencing unpredictable panic attacks. Due to her fears that these attacks will keep happening, she has been missing classes, has stopped driving, and is spending more and more time in her dorm room. She has considered taking a leave of absence from school.

- *Blaise* is a 28-year-old woman who has been attending a day treatment program for substance use recovery. She has been abusing cocaine for many years and has been arrested for a variety of drug-related charges, including possession, larceny, and prostitution. She finally decided to get sober this year. She is finding it difficult, however, and has experienced multiple lapses. She is becoming increasingly discouraged and depressed.

- *Johanna* and *Nick* are a married couple in their early 40s who feel that the love has gone out of their marriage. They seem to argue quite a bit and feel angry and resentful toward each other much of the time. Often, they go for long periods barely speaking to each other at all. Johanna and Nick are also having difficulty raising their son *James,* who has been showing increasingly oppositional behavior.

- *Elizabeth* is a 45-year-old woman who has been hospitalized more than 10 times for self-injurious behaviors, such as cutting or burning herself. She has been diagnosed with borderline personality disorder and experiences unstable moods, volatile relationships with others, and chronic thoughts of suicide. Her treatment was conducted in both an inpatient unit and a partial hospitalization program affiliated with the hospital.

- *Bethany* is a 17-year-old girl with obsessive–compulsive disorder (OCD). She has several irrational fears, such as that she will be contaminated by germs and contract a disease and that she will be seized with an uncontrollable urge to harm others. As a result, she engages in several compulsive rituals, such as washing, praying, and repeating actions.

- *William* is a 52-year-old gay man whose husband insisted he see a therapist. For most of his life, William has been unable to initiate tasks on his own or make decisions for himself, constantly asking his husband for guidance and reassurance. His husband now has to do nearly all of the household decision making and management. William has also been diagnosed with fibromyalgia, and he experiences chronic physical pain which, in his view, severely limits his activities.

- *Lauren* is a 30-year-old woman diagnosed with schizophrenia, paranoid type. She experiences delusional thoughts that others are monitoring, harassing, or trying to harm her. At times, she believes that she hears the voices of other people whispering threatening messages into her ear. She is chronically unemployed, and her self-care has been inconsistent. She is being seen in a day treatment program for the chronically mentally ill.

- *Samuel* is a 50-year-old Hispanic man attending a specialty sleep disorders clinic. For several years, he has struggled with severe insomnia, which leaves him chronically fatigued. He has difficulty concentrating, and his work performance has been inconsistent, leading him to fear that he will lose his job.

- *Shari* is an 18-year-old woman who suffers from bulimia and is attending an intensive outpatient program for people with eating disorders. Nearly every day, she engages in binge eating, in which she will eat a large amount of food rapidly, and she feels that she is out of control. After these binges, she feels disgusted with herself and makes herself vomit. She often feels depressed and ashamed of herself.

As you can see, our clients represent a broad range of ages, backgrounds, presenting problems, symptom severity, level of functioning, and treatment settings. As you progress through this book, one thing I'd like you to notice is that the same principles can be applied (to greater and lesser degrees) across diagnoses. The principles are, in many cases, exactly the same. Of course, that doesn't mean that CBT for schizophrenia will look exactly like CBT for social anxiety or couples' distress. But they have similar foundations, which we will discuss as we go.

Thinking Like a CBTer

Before we can do good CBT, we need to get into a CBT state of mind. That means that we make certain assumptions about psychological problems, why they occur, and how to treat them. Try these on for size.

A Good CBTer Sets Goals

Fundamentally, CBT aims to *do* something. Regardless of whom we're treating or why, it makes little sense to start treatment before we have a solid understanding of why we're doing it and what we hope to accomplish by doing it.

Of course, the desired outcome will vary depending on the client's presenting problem and goals. Clients can present with any number of treatment goals, such as:

"I'd like to feel less depressed."
"I'd like to stop drinking."
"I'd like to have better relationships."
"I'd like to be able to work again."
"I'd like to stay out of the hospital."

Sometimes the client has a hard time articulating his or her goals. Clarifying those goals therefore becomes part of our job as therapists. But regardless of whether the client comes into treatment with clearly stated goals or whether such goals have to be formulated during the therapy, we assume that there are indeed desired outcomes—we're not here "just to talk." Our treatment is explicitly designed to accomplish something.

Furthermore, as CBTers, we hold ourselves accountable for those outcomes and monitor our progress toward those outcomes along the way. If the treatment does not seem to be helping in a demonstrable way, we change what we are doing—we do not just keep doing the same thing over and over.

A Good CBTer Uses the Best Evidence

Numerous clinical trials have investigated the efficacy of various psychological treatments for various psychological problems or disorders. A central principle of our work is that this scientific work should serve as a guide for our clinical practice. The use of research findings to inform clinical practice is a major part of **evidence-based practice.** Evidence-based practice means that we start with the best research evidence for the presenting problem and then tailor the treatment (as needed) based on clinical expertise and client characteristics. Importantly, it doesn't mean that we have all of the answers, and it doesn't mean that the treatments are perfect (or even as good as they're going to get).

So what is the best evidence? This is not necessarily connected to any particular theoretical orientation, as there are some studies suggesting that psychodynamic and other psychological treatments can be effective for certain presenting problems (e.g., E. Frank & Levenson, 2010; Leichsenring & Rabung, 2008). So I'm not saying "CBT or nothing." But I am saying to go where the best evidence takes you—and when it comes to the sheer volume of solid evidence, CBT is, more often than not, the way to go. CBT is derived from well-documented principles of behavior and behavior change. Over the last several decades, basic scientists have taught us a lot about why thoughts, feelings, and behavior go haywire and how they can be changed. CBT builds upon that understanding. CBT, and the fundamental assumptions of CBT, are readily testable and therefore modifiable. This means that over time CBT evolves as scientific evidence accumulates, showing us what works and what does not. We routinely toss out things that don't work—indeed, if CBT were a highway, the roadside would be littered with old ideas that didn't pan out and got discarded. That's a good thing. It means we improve over time. CBT today is quite different from CBT a generation ago, and, hopefully, CBT a generation from now will be different from what we practice today.

It's also worth noting that over time CBT has incorporated some elements of other forms of therapy, and it's important to be open to that. A good idea is a good idea, and if there's evidence to back it up, we'll use it as long as it's not contraindicated by the other things we're doing. When done right, CBT is a flexible treatment. First and foremost, a good CBT therapist has to be a good psychotherapist. There is no manual or set of principles that will make up for lack of therapeutic skill. Good therapy is good therapy, and a good therapist is a good therapist. In Chapter 7, we'll talk about the elements that should be present in any good therapy, CBT or otherwise.

Should We Pick Elements from Various Schools of Psychotherapy?

It might surprise you, based on my previous mention that there are a lot of good aspects of non-CBT psychotherapy, to learn that I have real reservations about some forms of eclectic therapy (in which elements from multiple theoretical orientations are merged into a unified treatment). Yeah, I know that a lot of people like to include "CBT techniques" into an otherwise psychodynamic or humanistic therapy. And I can see the appeal of doing so. After all, there are good things about psychodynamic and humanistic therapies, and there are good things about CBT, so sampling the best from each ought to be as great as combining peanut butter and jelly, right? Well, sometimes it is, but I have heard of a lot of cases in which it was more like peanut butter and ketchup. They're great separately, but together, not so much.

There are two ways of introducing eclecticism into psychotherapy. The first of these, identified by Arnold Lazarus (e.g., A. A. Lazarus, 1967; A. A. Lazarus, Beutler, & Norcross, 1992), is *technical eclecticism,* in which we use strategies derived from different models of psychotherapy without necessarily subscribing to their underlying theory. Strategies are selected solely because they work. You'll see examples of technical eclecticism throughout this book. As just a few examples, I'll borrow interpersonal strategies derived from Rogers's (1957) client-centered therapy and techniques from Perls's (1973) gestalt therapy. In this book you'll see elements of motivational interviewing (W. R. Miller & Rollnick, 2002), cognitive therapy (A. T. Beck, 1976), behavior therapy (Wolpe, 1990), and mindfulness (Kabat-Zinn, 1994). This technical eclecticism is, in my opinion, helpful. I'm less concerned with who developed an idea, and whether they called it "CBT," than I am about whether it works within the overall framework of what I'm trying to accomplish.

But this kind of eclecticism works only because I'm always working as a CBT therapist, no matter what strategy I am using. I have a coherent, evidence-based model of why the client is suffering, and from that model I derive hypotheses about what's likely to work for that client. Remember, CBT is more than a set of techniques. It's a comprehensive understanding of why people suffer, how to interact with them, and how to intervene.

If I didn't have that coherent model, I would be at risk of the other kind of eclecticism, *theoretical integrationism* (Norcross, 1986), in which the clinician merges the theoretical models or worldviews of different schools of therapy, creating a new hybrid understanding of the client from (for example) a cognitive–psychodynamic–behavioral–gestalt perspective. Theoretical integrationism is not a good recipe for successful therapy (A. A. Lazarus & Beutler, 1993). It leaves you thrashing around aimlessly, without a good sense of what you're doing and why. Indeed, there are times when the theory behind one approach will directly conflict with the theory behind another approach. As just one example, think of OCD. The psychoanalytic model of OCD posits that obsessive thoughts represent unresolved conflicts from early stages of psychological development and that the person's compulsive behaviors represent an unconscious struggle for control over drives that are unacceptable at a conscious level. The CBT model of OCD, on the other hand, posits that strange thoughts are entirely normal, occurring in most people, and that the problem in OCD stems from the fact that the person takes these thoughts seriously, believes them to be true or dangerous, tries unsuccessfully to suppress them, and feels a need to do something about them. Now imagine talking to a client who is having, say, obsessive thoughts about harming his family and trying to somehow "blend" the psychoanalytic and cognitive-behavioral explanations for what's going on. Probably, you'll end up with a confusing mess.

Maybe you have the skill to pull off theoretical integrationism. I certainly don't. So I choose to do CBT and do it really well, even though I might include some technical eclecticism. As you go through this book, I encourage you to try doing the same. Jump in with both feet. We'll be open to new ideas and not unnecessarily dogmatic, but we'll keep our conceptualization firmly grounded in CBT. That is, we have good reason to believe that psychological problems are maintained by certain processes, and we always have those processes firmly in mind.

A Good CBTer Mixes Art and Science

We've discussed how the best treatment choices are based on scientific evidence of efficacy. That assumption sometimes leaves people wondering where we make room for the art of psychotherapy. I would suggest that our science and art are not mutually exclusive—in fact, they get along famously. Sometimes, people try to frame this as a conflict between the two, as if you have to choose one or the other. Rather, I suggest we think about science and art as being two important aspects of the complex task of psychotherapy, both of which are critical to success (see Figure 1.1). Artless science is probably not going to be helpful in providing psychotherapy, nor will scienceless art. The best practitioners use an artful application of scientifically derived principles. That's what we're shooting for here. Being a scientific artist (or an artistic scientist, whichever sounds best to you) is not an easy task, but it's an important one if you're going to do good CBT.

Combining Evidence to Fit Your Client

It's important for us to recognize that, if you have a client in front of you, and you go to the scientific literature looking for explicit guidance about what to do with this exact client, you might come away disappointed. Much of the scientific evidence comes from tightly controlled clinical trials, the participants in which may or may not match your clinic clients. For example, in most clinical trials only one diagnosis was being treated; there is usually little attention to the treatment of multiple problems simultaneously. You probably won't find, for example, much research that will show you clinical outcomes for clients who are simultaneously depressed and have drinking problems and personality disorders and chaotic living environments.

So how do we capitalize on the best available research evidence, given these limitations? We *start with the evidence* that seems to come closest to what we're trying to accomplish and make a (scientifically informed) best guess. Let's say I'm treating a client with a really bad case of panic disorder, who also suffers from a significant amount of depression. I know from the available literature that panic disorder can be effectively treated using

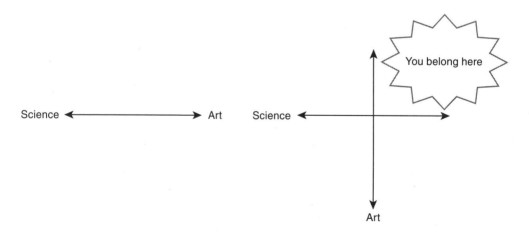

FIGURE 1.1. Science and art in psychotherapy. They are not opposite poles (left). Rather, they are two different constructs (right).

the CBT interventions of *interoceptive exposure, in vivo exposure,* and *cognitive restructuring* (more on these interventions later). That research didn't really address depression, but at least it's a start. So I will use that as my basic platform of treatment. I also know from the literature that *activity scheduling* is an effective treatment for depression. So I will think of ways to incorporate elements of this intervention into my treatment package.

A Good CBTer Uses the Clinic as a Laboratory

As part of this science-based thinking, we *treat every client as an experiment.* That doesn't mean our clients are guinea pigs, nor does it mean we just try whatever comes to mind in hopes that something will work. It's really just an honest way of dealing with reality: There is always an open question as to whether any intervention or combination of interventions will work for any given client. Therefore, we must take a scientifically informed educated guess, test whether our guess is right, and modify the plan as needed.

It is critical, therefore, to take repeated measures of the clients. We need to see, on an ongoing basis, whether they are getting better or not. Self-report is often just fine, and it's usually the most convenient thing we can do, although measurement need not be limited to self-report. For a given client, I could measure *outcomes,* such as symptoms of the disorder, daily functioning, quality of life, or other relevant variables (e.g., the number of drinks consumed per day). I could also measure hypothesized *mechanisms* of the problem—the variables that I think influence the outcomes—using measures of emotions or distorted thought patterns, physiological measures (e.g., heart rate during symptom provocation), overt behaviors (e.g., performance-based tests in session), or other relevant variables (e.g., the number of arguments with his or her spouse).

A Good CBTer Looks beyond the Label

Many of us are accustomed to using the fifth edition of the *Diagnostic and Statistical Manual of Mental Disorders* (DSM-5; American Psychiatric Association, 2013) in our work. The DSM has its uses. We need diagnoses to get paid for our work, and a diagnosis can often serve as a useful "shorthand" to communicate information about a client. But as a guide for treatment, it leaves much to be desired. You don't treat a diagnosis; you treat a person. The treatment for two people with the same diagnosis might be different, whereas treatment for two people with different diagnoses might be quite similar. And the number of diagnoses in there is so huge that there's no way we could hope to accumulate a decent scientific basis for the treatment of each diagnosis (let alone for combinations of diagnoses).

It's helpful, therefore, to focus less on diagnoses than on *syndromes of psychological problems.* Think of it this way: There are a limited number of syndromes (e.g., "depression," "fear"), that may range from mild to severe and that may occur alone or in combination. That is, it's less important to know the name of the problem than it is to understand what's going on.

My general dislike of labels extends to the labels slapped on CBT interventions as well. These days, it seems like everyone has come out with their own brand of CBT, all with different names and treatment manuals. I don't think a good CBTer needs to know every CBT package that has been developed or needs to memorize a treatment manual for everything. If you tried, your head would explode. What is important is that you understand the fundamental *ingredients* of these therapies. You'll find, once you start looking, that the number of actual working ingredients is much smaller than the number of treatment packages out there.

So we have a finite number of interventions for a finite number of syndromes. When we do the necessary conceptualization work, we'll see that any presenting problem can be broken into component parts, and we have effective core interventions to address those parts. That's how this book is arranged. Of course, for specific presenting problems you might want to look at manualized treatments to get a better sense of how treatment can be implemented. There are a lot of good CBT manuals out there that are worth a look; Appendix A will direct you to some of my favorites. But with the information you'll learn here, you'll find that you can anticipate what's going to be in most CBT manuals before even opening them. Should you opt to use treatment manuals in your practice, having a solid foundation in the principles and practice of CBT will help you use those manuals in a flexible manner, adapting them to meet the needs of your clients.

A Good CBTer Is Willing to Be Wrong

Thomas Huxley (1825–1895) wrote that "the great tragedy of science [is] the slaying of a beautiful hypothesis by an ugly fact." I can come up with a great conceptualization of the client's problem and think I have nailed down perfectly why it is happening . . . and then I learn more about the client, and my conceptualization falls apart. I don't like when that happens, and you probably won't, either. After all, being right feels a lot better. But central to thinking scientifically is a recognition that a lot of your ideas will turn out to be wrong. A good CBTer is open to the possibility of wrongness, even looking for signs of wrongness along the way. We can always modify our ideas as we learn new facts. We run into trouble when we start ignoring the facts that don't conform to our ideas. The tendency to do so is, unfortunately, human nature, and it applies as much to ourselves as to our clients. In Chapter 3 we'll talk about how these kinds of *information-processing biases* come into play in psychological problems.

What Is CBT?

Fundamentally, CBT is a way of *thinking* about psychological problems and their treatment. More than anything, it is an approach to case conceptualization that guides our understanding of *why* someone is suffering and *how* we can help him or her. Here are some elements that make CBT unique.

- As an intervention, CBT tends to be *focused*. That is, we spend most of our time discussing and working on the target problem.

- CBT tends to be *time-limited*, at least compared with many other treatments. Some CBTs are really short (e.g., one-session CBT for specific phobias [Öst, 1989]), and some CBTs are really long (e.g., two-year CBT for borderline personality [Linehan et al., 2006]), but generally speaking CBT tends not to be a forever, Woody Allen–style treatment.

- Unlike some other forms of psychotherapy, CBT, in most cases, is *present-oriented*. That is, we spend more time talking about the current situation than about historical events. When we ask the question, "Why is this person suffering?," that question could be interpreted as asking about *etiology* ("How did this person begin suffering?") or about *maintenance* ("Why, on a day-to-day basis, does this person continue to suffer?"). We are interested in etiology, but our therapy is most effective when we identify the factors that maintain the problem and then work to change those factors. That's true even when the etiology is really striking. Take, for example, our client Melissa, who has PTSD. Her childhood traumas were really awful and clearly were the initial source of her psychological suffering. And we are indeed interested in that and want to talk to Melissa about that. But ultimately what's going to get her feeling better is addressing the day-to-day factors that cause her suffering to persist.

- CBT tends to be *active*. CBT is about doing things, and the client will have new things to try throughout the course of therapy. In many cases, the therapist will do these things right along with the client, often outside of a traditional office setting.

- CBT is *directive*. Unlike some more humanistic and supportive forms of psychotherapy, in CBT the therapist takes a leadership role and helps set an agenda for the therapy and for each session. In many respects, the CBT therapist acts as a coach for the client.

- In keeping with its scientific foundations, CBT emphasizes *measurable gains* and *testable hypotheses*. We set clear goals for our desired outcomes, we take educated guesses about what will work, and then we check in a systematic fashion to see whether it actually did work.

Let me also make a comment about what CBT isn't. Some people have misconceptions about this kind of treatment, so let's get them out on the table.

- *CBT as a toolbox, manual, or set of techniques.* There are a lot of unique interventions in CBT, and I've often heard people use a "toolbox" or "clinical armamentarium" analogy (e.g., "Hey, this book is great because it'll give me more tools in my toolbox!"). It is true that the interventions we'll discuss here are effective, and I have no doubt that they'll be useful for you and your clients. But the toolbox analogy misses the point. Think about the difference between a cook and a chef. A cook can follow a recipe and come up with something delicious. But a chef can actually create the recipe, adapting what he or she is doing to meet the specific needs of the diner. A good CBTer is a chef, not a cook. Following a published therapy manual is one thing; knowing how to figure out why any given client is suffering and coming up with an interventional strategy that is tailored to that client's individual needs is another thing altogether. The intervention is most helpful if it's applied within the broader theory of why the problem is there.

- *CBT as a Band-Aid.* First of all, let's not disparage the Band-Aid. It reliably stops bleeding, prevents infection, and promotes rapid healing, all for a few cents, and can be obtained virtually anywhere by anyone. We should be so lucky as to have something that good in mental health! More substantively, when people use this analogy they are implying that CBT does not address the *cause* of the problem, only the *symptoms* of the problem. This is not accurate. CBT does address the cause—the reason *why*—but our conceptualization of the cause is different from those used in other disciplines. We do not chalk psychological problems up to a chemical imbalance, as in pharmacotherapy, nor do we attribute them to unconscious conflicts rooted in early childhood, as in classic psychoanalytic theory (not that such things don't exist; they're just not all that helpful for our purposes). Rather, CBT posits that psychological problems are caused and maintained by a mixture of factors, both internal and external to the person, that include emotions and physiological sensations, thoughts and beliefs, behaviors, information-processing biases, behavioral contingencies, and behavioral skill deficits. Understanding how those factors interact to cause the problem is at the core of developing effective interventions.

- *CBT as a set of techniques independent from relationship.* This is a little bit like the (false) science and art distinction described earlier. There are some who will tell you that CBT therapists are all about doing a certain technique and don't care about the relationship. It may be true that early basic research on behavioral interventions left something to be desired, relationship-wise. But when we're talking about modern CBT, technique and relationship are not mutually exclusive (see Figure 1.2). The bottom line here is that the best practitioners apply proper techniques in the context of a positive relationship. In many ways, the therapeutic relationship is central to the CBT. As one example, **collaborative empiricism** forms the basis of the therapeutic relationship, in which the client and therapist collaboratively form and test hypotheses (more on this in Chapter 7). As another example, the therapeutic relationship is used as a vehicle for shaping and reinforcing healthy behaviors in session (see Chapter 9).

I view good CBT as having three basic ingredients: (1) *good therapy,* (2) a *good CBT conceptualization,* and (3) specific *CBT techniques* (see Figure 1.3). All three ingredients are important; good CBT cannot occur unless each is present. Good therapy forms the foundation of the CBT. It represents a minimal set of criteria that must be present for therapy to be effective. A good CBT conceptualization is critical. Specifically, the therapist and client need to have a good working model of why the person is suffering. Technique is also critical. Often, if you have developed a good CBT case conceptualization within the context of good therapy, the specific techniques to be used become self-evident.

We'll spend a lot of time talking about the ins and outs of good CBT therapy in Chapter 7. Briefly, however, many of the elements of good therapy are independent of therapeutic orientation (e.g., J. D. Frank, 1974). Good therapy means *paying careful attention to the client.* That means we take the time to inquire about the person's symptoms, take a thorough history, learn about what is important to him or her, and understand his or her quality of life. It also means that we pay close attention to behaviors that the client exhibits in session, including how he or she interacts with the therapist.

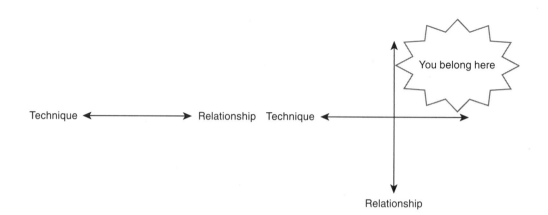

FIGURE 1.2. Technique and relationship in psychotherapy. They are not opposite poles (left). Rather, they are two different constructs (right).

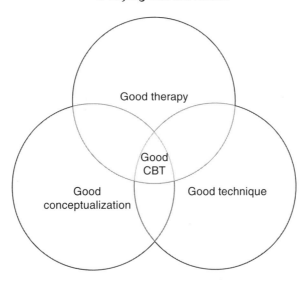

FIGURE 1.3. Elements of good CBT.

Good therapy means a *solid clinical relationship.* Carl Rogers (1957) was one of the first people to emphasize relationship factors in psychotherapy, and his ideas are still useful today. He suggested that good therapists display the following behaviors:

- *Empathy.* Good therapists routinely demonstrate, in words and in nonverbal cues, that they care about the clients' well-being and feel compassion for what they are going through.
- *Genuineness.* Good therapists act like themselves. They share, when clinically appropriate, their thoughts, ideas, and emotional reactions.
- *Unconditional positive regard.* Good therapists display a basic liking of their clients. They do not pass judgment or appear critical (though this does not preclude confronting the client when clinically appropriate). They respect the client as a person and believe that the client has a right to feel better.

Good therapy means *facilitating positive expectations and hope.* Of course, we should not oversell the benefits of therapy or lead clients to believe that we can perform miracles. But if we don't think that things will get better, then there's little reason for us to be doing therapy in the first place. So, using the best clinical judgment we have, we convey the message that the client's problem can be improved.

A good CBT conceptualization, which we address in detail over the next several chapters, means that we develop and share with the client a clear understanding of what is wrong and why. For each of our clients, our conceptualization is grounded in the idea that psychological problems consist of *cognitive* elements, *emotional* elements, and *behavioral* elements (see Table 1.1) and that the problem can be examined (and potentially addressed) by way of each of these elements and the interactions among them. *Cognitive* elements refer to the person's thoughts, beliefs, interpretations, and information-processing styles, as well as effortful mental strategies the person uses to try to cope. *Emotional* elements refer to subjective feeling states (e.g., sad, angry, scared) and associated physiological processes and sensations. *Behavioral* elements refer to the client's overt responses.

TABLE 1.1. Cognitive, Emotional, and Behavioral Elements of Selected Psychological Problems

	Cognitive	Emotional	Behavioral
Depression	Belief that I am worthless	Sadness, heavy sensation, low energy	Spend excessive time in bed
Mania	Belief that I am all-powerful	Excitement, high energy, decreased need for sleep	Impulsive sex, spending
Panic	Belief that I am dying	Fear, increased heart rate, dizziness	Avoidance, seeking reassurance
Borderline	Belief that others will abandon me and it will be devastating	All of the above at different times	Cutting, suicide threats, throwing things

So as CBT therapists, we're looking for these elements when we meet with our clients. From the start of therapy, the therapist is constantly asking questions (which we discuss in detail later), such as:

- Under what circumstances does this problem occur?
- What are the *behavioral* elements of the problem (see Chapter 2)?
- How do external and internal *contingencies* (e.g., reward and punishment) influence his or her behavioral responses?
- Does the person lack specific *behavioral skills* needed to adapt successfully to the environment?
- What are the negative effects of the person's behaviors?
- What are the *cognitive* elements of the problem (see Chapter 3)?
- To what extent does this person have *interpretations* that are unhelpful?
- To what extent do this person's *core beliefs* shape his or her thinking in difficult situations?
- To what extent do *information-processing biases* distort how information is attended to and remembered?
- To what extent does this person engage in *maladaptive mental coping strategies*?
- What are the *emotional* elements of the problem (see Chapter 4)?
- What are the subjective feeling states experienced?
- What physiological sensations are associated with those emotions?
- To what extent have emotional responses been *classically conditioned* through paired associations?
- How has the person's *learning history* shaped his or her thoughts, emotions, and behaviors?

Good conceptualizations make use of **Ockham's razor,** also known as the *principle of parsimony.* William of Ockham (c. 1285–1349) said: "One should not increase, beyond what is necessary, the number of entities required to explain anything." In plainer language, Ockham was telling us that we should avoid assumptions that cannot be examined, tested, or falsified, especially if our conceptualization works fine without them. So as we try to understand why a client is suffering, we'll be most effective if we start with the simplest and most straightforward explanation, trying our best to avoid making assumptions about unconscious processes that we'll never be able to evaluate. I'm talking to you, Freud.

Our conceptualization also hinges on the idea that the emotional, cognitive, and behavioral elements of psychological problems can mutually influence each other. An example of this interaction for our client Anna, who has panic disorder, is shown in Figure 1.4. As you can see, when she's feeling panicky, Anna has an *emotional response* (increased heart rate and a subjective feeling state of fear), a *cognitive response* (the thought "I'm dying!") and a *behavioral response* (avoidance and seeking reassurance from others). These

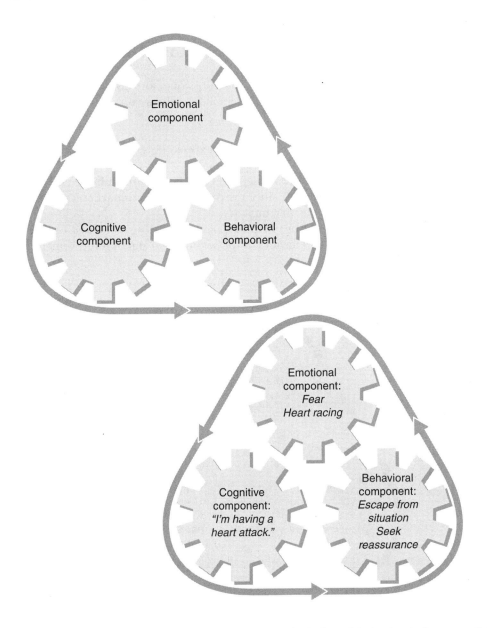

FIGURE 1.4. Reciprocal influence of cognitive, physiological, and behavioral elements of the core pathological process, in general (top) and for Anna, our patient with panic disorder (bottom).

three elements—cognitive, emotional, and behavioral—all fuel each other, causing the entire process to get worse and worse. The reciprocal escalation of these factors forms what I call the **core pathological process.** It's a snowball effect, such that as one element gets worse, the others get worse, too. Fortunately, this can also work the other way—which is what we strive to do in therapy (see Figure 1.5). In this case, Anna's decrease in physiological sensations (slower heart rate and less dizziness), decreased belief that she is dying, and decreased avoidance and reassurance-seeking behavior all deescalate each other, causing the entire process to get better and better. We can push the snowball in a healthy direction.

What Does a CBT Session Look Like?

As you might guess, there's no formula that is set in stone, and so one CBT session may not look much like another. However, in many CBT sessions you're likely to see several elements, including the following:

- The therapist actively listens to the client, expressing empathy, genuineness, and unconditional positive regard.
- The therapist collaboratively sets an agenda for the session with the client.
- The therapist reviews the events since the past session, with particular emphasis on any homework the client was to complete.
- The therapist makes liberal use of praise, congratulating the client on his or her efforts to get better or on behaviors in the session that signal improvement.

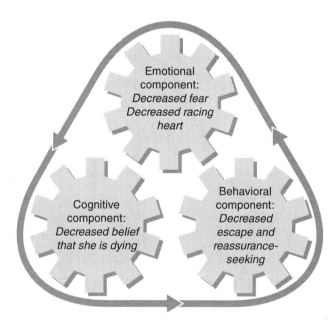

FIGURE 1.5. Reciprocal influence of cognitive, emotional, and volitional elements during Anna's recovery from panic disorder.

- The therapist and client discuss an aspect or instance of the problem by breaking it down into cognitive, emotional, and behavioral features.
- The therapist uses psychoeducation to help the client better understand the problem and why it is occurring.
- The therapist and client work together on a strategy or exercise that aims to help improve the problem.
- The therapist takes time to ensure that the client understands and agrees with the conceptualization and interventions.
- The therapist assigns homework for the client to continue to work on the problem until the next session.

What Does CBT Look Like over Time and across Sessions?

Nothing is set in stone, and the course of therapy will necessarily vary from client to client. However, one fairly typical progression might proceed as follows:

- The therapist assesses the client, gaining an understanding of the target problem(s).
- The therapist collaborates with the client to develop a cognitive-behavioral conceptualization (see Chapter 5) of the problem(s).
- The therapist and client agree on the goals of therapy, stated as explicitly as possible. They also agree on general principles such as the duration and frequency of treatment, expectations of the therapist and the client, time frame for reassessment and reevaluation of the plan, and so forth.
- The therapist works with the client on ways to improve the problem(s) effectively and efficiently. Depending on the problem(s) and the client characteristics, initial steps might involve directed behavioral change, skill training, cognitive restructuring, emotion regulation, or other strategies.
- The therapist and client routinely track progress and modify the treatment plan as needed. They openly discuss how the treatment is going, and whether changes need to be made.
- As therapy progresses, the discussion might turn to broader issues such as *core beliefs* (see Chapter 3) or long-standing maladaptive behavioral patterns.
- As the client nears his or her treatment goal, the therapist and client begin to discuss termination and relapse prevention.
- When it is agreed that the goals have been met and no additional treatment is needed, the treatment ends with the understanding that the client may initiate treatment again if needed in the future.

Learning CBT by Applying It to Yourself

As you go through this book, you might find it helpful to try out some of our concepts and interventions on yourself. As a learning exercise, I invite you to select a *personal target* that you'd like to work on. Ideally, your personal target would be an analogue (perhaps subclinical) of something for which people might seek treatment. A fear of spiders or public speaking, moodiness, irritability or crankiness, difficulty getting along with someone, overuse of caffeine or nicotine, perfectionism, nail biting, and overeating are all fairly common concerns that have some overlap with more severe clinical problems.

After many of these chapters, I'll encourage you to try out what we've been discussing on your personal target. Try to understand why the target is there, based on the principles in the chapter, and try various interventions to get a feel for how to implement them and how they work for you.

THE ESSENTIALS

✳ A good CBT therapist sets reasonable and meaningful goals for treatment.

✳ A good CBT therapist uses the best scientific evidence in understanding the problem and selecting treatments and mixes that science with the art of psychotherapy.

✳ A good CBT therapist looks beyond the diagnosis and tries to understand why this client's problem is persisting.

✳ A good CBT therapist always frames his or her ideas as hypotheses and is willing to be wrong.

✳ CBT is primarily a way of thinking about psychological problems.

✳ Good CBT comes from the interaction of good therapy, good conceptualization, and good technique.

✳ In general, CBT tends to be focused, time-limited, present-oriented, active, and directive, emphasizing measurable goals and testable hypotheses.

✳ CBT conceptualizations start with identifying the core pathological process: the interaction among maladaptive behaviors, thoughts, and emotions.

KEY TERMS AND DEFINITIONS

Case formulation approach: A hypothesis-testing approach to clinical assessment, formulation, and intervention.

Collaborative empiricism: An approach to the therapeutic relationship in which the therapist and client act as partners, forming and testing hypotheses about the causes of the problem and how to address it.

Core pathological process: An interaction of cognitive, emotional, and behavioral responses that become maladaptive or unhelpful.

Evidence-based practice: A treatment approach based on scientific evidence, filtered through clinical expertise and client characteristics.

Ockham's razor: The idea that explanations should make the fewest possible assumptions.

Definition of the Personal Target

Below please describe your personal target. Remember that ideally your personal target has some overlap with the kinds of things for which someone might seek therapy—for example, a problem related to mood or anxiety, a behavior that isn't well controlled, an interpersonal problem, and so on.

My Personal Target

What is your personal target? _____

_____

_____

What *behaviors* does your personal target include? _____

_____

_____

_____

What *thoughts* come before and after the behavior? _____

_____

_____

_____

What *emotions or physical sensations* come before and after the behavior? _____

_____

_____

_____

Under what *circumstances* does this target occur? _____

_____

_____

_____

From *Doing CBT* by David F. Tolin. Copyright © 2016 The Guilford Press. Permission to photocopy this worksheet is granted to purchasers of this book for personal use only (see copyright page for details). Purchasers can download enlarged versions of this worksheet (see the box at the end of the table of contents).

PART I

Why Do People Suffer?

CBT begins with understanding the reason *why*. Why is this person depressed? Drinking too much? Having anxiety attacks? Getting into fights? Attempting suicide?

Within the CBT perspective, we answer the question *why* by understanding several different factors, putting them together like pieces of a jigsaw puzzle. We emphasize *maintenance* of the problem—that is, the factors that cause the problem to keep occurring.

We can think about virtually any psychological problem as having three components:

1. The *behavioral system,* which reflects what the person does.
2. The *cognitive system,* which reflects what the person thinks and how the person processes information.
3. The *emotional system,* which reflects how the person feels.

Often, a disturbance in one of these systems is easier to spot than is a disturbance in the others. For example, when a client comes in with a complaint of feeling depressed all of the time, that's a fairly obvious disturbance in the *emotional system* (how the client feels). It might be harder to spot the disturbances in the *behavioral system* and the *cognitive system*. Alternatively, for the client who is drinking too much, we can easily see the problem in the *behavioral system* (what the client does), but the disturbances in the *cognitive system* and the *emotional system* might not be so apparent. As you'll see, part of our job as therapists is to look for all of the elements of this triad and to understand how they fit together.

In the next three chapters, we talk about each system in detail. After that, we discuss how these three systems interact with each other and how you can use that information to create a road map for your treatment.

CHAPTER 2

Oh, Be*have!*

The Behavioral System and How It Can Go Wrong

Defining behavior is like trying to nail Jell-O to a wall. In 1965, Ogden Lindsley famously remarked, "If a dead man can do it, it ain't behavior, and if a dead man can't do it, then it is behavior." That definition suggests that just about everything is a behavior, except for being very still and decomposing. B. F. Skinner (1974), one of the pioneers of behavioral theory, argued that the things we call thoughts and feelings were forms of behavior. Many contemporary behavioral theorists would make that same argument—that everything we do, think, and feel is a behavior. And this conceptualization is true, to a certain extent. After all, what we call thoughts, feelings, and actions are all basically responses that come out of our brains and get experienced and expressed in different ways.

However, from a therapist's perspective, it remains helpful to have a definition of behavior that is a bit narrower than Lindsley's dead-man test. We'll talk about the "behaviors" of thinking and feeling in the next couple of chapters. But for now, I'll define **behavior** as motoric acts. That is, I'm going to limit my definition to those acts that involve the skeletal muscles—anything you do with your hands, feet, mouth, face, and so forth. Avoiding things is a behavior. Drinking is a behavior. Cutting oneself is a behavior. Arguing is a behavior.

What Makes a Behavior Maladaptive?

We consider the behavioral system to be *maladaptive* when it gets in the way of the person's functioning or quality of life. Behaviors can be maladaptive for any number of reasons: The person might prioritize feeling better over doing better. The person might be stuck on the short-term payoff from the behavior without recognizing the longer-term costs. The person's behavioral response might be inflexible or inappropriate to the situation. Or the behavior might be technically "correct," but performed poorly.

Behavioral Excesses and Deficits

Some behaviors are maladaptive because they happen too frequently. We would call this a **behavioral excess.** For example:

- Samantha, our young client with trichotillomania, pulls her hair out.
- Lauren, our client with schizophrenia, shouts at people whom she (incorrectly) believes are harassing or following her.
- Blaise, our client struggling with substance use, continues to use cocaine despite serious consequences.
- Shari, our bulimic client, engages in bingeing and purging behaviors.

All of these clients have something in common: They are all engaging in a maladaptive behavior too frequently.

Conversely, some behaviors are maladaptive because they happen too *in*frequently. We would call this a **behavioral deficit.** For example:

- Scott, the socially anxious client, doesn't go out with coworkers, strike up conversations with others, or go to parties.
- Christina, our client with depression, stays home by herself all day watching TV rather than engaging in potentially more rewarding activities.
- William, who is highly dependent on others, rarely makes decisions for himself or initiates activities.

Why Do Behavioral Excesses and Deficits Occur?

Trying to Feel Better Instead of Trying to Do Better

Often, when someone has a behavioral excess or a behavioral deficit, we find that the person is engaging in these behaviors (in the case of behavioral excess) or not engaging in these behaviors (in the case of behavioral deficit) as a way of trying to feel better. The person selects a particular behavior or set of behaviors not because they are objectively helpful but because the person predicts (correctly or incorrectly) that the behaviors will help him or her reduce uncomfortable feelings. Some examples are:

- *Unnecessary avoidance.* When something makes us feel afraid, we're usually motivated to avoid it. That's fine, if the thing we're avoiding is actually dangerous. But when it's not dangerous, avoidance behavior can become part of the problem.
- *Shutting down.* It's natural to want to retreat in the face of overwhelming stressors. When a person starts withdrawing from important areas of life, such as school, work, friends, or family, as a way of coping with unpleasant feelings such as sadness, the problem can worsen.
- *Numbing.* Some people use alcohol or drugs to "dull the pain" when feeling unhappy, anxious, or tense. Others engage in excessive, even frantic, efforts to keep themselves busy and distracted so that they don't have to think about unpleasant things or feel unpleasant emotions.
- *Reactive aggression.* When angry, some people "lash out" in an almost reflexive manner. They might yell, throw things, hit someone, or even hurt themselves as a way of trying to get their anger out.

Does this mean that all efforts to feel better are maladaptive? Definitely not. There is an important role in our lives (and in CBT) for *emotion regulation,* a topic we'll discuss in detail in Chapter 19. But notice that all of the preceding examples involve desperate attempts to feel better by engaging in behaviors that have the potential to make the problem worse rather than better.

By contrast, adaptive behaviors often involve some attempt to make a bad situation better. As we'll discuss later in this chapter, some examples of adaptive behaviors include *problem solving* and application of appropriate *social skills.*

Again, however, there are exceptions. Not all efforts to make a problem better are adaptive. One could imagine, for example, that a client who constantly tries to solve an unsolvable problem, or tries over and over to improve a situation that cannot be improved, is not functioning in an adaptive manner. Behaviors such as problem solving and other skills are adaptive when they are likely to be helpful.

So what really makes a behavior adaptive or maladaptive is whether it's likely to improve things. Desperate attempts to avoid feeling bad are probably maladaptive, but some strategies to regulate intense emotions might be adaptive. The use of problem-solving and other skills is usually adaptive, but if these strategies are performed inflexibly in situations in which they're unlikely to help, they become maladaptive. A healthy person has to be able to size up the situation, make a reasonable decision about what behaviors are called for, and implement those behaviors.

Short-Term Gain, Long-Term Pain

Maladaptive behaviors often involve an unfavorable trade-off between short-term and long-term consequences. That is, many people will engage in behaviors that produce a short-term benefit, but at an unacceptable long-term cost. We refer to a behavior as *impulsive* when it is appetitive (pleasurable) and the person seems to be unable or unwilling to apply the brakes to the behavior. Problem gambling, excessive shopping, binge eating, and risky sexual behaviors are all examples of impulsive behaviors. They can give the person a short-term sense of satisfaction or excitement, but the long-range consequences of those behaviors can be damaging to the person.

Try This

Which would you rather have?

- $1.00 today, or $2.00 a week from now?
- $5.00 today, or $10.00 a year from now?
- $50.00 today, or $100.00 ten years from now?

These questions relate to the phenomenon of *delay discounting.* The longer we have to wait for a reward, the more likely we are to select a smaller but more immediate reward (Bickel & Marsch, 2001). All of us are prone to delay discounting; however, delay discounting is evident to a much greater extent among clients with poor impulse control. They can't get past the excitement of the immediate rewards and have difficulty delaying gratification, even when doing so would be in their best interest.

Our client Blaise, who is dependent on cocaine, is a good example of short-term gain and long-term pain. When she uses drugs, she feels good in the moment, but the behavior is ultimately self-destructive.

When the Behavior Is Just Wrong

Sometimes, clients' maladaptive behavior isn't well conceptualized as an excess or a deficit—that is, they are not necessarily doing something too much or too little, but rather they are just performing the wrong kinds of behaviors at the wrong times. These clients might be considered to have a **deficient behavioral repertoire** (Goldfried & Davison, 1994). That is, they are having difficulty selecting the appropriate behaviors, or are having difficulty carrying those behaviors out in an appropriate manner.

Why Do Deficient Behavioral Repertoires Occur?

Being Inflexible

Deficient behavioral repertoires are sometimes associated with a lack of flexibility—that is, the person is unable to adapt his or her behavior to the circumstances. Inflexibility of behavior is perhaps most clearly seen in the difficulty adapting to contextual changes in individuals with autism spectrum disorders (D'Cruz et al., 2013); however, the phenomenon operates at varying levels across many mental disorders. In many cases, it seems that the person's behavior is responsive less to the situation than to (often unspoken or unacknowledged) "rules" that the person feels that he or she should follow (Hayes, 1989). For example, strictly following the "rule" that says "never let anyone take advantage of you" can lead the person to miss the nuances of the situation and engage in an inflexible pattern of hostile or aggressive behavior. Adaptive behaviors, on the other hand, are flexible. That is, the person is able to adapt his or her behavior to the circumstances. We have a different behavioral response to a disagreement with a colleague, for example, than we have to a belligerent drunk in a bar. That flexibility allows us to modulate our response so that it is appropriate to what's going on.

Failing to Match the Behavior to the Situation

Often, a behavior that is perfectly fine in one situation is maladaptive in another. Some clients may fail to engage in the behavior needed for a given situation (e.g., fail to do a needed task), engage in a behavior that is not called for by the situation (e.g., do something impulsive, superstitious, or strange), or engage in the behavior at a level that is too high or low for the situation (e.g., overreact to stressful events). Our client Lauren, who has schizophrenia, talks when no one else is in the conversation, often drawing wary looks from passersby. That's a perfect example of a behavior that is not well matched to the situation. Talking and having a conversation are perfectly fine behaviors, but only when there's someone else involved with the conversation.

Performing Poorly

Even when the behavior is appropriate to the situation, behaviors can be maladaptive when they are poorly performed. The person may attempt to engage in the behavior that is called for by the situation; however, he or she may do so in a manner that does not work very well. One example might be Scott, our socially anxious client. He avoids social situations whenever he can (a behavioral deficit). When he does try to interact with others, however, his social performance is unskilled. There are long pauses in his speech, and he doesn't make good eye contact. He appears nervous and unconfident to others.

Where Do Behaviors Come From?

Behavioral change is a major focus in CBT. It's therefore helpful for us to review some basic facts about where behaviors come from, so that we can design interventions that can help modify those behaviors. Fundamentally, the CBT model posits that maladaptive behaviors are learned, in one way or another. Broadly speaking, therefore, we would say that a person gets into fights because he or she has learned to get into fights and that another person cuts himself or herself because he or she has learned to do so. There are some notable exceptions to this rule—simple motor tics, for example, are probably not learned—but the complex behaviors most of our clients describe are there because, one way or another, they learned to do them. In this section we talk about how maladaptive behaviors are learned, and in later chapters we discuss how to create new learning experiences that will help our clients adopt healthier and more adaptive patterns of behavior.

As we know from the core pathological process described in Chapter 1, psychological problems are a mutually escalating relationship among cognitive, emotional, and behavioral processes. Behaviors, therefore, have a strong impact on both emotions and thoughts (see Figure 2.1).

I'll preface this part by revisiting a point I raised in Chapter 1: The *etiology* of a behavior and the *maintenance* of that behavior can be quite different. So as we try to understand any particular behavior, we need to differentiate the factors that started the behavior in the first place (etiology) from the factors that cause the behavior to persist (maintenance). In a CBT model, we usually find that the maintaining factors are most critical, because they are the things that we have the potential to change.

Behaviors Are Influenced by Thoughts and Emotions

Emotions are associated with various **action tendencies:** a motivation to engage in certain behaviors based on a felt emotion. Frijda (1987, p. 133) identified 18 emotional action tendencies:

1. Approach: tendency to get closer in order to possess, use, enjoy, or inspect.
2. Avoidance: tendency to avoid, flee or protect oneself.
3. Being-with: tendency to stay in proximity of.
4. Attending: tendency to observe, watch, or think about.

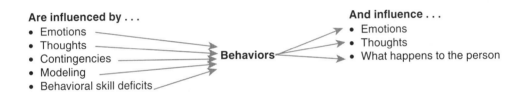

FIGURE 2.1. Inputs and outputs for behaviors.

5. Rejection: tendency to reject or break contact.
6. Indifference: tendency not to pay attention to or absence of tendency to attend to.
7. Antagonism: tendency to remove obstacle, hurt, oppose, or resist.
8. Interruption: tendency to interrupt ongoing action.
9. Dominance: tendency to control.
10. Submission: tendency to submit to control.
11. Apathy: generalised absence of action readiness and lack of responsivity.
12. Excitement: tendency towards action that has no direction.
13. Exuberance: free activation, increased and generalized action readiness.
14. Passivity: absence of goals for action.
15. Inhibition: presence of action readiness but absence of action.
16. Helplessness: action readiness but uncertainty about the direction it could take.
17. Blushing: blushing or felt tendency to blush.
18. Rest: absence of action readiness and acceptance thereof.

We can draw direct links between these action tendencies and certain emotional experiences. For example, feeling afraid is associated with avoidance and inhibition. Feeling angry is associated with antagonism. Feeling sad is associated with apathy. Feeling happy is associated with being-with and exuberance (Frijda, 1987).

And these action tendencies often work in our favor. It's good to avoid dangerous situations, for example. Certain threats warrant an antagonistic response. Slowing down when sad things happen can allow us to look more carefully at situations.

On the flip side, however, there are times that our action tendencies don't work well at all. For example, although fear is associated with the action tendency to escape from threat, that behavior wouldn't make sense when the threat is imagined rather than real. Although anger is associated with the action tendency to attack what's bothering us, if we do that whenever we're annoyed at a coworker, we're going to get into trouble. That means that sometimes in order to live well we have to override the natural action tendencies associated with an emotion. In Chapters 3 and 4, we'll talk more about how one's thoughts and emotions affect behavior.

Behaviors Are Influenced by Contingencies

Operant conditioning is a learning process that can contribute to both the etiology and the maintenance of behaviors. Operant conditioning, described by E. L. Thorndike (1901) and later elaborated by B. F. Skinner (1938), means that behavior is at least partially controlled by **contingencies.** Contingencies are defined as the context in which a behavior occurs, importantly including whatever *follows* the behavior, thereby increasing or decreasing the likelihood that the behavior will happen again.

The Four Contingencies: Reinforcement, Escape, Punishment, Penalty

Contingencies can be **positive** (meaning something is added to the person's experience that was not there before the behavior) or **negative** (meaning something is taken from the person's experience after the behavior). It's important not to confuse the terms *positive* and *negative* with *good* and *bad*. They just mean "*added* after the behavior" or "*withdrawn* after the behavior."

Contingencies can also be **reinforcers** (meaning that the behavior is more likely to happen again after the contingency is administered) or **punishers** (meaning that the behavior is less likely to happen again after the contingency is administered). Again, it's important not to confuse the terms *reinforcer* and *punisher* with *good* and *bad*. They just mean "*increases* the likelihood of the behavior happening again" or "*decreases* the likelihood of the behavior happening again."

So we can therefore imagine a two-by-two table of contingencies, as shown in Table 2.1. Some of these processes are heavily implicated in the etiology and/or maintenance of mental disorders.

Reinforcement (which Skinner called *positive reinforcement*; shown on the top left of Table 2.1) occurs when the behavior is followed by something that is added (positive), causing the behavior to subsequently increase (reinforcement). In a basic operant conditioning experiment, reinforcement would be demonstrated when a rat would receive a food pellet for pressing a lever, which would result in the rat pressing the lever more frequently. In this case, the food pellet is *positive* (it is added following the behavior) and a *reinforcer* (it increases the likelihood that the behavior will occur again). We can see the same phenomenon happening in the maintenance of maladaptive human behavior as well:

- While she was in the hospital, Elizabeth cut her wrists superficially in the day room. This resulted in her receiving increased attention from unit staff. As a result, Elizabeth cut herself more frequently. The behavior went up over time (reinforcer) because it had been followed by getting something (positive).
- Nick uses yelling to control Johanna. When he yells, Johanna complies. As a result, Nick yells more frequently. The behavior went up over time (reinforcer) because it had been followed by getting something (positive). Johanna's behavior is being influenced by contingencies, too—although in her case, the contingencies are different (see below).
- Samantha, who has trichotillomania, finds the experience of hair pulling to be pleasurable. As a result, she pulls her hair more frequently. The behavior went up over time (reinforcer) because it had been followed by getting something (positive).

Escape (which Skinner called *negative reinforcement*; shown on the bottom left of Table 2.1) occurs when the behavior is followed by something that is withdrawn (negative), causing the behavior to subsequently increase (reinforcement). In a basic operant conditioning experiment, escape would be demonstrated when a loud noise continuously sounds inside a rat's cage until it presses a lever, upon which the loud noise is removed for 30 seconds, resulting in the rat pressing the lever more frequently. In this case, the noise is *negative* (it is withdrawn following the behavior) and a *reinforcer* (it increases the likelihood that the lever-pressing behavior will occur again). The rat learns that it can terminate an aversive

TABLE 2.1. Contingencies in Operant Conditioning

	Reinforcer (increases the likelihood that the behavior will occur again)	Punisher (decreases the likelihood that the behavior will occur again)
Positive (something is added following the behavior)	Positive reinforcement (reinforcement)	Positive punishment (punishment)
Negative (something is withdrawn after the behavior)	Negative reinforcement (escape)	Negative punishment (penalty)

stimulus by engaging in the behavior. This phenomenon is happening in our clients as well:

- Blaise finds that when she is not using drugs, her feelings of withdrawal are intolerable. When she uses, the intolerable feelings subside and she feels more "normal." As a result, she uses more frequently. The behavior went up over time (reinforcer) because it was followed by escape from something (negative).
- Anna experiences panic symptoms at the shopping mall. She leaves the mall, resulting in relief from the panic symptoms. As a result, Anna leaves threatening situations more frequently. The behavior went up over time (reinforcer) because it was followed by escape from something (negative).
- As mentioned previously, when Nick yells, Johanna complies—and therefore Johanna is *positively reinforcing* Nick's yelling behavior. At the same time, from Johanna's perspective, when she complies, Nick stops his yelling. So her compliance behavior goes up over time (reinforcer) because it was followed by escape from something (negative). So Nick's behavior is influenced by *reinforcement,* while Johanna's behavior is influenced by *escape.* It gets tricky when dealing with family systems!
- At home, Elizabeth is experiencing strong feelings of sadness and anger. She cuts her wrists superficially, and the feelings of sadness and anger decrease as she is (momentarily) distracted from them. As a result, Elizabeth cuts herself more frequently. The behavior went up over time (reinforcer) because it was followed by escape from something (negative).

I put that last one in there on purpose. Note that at one time, Elizabeth's cutting behavior was *positively* reinforced; at another time, it was *negatively* reinforced. The same behavior can be maintained by more than one contingency, simultaneously or at different times.

Punishment (which Skinner called *positive punishment*; shown on the top right of Table 2.1) occurs when the behavior is followed by something that is added (positive), causing the behavior to subsequently decrease (punishment). In a basic operant conditioning experiment, positive punishment would be demonstrated when a rat would hear an unpleasant loud noise whenever it presses a lever, which would result in the rat pressing the lever less frequently. In this case, the noise is *positive* (it is added following the behavior) and a *punisher* (it decreases the likelihood that the behavior will occur again). Punishment shows up in many cases in which a desired behavior is low or suppressed:

- William tells us that while growing up, he attempted to be assertive and express his wishes to his parents. When he attempted to act assertively with a parent, he would often be slapped and told to shut up. As a result, William became unassertive (i.e., he now uses assertive behavior less frequently). The behavior went down (punisher) because of a history of bad consequences (positive).
- Scott works up the courage to introduce himself to a stranger at a party. The person makes a snotty and condescending remark to Scott, leading him to feel embarrassed. As a result, Scott approaches others less frequently. The behavior went down (punisher) because of a history of bad consequences (positive).

You might wonder, looking at some of our clients, why some things that we might call "punishment" don't actually decrease the behavior. For example:

- Every time she binge-eats, Shari makes herself throw up. Why doesn't the unpleasantness of throwing up make her stop binge eating?
- After a night of drug use, Blaise feels awful. She's hung over and is confronted with what a mess her life has become. So why doesn't that stop the drug use?
- Elizabeth sometimes says she cuts herself in order to "punish" herself for making mistakes in judgment, such as going home with a stranger. Why doesn't that "punishment" lead her to consider her choices more carefully?
- When Nick and Johanna's son James gets a bad grade in school, they "punish" him by sending him to his room and taking away his video games. So why doesn't that make him do better in school?

At the risk of talking in circles, these things are not "punishers" in the technical sense of the word. In CBT, we call something a punisher only if it actually reduces the likelihood that the behavior will happen again. Most of these unwanted behaviors, from Shari's purging to Blaise's drug use to James's bad school habits, are under the control of more immediate reinforcers (short-term payoffs). They all get something out of the behavior; either an increase in something desired (positive reinforcement) or a reduction in something not desired (negative reinforcement). Administering aversive consequences after the fact, without attending to the reinforcers, is a losing battle. This is why a hacking cough doesn't usually stop people from smoking and why weight gain doesn't usually stop people from eating junk food. We are all slaves to the immediate, unless we force ourselves not to be.

Penalty (which Skinner called *negative punishment*; shown on the bottom right of Table 2.1) occurs when the behavior is followed by something that gets taken away (negative), causing the behavior to subsequently decrease (punishment). In a basic operant conditioning experiment, negative punishment would be demonstrated when a rat would have food pellets taken away from its supply whenever it presses a lever, which would result in the rat pressing the lever less frequently. In this case, the removal of food pellets is *negative* (they are taken away following the behavior) and a *punisher* (it decreases the likelihood that the behavior will occur again).

On Intentionality and Contingencies

It's often tempting to infer that because contingencies are present, the person must be deliberately acting in a manner to get certain contingencies or avoid other ones. For example, we saw that at times Elizabeth's cutting behavior increased when she received more attention from others. Some would look at that pattern and conclude that Elizabeth was being "manipulative"; that is, she knew she would get more attention by cutting, so she did it. Elizabeth had certainly heard that accusation from family members and unit staff. But was the accusation true?

It's important to recognize that contingencies work *whether or not we are aware of them*, and they work *whether or not we intend them to*. Our behavior is nudged and molded by myriad contingencies, and in many cases the effect of the contingencies has nothing to do with our wishes or even our awareness. So did Elizabeth know that cutting was a way to get attention from others, and did she actively decide that this was how she wanted to get attention? Maybe, maybe not. It is just as likely that the attention from staff increased her cutting behavior over time without her or the unit staff even being aware of it. Flip the equation: Did the staff mean to make Elizabeth cut more? Did they get together and decide that the way to get her to cut more was to lavish her with attention whenever she

The Science behind It

Couples' distress is viewed, in part, as a mutual failure of reinforcement. Distressed couples routinely exhibit high rates of displeasing behavior and/or low rates of pleasing behavior toward each other (Gottman, Markman, & Notarius, 1977). Whereas satisfied couples primarily use reinforcement to modify each other's behavior, distressed couples primarily rely on escape (negative reinforcement) and punishment as a means of behavioral influence (N. S. Jacobson & Margolin, 1979). Couples also appear to match each other's contingencies in a "tit for tat" manner (sometimes called *reciprocity*), such that reinforcement from one member is usually followed by reinforcement from the other, and punishment from one member is usually followed by punishment from the other (Gottman et al., 1977). Over time, the contingencies between members of the couple balance out (Gottman et al., 1976), such that "a spouse who gives a lot, gets a lot; a spouse who gives a little, gets a little" (N. S. Jacobson & Margolin, 1979, p. 15).

Relatedly, family distress, particularly in the case of a child who demonstrates oppositional or antisocial behavior, is frequently associated with a *coercive family process*. When we observe these families, we often see that the discipline is harsh and inconsistent, with little positive interaction among family members (Patterson, DeBaryshe, & Ramsey, 1989). Behavioral explanations don't negate the presence of basic child temperamental factors; however, they emphasize that child behavior problems develop within the context of interactional systems, such as the family and the school, and therefore that there is an interaction between the child's basic tendencies and the contingencies for desired and unwanted behaviors (Strand, 2000). It has been suggested that within these family systems, family members train the child to engage in rotten behavior—sometimes through positive reinforcement, but usually through escape (negative reinforcement), in which the child uses rotten behavior to stop other family members' aversive intrusions. The child, in turn, is training the family members to escalate their aversive behaviors. For example, Johanna and Nick's marital distress often "spills over" into their interactions with their son James, as they frequently yell at him and nag him. He acts out, which temporarily gets them to stop their nagging. They also pay more attention to him after he engages in bad behavior. So James is learning that he can control Johanna and Nick by acting out. Johanna and Nick, not aware of the contingencies that are in place, feel that their only option is to yell and nag even more—so both parents and child get locked into a cycle of escalation. Simultaneously, positive (prosocial) behaviors are ignored or even punished (Kazdin, 2008; Patterson, 1982). Johanna and Nick do not consistently reinforce James for asking for permission, doing his homework, cleaning his room, and so on, so he is less likely to do those behaviors. The coercive family process seems to worsen under conditions of family stress, such as unemployment, marital discord, and divorce (Conger, Ge, Elder, Lorenz, & Simons, 1994). Sadly, this pattern seems to continue across multiple generations, as one generation uses the poor parenting they witnessed as kids on their own children (Elder, Caspi, & Downey, 1983).

did it? I seriously doubt it. But the contingencies were there nevertheless. So rather than jumping to the conclusion that Elizabeth was being *manipulative,* I think it's more accurate to say that both Elizabeth and the unit staff were being *manipulated* by contingencies. They were locked into an unhealthy system of reciprocal reinforcement that they didn't fully understand and couldn't fully control.

Schedules of Reinforcement

The frequency of reinforcement plays an important role in the acquisition and maintenance of behavior. Skinner (1938) identified several distinct schedules, including continuous, fixed interval, fixed ratio, variable interval, and variable ratio. For our purposes, however, we'll consolidate these into two basic groups: *continuous reinforcement* and *intermittent reinforcement.*

Continuous reinforcement occurs when the reinforcement *always* follows the behavior. For example, the rat receives a food pellet every time it presses the lever, or the client receives increased attention from others every time he or she cuts him- or herself.

The most important effect of continuous reinforcement is that it makes behavior increase rapidly—that is, it is most heavily implicated in the *etiology* or acquisition of the behavior. So a lot of maladaptive behaviors will start under a continuous reinforcement schedule. Elizabeth's cutting, Blaise's substance use, Samantha's hair pulling, and Bethany's compulsions all began under a schedule of continuous reinforcement, so the behaviors were acquired and escalated rapidly.

Intermittent reinforcement occurs when the reinforcement *sometimes* follows the behavior. For example, the rat receives a food pellet only some of the times it presses the lever, or the client wins money only some of the times he or she gambles.

The most important effect of intermittent reinforcement is that it makes the behavior "stick," even when no reinforcer is provided. When the behavior is not followed by a reinforcer, the person knows that if he or she keeps at it, the reinforcer will come eventually. Intermittent reinforcement, therefore, is implicated in the *maintenance* or persistence of the behavior. So a lot of maladaptive behaviors may have *started* under a continuous reinforcement schedule, but they *persist* under an intermittent reinforcement schedule (see Figure 2.2). Suzanne, for example, constantly checks the doors and windows in her home

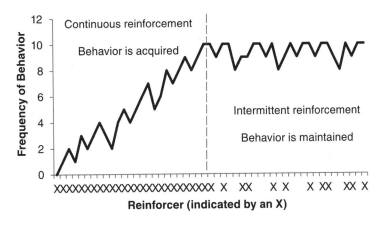

FIGURE 2.2. An example of the effect of continuous and intermittent reinforcement on behavior.

to make sure they are locked. Every so often, she finds one unlocked. This intermittent reinforcement ensures that she will keep checking, regardless of what she finds. Nick can sometimes (but not always) get Johanna off his back by yelling at her, so he'll keep at it, even when it's clearly not working.

Extinction

In addition to reinforcement and punishment, there are some other important principles from operant conditioning that play a key role in mental disorders. **Extinction** occurs when a behavior that had previously been reinforced no longer results in reinforcement. In a basic experiment, for example, after teaching a rat to press a lever in order to obtain food pellets, we stop providing the pellets (i.e., the behavior is no longer effective). Two things are likely to happen in this case (see Figure 2.3):

First, the rat will probably do *more* of the behavior in order to try to get the reinforcement coming again. This is called an **extinction burst.** When that doesn't work, the rat will press the lever less and less frequently, and eventually stop. The behavior is now said to be *extinguished*.

Extinction can contribute to human psychological problems. Imagine, for example, that a child of a depressed mother tries to engage the mother to play. She is unresponsive (i.e., does not reinforce the child's behavior). As a result, the child stops trying to engage the mother and has less interest in playing, eventually taking on some of his or her mother's signs of depression.

Avoidance Learning

Avoidance learning occurs when the person engages in a behavior in *anticipation* of a stimulus, thus preventing the stimulus from occurring. Note that this is slightly different from escape. In escape, the person engages in a behavior in order to terminate an unpleasant stimulus, whereas in avoidance the behavior is used to prevent the stimulus from occurring in the first place.

Avoidance behavior is strongly implicated in the maintenance of conditioned emotional reactions. In a classic experiment, Solomon, Kamin, and Wynne (1953) trained

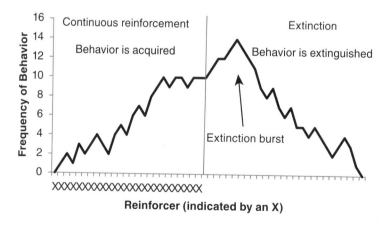

FIGURE 2.3. An example of extinction.

dogs to fear a light by pairing it with an electric shock (see discussion of *classical conditioning* in Chapter 4). The experimenters would flash a light and then administer an electric shock through the metal floor of the dogs' cage. The dogs quickly developed a fearful reaction to the light, even though the shocks were terminated. They then examined the process of fear extinction. Some of the dogs were given the opportunity, once the light flashed, to jump over a small fence and get away from the metal floor that had previously shocked them. When the dogs had the ability to avoid the thing that was scaring them (the light), their fears persisted indefinitely. Dogs that were blocked from jumping over the fence, on the other hand, showed reduction of fear. Therefore, avoidance behaviors cause fear to persist.

And the same phenomenon shows up in our clients, as well.

- Scott, our socially anxious client, avoids public speaking by selecting a job that doesn't require him to speak in front of other people, by not volunteering to give the toast at weddings or parties, by not being a reader in church, and by not leading activities in his child's scout troop. His public speaking fear persists over time.
- Melissa, who has PTSD, is afraid to remember the details of her traumatic experiences because of the painful feelings associated with those memories. Therefore, she goes out of her way to avoid talking about the traumas, seeing people or places that are objectively safe but that might remind her of the traumas, seeing things on TV that might bring up memories of the traumas, and so on.
- Suzanne, who has GAD, engages in excessive worrying in order to prevent being "caught off guard" by a disaster. At times, she drinks or uses substances as a way of feeling more "numb." These avoidance behaviors cause her intolerance of uncertainty to persist.

Behaviors Are Influenced by Modeling

Behaviors can also be acquired through **modeling.** In a classic experiment, children who watched an adult model aggressively beat on a doll were, when mildly frustrated and given access to a similar doll, more likely to behave aggressively toward the doll themselves than were children who did not watch the adult model beat the doll (Bandura, Ross, & Ross, 1963a). In addition, children were much more likely to imitate the aggressive behavior when they witnessed the adult being reinforced for his or her aggression (Bandura, Ross, & Ross, 1963b). Thus, we can acquire behaviors by watching someone else engage in those behaviors, and the imitative process is amplified when we see someone else be reinforced or punished for a behavior.

There are all kinds of ways that modeling might be implicated in the etiology or maintenance of our clients' maladaptive behaviors.

- Suzanne tells us that her mother was a highly nervous person who constantly telephoned Suzanne and Suzanne's father to make sure that they were all right and would triple-check the door and window locks on the house.
- Shari, who is diagnosed with bulimia, initially started purging after learning that other members of her peer group—the "cool girls"—were doing it.
- While hospitalized, Lauren, who is diagnosed with schizophrenia, engages in disruptive behavior after seeing another client receive attention for similar behaviors.
- Nick and Johanna's son James learns, by watching his parents, that yelling and other forms of aggression pay off. His behavior becomes increasingly aggressive.

Behaviors Are Influenced by the Presence of Behavioral Skill Deficits

Sometimes people engage in a behavior because they don't know what else to do, or because they are not good at other, more adaptive behaviors. We refer to these as **behavioral skill deficits.** Examples of common behavioral skill deficits include *social skill deficits* and *problem-solving deficits.*

Social Skill Deficits

Social skills refers to a complex set of behavioral skills that include verbal (what to say, how to phrase it, when to say it, how long to speak, etc.) and nonverbal (tone of voice, volume, body posture, facial expression, interpersonal distance, etc.) aspects. Complicating the process is the fact that different settings call for different skills (e.g., the skills you use in a meeting with your boss may differ from those you use with your friends) and that different cultures have different norms (e.g., the degree of interpersonal distance during conversation is different between the United States and parts of the Middle East). It is hardly surprising, therefore, that some people might exhibit a deficit in one or more aspects of social skill. Imagine:

- Scott tries to make conversation with others at a party. However, he makes poor eye contact, speaks very quietly, and is silent for long periods. We could easily imagine that this scenario is not likely to end with Scott being reinforced for his efforts.
- Elizabeth feels like her partner has treated her unfairly. However, engaging in assertive behavior (e.g., expressing how she feels and asking the partner to change his behavior) is too difficult. Without a healthy way to get the partner to change, Elizabeth engages in aggressive behaviors such as screaming and throwing things. We could easily imagine that these maladaptive behaviors would be reinforced (e.g., by getting others to take notice of her or to leave her alone), thus leading to further atrophy of Elizabeth's assertion skills.

The Science behind It

Lots of clients will have social skill deficits of varying degrees. For example:

- The poor interpersonal functioning seen in *personality disorders* can be conceptualized in part as a skill deficit. For example, self-injurious clients with borderline personality disorder show skill deficits in the area of emotional communication, both in terms of expressing emotions and in the interpretation of emotional communication from others (McKay, Gavigan, & Kulchycky, 2004). When social performance tests such as mock conversations are used, individuals with a range of maladaptive personality features show deficits in the areas of initiating social interactions, assertive behavior, and self-disclosure (Muralidharan, Sheets, Madsen, Craighead, & Craighead, 2011; Waldeck & Miller, 2000).

- *Autism spectrum disorders,* by definition, are associated with impaired interpersonal behavior. Observations of clients with autism spectrum disorders indicate that their interpersonal communication is often overly verbose and perseverative on fixed topics of interest.

They often display a lack of interest in the other person and have difficulty taking turns in conversation (Mandelberg et al., 2014).

- Individuals with *schizophrenia* show marked deficits in both the verbal and nonverbal aspects of interpersonal communication (Bellack, Morrison, Wixted, & Mueser, 1990). Among people with schizophrenia, poor social skill is associated with poorer psychosocial functioning both before and after the onset of the illness (Mueser, Bellack, Morrison, & Wixted, 1990).

- Many authors have suggested the presence of social skill deficits in *depression*. Interpersonal theories of depression suggest that poor social skill leads to rejection from others (Coyne, 1976) and less positive social reinforcement (Lewinsohn, 1974). Research suggests that poor social skill is both a vulnerability factor for and a consequence of depressed mood (Segrin, 2000). Observation studies of people with depression compared with those without suggest that those with depression display less variation in pitch and facial expression, have prolonged silences, have decreased eye contact, spend less time talking, and focus on negative themes in conversation (Segrin, 1990, 2000; Tse & Bond, 2004). The impact of depressive social behavior on others is notable and immediate: Within the first few minutes of talking to a depressed individual, even nondepressed people show less pleasant facial expressions, talk about less positive and more negative content, and make fewer statements of direct support (Gotlib & Robinson, 1982). It's worth noting that depressed people typically rate their own social skills as poorer than they actually are (Gotlib, 1983), which is not surprising given the cognitive distortions and information-processing biases in depression (see Chapter 3). Conversely, nondepressed people tend to rate their own social skills as better than then actually are (Lewinsohn, Mischel, Chaplin, & Barton, 1980). Most likely, depressed people's negative views of their own social skills are due to a combination of negative processing biases and actual performance deficits (Dykman, Horowitz, Abramson, & Usher, 1991).

- *Socially anxious* people are frequently inhibited around others. People with social anxiety have been observed to display poor eye contact (Baker & Edelmann, 2002; Horley, Williams, Gonsalvez, & Gordon, 2003) and appear anxious (Alden & Mellings, 2004). Even when speaking with their romantic partners, socially anxious people show less eye contact, less smiling, fewer prompting sounds such as "uh-huh," fewer head nods, fewer gestures, less touching, more fidgeting, and quieter speech (Wenzel, Graff-Dolezal, Macho, & Brendle, 2005). Impaired social skill appears particularly strong among individuals with avoidant personality disorder (Turner, Beidel, Dancu, & Keys, 1986) and when the social situation is less structured (S. Thompson & Rapee, 2002). These impaired social behaviors can exert a profound but often undetected influence on others' perceptions of the socially anxious individual: They tend to rate him or her as less likeable (Alden & Wallace, 1995) and even less intelligent (Paulhus & Morgan, 1997). They also tend to respond to the socially anxious person in a negative manner that furthers his or her social withdrawal (Creed & Funder, 1998; Paulhus & Morgan, 1997)—a classic self-fulfilling prophecy. In social anxiety, we see a similar cognitive bias to that we saw in depression. Socially anxious people tend to rate their social skills as lower than they actually are (which does not negate the presence of an actual skill deficit). They tend to grade their social performance less on their actual behavior than on the amount of anxiety they feel (Alden & Mellings, 2004)—which is related to the concept of *emotional reasoning* that we'll discuss in Chapter 3 ("If I feel anxious, I must be doing a bad job").

- Children and adolescents with *attention-deficit/hyperactivity disorder* display poorer knowledge of social skills than do their unaffected peers. Their interpersonal behavior is frequently described as inappropriate or aggressive, leading to peer rejection (Frederick & Olmi, 1994).

Social skills can go wrong for several reasons, including:

- **Acquisition deficit.** The person simply does not know the appropriate social skill.
- **Performance deficit.** The person knows the appropriate social skill but is inhibited from enacting the skill due to cognitive or emotional factors.
- **Fluency deficit.** The person knows the appropriate social skill but has difficulty performing it smoothly and naturally.

These three different kinds of deficits are all amenable to social skill training, but they will influence the kind of training you provide (see Chapter 12).

The Science behind It

Social skill deficits play a strong role in distressed interpersonal systems such as couples and families. Even though the members of the system might *know* the appropriate skills to use, they have difficulty *implementing* those skills in a consistent manner.

Distressed couples frequently fall into patterns of unskilled interpersonal behavior. Even though they might know the appropriate behaviors, they display a performance or skill deficit in how they interact with each other. Gottman (1999) notes that four categories of interpersonal behavior, which he termed the "Four Horsemen of the Apocalypse," predicted later divorce:

- *Criticism:* Making statements implying that something is globally wrong with the partner, rather than addressing a specific behavior (e.g., "You forgot to pay the phone bill again. How could you be so stupid?").
- *Contempt:* Words, actions, or expressions that imply that one is superior to one's partner in some way (e.g., "Well, I guess I just prioritize the kids more than you do, because somehow I found the time to go to their school functions").
- *Defensiveness:* Denying responsibility or otherwise attempting to ward off a perceived verbal attack from the partner (e.g., "But I'm trying! It's not my fault! Why blame me?").
- *Stonewalling:* "Checking out" of the conversation or interaction (e.g., minimizing interactions with one's partner, or not attending to the discussion).

Distressed families can also fall into negative interactional patterns. One important example is the phenomenon of *expressed emotion* (Hooley, 1985; Leff & Vaughn, 1985) in families of clients with psychiatric disorders. Expressed emotion (which might sound like a nice thing, but it isn't) refers to negative interpersonal behaviors on the part of family members. Expressed emotion includes (Chambless, Bryan, Aiken, Steketee, & Hooley, 1999):

- *Criticism* (described above).
- *Emotional overinvolvement:* Being overly intrusive or overprotective, using excessive praise or blame, showing exaggerated emotional reactions, or taking over too many tasks for the client.
- *Low rates of positive or warm interaction.*

The degree of expressed emotion in a family is a strong predictor of relapse after hospitalization for clients with various mental illnesses such as schizophrenia, mood disorders, and eating disorders (Butzlaff & Hooley, 1998) and may similarly predict poor outcome of individual treatment for mood and anxiety disorders. Among adolescents, expressed emotion in the family appears to also be a vulnerability factor for externalizing symptoms (Nelson, Hammen, Brennan, & Ullman, 2003) and suicidal thoughts and behaviors (Wedig & Nock, 2007).

Problem-Solving Deficits

Effective **problem solving** generally involves (1) a positive general orientation toward problem solving (e.g., a belief that problems are normal and can be dealt with); (2) defining the problem and attempting to understand its cause; (3) generating multiple possible solutions to the problem; (4) deciding on a particular solution; and (5) determining whether the solution was effective (D'Zurilla & Goldfried, 1971). This sequence can go awry in several ways. An individual may not adequately define the problem, may choose the first solution that comes to mind without evaluating alternatives, may be unable to decide among several possibilities, or may not reflect on whether the chosen solutions were actually effective. Depending on where the deficit occurs in the sequence, various maladaptive behaviors can emerge or persist due to problem-solving deficits. Imagine:

- Suzanne, who has GAD, knows that she will not have enough money to pay the electric bill this month. She engages in excessive worry as a form of pseudo–problem solving, thinking about all of the potentially disastrous consequences of not paying the bill. However, she does not generate multiple solutions to the problem, weighing the pros and cons of each, and decide on a course of action. As a result, she remains stuck in the cycle of worry.
- William, who is dependent on others, is having difficulty at work. However, he has a poor problem orientation (i.e., instead of believing that problems are normal and can be dealt with, he believes that this problem is unique and unresolvable). Instead of engaging in problem-solving efforts, he feels hopeless and does not take adaptive action.

The Science behind It

Deficient problem solving, in one form or another, is fairly ubiquitous across mental disorders (Thoma, Friedmann, & Suchan, 2013; Tisdelle & St. Lawrence, 1986). Here are just a few examples:

- Individuals with *schizophrenia* and acute *bipolar disorder* show demonstrable social problem-solving deficits. They generate poor solutions to problems, which are less feasible and less likely to be effective. They have difficulty implementing effective problem-solving strategies in conversations with others. They are also less persistent in defending their point of view, with unclear arguments and diminished ability to negotiate solutions to problems (Bellack, Sayers, Mueser, & Bennett, 1994).

• *Depression* may also be characterized by problem-solving deficits. The presence of a negative problem orientation is associated with hopelessness, depression, and suicidal ideation (D'Zurilla, Chang, Nottingham, & Faccini, 1998), and individuals with poor problem-solving skills tend to have lower self-worth and attachment insecurity (Davila, Hammen, Burge, Daley, & Paley, 1996). One's problem-solving ability appears to moderate one's depressive reaction to major negative events (Nezu, Nezu, Sarayadarian, Kalmar, & Ronan, 1986), as well as daily stressors (Nezu & Ronan, 1985). Thus, individuals with poor problem-solving skills seem more vulnerable to developing depression under stressful circumstances.

• Problem-solving deficits have also been implicated in *suicidality* and *self-harm*. A negative problem orientation among suicidal individuals has been identified. Labeled the "Three I's" (Chiles & Strosahl, 1995), this orientation assumes that physical or emotional pain is *intolerable,* the person's life situation is *interminable,* and the situation is *inescapable.* Clients with suicidal ideation show less active problem solving than do other psychiatric clients (Linehan, Camper, Chiles, Strosahl, & Shearin, 1987), generate less than half as many potential solutions to interpersonal problems, focus on the negatives of potential solutions, and implement fewer alternatives (Schotte & Clum, 1987). Suicidal or self-injurious adolescents similarly show poor social problem-solving ability (Speckens & Hawton, 2005), characterized in particular by choosing negative solutions to problems and having low self-efficacy for performing adaptive solutions (Nock & Mendes, 2008).

• Problem solving, including social problem solving, breaks down in *distressed couples*. It is thought that the couple's usual problem-solving abilities become clouded by high levels of negative affect and cognitive distortions such as overgeneralization. For example, a conversation that begins as a disagreement between spouses about whose turn it is to watch the kids can quickly spiral into an argument about larger, potentially unresolvable issues such as selfishness and love (D'Zurilla & Nezu, 1982). Distressed couples have been noted to engage in "cross-complaining," in which one member's complaint is matched with another member's complaint that may or may not be directly related to the original complaint (Gottman et al., 1977). In such a case, actual problem solving never gets off the ground, and problems persist.

What Do Behaviors Do?

Behavior Affects Emotions

Our behaviors can have a strong influence on our emotions. For example:

• Scott, who is socially anxious, avoids going to parties or interacting with people he doesn't know well. His avoidant behavior, temporarily relieving as it may be, has contributed to the maintenance of his fear. By avoiding, he deprives himself of the opportunity to receive corrective information about social interactions.
• Elizabeth, who feels sad and despondent much of the time, will isolate herself in her room and will, at times, engage in self-injurious behaviors. Those behaviors give her a bit of short-term relief from her distress, but over time they cause her feelings to worsen as she feels worse and worse about herself.
• Shari, who struggles with bulimia, engages in binge-eating behaviors, which lead

her to feel disgusted and ashamed of herself and to get anxious about gaining weight. She then tries to compensate by making herself throw up. Although the vomiting helps reduce her fear of weight gain, she feels even more ashamed and out of control.

- Bethany, who has OCD, engages in compulsive hand washing when she is anxious about contamination. Her hand washing is temporarily relieving but only serves to prolong her fear because she does not get the opportunity to learn that dirty hands are unlikely to harm her.
- Nick "blows up" at Johanna during an argument, yelling at her and slamming the door on the way out of the room. He finds that as he does so, his angry feelings only get worse.

Imagine what would have happened to these clients' emotions if they had chosen different behavioral responses. What would have happened if Scott had pushed through his fear and interacted with people? What would have happened if Elizabeth had left her room, even though she was feeling sad, and engaged in activities that gave her a sense of pleasure or accomplishment? What would have happened if Shari, after an eating binge, had worked through her feelings of disgust rather than making herself throw up? What would have happened if Bethany had refrained from washing her hands, even though she felt contaminated? What would have happened if Nick, despite his angry feelings, had opted to talk to Johanna in a calm and gentle manner? Over time, their emotions would adjust. That's one of the central tenets of CBT: **Doing better in order to feel better.** We'll talk a lot more about this principle in Part II of this book.

The Science behind It

Research studies have demonstrated that asking people to change their facial expressions leads to a shift in their moods (Levenson, Ekman, & Friesen, 1990). The participants were given specific instructions about which facial muscles to move and how. For example: "(a) pull your eyebrows down and together; (b) raise your upper eyelid; (c) push your lower lip up and press your lips together" (p. 365). Importantly, the participants weren't told to mimic any specific emotion (in this case, anger). Yet, when asked how they were feeling, participants making that facial expression were more likely to describe themselves as feeling angry than were participants instructed to make other facial expressions. Similarly, they showed greater evidence of anger-related physical arousal in terms of their heart rate, skin conductance (moisture), and finger temperature.

It is also likely that avoiding a particular stimulus makes it seem scarier. In one study, participants were asked to avoid contamination for 1 week by engaging in behaviors such as taking two or more showers a day, carrying hand sanitizer, avoiding touching money, and so on. After a week of these avoidance behaviors, participants reported an increase in their fears of contamination, as well as an increase in their beliefs about the dangerousness of contamination (Deacon & Maack, 2008). In a similar study, after a week of being instructed to perform a lot of health-related safety behaviors such as monitoring heart rate, checking websites for health information, and so on, participants reported an increase in health-related anxiety and hypochondriacal beliefs (Olatunji, Etzel, Tomarken, Ciesielski, & Deacon, 2011).

Things That Might Bug You about This

Many of us were taught that it's a good idea to "blow off steam" when we feel upset or angry by engaging in aggressive, yet harmless, behaviors. This idea is based on the theory of *catharsis,* which goes all the way back to Breuer and Freud (1893–1895/1955). For example, a popular self-help book on managing anger advises:

> *Punch a pillow or a punching bag. Punch with all the frenzy you can. If you are angry at a particular person, imagine his or her face on the pillow or punching bag, and vent your rage physically and verbally. You will be doing violence to a pillow or punching bag so that you can stop doing violence to yourself by holding in poisonous anger.* (Lee, 1993, p. 96)

Based on what you know about the reciprocal relationship between behavior and emotion, does this seem like a good idea or a bad idea? If you guessed "bad idea," you're right. It's long been known that aggressive behavior breeds anger and more aggression (Bandura, 1973). As one example, when research participants were made angry and then given the opportunity to hit a punching bag, they ended up feeling more angry than did participants who did not hit a punching bag (Bushman, 2002). Other research, similarly, shows that such "cathartic" aggressive behavior toward inanimate objects actually increases the likelihood that research participants will behave aggressively toward other people (Bushman, Baumeister, & Stack, 1999; Geen, Stonner, & Shope, 1975). Emotions aren't something that you "let out," like vomiting or removing a tumor. They're something that you work with in a healthy or unhealthy way.

Behavior Affects Thoughts

Behaviors affect how we perceive and interpret things. That is, acting a certain way can actually influence what you think. A great example of this is Festinger's (1962) concept of **cognitive dissonance.** The basic idea of cognitive dissonance (at least one aspect of it) goes something like this:

"I believe X."
"However, I am behaving in a way Y that is not consistent with X."
"It's uncomfortable to believe X yet behave like Y."
"Therefore, I am motivated to either change behavior Y or, if that's too difficult, to change belief X."

Imagine all of the ways that cognitive dissonance could shape our beliefs and attitudes. For example:

"I believe I am a decent person."
"However, I am engaging in undesirable behaviors, which is not consistent with the belief that I am a decent person."
"It's uncomfortable to believe that I am a decent person yet engage in undesirable behaviors."
"Therefore, I am motivated to either engage in fewer undesirable behaviors, or, if that's too difficult, to either believe that I am less decent, or to convince myself that my undesirable behaviors were justified and therefore not so undesirable after all."

Or . . .

"I believe that people are basically good."
"However, I am behaving aggressively, which is not consistent with the belief that people are basically good."
"It's uncomfortable to believe that people are basically good, yet act aggressively."
"Therefore, I am motivated to either act less aggressively or, if that's too difficult, to believe that people are less good, or to convince myself that my aggressive behavior was OK (e.g., the victim had it coming)."

Or even . . .

"I believe the world is basically safe."
"However, I am behaving in an avoidant manner, which is not consistent with the belief that the world is basically safe."
"It's uncomfortable to believe that the world is basically safe, yet behave in an avoidant manner."
"Therefore, I am motivated to either behave in a less avoidant manner, or, if that's too difficult, to believe that the world is less safe, or perhaps to convince myself that I'm not really avoiding and that my behavior is perfectly normal."

It kind of blows your mind to think that we can adjust our beliefs based on our behavior. But it happens all the time. We change what we think in accordance with our behavior. Our behavior exerts a powerful influence (of which we are often unaware) on how we view ourselves, other people, and the world—for better or for worse.

 ## The Science behind It

We will often adjust our beliefs so that they "fit" our behaviors better. In one study of cognitive dissonance, research participants were shown two items and were then asked to pick only one that they could take home. Their ratings of the desirability of the items that they picked subsequently increased, and their ratings of the desirability of the items that they did not pick subsequently decreased (Brehm, 1956). Liking something that you had rejected is uncomfortable, and because they couldn't change the behavior, they changed the belief.

Hazing in college or other organizations is a good example of cognitive dissonance at work. The more we suffer to get into an organization, the more we tend to value that organization (Keating et al., 2005). And the more we "volunteer" to be hazed, the greater the dissonance, and the more we are motivated to resolve that dissonance, either by minimizing the negative aspects of the hazing (e.g., "It wasn't degrading; it was fun!"), overvaluing the group (e.g., "Belonging to this group is so worthwhile that it is worth suffering in order to become part of it"), or both. In some classic experiments, participants who underwent an embarrassing induction found fellow group members to be more attractive than did participants who experienced a mild induction (Aronson & Mills, 1959), and participants given intense electrical shock during initiation into a group exhibited greater liking for their group than did those who received mild shock (Gerard & Mathewson, 1966). Our beliefs are easily influenced by what we're doing, as we try to explain ourselves to ourselves.

Another way in which behavior affects thoughts is in the fact that maladaptive behaviors *allow maladaptive beliefs to persist.* As an example, let's look at Bethany, who has OCD. One of her obsessive beliefs is that she will become contaminated and contract a disease. As shown in Figure 2.4, we see that her behavioral response includes avoiding anything that looks "dirty" and washing her hands over and over. Those behaviors serve to strengthen her belief that she is at risk of dying from disease. The fact that she *doesn't* die actually seems to prove her point that the avoidance and washing were necessary. In essence, her behaviors have created a situation in which she is unable to learn anything different. The reality is that she wouldn't have died even if she had dropped the avoidance and washing—but she'll never know that until she changes her behavior.

Imagine, just for a moment, what would happen if Bethany adopted a different behavioral response. Let's say she didn't avoid touching things that looked dirty, and she didn't engage in excessive hand washing. What would happen? For starters, we might predict that she'd feel more anxious. But what then? Most likely, she would realize that she was not dying. Her beliefs would start to change. As that happened, she would probably notice herself feeling less anxious as well. She would have set into motion a pattern of **acting the opposite:** behaving in a manner that has the potential to disconfirm her beliefs, rather than continuing the same confirmatory pattern.

Things That Might Bug You about This

We're used to thinking about behavior as being the end result of something. It makes sense, right? It fits with most common ways of thinking about behavior, and sometimes it's been drummed into our heads during our training. It can be hard to think about it any other way.

In the worst cases, we point to a diagnosis as the cause of behavior. That person attempted suicide *because* he has depression. That person is drinking *because* she is an alcoholic. That person cut herself *because* she has borderline personality disorder. This way of thinking is based on a medical model, in which there is an underlying disease (e.g., depression) and the behavior (e.g., suicide attempt) is a symptom of that disease. But that's not really how it works. Psychiatric diagnoses are purely descriptive: They describe clusters of emotional, cognitive, and behavioral problems, but they are not disease states that "cause" behaviors to occur.

Even when we get outside of the diagnosis, we often think about clients' problems as if they were a linear process. For example, some would argue that the order goes like this: thought → emotion → behavior. That is, thoughts cause emotions, and emotions cause behavior. But it ain't always so. In this chapter, we see that all of the relationships inside the core pathological process are reciprocal. Yes, thoughts and feelings can influence behavior, but behavior can also influence thoughts and feelings. This issue will be important for us later, because we'll see that many of our interventions focus on changing behavior in the service of helping the person feel better.

So does alcohol addiction cause drinking? Partly, but drinking is also the primary maintaining factor in alcohol addiction. Do depressed thoughts and feelings cause suicide attempts? Partly, but suicide attempts also maintain depressed thoughts and feelings. Does the constellation of emotional dysregulation and poor self-concept associated with borderline personality cause cutting? Partly, but cutting also maintains that emotional dysregulation and poor self-concept.

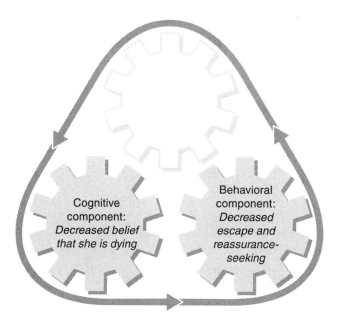

FIGURE 2.4. The reciprocal relationship between Bethany's thoughts and behaviors.

Behavior Affects What Happens to the Person

So we see that inside the core pathological process, maladaptive behavior affects both emotions and thoughts. Maladaptive behaviors have other negative effects as well (see Figure 2.5). First, behavior affects the person's experience of contingencies, as discussed previously. Christina, our depressed client, believes that she is unlovable and that no one likes her. So she gets in bed or lies down on the couch and spends the day at home by herself. There's been no real *reinforcement* (Ferster, 1973; McDowell, 1982) in her day. By sitting around the house, Christina is unable to receive any reinforcement for going out and being active, and therefore she is not particularly likely to go out the next day, either. The absence of positive reinforcement in one's life has been identified as a significant maintaining factor in depression (Lewinsohn, 1974). As Christina isolates herself more and more, she loses touch with others, and some of her friends have indeed drifted away. Some of those she still speaks to may react more negatively to her (Coyne, 1976). So social interaction becomes less reinforcing for Christina and potentially more punishing, and she becomes less and less likely to engage with others (and it would also not be surprising to learn that Christina's behavior also influenced her thoughts—the more time she spent alone, the more she became convinced that she was unlikeable and no one would want to spend time with her).

Imagine what would have happened if, instead of lying around her apartment, Christina went out and interacted with people. She might encounter some friendly people, who would smile and be nice to her. Those little experiences would *reinforce* Christina's going-out behavior, potentially lifting her spirits and making her more likely to go out again the next day.

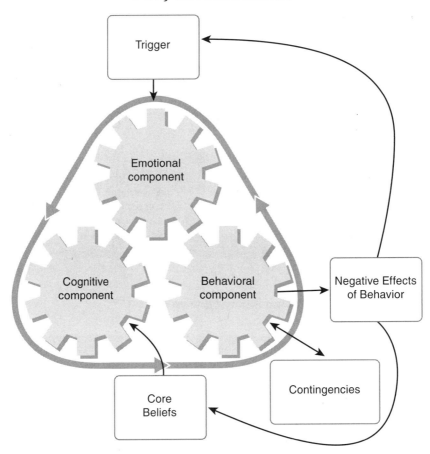

FIGURE 2.5. Effects of behavior.

Behaviors can also cause *further aversive events* to occur. This part is often overlooked. We spend so much time examining how the client *reacts to* his or her environment that we sometimes fail to pay attention to how the client *influences* his or her environment. As an example, consider our client Johanna, whose marriage to Nick is in trouble. One day, she comes home, and Nick gives her what she considers to be a strange look. Her behavioral response will greatly influence how the rest of the encounter goes. In this example, she shot Nick a dirty glare and walked out of the room without saying anything. The events of the evening have now been set into motion, and it's not going to be pleasant. We don't know what Nick's intentions were at the beginning of this encounter, but after Johanna's behavioral response of glaring and leaving the room, it's a good bet that Nick's next behaviors toward Johanna will be hostile. Imagine what would have happened if Johanna had chosen a different behavioral response. Had she ignored the perceived slight of Nick's facial expression and instead greeted him or asked him what was wrong in a nonconfrontational manner, Nick's subsequent behaviors would likely have been more pleasant.

So we see that behaviors influence emotions, allow negative beliefs to persist, and change what happens to the person. We've discussed some of our clients in detail, but I want to also point out that we can see similar patterns for all of our clients. For example:

- Scott avoids interacting with people he doesn't know well. When he does interact with others, he does so in an unskilled manner. These behaviors exacerbate his fears, maintain his prediction that he will be terribly embarrassed, lead him to be reinforced for avoidance, deprive him of reinforcement for social interaction, and result in a minimal social life.
- Anna avoids going to crowded places, driving by herself, and allowing her heart rate to go up too much. These behaviors increase her fears of those activities or situations, maintain her belief that she is at risk of having a heart attack, lead her to be reinforced for avoidance, and cause her life to become more and more restricted.
- Blaise uses drugs when she feels bored or upset, or when she experiences cravings. That behavior maintains her belief that using is the only way she can feel better, causes her to rely on drugs for reinforcement, and puts her in increasingly unpleasant and dangerous situations.
- William, who is interpersonally dependent and experiences chronic pain, relies on his husband for virtually all household tasks and decision making. That behavior makes him feel even more dejected, strengthening his belief that he is incompetent and fragile. He does not obtain reinforcement for doing things on his own.

One thing to note is that a lot of the maladaptive behaviors associated with psychological problems have some payoff in the short term and adverse long-term consequences. As shown in Figure 2.6, Christina's behavioral response of going to bed and staying home alone for the evening results in her having decreased social interaction and potential for positive social experiences, which will likely contribute to her persistent feelings of sadness. Note as well that her behavioral response also serves to strengthen her belief that she is worthless and unlovable—after all, she's spending yet another evening home alone, so that seems to confirm her existing beliefs. And around we go in a vicious cycle.

You might notice a pattern here that cuts across psychiatric diagnoses. In many (though not all) cases, clients behave in a manner that creates a **self-fulfilling prophecy**. It's human nature to do so. We tend to assume that our beliefs are correct, so we behave accordingly, which in turn creates changes in our environment. Interpersonally, our behavior exerts a "pull" on other people so that they act in a manner that is consistent with our beliefs and expectations (Curtis & Miller, 1986; Strupp & Binder, 1984). So Christina behaves in a manner that seems to affirm, rather than disconfirm, her beliefs about how worthless and unlovable she is. She withdraws from her friends and family and acts in a manner that others consider to be negative and pessimistic. As a result, people don't want to spend as much time with her, and they react less sympathetically to her—thus seeming to confirm Christina's beliefs about herself. Joanna interprets Nick's facial expression as a sign of hostility, so she responds in kind, which sets off a cycle of nastiness—serving, in her mind, to confirm her belief.

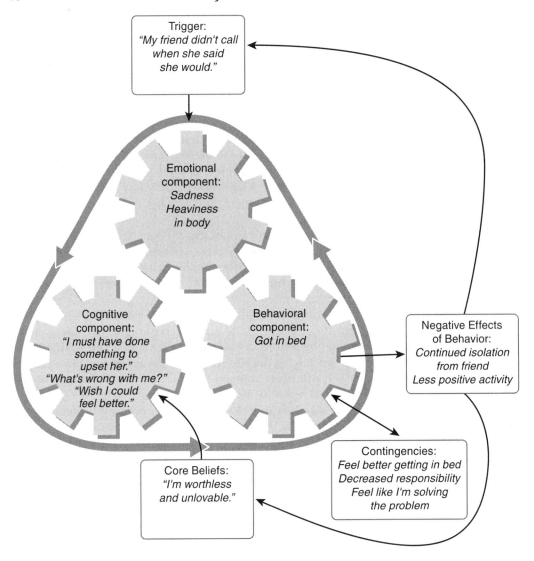

FIGURE 2.6. The effects of Christina's behavior.

THE ESSENTIALS

* Behaviors (motoric acts) are maladaptive when they impair the person's functioning or quality of life.

* Maladaptive behaviors can be categorized as behavioral excesses, behavioral deficits, or deficient behavioral repertoire.

* Behaviors are influenced by our thoughts and emotions.

* Contingencies exert a powerful influence on the acquisition and maintenance of behaviors. The contingencies leading to behavioral excesses are reinforcement and escape. The contingencies leading to behavioral deficits are punishment and penalty.

✳ Contingencies can be continuous or intermittent and have different effects on behavior.

✳ Extinction can result in behavioral deficits.

✳ Avoidance learning can result in behavioral excesses or deficits.

✳ Behavior can be influenced by modeling.

✳ Behavior can be influenced by the presence of behavioral skill deficits, such as problems of problem solving or social skill.

✳ Behaviors influence our thoughts and emotions.

✳ Behaviors influence the environment and subsequent experiences.

KEY TERMS AND DEFINITIONS

Acquisition deficit: A skill deficit in which the person does not know the appropriate skill.

Acting the opposite: Behaving in a manner that challenges beliefs, rather than confirming them.

Action tendency: An emotionally driven motivation to engage in certain patterns of behavior.

Avoidance learning: Learning to perform a behavior in anticipation of an aversive stimulus with the aim of preventing it.

Behavior: Defined here as a motoric act involving the skeletal muscles.

Behavioral deficit: An adaptive behavior that occurs too infrequently.

Behavioral excess: A maladaptive behavior that occurs too frequently.

Behavioral skill deficits: A lack of knowledge of, poor implementation of, or inconsistent use of, behavioral skills that would help the individual interact successfully with the environment.

Cognitive dissonance: Adjusting beliefs so that they "fit" our behaviors.

Contingencies: The context in which a behavior occurs, including rewards and punishers that follow a given behavior, thus increasing or decreasing its future likelihood of occurrence.

Continuous reinforcement: Reinforcement that always follows the behavior.

Deficient behavioral repertoire: An inability to select and/or perform the required behavior in the appropriate circumstance.

Doing better in order to feel better: Using behavioral change in order to affect emotions and thoughts.

Escape (negative reinforcement): A contingency that subtracts something (unwanted) from the client's experience, thus increasing the likelihood that the behavior will occur again.

Extinction: The removal of reinforcement for a behavior.

Extinction burst: The initial increase in behavior following removal of reinforcers.

Fluency deficit: A skill deficit in which the person knows the appropriate skill, but is unable to perform it in a smooth a natural manner.

Intermittent reinforcement: Reinforcement that sometimes follows the behavior.

Modeling: The development of behavior or beliefs through observing others.

Negative contingency: Something is withdrawn from the person's experience, following the person's behavior, that was there before the behavior.

Operant conditioning: The learning of behavior patterns via contingencies.

Penalty (negative punishment): A contingency that subtracts something (wanted) from the client's experience, thus decreasing the likelihood that the behavior will occur again.

Performance deficit: A skill deficit in which the person knows the appropriate skill, but is inhibited from enacting the skill due to one or more factors.

Positive contingency: Something is added to the person's experience, following the person's behavior, that was not there before the behavior.

Problem solving: Addressing problems in living with a positive orientation toward problem solving, defining the problem and attempting to understand its cause, generating multiple possible solutions to the problem, deciding on a particular solution, and determining whether the solution was effective.

Punishers: Contingencies that decrease the likelihood that the behavior will occur again.

Punishment (positive punishment): A contingency that adds something (unwanted) to the client's experience, thus decreasing the likelihood that the behavior will occur again.

Reinforcement (positive reinforcement): A contingency that adds something (wanted) to the client's experience, thus increasing the likelihood that the behavior will occur again.

Reinforcers: Contingencies that increase the likelihood that the behavior will occur again.

Self-fulfilling prophecy: Behaving in a manner that affects subsequent events, such that one's beliefs seem to be confirmed.

Social skills: A complex set of behavioral skills that include verbal and nonverbal aspects of social interaction.

Understanding Your Behavioral System

Using a *recent* occurrence of the personal target, identify any *unhelpful* behavior(s) you engaged in, or any behaviors that you did *not* do but should have.

Situation: _____

_____

Unhelpful behavior(s) or lack thereof: _____

_____

Which of the following do you think best characterizes the unhelpful behavior(s)? (You can select more than one)

- ☐ Behavioral excess: a behavior that occurs too frequently.
- ☐ Behavioral deficit: a behavior that occurs too infrequently.
- ☐ Deficient behavioral repertoire: An inability to select and/or perform the required behavior in the appropriate circumstance.

Where do you think this/these responses come from? Check all that apply, and explain.

Contribution	Explanation
☐ Reinforcement (positive reinforcement): *The behavior increased over time because something desirable was added after doing the behavior.*	
☐ Escape (negative reinforcement): *The behavior increased over time because something undesirable was taken away after doing the behavior.*	
☐ Avoidance learning: *You avoid doing something in order to prevent an unwanted outcome (that may or may not actually happen).*	
☐ Punishment: *The behavior decreased over time because something undesirable was added after doing the behavior.*	

(continued)

From *Doing CBT* by David F. Tolin. Copyright © 2016 The Guilford Press. Permission to photocopy this worksheet is granted to purchasers of this book for personal use only (see copyright page for details). Purchasers can download enlarged versions of this worksheet (see the box at the end of the table of contents).

Contribution	Explanation
☐ Extinction (failure to reinforce appropriate behavior): *The behavior decreased over time because it was not reinforced.*	
☐ Continuous schedule of reinforcement: *The behavior increased over time because reinforcement always followed the behavior.*	
☐ Intermittent schedule of reinforcement: *The behavior persisted over time because reinforcement sometimes followed the behavior.*	
☐ Modeling: *You imitated the behavior of someone else.*	
☐ Behavioral skill deficit (e.g., social skill or problem-solving deficit): *You engaged in a behavior, or did not engage in a behavior, because you did not know or were unable to perform the appropriate behavior.*	

What was/were the effect(s) of your response? Check all that apply, and explain.

Effect	Explanation
☐ Exacerbated or maintained negative emotion.	
☐ Allowed maladaptive belief to persist.	
☐ Changed your experience of reinforcement and punishment.	
☐ Caused further aversive events.	

CHAPTER 3

Stinkin' Thinkin'

The Cognitive System
and How It Can Go Wrong

The cognitive system encompasses a lot of mental processes that maintain psychological problems in different ways. We can divide these mental processes into three general categories: automatic cognitive processes, semi-automatic cognitive processes, and effortful cognitive processes. Table 3.1 shows the various elements we'll be discussing in this chapter.

What Makes Cognition Maladaptive?

Cognitive factors are adaptive when they are reasonably accurate and provide a reasonable perspective on reality. I say "reasonably" because no one's cognitive factors provide us with a 100% accurate representation of how things are. That's just not how the brain works; it's not a computer. Rather, the brain uses various shortcuts so that we can process information quickly and be right more often than we are wrong. We reconstruct memories based on what we think most likely happened. We allocate attention to the things we think are most relevant. We make interpretations based on limited information and "rules of thumb" and make the best guesses that we can. So everyone's cognitive factors are wrong some of the time. In most cases, the errors we make are semi-random, so they don't

TABLE 3.1. Automatic, Semi-Automatic, and Effortful Cognitive Processes That Contribute to the Maintenance of Psychological Problems

Automatic cognitive processes	Semi-automatic cognitive processes	Effortful cognitive processes
• Attentional bias • Memory bias • Intrusions	• Interpretations • Core beliefs	• Thought suppression • Worry • Rumination

consistently pull our emotions and behaviors in any particular direction. That's about as good as it can get. Note that I don't say that positive thoughts are necessarily adaptive, nor are negative thoughts necessarily maladaptive. The critical issue is their accuracy. Maladaptive cognitive factors are those in which we tend to make the same kind of errors over and over again. When that happens, the net result is that our emotions and behaviors start to get pulled in a particular (often negative) direction.

Automatic Cognitive Processes

Automatic cognitive processes are those mental activities that happen completely involuntarily. That is, the person is not trying to have this happen; it just happens. Two categories of automatic cognitive processes are particularly important for our purposes: *information-processing biases* and *intrusions.*

Information-Processing Biases

Information processing refers to the ways in which the brain filters, processes, retains, and recalls information. Information processing is never perfect. For example, there is ample evidence that memory is highly fallible. Experiences aren't stored in the brain the way video is stored inside a camera. Rather, we reconstruct our memories based on bits and pieces of information that have been encoded throughout the brain. Where there's a gap in the information, the brain seeks to fill the gap as best it can with whatever seems most reasonable (whether it is factual or not). Memories can be reconstructed in a highly selective manner, can be only partially accurate, or can even be completely false. Similarly, attention is imperfect. Think of attention like a camera with a shallow depth of field: Only a few things can be in focus at any one time. The rest is blurry. So at any given time, only a tiny fraction of the available sensory information gets attended to and processed.

Of the different aspects of information processing, attention and memory seem most directly implicated in psychological problems (J. M. G. Williams, Watts, MacLeod, & Mathews, 1997). Specifically, when attention and memory start processing information in a way that is distorted—that is, favoring some information over other information—we refer to this as an **information-processing bias.**

A classic diagram of cognitive processes (Atkinson & Shiffrin, 1968) is shown in Figure 3.1. We receive a wide range of *sensory input.* This includes vision, hearing, smell, taste, and touch, as well as *interoceptive* information (information about body sensations). Out of all of that sensory information, we can only pay **attention** to some of it. The brain, through

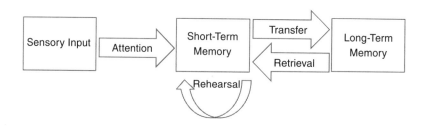

FIGURE 3.1. A schematic diagram of attention and memory processes. Based on Atkinson and Shiffrin (1968).

various mechanisms, determines what we should pay more attention to, what we should pay less attention to, and what we should ignore altogether. Your ability to focus on a particular conversation at a crowded party is an example of selective attention—your brain pays attention to the voice of the person you're talking to, while seeming to "muffle out" the voices of everyone else. So right off the bat, only a little bit of the available information gets into your brain at all.

The tiny fraction of available sensory information that you paid attention to is encoded in **short-term memory.** Short-term memory is a limited-capacity "holding" area for information. Information in short-term memory doesn't tend to last long, and it's quickly forgotten unless you engage in **rehearsal** of the information. When someone tells you his or her phone number, you probably have to repeat it to yourself over and over. That rehearsal process prevents the information from being forgotten.

Rehearsal also facilitates the transfer of the information from short-term memory to **long-term memory.** Long-term memory can contain much more information, and once information is in there, it seems to be relatively permanent (this doesn't mean that forgetting can't occur—it does, but the memories can be **retrieved** again with certain contextual cues or "hints").

Look at Figure 3.1 and think of all of the things that could potentially distort the information being processed. You might not receive appropriate *sensory input* (e.g., you fail to see or hear something). You could pay *attention* to the wrong part(s) of the sensory information (e.g., you focus on a detail that does not adequately capture the situation). You could *rehearse* the wrong information (e.g., you could repeat selective elements over and over, causing them to be transferred from short-term to long-term memory). You could *retrieve* long-term memories selectively (e.g., you could retrieve only parts of the information, or could even fill in missing information with best guesses that are indistinguishable from actual memories). There's a lot that can go wrong.

As an example, let's look at our client Scott, who is socially anxious. As Scott tells us about his recent experience giving a presentation at work, we can hypothesize several different kinds of problems with his information processing:

- Scott disproportionately paid *attention* to the audience members who seemed least interested in, or pleased with, his presentation, ignoring those who were attentive and receptive. He also paid excessive attention to himself, trying to detect how his voice was sounding and whether his face was feeling hot.
- After Scott made a minor error in his presentation, he *rehearsed* that error in his mind over and over again, causing that experience of the error to be transferred from short-term to long-term memory.
- Later, when recalling his presentation, Scott selectively *retrieved* the worst elements of it. He recalled all of the unhappy or uninterested faces in the audience, how hot his face felt, and the "terrible" error he made.

These kinds of information-processing errors happen to all of us, much of the time. Again, no one's brain is perfect. However, we run into real problems when we make the same kinds of errors over and over again. We would then call this not just information-processing errors, but an *information-processing bias.* When an information-processing bias is present, the net result is that our emotions and behaviors start to get pulled in a particular direction.

I live in Connecticut. In our small state, there is a pervasive belief that people from Massachusetts are bad drivers (friends from Massachusetts, don't blame me; I didn't start this). Everyone knows that "Massholes," as they are sometimes called, tailgate, drive too fast, change lanes without signaling, and are generally obnoxious in every possible way on the road. And, sure enough, my experience seems to bear that out. I see rotten drivers with Massachusetts license plates all over the place, terrorizing the gentle and respectful Connecticut drivers like myself. So the stereotype must be true, right?

Or . . . is there an information-processing bias at work here? When I see a rotten driver, I'm now in the habit of looking at the license plate. When it's from Massachusetts, I think to myself, "Yup, I knew it." But what happens when that license plate is *not* from Massachusetts? I'll tell you what I *don't* do; I don't think to myself, "Goodness, I must have been inaccurate in my beliefs about Massachusetts drivers. Perhaps there are good and bad drivers all over the country. I will be sure to take a more balanced perspective from now on." Nope, not me. Instead, I quickly forget about it and go looking for the next Masshole.

And on the flip side, notice that I only check the license plate once I've identified the driver as being rotten. I don't check the license plates of people who seem to be driving just fine. So, on any given day on the highway, I might see 1,000 cars. And if one of them is driving badly, I check that one's license plate and ignore the other 999.

So you can see here how my beliefs play a powerful role in how I process information. I selectively attend to information that seems to be consistent with my beliefs, ignoring information that contradicts my beliefs. That's called an **attentional bias.** And, when I think back on all of the other drivers that I've seen recently, I will disproportionately recall information that is consistent with my beliefs and fail to recall information that is inconsistent with my beliefs. That's a **memory bias.** I am constantly "proving" myself right by (involuntarily) diverting my attention and memory toward information that's consistent with what I already think to be true. And so with each bad Massachusetts driver I see, I become even more convinced that the stereotype is true. That is, information-processing biases tend to *strengthen* our beliefs rather than change our minds. So we believe what we believe, more and more strongly, over time.

Globally, these information-processing biases have been described as **confirmation biases.** We search for, interpret, and recall information in a way that confirms our existing beliefs. In psychological problems, once the person has an unhealthy mind-set, he or she will unintentionally distort incoming information in order to make it conform to the mind-set. Attentional biases are present when a person disproportionately allocates attention toward stimuli that are relevant to his or her negative beliefs or mood. This phenomenon is well documented in anxiety-related problems, in which clients show selective attention toward the things they fear or things that could potentially be associated with the things they fear. For a moment, try walking in the shoes of our client Anna, who has panic disorder. As you go through life, you're constantly paying attention to your body sensations. At times it seems like all you can hear is the beating of your own heart. What would the impact be on you? First, you'd probably notice a lot more irregularities and odd bodily sensations because you're so focused on them. That would probably serve to confirm your belief that there is something wrong with your body. It would also probably keep you in a chronically anxious and tense state. Because attention has limited capacity, you'd also probably notice that your ability to pay attention to routine matters is diminished. And so it is with Anna. She's chronically focused on her own body, looking for signs of disaster, and so she's constantly detecting worrisome signs and feeling anxious. She also tells us that her ability to focus on anything else, such as school, is seriously compromised. And it's no wonder.

The Science behind It

Anxious people show an automatic attentional bias toward threatening stimuli. As an example, someone with a fear of spiders will disproportionately allocate attention toward spider-related cues in the environment (Watts, McKenna, Sharrock, & Trezise, 1986). People with panic disorder characterized by a fear of medical disaster show increased monitoring and detection of their own heart rates (Ehlers & Breuer, 1992). People with social anxiety disorder pay more attention to audience members who react negatively (Perowne & Mansell, 2002) and will also allocate excessive attention toward themselves and their own outward presentations, as if they were viewing themselves (Spurr & Stopa, 2002). People with PTSD allocate attention toward trauma-related stimuli (Bryant & Harvey, 1995), consistent with the DSM-5 diagnostic criterion of *hypervigilance*.

The phenomenon isn't limited to anxiety-related disorders, however. Clients with eating disorders disproportionately allocate attention toward high-calorie foods (Shafran, Lee, Cooper, Palmer, & Fairburn, 2007). Cocaine-dependent clients allocate attention toward drug-related stimuli (Hester, Dixon, & Garavan, 2006). Clients with paranoid schizophrenia show an attentional bias toward stimuli consistent with their persecutory delusions (Moritz & Laudan, 2007).

Attentional bias even shows up when working with couples and families, such that family members selectively attend to unpleasant behavior on the part of other members while failing to attend to their desired behaviors (N. B. Epstein, Baucom, & Rankin, 1993). In each case, notice how the attentional bias is toward stimuli that confirm maladaptive beliefs or strengthen negative emotions.

Memory biases, in which belief- or mood-congruent information is disproportionately retrieved from long-term memory, also play a significant role in maintaining psychological problems. Imagine that you are our client Christina, who is severely depressed. As you look back over your life, what kinds of things would come to mind? Most likely, all of your failures and negative experiences would seem prominent. It would be hard for you to come up with specific examples of things that have gone right. Even as you think back on the events of the past week, you'd tend to remember more of the bad than the good, leading you to conclude that this was "another terrible week." What would the impact of that memory bias be on you? Most likely, it would seem to affirm your basic belief about your own worthlessness. It would also probably contribute to keeping your mood low. An inability to come up with clear positive examples would also make it difficult for you to solve current problems effectively (solving problems requires you to recall what worked before). This is exactly what happened to Christina. She primarily retrieved mood-congruent (negative) information from long-term memory, and the smidgen of positive information she could retrieve was vague. As a result, she felt even worse about herself and couldn't solve problems well.

Intrusions

Some thoughts seem to "pop" into our heads automatically. I know that when I'm feeling hungry, it might not be unusual for an image of a sandwich to come to mind. That's an

The Science behind It

Emotions can exert a profound impact on memory. In laboratory research, when people learn lists of words in an emotional state (positive or negative), they are better at remembering those words when they are in the same emotional state. When asked to recall events of the previous week, people in a positive mood tend to recall more positive events and rate them more positively; people in a negative mood tend to recall more negative events and rate them more negatively (Bower, 1981).

When asked to remember past experiences, people who are clinically depressed tend to remember negative experiences very well. But when asked to recall positive experiences, they often find this quite difficult, and the memories retrieved tend to be overly general rather than specific experiences (Moore, Watts, & Williams, 1988)—for example, a person might be able to come up with something vague, such as "I had a good relationship with my sister," but have a hard time coming up with any actual, specific memories of that good relationship.

intrusion, which is an involuntary process—in fact, if I'm hungry enough, the sandwich image might pop into my mind even though I'm trying to focus on something else (like, say, writing this book). An intrusion might be a mental picture, like my sandwich, or it could be words, such as thinking, "Oh no, I forgot to pack my lunch!" after I've left the house. In either case, it's an involuntary process.

Intrusions happen in all kinds of psychological problems. A classic kind of intrusion is an *obsession,* which is a thought or image that comes to mind automatically and causes the person to feel distressed. Bethany, our client with OCD, has lots of intrusions. For example, whenever she sees a knife or another sharp object, an image pops into her mind of picking it up and stabbing someone with it. It's not that she's a violent person; in fact, she finds the image repugnant and scary. But the intrusion enters her mind anyway.

In Bethany's case, her intrusion is about something that hasn't happened and likely never will. But intrusions can also be about actual things that have happened. Our client Melissa, for example, suffers from PTSD due to a history of childhood sexual abuse. She experiences *intrusive memories,* in which she remembers bits of her abuse as if they were movies playing in her head. At times, the memories can be so vivid that they are experienced as *flashbacks,* in which she has not only the memory but also a number of associated body sensations and feels as if the traumatic event is happening again.

Our client Lauren, who is diagnosed with schizophrenia, has intrusions, too. In her case, some of the intrusions take the form of *hallucinations.* For example, she might hear the sound of people whispering or talking; usually saying things that are derogatory or threatening toward her. Lauren doesn't always recognize that these sounds are actually the product of her own mind, but they are intrusions nevertheless. They are involuntary, automatic cognitive processes.

What's the relationship between intrusions and psychological problems? The answer depends very much on how the person responds to or copes with the intrusions. The intrusions themselves don't maintain the problem, although they can be a result of the problem. Some responses to intrusions are healthy, and other responses are unhealthy. We'll talk more about that topic later when we get to effortful cognitive processes.

The Science behind It

Intrusions are extremely common and are not necessarily accompanied by emotional or behavioral disturbance. In fact, in all likelihood, you've experienced intrusions. Me, too. Ordinary people have intrusive impulses to hurt themselves or other people, bizarre sexual thoughts, images of loved ones dying, thoughts that they have a severe health problem, and other strange thoughts (Freeston et al., 1994; Rachman & de Silva, 1978). They experience intrusive memories of distressing events (Brewin, Christodoulides, & Hutchinson, 1996; Bywaters, Andrade, & Turpin, 2004; Newby & Moulds, 2011). Over one-third of the population reports having experienced hallucinations (Ohayon, 2000).

If intrusions are so common, why do some people become disturbed and others don't? One possibility is that some people have more negative *interpretations* of their intrusions than do others (Salkovskis, 1985). Some people interpret their intrusions to be immoral or shameful (Valentiner & Smith, 2008), to be a reminder of their personal inadequacies (Newby & Moulds, 2010), or to be threats to their sense of self (Rowa & Purdon, 2003). In some cases, they believe that their thoughts may come true, or that the presence of intrusions means something is terribly wrong with their minds (Foa, Ehlers, Clark, Tolin, & Orsillo, 1999; Morillo, Belloch, & Garcia-Soriano, 2007). Many believe that it's critical to gain control over their thoughts (Newby & Moulds, 2010; Tolin, Woods, & Abramowitz, 2003). Some people display a phenomenon called *thought–action fusion* (Rachman, 1993), in which they appraise a thought as being morally or realistically equivalent to its behavioral manifestation—for example, that thinking about hurting someone is as bad as actually hurting someone.

We also see that some people use *maladaptive strategies* to deal with their intrusions. Avoidance of intrusions, in particular, appears to increase vulnerability for a range of psychological problems, including depression (Newby & Moulds, 2011), PTSD (Ehlers, Mayou, & Bryant, 1998), generalized anxiety disorder (P. R. Gross & Eifert, 1990), and OCD (Purdon, Rowa, & Antony, 2005). Although avoidance strategies differ, they all relate to the general theme of trying to feel better by trying to make "bad" thoughts go away or to think "good" thoughts. *Thought suppression* is a commonly used avoidance strategy; a wealth of research shows that this can increase both the frequency and the aversiveness of the intrusions (Marcks & Woods, 2007; Wegner, Schneider, Carter, & White, 1987; Yoshizumi & Murase, 2007). Depressed people may engage in *rumination* about their intrusions (Newby & Moulds, 2010; Starr & Moulds, 2006), which, as we'll see, can worsen negative mood (Nolen-Hoeksema & Morrow, 1993). So one's cognitive and behavioral *response* to intrusions may be more of a problem than the intrusions themselves.

Semi-Automatic Cognitive Processes

Somewhere between automatic and effortful cognitive processes lies a category of mental activity that is not truly involuntary but that can easily go on "auto-pilot." So we do them mindlessly most of the time, although we can, with some effort, exert control over them. The semi-automatic cognitive processes we'll focus on are *interpretations* and *core beliefs*.

Interpretations

As we encounter various stimuli and situations, we make meaning of them. Imagine that you see a friend across the street and call out "hello." But your friend doesn't respond.

The Science behind It

There has been a lot of research and debate on the topic of which cognitive functions are automatic and which are effortful (Bargh & Ferguson, 2000; Moors & De Houwer, 2006). Many modern cognitive scientists believe that automaticity exists on a continuum, from "totally automatic" to "totally controlled" and everything in between (Moors, 2010). Aspects of basic information processing, such as attention and memory, are closer to the "totally automatic" side of that continuum: They are quite fast and efficient, and the person is unaware of the process, does not intentionally engage the process, and usually has little ability to control it directly (Bargh, 1992). Thoughts, in the usual sense of the word, are less automatic. Some very basic snap judgments, such as gross estimation of whether something is good or bad, occur within a fraction of a second, without intent or awareness (Bargh, Chaiken, Govender, & Pratto, 1992), and can therefore be considered automatic. However, more complex interpretations and appraisals—the kind we typically talk about in therapy—have some elements of automaticity (e.g., they are usually unintentional), but they have other elements suggestive of a controlled process. The person might be initially unaware of his or her thoughts and appraisals, but once his or her attention is directed to them, he or she can identify them and correct them. Although some cognitive therapists have referred to interpretations as "automatic thoughts," from a cognitive science perspective they are not completely automatic.

What meaning would you make of that? You could think that the friend simply didn't hear you. Or you could think that the friend was deliberately ignoring you. Your **interpretation** would likely exert a substantial influence on how you felt and what you did next.

Some have used the term *automatic thoughts* in this context. I find that term a bit confusing, because interpretations are really only semi-automatic. They are often fleeting and often are not noticed at all; however, they're not completely automatic. The person can usually identify them with appropriate questioning (e.g., "What just went through your mind?" or "What did you make of that?"). Further, in some cases people have referred to quite effortful mental processes as "automatic thoughts" as well. So I'm going to use the term *interpretations,* which captures the phenomenon a bit more accurately. And, as you'll see in Chapters 13–15, the distinction between automatic, semi-automatic, and effortful cognitive processes has some significant implications for our selection of interventions.

Sometimes, interpretations reflect what the person truly believes; other times, once the person takes a good look at them, he or she doesn't believe them. But the fact that they occur so rapidly and habitually makes them *feel* real.

Where Do Interpretations Come From?

Figure 3.2 shows some of the complex inputs and outputs of interpretations. As we saw with behaviors in Chapter 2, interpretations influence, and are influenced by, other parts of the core pathological process.

INTERPRETATIONS ARE INFLUENCED BY EMOTIONS

Interpretations can be affected by the person's *emotions* and *physiological sensations.* Figure 3.3 shows an example for our client Anna, who is experiencing panic attacks. As she

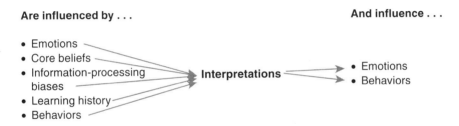

Are influenced by . . .   And influence . . .

- Emotions
- Core beliefs
- Information-processing   **Interpretations**   • Emotions
  biases   • Behaviors
- Learning history
- Behaviors

FIGURE 3.2. Inputs and outputs for interpretations.

experiences the emotion of fear and the physiological sensation of a racing heart, she thinks, "I'm having a heart attack!"

Put yourself in Anna's shoes. Imagine that you're just sitting there, minding your own business, and for reasons you can't understand, you start noticing your heart racing, feeling dizzy, and feeling an intense fear. Might the thought of dying cross your mind? I bet it would. So how you feel can have an impact on what you think.

In fact, how we feel plays a strong role in how we interpret all kinds of events or situations. For example:

- Scott, our socially anxious client, feels anxious and tense at a party. He searches for a reason for his anxiety and infers that others are looking at him and judging him negatively.
- Melissa, our client with complex PTSD, feels the hair on the back of her neck

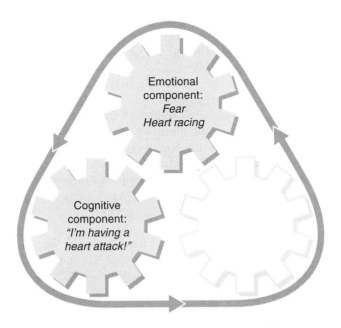

FIGURE 3.3. Reciprocal relationship between interpretations and emotions for Anna.

standing up as she is walking outside. She determines that the situation must be dangerous.

- Johanna feels irritated toward Nick. She reasons that Nick must have done something wrong, even if she can't recall what it was.
- When William, our client with dependency and pain issues, needs to do a chore, he feels some pain and uneasiness. He thinks, "I just can't do it today. I'm not strong enough."

INTERPRETATIONS ARE INFLUENCED BY CORE BELIEFS

Interpretations can be fueled by the person's *core beliefs*, which we discuss in more detail below. Briefly, how one responds mentally to an event is partly due to the event itself and partly due to one's beliefs. Going back to our example of seeing your friend who does not respond to you, you might have the interpretation "He's ignoring me," or you might think "He didn't hear me." Why would you think one of these, but not the other? It's based, in part, on your *core beliefs*. Are you prone to thinking that people generally don't like you, or that you're not likeable? If so, you're more likely to interpret your friend's silence as deliberate ignoring. On the other hand, if you generally believe that you are likeable and that people like you, you're more likely to interpret the silence as reflecting the fact that your friend simply didn't hear you.

INTERPRETATIONS ARE INFLUENCED BY INFORMATION-PROCESSING BIASES

Our interpretations are influenced by our processes of attention and memory. We have to pay attention to something in order to interpret it, and our interpretations depend on what we can recall that relates to what we're interpreting. If you didn't pay attention to your friend's response, there would be nothing to interpret. Assuming that you do pay attention, your interpretation will be guided by your memories of previous encounters with that friend. Does he usually respond to you when you say hello? Has there been friction between you? Is he hard of hearing? All of these memories influence how you'll interpret the situation.

Now imagine how an information-processing bias can affect the interpretation. For example, imagine that you have an *attentional bias* for grumpy-looking faces or other signs of interpersonal rejection, and you key in on the fact that your friend's brow is furrowed. Or imagine that, while you search your memory, you have a *memory bias* in which you selectively recall every negative interaction you've ever had with that friend while failing to recall all of the positive interactions. Those biases are going to substantially increase the likelihood that you'll make a more negative interpretation of your friend's silence.

INTERPRETATIONS ARE INFLUENCED BY LEARNING HISTORY

Interpretations can also derive from the person's *learning history*. Staying with the example of your friend across the street, over the course of your life you've had countless interactions with other people, some friendly, some not. Your history of those events will strongly influence what interpretation you make. Remember, of course, that your memory system (like everyone else's) is highly imperfect, as we discussed earlier. So what you do and do not recall, and the interpretations you subsequently make, will likely be influenced by your present emotional state (see, it's complicated).

INTERPRETATIONS ARE INFLUENCED BY BEHAVIOR

How we act also influences how we perceive things. As we discussed in Chapter 2, there is ample evidence to suggest that we reinterpret situations so that our interpretations are consistent with our behaviors. Avoiding things, for example, makes it more likely that you will interpret those things as being dangerous (Deacon & Maack, 2008; Olatunji et al., 2011). Similarly, withdrawing from activities can, over time, lead you to interpret those activities as being less desirable or rewarding than you would otherwise. Behaving in an aggressive manner can make you more likely to interpret others' actions as being hostile.

What Do Interpretations Do?

INTERPRETATIONS AFFECT EMOTIONS

Interpretations can exert a powerful influence our emotions. The Stoic philosopher Epictetus (55–135 C.E.) is quoted as saying, "Man is disturbed not by things, but rather by the view he takes of them." Another way of saying this is that events do not cause unhappiness. Rather, the person's *interpretations* of those events are viewed as the cause of the unhappiness. We can see several examples of this phenomenon in our clients:

- Anna, our client with panic disorder, experiences an increase in her heart rate and has the interpretation "I'm going to have a heart attack." As a result of this interpretation, she experiences a feeling of fear, as well as an increase in the physiological sensations of arousal (see Figure 3.3). So the interpretation that she is having a heart attack is part of what is driving the fear and the eventual panic attack.
- Christina, our client with severe depression, experiences a minor setback and has the interpretation "I can't do anything right." As a result of this interpretation, she feels even sadder. Her thought that she can't do anything right is causing her depression to deepen.
- Elizabeth, our client with borderline personality disorder, experiences disappointment in a therapy session and has the interpretation "My therapist doesn't care about me at all." This interpretation leads her to feel frustrated and angry. Left unchallenged, this belief festers, and her working relationship with the therapist worsens.
- Lauren, our client with schizophrenia, experiences unusual thoughts and has the interpretation "Someone is trying to control my mind." She feels increasingly fearful because of this interpretation.
- Nick, whose marriage with Johanna is in distress, is experiencing some problems with child rearing and has the interpretation "This is all Johanna's fault; she is trying to make my life miserable." As he makes this interpretation, he feels angry.
- Samuel, who suffers from insomnia, lies in bed and thinks, "If I can't fall asleep, I'll never be able to function and my day will be ruined. Maybe I'll even get fired." This interpretation leads him to feel increasingly anxious.

INTERPRETATIONS AFFECT BEHAVIORS

Interpretations also affect what we do. We adjust our behavior based on the perspective we take about events. For example:

- Shari, our client with bulimia, has an episode of binge eating and thinks, "I'm so disgusting and fat." She responds to this interpretation by making herself throw up.
- Blaise, who has a substance use disorder, has urges to use and has the interpretation "If I can't use right now, I'll never be able to feel better." Her response to this interpretation is to use cocaine.
- Scott, who is socially anxious, is talking to someone for the first time. He thinks, "This person can see how anxious and awkward I am, and is judging me negatively." He responds by ending the conversation as quickly as possible.
- Bethany, our client with OCD, touches a doorknob and thinks, "I have germs on me. I'm going to get a terrible disease now and die." Her response to that interpretation is to wash her hands over and over.

Cognitive Distortions

Sometimes our interpretations are accurate. Sometimes they are not. When interpretations are not accurate (meaning they do not accurately reflect reality), we call them **cognitive distortions.** Some common cognitive distortions are listed in Table 3.2. They all reflect a mismatch between the interpretation and the reality.

- When Anna thinks, "I'm going to have a heart attack!," that's *probability overestimation.* In reality, the likelihood of her having a heart attack is extremely small.
- When Scott thinks, "If people can see I'm nervous, I'll have a complete meltdown and I'll never be able cope with it or show my face in public again!," that's *catastrophizing.* In reality, the consequences of having people see he's nervous are not nearly that devastating.
- When Melissa thinks, "I can't trust anyone because everyone's a potential threat," that's *overgeneralizing.* Some people are indeed threatening, but most aren't.
- When Lauren thinks, "That person's smiling because she's ridiculing me," that's *personalizing.* In reality, the person's smile had nothing to do with Lauren.
- When Elizabeth thinks, "My therapist doesn't respect me because he didn't validate what I just said," that's *all-or-nothing thinking.* In reality, the therapist respects her very much, and the lack of validation was a momentary slip.
- When Nick thinks, "Johanna should ask me how my day was whenever I come home," that's a *"should" statement.* In reality, although Nick might prefer it that way and wish that it were so, there is no rule about what Johanna is supposed to ask him.
- When Johanna thinks, "Nick just said that because he wants to make me miserable," that's *mind reading.* In reality, Johanna has no way of really knowing what Nick is thinking.
- When Suzanne thinks, "I'm just sure something bad's happened to my husband because I have this sinking feeling in my stomach," that's *emotional reasoning.* In reality, the sinking feeling in her stomach is just a feeling, not an indicator of external events.
- When Blaise thinks, "I can use this one time and keep it under control," that's *minimizing.* In reality, Blaise has had numerous relapses that started just this way, and at present, she doesn't have much ability to stop.

Notice that Lauren's persecutory delusions are listed along with everyone else's cognitive distortions. In our model, we view delusional beliefs (such as those seen in clients

TABLE 3.2. Cognitive Distortions

Cognitive distortion	Examples
Probability overestimation: Predicting a low-probability event without evidence to support it (or in the face of contradicting evidence).	• "If I go to the mall, I'll have a heart attack." • "Everyone at the party is going to hate me." • "My plane will crash."
"Catastrophizing": Exaggerating the significance of an event; making mountains out of molehills.	• "If I faint in a public place, it will be the most humiliating thing ever and I will never be able to show my face in public again." • "My husband is late for dinner; he's probably lying dead in a ditch somewhere." • "If my partner leaves me, I'll be all alone forever and will never find love again." • "I had an argument with my spouse; therefore, I have a lousy marriage." • "My friend did not call me this weekend; therefore, no one cares about me."
Overgeneralization: Seeing isolated negative events as a global or never-ending pattern.	• "I failed a test; therefore, I can't do anything right and I'll never succeed." • "If I get anxious, I'll be anxious forever and will never be happy again."
Personalizing: Blaming yourself for external events, or believing that external events are in some way related to you.	• "My boss has a sour look on her face. I must have done something to make her mad." • "If I had just been a better parent, my kids would have received better grades in school."
All-or-nothing thinking: Seeing things in black-and-white categories.	• "If I can't do it perfectly, I'm a failure." • "If my family doesn't support everything I do, that means they don't love me."
"Should" statements: Making "rules" about how you or others should or must behave—and getting upset when the "rules" are broken—even if those rules aren't recognized by the rest of the world.	• "People should be nice to me all of the time." • "I should always put other people first, and I'm rotten if I fail to do so."
Mind reading: Inferring what someone else is thinking or feeling, without sufficient evidence.	• "I'm certain that they don't like me." • "My wife thinks I'm a lousy husband, even if she doesn't say so."
Emotional reasoning: Assuming that your emotions reflect the way things really are: "I feel it; therefore, it must be true."	• "This situation must be dangerous; otherwise, why would I feel so anxious?" • "I know my husband is a jerk because I'm so angry at him all the time."
Minimizing: Downplaying the significance of events, or making unrealistically "permissive" statements to oneself.	• "Just one drink won't hurt. I can keep it under control." • "I won't get caught this time." • "Everyone's making too big a deal out of this."

with schizophrenia) as being on a continuum with normal and "neurotic" beliefs. That is, a belief such as "The government is following me" is viewed as a distorted belief, as are the beliefs that we might find in our clients with depression, anxiety, marital discord, and so forth. Delusions are, therefore, simply viewed as a particularly strongly believed kind of cognitive distortion. Importantly, we do not draw a bright line between "neurosis" and "psychosis." Indeed, there is ample evidence that delusional beliefs can be modified (O'Connor et al., 2007), and that CBT can be effective for clients with psychotic disorders (e.g., S. Lewis et al., 2002).

Core Beliefs

Our interpretations are the verbal statements we make to ourselves in order to make meaning of stimuli or situations. Behind these interpretations are our **core beliefs,** which are basic assumptions and beliefs about oneself or the external world. These core beliefs don't necessarily flash through our minds in the same way that interpretations do. Rather, they serve as the underlying "program" that shapes how we respond to situations and what thoughts or images will come to mind.

Many schools of psychotherapy, including CBT, are interested in the idea that there is something larger and deeper underlying the symptoms with which clients present for treatment. This idea has long been a mainstay of psychoanalytic/psychodynamic thinking, in which unconscious wishes, drives, conflicts, and defenses are thought to stimulate the development of overt symptoms (e.g., Gabbard, 2014). Cognitive theorists have pointed to the concept of **schemas,** defined as broad and pervasive themes or patterns of core beliefs, memory, emotion, interpretations, and bodily sensations (A. T. Beck, Rush, Shaw, & Emery, 1979; Young, Klosko, & Weishaar, 2003). According to this model, a schema may be active (meaning it is exerting an influence on thoughts, feelings, and behaviors) or inactive, but it's always there.

In each of these theories, there is a common theme: that people have an underlying pattern or *modus operandi* that, when it is activated, repeats itself over time and across situations. A presenting set of symptoms, therefore, is viewed as one example of the pattern, although not necessarily the only example that will occur during the person's life. These underlying patterns are frequently discussed in the context of *character* or *personality,* although they need not reflect the presence of a DSM-5 personality disorder.

A corollary of this theory is that successful treatment of an individual should not solely focus on the presenting symptoms—for example, treatment of depression should not solely be about alleviating the client's depression. Rather, treatment should also address and correct the underlying pattern that makes the person vulnerable to developing symptoms.

Core beliefs form a person's basic view of themselves, other people, and the world. Like all other cognitive processes, they can be adaptive or maladaptive. Maladaptive core beliefs, when they interact with an event, elicit maladaptive and distorted interpretations, which, in turn, can contribute to negative emotions (see Figure 3.4). When core beliefs are healthy, stressful events do not result in negative interpretations, and our emotional response is fairly normal (see Figure 3.5). However, when core beliefs are unhealthy, stressful events combine with core beliefs to result in negative interpretations, and the emotional response is exaggerated or maladaptive (see Figure 3.6). Some examples of healthy and unhealthy core beliefs are shown in Table 3.3.

The Science behind It

There's reason to believe that long-standing, unexamined ways of viewing oneself and the world underlie vulnerability to developing psychological disorders. The presence of maladaptive personality traits is strongly predictive of the presence of what used to be called "Axis I" disorders, such as anxiety, mood, psychotic, and substance use problems (Coid, Yang, Tyrer, Roberts, & Ullrich, 2006); and personality features predict chronicity and recurrence of these disorders (Ansell et al., 2011; Grilo et al., 2010). Importantly, it has also been demonstrated that the presence of maladaptive personality features has a negative impact on the short- and long-term efficacy of treatment for "Axis I" disorders (Alnaes & Torgersen, 1997; Ilardi, Craighead, & Evans, 1997; Krampe et al., 2006; Verheul, van den Brink, & Hartgers, 1998).

Even beyond the common conceptualizations of personality, there has been a great deal of research demonstrating that certain people are more vulnerable to developing psychiatric disorders than are others, and that these vulnerabilities have cognitive features. For example, research on depression (Abramson, Metalsky, & Alloy, 1989) shows that people who are vulnerable to becoming depressed are those who (1) tend to attribute negative events to global and stable causes, (2) tend to anticipate negative consequences, and (3) view themselves as inherently flawed. Relatedly, studies of anxiety (Riskind, 1997) demonstrate that individuals vulnerable to anxiety tend to perceive threats as growing or escalating, rather than static. Research-based models of anxiety and depression jointly (which have collectively been termed *negative affect*) suggest that vulnerable individuals tend to perceive themselves as having a lack of control over events (Rotter, 1966) or as having poor ability to cope or solve problems (Bandura, 1982).

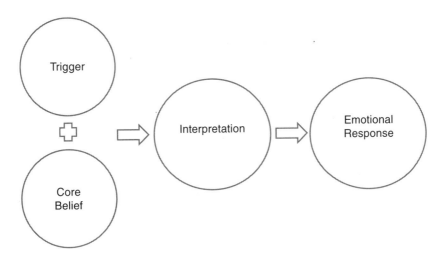

FIGURE 3.4. Core beliefs interact with events to give rise to interpretations and subsequent emotions.

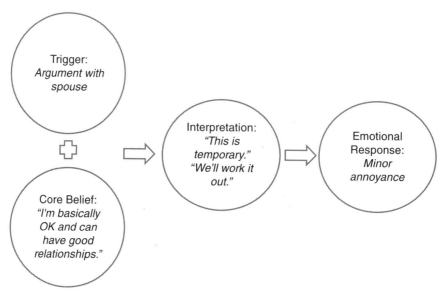

FIGURE 3.5. Adaptive core belief interacting with a stressful event to cause adaptive interpretations and emotion

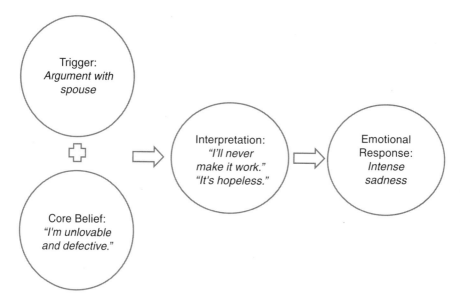

FIGURE 3.6. Maladaptive core belief interacting with a stressful event to cause maladaptive interpretations and emotion.

TABLE 3.3. Examples of Healthy (Adaptive) and Unhealthy (Maladaptive) Core Beliefs

Healthy core beliefs	Unhealthy core beliefs
Self	
• "I am competent."	• "I am incompetent."
• "I am worthy."	• "I am unworthy."
• "I am basically good."	• "I am basically bad."
Others	
• "People are basically decent."	• "People are basically rotten."
• "I can trust people."	• "I can't trust anyone."
World	
• "Efforts usually pay off."	• "Nothing ever changes."
• "The world is usually safe."	• "The world is dangerous."

Psychological problems are often associated with maladaptive core beliefs. Beck, Freeman, and Davis (2004) have hypothesized the presence of certain core beliefs that are linked to specific personality disorders. These include:

- *Dependent:* "I am helpless."
- *Avoidant:* "I may get hurt."
- *Passive–aggressive:* "I could be controlled."
- *Paranoid:* "People are dangerous."
- *Narcissistic:* "I am special."
- *Histrionic:* "I need to impress."
- *Obsessive–compulsive:* "I must not err."
- *Antisocial:* "Others are to be taken advantage of."
- *Schizoid:* "I need plenty of space."

Young et al. (2003) have characterized some of the maladaptive core beliefs seen in psychiatric clients. They frame these beliefs as part of broader schemas, but here I focus on the beliefs themselves. They include:

- *Abandonment/instability:* A belief that those available for support and connection are unstable or unreliable.
- *Mistrust/abuse:* An expectation that others will hurt, abuse, humiliate, cheat, lie, or take advantage.
- *Emotional deprivation:* An expectation that one's desire for normal emotional support (e.g., nurturance, empathy, protection) will not be adequately met by others.
- *Defectiveness/shame:* A belief that one is defective, bad, unwanted, inferior, or invalid, or that one would be unlovable if exposed.
- *Social isolation/alienation:* A belief that one is isolated from the rest of the world, is different from other people, or does not belong to any group or community.
- *Dependence/incompetence:* A belief that one is unable to handle everyday responsibilities in a competent manner without considerable help from others.

- *Vulnerability to harm or illness:* A belief that imminent catastrophe will strike at any time and that one will be unable to prevent it.
- *Enmeshment/underdeveloped self:* A belief, associated with excessive emotional involvement and closeness with another person at the expense of full individuation, that at least one of the enmeshed individuals cannot survive or be happy without the constant support of the other.
- *Failure:* A belief that one has failed, will inevitably fail, or is fundamentally inadequate in areas of achievement.
- *Entitlement/grandiosity:* A belief that one is superior to others, is entitled to special rights and privileges, or is not bound by the rules of reciprocity that guide normal social interaction.
- *Insufficient self-control/self-discipline:* A belief that one should be able to feel better, or have what one wants, right now.
- *Subjugation:* A belief that one has been coerced into surrendering needs or emotions to others and that one's own desires, opinions, and feelings are not valid or important to others.
- *Self-sacrifice:* A belief that one should voluntarily meet the needs of others in daily situations at the expense of one's own needs.
- *Approval-seeking/recognition-seeking:* A belief that one must obtain approval, recognition, or attention from others, or that one must fit in, at the expense of developing a secure sense of self.
- *Negativity/pessimism:* A pervasive focus on the negative aspects of life, while minimizing the positive aspects. Includes a belief that things will eventually go seriously wrong or that aspects of one's life that seem to be going well will ultimately fall apart.
- *Emotional inhibition:* A belief that one should inhibit spontaneous action, feeling, or communication in order to avoid disapproval by others, feeling ashamed, or losing control of one's impulses.
- *Unrelenting standards/hypercriticalness:* A belief that one must strive to meet very high internalized standards of behavior and performance, often in order to avoid criticism.
- *Punitiveness:* A belief that people, often including oneself, should be harshly punished for making mistakes.

Now, there is no need to limit your conceptualization to these specific core beliefs—these are examples. The idea is that a client may have persistent and maladaptive beliefs about themselves, about others, or about the world that interact with external events to lead to maladaptive interpretations, emotions, and behaviors. It is also noted that although this theory was originally developed with personality disorders in mind (Young, 1999), there's no need to limit this conceptualization to the DSM personality disorders. We don't draw a bright line between "Axis I" and "Axis II," to use slightly outdated terminology.

Where Do Core Beliefs Come From?

Fundamentally, we believe core beliefs are *learned*. This learning process usually doesn't happen all at once; rather, the core beliefs are molded and shaped over time. Some ways in which core beliefs can be learned (shown for Christina in Figure 3.7) include:

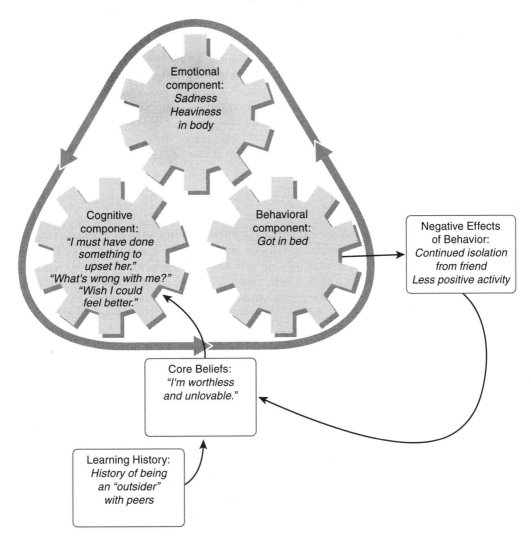

FIGURE 3.7. The causes and effects of Christina's core beliefs.

EXPERIENCE

Some people have a string of adverse life circumstances that shape their core beliefs. In many cases, these circumstances occur during periods of particular developmental sensitivity—for example, a child who is repeatedly abused may develop maladaptive core beliefs, persisting into adulthood, about his or her self-worth, the dangerousness of the world, and so on.

However, we also recognize that the development of core beliefs is an ongoing process that occurs over the lifespan. Therefore, experiences in adulthood can also impact core beliefs. Being sexually assaulted in adulthood, for example, could also distort one's core beliefs about one's self-worth, the dangerousness of the world, and so forth.

It is also worth noting that not all experiences shaping core beliefs need be "traumatic" in the classic sense of the term. More routine adverse experiences, such as receiving constant disapproval by parents, teachers, or peers; being rejected by others or having little positive social interaction; having unpredictable or inadequate parenting; or failing to receive adequate positive feedback about one's accomplishments are all examples of experiences that are not commonly considered "traumas" but that nevertheless can have a powerful impact on core beliefs. In the model shown here, Christina has a long history, dating back to childhood, of being an "outsider" with peers. This history of peer rejection and failing to find a normative social group helped shape her core belief that "I'm worthless and unlovable."

THE EFFECTS OF ONE'S OWN BEHAVIOR

People tend to behave in ways that strengthen, rather than disconfirm, their core beliefs. That is, once a core belief has been established, we usually act in a manner that is concordant with that belief, creating a self-fulfilling prophecy. Those behaviors, in turn, lead us to experience our environments differently, which seems to confirm the belief. In Christina's case, we see that her behavioral responses include spending excessive amounts of time in bed, not interacting with others. We might therefore hypothesize that Christina has little opportunity for positive social experiences. This isolation, in turn, serves to strengthen her core belief "I'm worthless and unlovable." Christina doesn't stop to consider the likelihood that her own behavior is the real reason for the isolation.

MODELING

We can develop core beliefs through the process of observing and interacting with others. Over time, we can begin to acquire similar beliefs. A visibly and chronically anxious parent, for example, might "transfer" to his or her child the core belief that the world is a dangerous place. I've seen lots of anxious clients who recall that their parents routinely took them to unnecessary doctor's visits for routine sniffles, constantly checked on them, or were reluctant to let them go outside and play. Perhaps it's no surprise, then, that over time these clients developed a rather skewed view of the world.

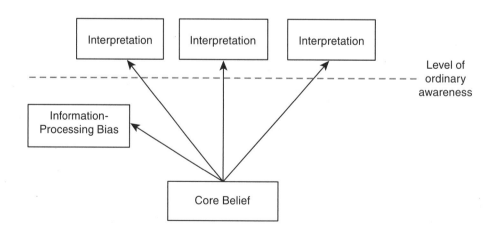

FIGURE 3.8. Core beliefs influence interpretations and information-processing biases.

What Do Core Beliefs Do?

Core beliefs influence other cognitive processes. As shown in Figure 3.8, core beliefs contribute to interpretations and information-processing biases. Note that core beliefs and information-processing biases are below the threshold of ordinary awareness. This does not mean that they are "unconscious" in the same sense that psychodynamic therapists use the term (i.e., they are not repressed or otherwise kept from consciousness by ego defenses). Rather, it means that the person is not used to paying attention to them and is therefore largely unaware of their role in maintaining the problem.

Figure 3.9 shows an example of how these cognitive factors look for our client Suzanne, who is diagnosed with GAD characterized by chronic worry and tension. As you can see, she has a core belief that the world is a dangerous place. That core belief fuels the presence of an attentional bias toward threat-related cues, so she is more likely to detect scary things. The core belief and attentional bias are below her ordinary level of awareness. What she does notice, however, are the interpretations that come into her mind: "Something bad must have happened to my husband" when he is late coming home, "I must have a tumor" when she has a headache, and "Someone's going to break into the house" when she hears noises at night.

Figure 3.10 shows another example, this time for our client William, who is highly dependent on others. William's core belief is that he is incompetent. That core belief leads to a memory bias: As he looks back on his life, he disproportionately recalls instances of personal failure, failing to remember the times that he acted competently. As was the case with Suzanne, William is not particularly aware of the presence of these core beliefs and information-processing bias. However, he is aware of his interpretations of various stressful situations: "I can't do this without help" when he has to do a chore, "My husband knows better than I" when he has to make a decision, and "It's too risky" when pondering making a change in his life.

Core beliefs also exert an impact on our behaviors. Young et al. (2003) have an intriguing idea about how schemas can shape behavior (again, I will focus on the core

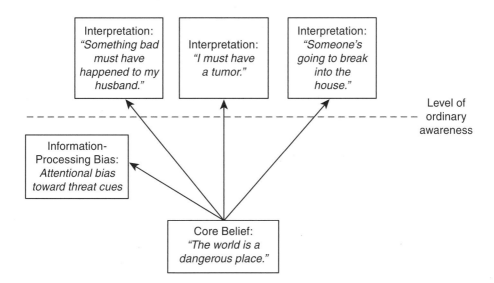

FIGURE 3.9. Core beliefs, interpretations, and information-processing biases for Suzanne.

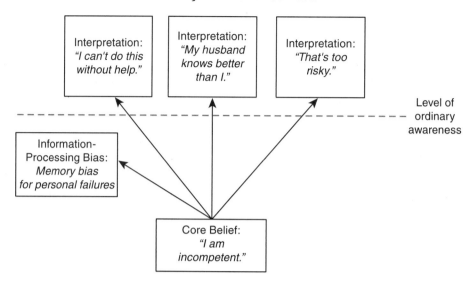

FIGURE 3.10. Core beliefs, interpretations, and information-processing biases for William.

belief aspects of their theory). Specifically, when a core belief is present, they suggest that one of three things can happen:

1. *Surrender.* The person yields to the core belief and does not try to fight it. He or she acts in ways that confirm the core belief. As one example, an individual surrendering to an abandonment/instability core belief (i.e., that those available for support and connection are unstable or unreliable) might habitually select partners who cannot make a commitment, assuming that it's pointless to even try to have a stable relationship with a supportive person.

2. *Avoidance.* The person tries to arrange his or her life so that the core belief is never activated. He or she avoids thinking about it and avoids situations that might trigger the belief. As one example, an individual avoiding an abandonment/instability core belief might avoid intimate relationships altogether and drink heavily when alone.

3. *Overcompensation.* The person tries to think, feel, and behave as if the opposite of the core belief were true, trying to be the polar opposite. As one example, an individual overcompensating for an abandonment/instability core belief might cling to and "smother" partners to the point of pushing them away.

On Awareness and Maladaptive Cognitive Processes

To varying degrees, the maladaptive automatic and semi-automatic cognitive processes can occur outside of our awareness. We are usually not aware that we have an attentional bias toward threat or that we are selectively recalling sad memories. We might not be aware that we have a particular interpretive style or that we have certain negative core beliefs about ourselves, other people, or the world. Although CBT doesn't share the traditional psychoanalytic concept of the unconscious, we nevertheless recognize that much of our cognitive activity occurs outside of our usual scope of awareness. What we do share with our psychoanalytic colleagues, however, is a belief that by making the person aware of these processes, we can help them to recognize and change them. We discuss specific ways to help bring these cognitive processes to awareness in Chapter 13.

Effortful Cognitive Processes

Unlike information-processing biases and intrusions, which occur automatically, and interpretations and core beliefs, which are semi-automatic, some mental processes are purposeful and effortful. **Effortful cognitive processes** are those in which the person *attempts* to think a certain way, or to think (or not think) about certain things. In many cases, the person is trying to influence his or her thoughts in an effort to cope with distress—for example, someone might try not to think about upsetting things, might try to mentally kick him- or herself in the butt in order to try to snap out of a bad mood, or might think about certain things again and again to try to make them better. The term *experiential avoidance* has been used to describe maladaptive efforts to control, suppress, or get away from uncomfortable thoughts or feelings (Hayes, Strosahl, & Wilson, 2012).

Effortful cognitive processes, like everything else, can be adaptive or maladaptive. Adaptive effortful cognitive processes often involve efforts to solve problems, including defining the problem, generating multiple possible solutions to the problem, and deciding on a particular solution (D'Zurilla & Goldfried, 1971). Adaptive effortful cognitive processes often involve some degree of **acceptance.** In Alcoholics Anonymous, members repeat the "Serenity Prayer": "God, grant me the serenity to accept the things I cannot change, the courage to change the things I can, and the wisdom to know the difference." Changing things—the goal of most psychotherapy—requires understanding which things are changeable and which are not. We cannot, for example, change the fact that a loved one has died, that we have a serious or painful medical condition, or that we are experiencing auditory hallucinations, but we can change how we react to those things. We may not be able to change the fact that we feel angry or sad or fearful about something, although we can prevent those feelings from overwhelming us and dictating our behavioral response. When our effortful cognitive processes are adaptive, we accept reality as it is and focus on our responses.

Maladaptive effortful cognitive processes, on the other hand, are those that often start as efforts to feel better, but they frequently end up backfiring and making things worse. Common maladaptive effortful cognitive processes include *rumination, worry, thought suppression,* and *mental compulsions.*

There's a back-and-forth relationship between intrusions and effortful cognitive processes. As shown in Figure 3.11, clients often experience intrusions such as unpleasant memories, frightening mental images, or unpleasant, sometimes personally repugnant, thoughts. They then respond to these intrusions with maladaptive effortful cognitive processes. However, as you see in Figure 3.11, the maladaptive effortful cognitive process often increases the frequency or the intensity of the intrusions over time.

Rumination

The word *rumination* brings to mind an image of a cow chewing its cud. The cow swallows food, regurgitates the food, chews it, and swallows it again. Now imagine that same process of regurgitating and rechewing as a mental activity. In **rumination,** the person thinks about the same negative thing over and over again. In the case of *depressive rumination,* sometimes called "brooding," the person repeatedly thinks about his or her upsetting

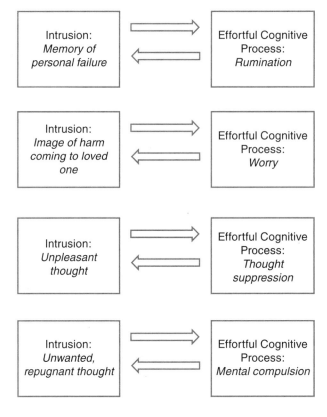

FIGURE 3.11. The interaction of intrusions and effortful cognitive processes in psychopathology.

symptoms and the causes and consequences of those symptoms, while failing to initiate the active problem solving that might alter the cause of that distress (Nolen-Hoeksema, 1991). In the case of *postevent rumination,* the person rehashes details about an event that has occurred, including critical evaluations of his or her own performance (Kashdan & Roberts, 2007).

Note that rumination is not the same thing as problem solving, working through an issue, or figuring things out. Unlike these (potentially) more productive forms of thinking, rumination is characterized not only by the presence of negative thoughts but also by a tendency for those thoughts to be perseverative (i.e., the same subset of negative thoughts are repeated over and over). Over time, the content of ruminative thought can become increasingly negative (which also helps us distinguish it from actual problem solving).

Over time, rumination causes *exacerbation of negative mood.*

- Christina experiences a feeling of sad mood. She thinks, "Why am I so depressed? Why can't I feel better? Why do other people seem to feel so much better than I do?" She becomes increasingly unhappy and hopeless as she realizes how out of control the mood is.
- As Nick ponders the state of his marriage with Johanna, he thinks, "Why can't I just snap out of it? Everyone else's marriage seems to be so much better than mine. Why can't we just be a happy couple like everyone else?" This thinking pattern makes him feel increasingly discouraged.

The Science behind It

Rumination requires one to focus attention on one's own feelings and the mental search for their causes and consequences. As a result, the individual has less attentional resources available to allocate toward (potentially) more adaptive responses to negative mood, such as complex problem solving or other forms of problem-focused coping (Hong, 2007; Nolen-Hoeksema, 1991).

Rumination increases the likelihood of negative automatic thoughts, such as believing that things will turn out poorly (Lyubomirsky & Nolen-Hoeksema, 1995), as well as core beliefs that one is worthless and incompetent (Rimes & Watkins, 2005).

Rumination also impairs cognitive processes: It makes people less effective at interpersonal problem solving (Lyubomirsky & Nolen-Hoeksema, 1995), impairs executive functioning (Watkins & Brown, 2002), and enhances memory bias for negative life events (Lyubomirsky, Caldwell, & Nolen-Hoeksema, 1998).

Interestingly, some individuals believe that rumination is a *good* way to manage emotions—they may believe, for example, that "Thinking about the causes of my sadness will help me prevent it," "If I dwell on my past mistakes, I can be a better person," or "Thinking about how bad I am will make me snap out of it" (Wells, 2009, p. 200). When studied over time, these people tend to ruminate more and to develop more symptoms of depression than do people who don't believe that rumination is an effective solution to problems (Weber & Exner, 2013).

Despite the fact that people engage in rumination in an effort to reduce negative emotions, research shows that ruminating actually causes these moods to worsen (Nolen-Hoeksema & Morrow, 1993; Wegner, Erber, & Zanakos, 1993). As people ruminate, they feel worse, which in turn causes more rumination, resulting in a downward spiral (Moberly & Watkins, 2008).

Worry

Another maladaptive effortful cognitive process is **worry.** Although worry can feel uncontrollable, it is, in fact, an effortful cognitive process. When intrusive and scary thoughts pop up, some people engage in worry, which is a form of quasi-problem solving in which the person repetitively rehearses a number of uncertain (or even unlikely) potentially catastrophic outcomes to current or potential future situations (Borkovec, 1994).

The effortful process of worry can cause *long-term maintenance of anxiety.*

- When Suzanne's husband is late coming home, she has an intrusive thought that something bad might have happened to him. She reacts by imagining all of the bad things that might have happened, mentally bracing herself for the worst. She feels chronically anxious.
- As Samuel lies in bed, unable to fall asleep, he begins thinking about all of the bad things that could happen if he can't get to sleep. He imagines being tired the next day, perhaps even getting fired because he can't concentrate. He tells himself that he *must* fall asleep, or else. Not surprisingly, this worrying only serves to keep him awake longer.

The Science behind It

Worry causes prolonged anxious and dysphoric mood (Brosschot, Gerin, & Thayer, 2006). When people worry, they experience greater negative affect (Llera & Newman, 2010), as well as prolonged cardiac signs of arousal (Pieper, Brosschot, van der Leeden, & Thayer, 2010). They have more negative interpretations, such as expecting negative outcomes and feeling unable to cope with those outcomes (Stapinski, Abbott, & Rapee, 2010); they also have decreased attentional resources available to allocate toward nonthreatening concerns needed for daily functioning (Stefanopoulou, Hirsch, Hayes, Adlam, & Coker, 2014) and have diminished executive functioning resources needed to solve problems and make decisions (Hallion, Ruscio, & Jha, 2014).

One might wonder: If worrying is so aversive, why do people do it? Despite the fact that worrying feels bad and is disruptive, some individuals believe that worry is a good idea—they may believe, for example, that worry motivates them to do better, prepares them for the worst, or prevents negative outcomes (Borkovec & Roemer, 1995; Davey, Tallis, & Capuzzo, 1996). People with GAD, a disorder in which excessive worry is the most distinguishing symptom, are particularly likely to endorse a belief that worrying helps distract them from more emotional topics (Borkovec & Roemer, 1995). It has been suggested, therefore, that "individuals with GAD use worry as a coping strategy because they prefer to feel chronically distressed in order to prepare for the worst outcome, rather than to experience a shift from a positive or euthymic state to a negative emotion" (M. G. Newman & Llera, 2011, p. 375). I'm not sure the word *prefer* is entirely accurate here. The person who worries doesn't necessarily *like* worrying, or *choose* to worry. Rather, he or she gets stuck in a pattern of worrying that makes him or her feel prepared, even though it's not truly preparing or helping him or her to deal with stressors.

Thought Suppression

Thought suppression is another maladaptive effortful cognitive process. When people experience unwanted, unpleasant thoughts, they will often attempt to make these thoughts go away by "clearing the mind" or trying to think about something else (Wenzlaff & Wegner, 2000). As we discuss later, these efforts can sometimes backfire, leading the thoughts to increase rather than decrease in frequency or intensity.

Thought suppression can cause *paradoxical thought increases.*

Try This

Try this exercise: for 1 full minute, try not to think about a white bear. What happened? If you're like most people, it was hard not to think about a white bear. You probably tried thinking about something else, but eventually thoughts of a white bear crept into your awareness. The reason for this is that the very act of suppression serves to remind you of what you are suppressing—thus making the white bear come to mind.

The Science behind It

The phenomenon of thought suppression causing the frequency and intensity of thoughts to increase is well documented in social psychology (Wenzlaff & Wegner, 2000). Specifically, when we try to suppress a thought, two things can happen: First, the act of thought suppression means that we intentionally search for a distracter thought but also automatically monitor our own thoughts for occurrences of what we are trying to suppress to "make sure" we're not thinking about the forbidden thought. This can cause an *immediate enhancement effect* in which we think about it more. Second, after we finish actively trying to suppress thoughts, we experience a *rebound effect*, in which the thoughts become more frequent for a period of time (Abramowitz, Tolin, & Street, 2001). Research also shows us that these paradoxical effects of thought suppression are particularly pronounced in people with mental disorders characterized by intrusive thoughts, such as OCD (Tolin, Abramowitz, Przeworski, & Foa, 2002) and PTSD (Shipherd & Beck, 1999), though they are certainly not limited to those disorders.

We also see that when people try (and fail) to suppress unwanted thoughts, they become more distressed by those thoughts than they would have had they not attempted to suppress (Marcks & Woods, 2005). They also show increased physiological arousal (Campbell-Sills, Barlow, Brown, & Hofmann, 2005) and increased memory bias for the material they are trying to suppress (Kircanski, Craske, & Bjork, 2008). In some cases, they interpret their thought suppression failures as confirming the idea that they are mentally defective or that the thought is particularly important (Tolin, Abramowitz, Hamlin, Foa, & Synodi, 2002).

- Melissa experiences intrusive, unwanted memories of a previous traumatic experience. She tries hard not to think about it, talk about it, or be reminded of it. These efforts are not successful, and the intrusive memories become more intense and frequent.
- Bethany has the intrusive thought that she might lose control of herself and hurt someone. She tries to get that thought out of her head by thinking of something else. But the intrusive thought just keeps popping up, despite her efforts.

Mental Compulsions

Finally, **mental compulsions** are an effortful, maladaptive cognitive process. The role of mental compulsions is well documented in OCD, in which clients might say a specific prayer over and over, count up to a certain number, and so on (Foa et al., 1995). Though mental compulsions might be most easily identified in OCD, the phenomenon is likely not limited to that disorder: many clients, regardless of diagnosis, may engage in mental strategies that are essentially aimed at making them feel better or warding off some feared outcome.

Mental compulsions can cause the intrusion to increase in persistence and scariness.

- When Bethany has the intrusive thought that she might lose control of herself and hurt someone, one of her habitual responses is to say prayers to herself over and over, in an effort to make sure she remains safe. Over time, however, the intrusive thought feels increasingly real to her.

On Intentionality and Effortful Cognitive Processes

Because processes such as rumination, worry, thought suppression, and mental compulsions are effortful (rather than automatic), one might guess that the person has made a deliberate and calculated decision to engage in the process. Suzanne's husband once became exasperated with her worrying and shouted, "I think you just *want* to be worried and miserable all the time!" And it's easy to see how he could reach that conclusion. However, often that conclusion is inaccurate. For example, Christina didn't decide, "I'm going to ruminate now so that I can stay miserable." Sam didn't think, "I bet worrying will help me fall asleep better." These processes are effortful, but they are not entirely deliberate.

Think back to our discussion of *contingencies* in Chapter 2. When something pays off in the short term, we tend to do more of it—and often that has little to do with our awareness or our intentions. Maladaptive effortful cognitive processes pay off in the short term. By ruminating, Christina feels as if she is solving problems and helping herself feel better. By worrying, Sam feels as if he is preparing himself for bad things that might happen. By trying to suppress her intrusive memories, Melissa gets momentary relief from the aversive images. By praying, Bethany feels as if she is becoming less dangerous. So these effortful cognitive processes are *reinforced*, either positively (*reinforcement*) or negatively (*escape*). Over time, they can become mental "habits" that are hard to break, even though they are clearly not helping and are even making the problem worse in the long run. Remember, we are all slaves to the immediate, unless we force ourselves not to be.

THE ESSENTIALS

* Cognitive processes become maladaptive when we make the same kinds of errors over and over.

* Maladaptive automatic cognitive processes include confirmatory biases in information processing (particularly attention and memory) and intrusions (for example, intrusive thoughts and memories, hallucinations).

* Maladaptive semi-automatic cognitive processes include interpretations (what we think about our experiences) and core beliefs (our pervasive beliefs about ourselves, other people, and the world).

* Cognitive distortions are errors in interpretations that give us a skewed version of reality.

* Interpretations are influenced by our emotions, behaviors, core beliefs, information-processing biases, and learning history.

* Interpretations influence our emotions and behaviors.

* Core beliefs are influenced by our experience, the effects of our own behavior, and modeling.

* Core beliefs affect our interpretations and behaviors.

* Maladaptive effortful cognitive processes include rumination, worry, thought suppression, and mental compulsions.

* Maladaptive effortful cognitive processes tend to backfire and cause persistence of the emotion or thought we are trying to control.

▰▰▰▰▰▰ KEY TERMS AND DEFINITIONS ▰▰▰▰▰▰

Acceptance: A willingness to experience certain thoughts or feelings.

Attention: The mental process that allows sensory information into awareness.

Attentional bias: A tendency to allocate attention disproportionately toward stimuli that are consistent with current mood or beliefs.

Automatic cognitive processes: Mental activity that happens involuntarily, sometimes without the person's awareness.

Cognitive distortion: An inaccuracy in interpretations.

Confirmation bias: A tendency to search for or interpret information in a way that confirms one's preconceptions.

Core belief: A belief that serves as an (often unrecognized or unacknowledged) "program" for how the individual responds to stressors or other triggers.

Effortful cognitive processes: Cognitive processes done volitionally, often representing efforts to cope with distress.

Information processing: How the brain filters, processes, retains, and recalls information.

Information-processing bias: Biased or distorted filtering, process, retention, and recall of information.

Interpretations: Semi-automatic cognitive processes that make meaning of stimuli or situations.

Intrusions: Images, ideas, words, or urges that come to mind automatically and involuntarily.

Long-term memory: A much larger storage of information that is kept in the brain on a relatively permanent basis.

Memory bias: A tendency to disproportionately recall information that is consistent with current mood or beliefs.

Mental compulsions: Volitional mental responses aimed at trying to neutralize a potential threat or to make the person feel better.

Rehearsal: In information processing, mentally repeating information in order to transfer it from short-term memory to long-term memory.

Retrieval: The act of pulling information out of long-term memory.

Rumination: An effortful mental response that involves thinking about the same thing over and over without actual problem-solving.

Schema: A broad and pervasive theme or pattern of core beliefs, memory, emotion, interpretations, and bodily sensations.

Short-term memory: A limited-capacity "holding" area for information that usually requires rehearsal to maintain the information.

Thought suppression: An effortful mental response that involves trying not to have certain thoughts.

Worry: An effortful mental response that involves thinking about a number of catastrophic outcomes under conditions of uncertainty.

Listing Interpretations

Using a *recent* occurrence of the personal target, identify your interpretations and the emotions that followed.

Situation	Interpretation(s)	Emotion(s) (rate intensity from 0 to 100)
Example: *Late for work*	*I'll never succeed in this job*	*Sadness 65*

Next, check whether any of the following cognitive distortions are present in your interpretations, and briefly indicate *why* you think those distortions apply.

Probability overestimation _____

Catastrophizing _____

Overgeneralization _____

Personalizing _____

All-or-nothing thinking _____

"Should" statements _____

Mind reading _____

Emotional reasoning _____

Minimizing _____

From *Doing CBT* by David F. Tolin. Copyright © 2016 The Guilford Press. Permission to photocopy this worksheet is granted to purchasers of this book for personal use only (see copyright page for details). Purchasers can download enlarged versions of this worksheet (see the box at the end of the table of contents).

CHAPTER 4

I Got a Bad Feeling about This

The Emotional System
and How It Can Go Wrong

Emotion is a broad label that is sometimes used to refer not only to feelings but also to their associated cognitive and behavioral processes. For our purposes, however, we'll use a narrower definition so that we can separate out the various components of the core pathological process. We'll use two factors to define an **emotion:** a *subjective emotional state* (how we "label" what we are feeling—sad, scared, angry, etc.) and *physiological sensations* (what we experience in our bodies—heaviness, racing heart, muscle tension, etc.). Subjective emotional states and physiological sensations tend go together in fairly predictable ways. Some common associations between subjective feeling states and physiological sensations are shown in Table 4.1.

There are, however, lots of noteworthy exceptions to this rule.

- Many people will experience physical sensations we associate with fear, such as racing heart, sweating, breathing hard, and so on, but will not subjectively label their feeling state as "fear."
- Many people will have a subjective feeling state, such as "angry," but do not exhibit the associated physiological sensations such as muscle tension, heart rate increase, and so on.
- Still other people will report one subjective feeling state, such as "anger," but will exhibit physiological sensations that seem consistent with another emotion, such as fear.

TABLE 4.1. Physiological Sensations Commonly Associated with Negative Subjective Feeling States

Subjective feeling state or label	Afraid or anxious	Sad or depressed	Angry or mad
Physiological sensations	• Heart racing • Sweating • Breathing hard • "Butterflies" in stomach • Tingling	• Heavy feeling • Fatigue • Headache • Upset stomach	• Heart racing • Face getting hot • Muscles tensing

Sometimes these discrepancies are socially moderated, such as when "macho" guys don't want to admit to feeling afraid (Pierce & Kirkpatrick, 1992). At other times, the discrepancy occurs because we're not always good at identifying and labeling exactly how we feel. At still other times, the discrepancy occurs because the subjective states and the physiological sensations are only loosely correlated. It's just not a perfect match.

So the presence of certain physiological sensations might raise a hypothesis about an emotional state, but we wouldn't want to fall into the trap of assuming that the presence of certain physiological sensations (such as increased heart rate and sweating) "proves" that the person is experiencing an emotion (such as fear). The subjective feeling state and the physiological sensations are both important, and although they often line up together in intuitive ways, sometimes they don't. Neither one is necessarily more "right" than the other; they are just different aspects of the emotional experience that need to be taken into consideration.

Emotion researchers have suggested that all humans have a set of innate *basic emotions* that include happiness, sadness, fear, anger, and disgust (Ekman, 1992a; Izard, 1977). These basic emotions are associated with distinct patterns of neural activity (L. F. Barrett & Wager, 2006), physiological activity (Levenson, 1992), and facial expressions (Ekman, 1992b). As we grow and develop greater self-awareness, we acquire more complex emotions, such as embarrassment, envy, and empathy. As we mature further and develop an understanding of societal rules and expectations, we develop still more complex emotions, such as pride, shame, and guilt (for a review, see M. Lewis, 2000).

What Makes Emotions Maladaptive?

It might be tempting to think that unpleasant emotions such as fear, sadness, and anger are inherently maladaptive and that pleasant emotions such as happiness are inherently adaptive. But this isn't necessarily true: Spend some time with a client in a manic episode and you'll get a good look at maladaptive happiness. It's more useful to think about whether the emotion helps the person function better (adaptive) or gets in the way of the person's functioning (maladaptive).

Impairing Function, Rather Than Helping It

Adaptive emotions can improve our performance. A classic example of this phenomenon is the century-old *Yerkes–Dodson* law (Yerkes & Dodson, 1908). According to this principle, emotional arousal can improve one's performance, likely by increasing one's interest, focus, and motivation. After all, very low emotion could manifest as boredom or lack of interest, which is likely to make one not perform well. However, this is true only up to a point: When arousal levels get too high, performance decreases as attention, memory, and problem solving begin to suffer. As an example, many performers report that a little bit of "stage fright" actually helps them do a better job. Their anticipatory anxiety energizes them, focuses them on the task at hand, and motivates them to do their best. But as we increase the level of that emotion, some people suffer from more crippling forms of performance anxiety; in such cases, their anxiety tends to lead them to forget what they're supposed to be doing, draws their attention away from the task and onto more anxiety-provoking stimuli, and leads them into avoidant behavioral patterns. This curvilinear relationship between emotion and performance is shown in Figure 4.1.

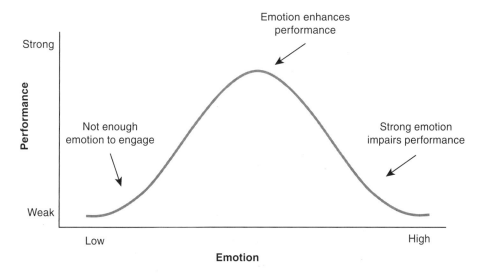

FIGURE 4.1. Graphical depiction of the Yerkes–Dodson law.

Being Inflexible or Out of Proportion

Maladaptive emotions may wax and wane somewhat, but they often do not remit with a change of circumstances (e.g., a pleasant event may create a momentary decrease in sadness but will not eliminate it). As an example, people with major depressive disorder show less emotional reaction to positive *or* negative stimuli, compared with nondepressed people (Rottenberg, Gross, & Gotlib, 2005). Their emotions are less sensitive to external influence. By contrast, adaptive emotions fluctuate more readily according to circumstances (e.g., a pleasant event will make us happier, and an unpleasant event will make us sadder). The intensity of adaptive emotions is appropriate to the situation (e.g., our level of sadness will vary depending on whether we have lost $5 or whether a loved one dies). Emotions can become maladaptive when they are out of proportion to the situation (e.g., we feel intensely sad even when the negative event would be considered minor by most people).

Maladaptive emotions often play a significant role in mental disorders. So, for example:

- Anna, who suffers from panic attacks, experiences maladaptive *fear.*
- Christina, our depressed client, experiences maladaptive *sadness.*
- Elizabeth, who is diagnosed with borderline personality disorder, experiences maladaptive *fear, sadness,* and *anger* at varying times.
- Lauren, our client with paranoid schizophrenia, experiences maladaptive *fear.*
- Blaise, who is struggling with addiction, experiences physiological sensations of *arousal,* even though she might not subjectively label it as a feeling state.
- Shari, our bulimic client, feels maladaptive *disgust* after an episode of binge eating.

Your clients might have these same emotional patterns, or they might not. The client's diagnosis might help us generate a hypothesis about the person's emotions, but it doesn't guarantee it. Some people with major depressive disorder, for example, don't subjectively report feeling sad.

Where Do Emotions Come From?

Remember that the *core pathological process* is the interplay among cognitive, emotional, and behavioral factors. Everything affects everything within that process (see Figure 4.2).

Emotions Are Influenced by Interpretations

As we discussed in Chapter 3, what we think can greatly affect how we feel. Thoughts about threat are likely to lead to the emotion of *fear*. Thoughts about loss are likely to lead to the emotion of *sadness*. Thoughts about past errors are likely to lead to the emotion of *guilt*. Thoughts about others' perceived misdeeds are likely to lead to the emotion of *anger*. If one's thoughts habitually revolve around these themes, the emotions tend to persist and become more intense.

However, it's a mistake to conclude that *all* emotions are caused by thoughts. There are other roads to emotion (Zajonc, 1984). As we'll discuss further later in this chapter, it is quite likely that emotions are sometimes generated by thoughts (e.g., the activity of the frontal lobes of the brain), whereas at other times the frontal lobes are bypassed and the sensory information goes straight to emotion-producing parts of the brain such as the amygdala (LeDoux & Phelps, 2000). That's important for our case conceptualizations. Sometimes, feelings just show up, and sometimes they are the result of our interpretations.

Emotions Are Influenced by Behaviors

As we discussed in Chapter 2, our behaviors affect how we feel. Avoidance breeds fear. Withdrawal breeds sadness. Aggression breeds anger. Just as our emotions can change our behavior, so can our behavior change our emotions.

Emotions Are Influenced by Information-Processing Biases

In Chapter 3, we reviewed how biases in attention and memory can exert a strong impact on how we feel. Selectively attending to threatening stimuli while failing to attend to more benign stimuli can elicit and increase feelings of fear and anxiety. Selectively recalling disappointing or unfortunate experiences while failing to recall happier experiences can elicit and increase feelings of sadness.

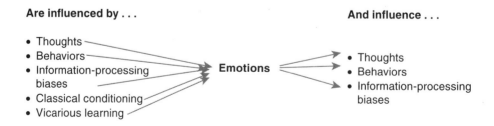

FIGURE 4.2. Inputs and outputs for emotions.

Emotions Are Influenced by Classical Conditioning

One important (yet easily overlooked) road to emotion is **classical conditioning.** In Chapter 2 we talked about *operant conditioning*, which is one process by which overt behaviors can be learned. *Classical conditioning*, conversely, refers to a process by which emotions and physiological reactions can be learned. In essence classical conditioning occurs when a reflexive physiological response (e.g., an emotional reaction) becomes paired (associated) with a stimulus that did not previously elicit that reaction.

Ivan Pavlov (1927/1960) conducted the original studies on classical conditioning using dogs (scc Figure 4.3). Dogs have a natural (reflexive) tendency to salivate when presented with food. Food is therefore called an **unconditioned** (meaning "not learned") **stimulus**, and salivating is called an **unconditioned response** (see Figure 4.3, row 1). Dogs do not naturally salivate when you ring a bell (see Figure 4.3, row 2). Pavlov *paired* the two stimuli (the food and the bell) by presenting them to the dogs at the same time, again and again (see Figure 4.3, row 3). Eventually, the dogs began salivating whenever the bell was rung, even though no food was being offered (see Figure 4.3, row 4). The bell was now called a **conditioned** (meaning "learned") **stimulus**, and salivating was now called a **conditioned response**. In short, to the dogs, the bell meant food, and food meant it was time to drool.

What does all of this saliva discussion have to do with emotions? Like physical reflexes such as salivation, emotions can occur reflexively toward some stimuli. If a vicious dog threatens me, for example, it's a natural reflex to feel afraid. No one has to teach me to be afraid of that. So the vicious dog is an unconditioned stimulus, and my fear is an unconditioned response. But after that happens, I now might feel fear even when looking at a picture of a dog or talking about a dog. Because of my learning experience, I now have the same kind of emotional response to words and pictures that I do toward an actual vicious dog who is threatening me. The words and pictures have become conditioned stimuli, and my fear has become a conditioned response.

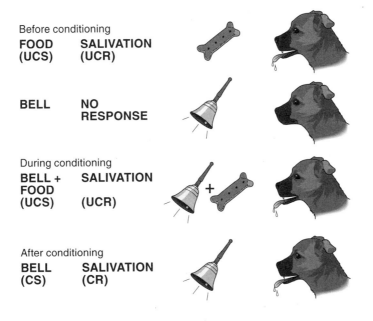

FIGURE 4.3. An example of classical conditioning.

Try This

You can see the effects of classical conditioning in yourself. Think about a lemon being squeezed. Say to yourself the word *lemon*. What do you notice happening physically? If you found yourself producing more saliva, that's classical conditioning in action. Lemons naturally cause salivation, so that is an unconditioned stimulus and an unconditioned response. But words and mental images don't naturally cause salivation. (Try saying the word *lemon* to an infant and see what happens. Nothing.) The reason this mental image and word cause you to salivate is because you have learned, through experience, to associate them with actual lemons. So now the word *lemon* and the mental image of the lemon are conditioned stimuli, and your salivation is a conditioned response.

Nearly a century ago, John Watson illustrated this phenomenon in a rather nasty way with an infant nicknamed "Little Albert." Albert initially showed no fear of a white mouse. When Watson made a loud noise at the same time that he presented a white mouse, Albert naturally became quite distressed. Eventually, Albert would become distressed whenever the mouse was presented, even when no noise was being made. Albert had developed a **conditioned emotional response,** in which the mouse was the conditioned stimulus and distress was the conditioned response (Watson & Rayner, 1920).

Now, it's easy for us to imagine how classical conditioning can work in the case of specific phobias, such as fears of mice or dogs or snakes. But it shows up in other emotional disorders as well (Mineka & Oehlberg, 2008).

• Our client Melissa was sexually abused by her stepfather, who would repeatedly assault her in her bed at night. Through classical conditioning, it's not difficult to imagine that she would develop a fearful response to her stepfather, or perhaps men that resembled him. We could probably imagine as well that she could have become fearful of being alone in her room at night. That's the straightforward part. But over time, Melissa's fears spread through a process called **stimulus generalization.** As she got older, she started to fear not only her stepfather and men who resembled him, but also men in general. Over time she even became fearful and mistrustful of all people. And her fears didn't stay confined to her childhood bedroom where she was assaulted. Over time, she became fearful of dark places in general, even being at home in the dark. She started to become fearful of being home alone, just at night at first but eventually during the day as well. (This happened to Little Albert, too: Over time, he became fearful not only of white mice, but also of similar objects such as a white rabbit, a dog, even a Santa Claus mask with a furry white beard.) Whenever Melissa experiences one of these things, she has a subjective feeling state of fear and a range of physiological symptoms of arousal. So, naturally, she started avoiding these things and became increasingly limited in her actions. Over time, she started to "shut down" as a way of trying to control her fear reactions.

• Blaise, who is addicted to cocaine, would always use with a particular group of friends, usually at one friend's house. The house has a particular look, smell, and sounds. So with repeated experience, Blaise started to associate the feelings she gets from cocaine with the look, smell, sounds, and so forth, of that house and with the people she uses with. It's not surprising, then, if being in that house, seeing those people, or smelling those smells triggered urges to use. The urge to use had become a conditioned response, associated with the conditioned stimuli of the friends and the house. Blaise would also use when she was feeling bored. Here comes classical conditioning again: Over time, the feeling of boredom became a conditioned stimulus, and her urge to use became a conditioned response.

- Nick and Johanna, our distressed couple, have had repeated arguments on the phone. Each time, they come away from the phone call feeling intensely angry. Now, when Johanna's phone rings and she sees it's Nick calling, she starts to feel her temper rising before she even answers the phone. The phone call from Nick has become a conditioned stimulus, and her anger has become a conditioned response.

Here's an experience I had a while back. My mother was visiting me, and for whatever reason I was really irritated at her. (I love my mom; don't judge me.) I went out to mow the lawn. I can remember rounding a particular tree in the yard and feeling really annoyed. The next week, when I was mowing the lawn again, I rounded that same tree and found myself feeling irritated again! The original source of my irritation had left, so why was I feeling that way? One possible answer is that the annoying experience with my mother was the unconditioned stimulus, the situation (mowing the lawn around that particular tree) served as a conditioned stimulus, and my emotional reaction was a conditioned response. So just being in a setting that has previously been associated with an emotion can elicit a similar emotional experience.

The twist here is that unlike Little Albert or someone with PTSD, classical conditioning wasn't the original *cause* of my emotion. My mom didn't beat me with a tree, causing me to have an emotional reaction to trees. However, classical conditioning was behind the *maintenance* of my emotion. Because I had happened to feel a certain way in a certain circumstance, later on that circumstance was able to elicit some of the same feelings.

We can see that process happening in some of our clients as well:

- Nick is often angry toward Johanna. As he drives from his work to his home (where Johanna is), he starts to feel his muscles tightening up, his teeth clenching, and his face contorting into a scowl. He has been angry at home so much that the stimuli associated with going home are eliciting a conditioned emotional response. Interestingly, when we ask Nick why he felt angry, he might give us an answer such as, "I think it was because I was just remembering how nasty she had been to me yesterday." But we can see that this isn't necessarily true. When we feel something, we tend to look for an explanation. Nick's anger in this particular moment was the result of a conditioning process, but since he wasn't aware of that, he created a **post-hoc rationalization** in which he identified a "reason" that was not the true cause of the emotion.

- Anna has experienced recurrent panic attacks, the first sign of which is increased heart rate. Now, it seems like every time her heart rate increases, she experiences more panic-like sensations. She has also had bad panic attacks at her local shopping mall; now, just being at the mall causes those panicky feelings to surface. As was the case with Nick, the fact that she has had strong emotions in one particular context is enough to trigger the same emotional response. Interestingly, when we ask Anna why she felt panicky, she replies, "I have no idea. The feelings just came from nowhere." But we can see that they didn't come from nowhere: They were the result of a conditioning process that had occurred outside of her awareness.

- Samuel, who suffers from insomnia, habitually lies awake in bed, worrying. Now, just getting in bed seems to increase his feelings of anxiety. Because he has paired the bed with worrying so frequently, the bed has now become a conditioned stimulus, and anxiety has become a conditioned response.

Emotions Are Influenced by Vicarious Learning

One doesn't have to be bitten by a dog in order to develop a fear of dogs. Just watching someone be bitten (in person or on television) or learning about someone who was bitten can be enough to develop a conditioned emotional response. Anyone who has watched the movie "Jaws" and then felt afraid to swim in the ocean knows what I'm talking about. We refer to "picking up" an emotional response by watching others as **vicarious learning.** In fact, just being around other people who display a particular emotional response to a given stimulus, especially during our developmental years, can lead us to pick up a similar response. Our client Suzanne, who has generalized anxiety, was raised by a chronically anxious parent. Her parent reacted to everything with an overexpression of fear, tension, or dread. Over time, Suzanne developed similar emotional responses.

What Do Emotions Do?

Emotions Affect Interpretations

We've discussed how thoughts can influence emotions, as shown for Anna in Figure 4.4. As Anna thinks "I'm having a heart attack," she experiences a greater amount of tachycardia, dizziness, and fear. Note, however, that the causation can go in both directions. Just as Anna's interpretations increase her physiological arousal, so too does her arousal influence her interpretations. The more physical arousal she experiences, the more she believes that she really is dying. It becomes a vicious cycle.

In this fashion, we see that a person's emotions can strengthen preexisting beliefs or "prove" them right. This is related to the cognitive distortion of *emotional reasoning* we discussed in Chapter 3: We believe something is true because we feel it.

Emotions Affect Behaviors

In Chapter 2, we discussed how emotions are associated with various *action tendencies.* These action tendencies often work in our favor. When we feel sad, we have an action tendency to slow down, allowing us to look more carefully at situations. Our affective expression of sadness (e.g., crying) signals to others that there is a problem, eliciting helping behavior. When we feel angry, we have an action tendency to engage in a strong and sustained response to difficult situations. The affective expression of anger may inhibit the bad behavior of others. When we feel fear, our action tendency is to escape from threat. Similarly, the affective expression of fear signals the presence of threat to others. Even an emotion like shame has a purpose. When we feel shame, our action tendency is to increase our social conformity and cohesion, to acquire better skills and competencies (for reviews, see Frijda, 1987; Izard & Ackerman, 2000; Lowe & Ziemke, 2011). So emotions and their associated action tendencies are basically a good thing. However, there are also times when we need to inhibit those action tendencies, so we don't run away from everything that seems scary or punch everyone who makes us angry. When we fail to override our emotional action tendencies, we often end up with either a *behavioral excess* or a *behavioral deficit.*

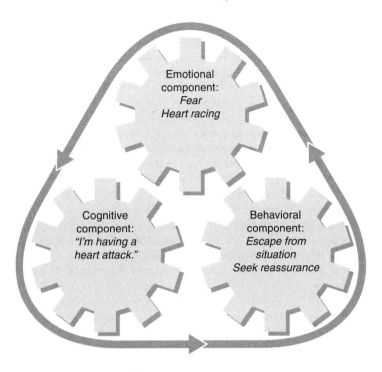

FIGURE 4.4. Anna's core pathological process.

The Science behind It

The idea that emotions are *caused* by thoughts and interpretations has been the mainstay of cognitive theory for a long time (e.g., A. T. Beck et al., 1979). The "primacy of cognition" has been the subject of a long-standing debate (e.g., R. S. Lazarus, 1984; Zajonc, 1984). Research tells us that sometimes thoughts do cause emotions, but not always.

There is good evidence that emotions can be elicited independently of cognitive appraisal (at least the kind of appraisal we talk about in therapy). Subliminal presentation of emotion-evoking stimuli (e.g., presenting a picture so quickly the person doesn't even consciously know what he or she saw) can elicit physiological arousal (Esteves, Parra, Dimberg, & Ohman, 1994) and influence behavior (Chen & Bargh, 1999). Interestingly, the "mystery moods" elicited by subliminal stimulus presentation can easily be misattributed to something else—for example, a person might mistakenly attribute his feelings of anger to his wife's behavior, when in fact his anger was elicited by something entirely different (Chartrand, van Baaren, & Bargh, 2006). When we feel something, we look for an explanation—and sometimes that explanation isn't accurate.

Neurobiological studies of one emotion—fear—demonstrate that there are two distinct information pathways in the brain to the amygdala, which resides in the limbic system and is commonly considered the "fear center" of the brain. One route, called the "slow route," goes from the thalamus (where perceptual information is routed) through the frontal cortex and then to the amygdala. The "fast route," on the other hand, goes directly from the thalamus to the amygdala, bypassing the frontal cortex altogether (LeDoux & Phelps, 2000). One could make the argument that this same basic setup exists for any given emotion: Sometimes, the emotion is mediated by thinking (the activity of the frontal cortex), and sometimes it is not—it just seems to "happen" for reasons that the person cannot understand, because the emotional centers of the brain are being triggered by other, more rapid, means.

The hypothesized one-way street from thoughts to emotions also turns out not to be true: Emotions have a distinct impact on thoughts. The *affect-as-information hypothesis* suggests that our emotions are a source of information that we use to determine what to think about things. So if something gives you a warm, fuzzy feeling in your body, you're likely to have favorable thoughts about it. On the other hand, if something raises the hair on the back of your neck and makes you clench your jaw, you're likely to have unfavorable thoughts about it. In one study, manipulations of fear versus anger during a discussion of the September 11, 2001, terrorist attacks led respondents to change their estimates of the risk of additional attacks, as well as their attitudes about retaliatory policies (Lerner, Gonzalez, Small, & Fischhoff, 2003). In another, just listening to sad music while standing at the bottom of a hill to be climbed led participants to overestimate the steepness of the hill (Riener, Stefanucci, Proffitt, & Clore, 2011)—literally, making mountains out of molehills.

At a biological level, the *somatic marker hypothesis* (Bechara & Damasio, 2007) suggests that feelings play a critical role in judgment and decision making. The ventromedial prefrontal cortex (VMPFC) transmits information about bodily sensations (feelings) to other regions of the brain that are involved in making decisions (thinking). When people have damage to the VMPFC—that is, when they don't have the capacity to incorporate information about feelings into their judgments—they often appear completely cognitively intact, yet they repeatedly make bad decisions (Bechara, Damasio, Damasio, & Anderson, 1994).

In many cases, behavioral excesses and behavioral deficits represent an attempt to feel better, or an attempt to make the thing we perceive as causing distress stop or go away. We can see an example of this in Anna's core pathological process (see Figure 4.4). Anna experiences the physiological sensation of increased heart rate, as well as the subjective feeling state of fear. Her behavioral response is to attempt some kind of escape from the situation (in this case, leaving the shopping mall). She also tried to reduce her distressed feelings by calling a loved one and seeking reassurance. At other times, Anna has tried to escape from the uncomfortable physiological sensations themselves by taking deep breaths, breathing into a paper bag, sipping water, or taking a benzodiazepine medication. In all of these cases, her behavioral response is a direct reaction to the maladaptive emotion and reflects her attempt to feel better or escape from the distressing stimuli.

Some common behavioral reactions to emotions are shown in Table 4.2. As with everything, however, remember that there are always exceptions. There isn't a one-to-one correspondence between emotion and behavior. Many people, for example, can feel afraid but will not engage in avoidance or escape behaviors. Similarly, many may engage

TABLE 4.2. Common Behavioral Reactions to Emotions

Subjective feeling state or label	Afraid or anxious	Sad or depressed	Angry or mad
Behavioral responses	• Avoidance • Escape	• Decreased activity	• Aggression • Agitation

in aggressive behavior but do not report the subjective feeling state of anger. So we can never assume the presence of an emotion from a behavior, nor can we assume the presence of a behavior from an emotion. At best, these common relationships help us generate hypotheses that must be checked out.

Emotions Affect Information Processing

Emotions create *information-processing bias*. You may recall the *mood-congruent bias* discussed in Chapter 3, in which emotions exert a strong impact on information processing. Specifically, there are well-documented effects of emotion on *attention, memory,* and *executive functions* (higher order cognitive processes such as reasoning, task flexibility, problem solving, and planning; R. Elliott, 2003). You can see this phenomenon happening in a lot of our clients:

- As Melissa, who suffers from PTSD, becomes increasingly fearful, her attentional bias for threat-related information increases.
- As Christina, our depressed client, becomes increasingly sad, her memory for past losses and failures becomes clearer, and she is less able to recall positive experiences.
- As Blaise, our substance-abusing client, feels more anxious and agitated, her ability to make plans decreases, as does her ability to inhibit impulses and think about the consequences.

Now, don't get me wrong. I'm not suggesting that emotions are bad, or that emotions necessarily cause cognitive function to break down. We're not robots, after all. Indeed, as we've discussed, emotions are critical to effective judgment and decision making. Remember the Yerkes–Dodson law: A moderate amount of an emotion can be adaptive and helpful, but when the "volume" of that emotion gets too high, performance begins to suffer.

The Science behind It

People are better at remembering information that is consistent with their current mood: People in a positive mood tend to recall more positive events and rate them more positively; people in a negative mood tend to recall more negative events and rate them more negatively (Bower, 1981; Eich, 1995).

Emotion can cause the person to disproportionately allocate attentional resources toward stimuli that are consistent with the emotion. An excellent example of this phenomenon is "weapon focus," in which people witnessing a crime scene tend to narrow their attention to the weapon in the perpetrator's hand to the exclusion of other, less threatening stimuli, such as the perpetrator's face (Loftus, Loftus, & Messo, 1987). Individuals who are hungry disproportionately allocate attention to food-related cues (Mogg, Bradley, Hyare, & Lee, 1998). The presence of a subjective feeling state or certain physiological sensations can cause an individual to be "on the lookout" for things related to his or her emotional state, creating an attentional bias.

Excessive emotional arousal has been demonstrated to adversely affect executive functions. Individuals in an aroused state tend to engage in poorer problem solving, reviewing alternatives less thoroughly and making impulsive decisions (Keinan, 1987). They tend to be less able to inhibit impulsive actions such as eating, smoking, shopping, and procrastination (Pham, 2007).

THE ESSENTIALS

* Emotions are both subjective feeling states and physiological sensations.
* Some degree of emotion is helpful, but emotions become maladaptive when they impair functioning.
* Emotions are influenced by interpretations, behaviors, and information-processing biases.
* Emotions can be acquired via classical conditioning, in which a previously neutral stimulus is paired with an emotionally evocative stimulus.
* Emotions can be influenced by vicarious learning.
* Emotions influence our thoughts, behaviors, and patterns of information processing.

KEY TERMS AND DEFINITIONS

Classical conditioning: A process of learned emotional responses, in which stimuli become associated with one another and can elicit the same emotional reaction.

Conditioned emotional response: An emotional response that is acquired through classical conditioning (pairing of one stimulus with another).

Conditioned response: A person's learned emotional or physiological reaction to a stimulus.

Conditioned stimulus: A stimulus that the person has learned to react to in a particular way.

Emotion: Defined here as a subjective feeling state and/or physiological sensation(s).

Post-hoc rationalization: Explaining an emotional response after the fact by creating a rationale for it.

Stimulus generalization: The process by which a broader range of stimuli develop the ability to elicit a conditioned emotional response.

Unconditioned response: A person's natural emotional or physiological reaction to a stimulus, without any prior learning.

Unconditioned stimulus: A stimulus that the person naturally reacts to in a particular way, without any prior learning.

Vicarious learning: Acquiring a conditioned emotional response by watching the experiences of another person.

Identifying Emotions

Using a *recent* occurrence of the personal target, identify your emotion(s) and the factors related to them.

Situation: _____

Subjective feeling state(s): _____

Physiological sensation(s): _____

Where did the emotion come from?

Interpretations: What interpretations did you have that preceded the emotion? _____

_____

Classical conditioning: What was the conditioned stimulus? _____

_____

How was that stimulus conditioned to elicit that emotion? _____

_____

Vicarious learning: What have you witnessed or learned of that contributed to the emotion? _____

_____

Your behavior: How did your behavior contribute to the emotion? _____

_____

What was the effect of the emotion? _____

_____

Interpretations: What effect did the emotion have on your thoughts and beliefs? _____

_____

Behavior: What effect did the emotion have on your behavioral responses? _____

_____

Information-processing bias: What effect might the emotion have had have on your selective attention or memory? _____

_____

From *Doing CBT* by David F. Tolin. Copyright © 2016 The Guilford Press. Permission to photocopy this worksheet is granted to purchasers of this book for personal use only (see copyright page for details). Purchasers can download enlarged versions of this worksheet (see the box at the end of the table of contents).

CHAPTER 5

Creating Meaty Conceptualizations

We've talked about how behaviors, cognition, and emotions can contribute to the maintenance of psychological problems. We've also seen how these factors interact with each other, so that a problem in one system contributes to problems in the others, resulting in a vicious cycle for our clients. So what do we do with this information?

We're aiming to create a **meaty conceptualization** of the client's problems. By *meaty*, I mean that our conceptual model should not just tell a story about the client. Rather, it should provide clear and actionable information about the processes by which the problem persists. The meaty conceptualization provides us with **targets** that become the basis of our selection of interventions. A major part of the meaty conceptualization is **functional analysis** of behavior, which means that we try to understand *why* a behavior does or does not occur by looking at the *antecedents* (what comes before the behavior) and the *consequences* (what comes after the behavior).

Any case has a wide range of potential targets. As shown in Figure 5.1, the client may come in to treatment complaining of a particular **symptom** (in the case shown, depressed

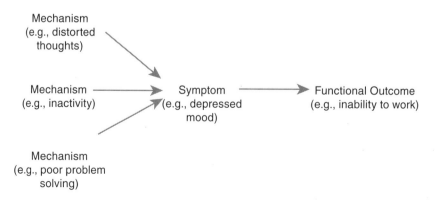

FIGURE 5.1. Potential targets include mechanisms, symptoms, and functional outcomes.

94

mood). From that symptom, we can look either upstream or downstream. When we look upstream, we find that there are several potential **mechanisms** that are causing the symptom to persist. In the case shown, we hypothesize that the client's depressed mood is being maintained by three mechanisms: distorted thoughts, behavioral inactivity, and poor problem-solving skills. When we look downstream, we see that the symptom of depressed mood is contributing to an important **functional outcome**. Functional outcomes refer to the person's ability to engage in important activities such as work, school, social relationships, family relationships, and so on.

So when it comes time to pick our targets, we have several options. This client is asking to feel less depressed, so depressed mood might become our direct target. But that's not our only option. As you can see in the figure, we can also influence that depressed mood by going upstream and effectively targeting one or more of the mechanisms that are causing the depressed mood to persist. For example, we might hypothesize that if we can get the person thinking in a less distorted and depressing manner, get him or her to be more active, or boost his or her problem-solving skills, the person's mood will improve. In other cases, we might opt to go downstream and target the functional outcome. For example, we might be able to find ways to help the person resume work despite the presence of depression.

Putting the Puzzle Together

For any given client, we can create a diagram that helps us understand how these various factors contribute to the problem. We saw in Chapter 1 how we can start by getting an understanding of the *core pathological process:* the interaction among emotional, cognitive, and behavioral elements of the problem.

Often, we are most effective when we diagram *episodes* of the problem, rather than trying to tackle the entire thing. Recall from Chapter 1 how we did this with Anna, our client with panic disorder. We took one episode of the problem (in her case, a panic attack) and separated its emotional, cognitive, and behavioral components (see Figure 1.4). Most psychological problems can be examined in terms of episodes: people with anxiety have periods when they feel especially anxious; depressed people have periods when they feel especially depressed; people with personality disorders have periods when their interpersonal functioning is particularly impaired; and so on. Once in a while I'll see a client who says that the problem is exactly the same, 24 hours a day, 7 days a week, with no fluctuations. But usually with a little bit of probing, we find that there are in fact some ups and downs. That gives us more to work with.

Anna's Trigger

As we try to understand one of Anna's panic attacks, we might start by asking, "Under what circumstances did this panic attack occur?" In other words, what was the **trigger** for the panic attack? That's not always easy to find out, and we'll talk more about how we get this information in Chapter 6. Many patients, including many with panic disorder, have a hard time identifying what set them off, so we have to do a bit of probing. In Anna's case, over the course of our conversation we found that the first thing she noticed was a slight feeling of dizziness and that the big cascade of panic symptoms started right after that. So we'll go with dizziness as our trigger for now. Remember that we're not looking for what started her panic disorder in the first place (although we are interested in that); for this part of our understanding we're just inquiring about what triggered *this* panic attack. Note as well that this particular trigger came from inside of Anna—it was a body sensation. Triggers can come from *inside* the person or from *outside* the person.

You might ask, however, "Why would a little dizziness be a trigger for Anna? Most of the time, if I have a little dizziness, I barely notice it." So why does Anna notice her body sensations when other people might not? The answer is, in part, that she has an *attentional bias* (see Chapter 3), in which she focuses excessively on her own bodily sensations. So she pays much more attention to how her body feels than the average person does. Therefore, when she does have some dizziness or another odd body sensation, she's much more likely to notice it, thus triggering the core pathological process (see Figure 5.2). Perhaps if she hadn't been so focused on her body, she wouldn't have noticed the dizziness and subsequently wouldn't have had the panic attack.

Anna's Emotional System

As we look at the emotional component of Anna's panic attack, we see that as she noticed (paid attention to) her dizziness, she experienced fear and racing heart. Why? After all,

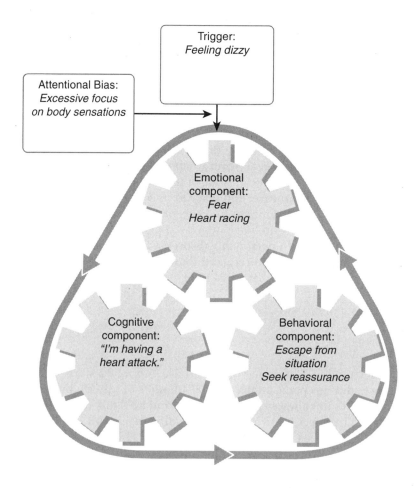

FIGURE 5.2. Anna's core pathological process, trigger, and attentional bias.

when you or I feel dizzy, that's probably not our reaction. There are probably a couple of reasons. First, as we know, the core pathological process is emotion, thought, and behavioral response all snowballing together. So we can guess that the more Anna thinks a certain way, and the more she behaves a certain way, the worse she's going to feel. And there's another piece we could add to this. *Classical conditioning* (see Chapter 4) could be behind her reflexive fear reaction. In the past, when Anna's felt dizzy, she's had a panic attack. So perhaps it's not surprising that she had a fearful reaction to her dizziness this time (see Figure 5.3).

Anna's Cognitive System

The cognitive component of Anna's panic attack consisted of her telling herself that she was going to have a heart attack. Why? You and I don't think that way, at least not if we don't have heart disease. When we feel anxious or dizzy, or notice our hearts racing, we don't interpret it as an oncoming heart attack. Again, we can guess that Anna's emotions and behaviors probably contributed to this thought. We can also add a couple of other elements. In later sessions, we learn that Anna carries around a basic *core belief* (see Chapter

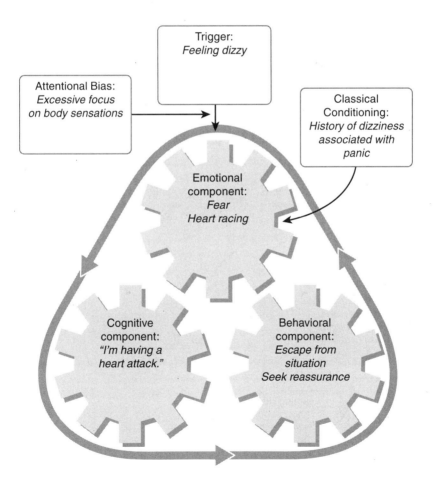

FIGURE 5.3. Classical conditioning as part of Anna's emotional response.

3) that she is constantly vulnerable to danger. So it's natural that when something vaguely threatening shows up, she jumps to the worst possible conclusion. She's had some **learning history** that might have helped shape that belief, as well; she's had some relatives and older friends die of heart attacks, and that's left her feeling vulnerable. In fact, as she noticed her heart starting to race, those loved ones who had died were exactly who came to mind for her. Importantly, she failed to remember all of the people who *didn't* die of heart attacks, or all of the times that she had felt this way and not had a heart attack—a *memory bias* (see Figure 5.4).

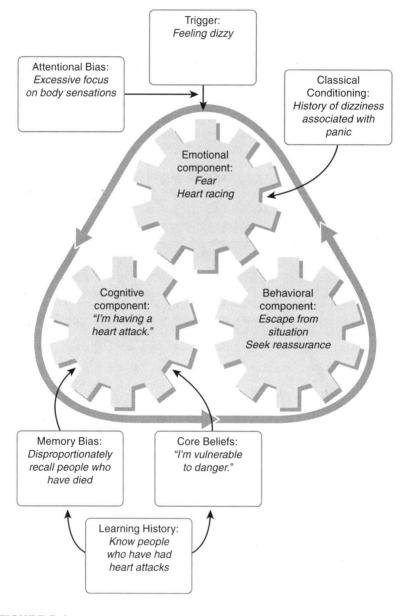

FIGURE 5.4. Understanding the cognitive component of Anna's panic attack.

Anna's Behavioral System

Let's take a look at the behavioral component next. Here, Anna's behavioral response consisted of escaping from the situation and seeking reassurance from another person. Just as we did with the emotional and cognitive components, we might well ask: Why those particular behaviors? I mean, not everyone who feels anxious engages in escape or reassurance-seeking behaviors. We can speculate that her selection of those behaviors is due, in part, to the influence of her thoughts (e.g., the idea that she was having a heart attack) and her emotions (the subjective feeling state of fear and her physiological sensation of racing heart). That helps us understand why Anna acted the way she did. It also seems that there are some powerful *contingencies* (see Chapter 2) associated with those behaviors. In this case, when Anna gets out of the situation and gets reassurance, she immediately feels a sense of relief. That's *escape* (negative reinforcement), which is a powerful contingency that helps "lock" that behavior into place. So the more she escapes, the more relief she gets—and the more relief she gets, the more she will want to escape next time this happens. We also see that Anna experiences *negative effects of her own behavior*. That is, Anna's behavior feeds back into the problem. Specifically:

- Her chronic avoidance is leading her to have academic problems, which in turn is making her life more stressful.
- Her avoidance prevents her from learning that her physical sensations are not a sign that she is dying or having some other medical disaster.
- Because Anna gets such immediate relief from avoidance and escape behaviors, she becomes increasingly dependent on those behaviors and needs to do more and more of them over time.
- As Anna avoids, she isn't practicing behaviors (such as staying in the situation and coping with her anxiety) that would be more beneficial to her in the long run.

So what the person *does* is really important to our understanding. In this case, by escaping from the situation, Anna never really absorbs the "truth" of the matter, which is that she's fine and this is just a temporary (albeit unpleasant) feeling. So she continues to fear her own body sensations. That ongoing fear, then, translates into an ongoing (or perhaps even stronger) vigilance for unpleasant body sensations, making the whole thing likely to happen again.

Anna's Full Conceptualization

So you can see from Figure 5.5 that the full conceptual model for one of Anna's panic attacks looks rather complicated, yet it consists of discrete and understandable components that interact with one another. If I had to articulate the whole thing verbally, I might say something like this:

Anna's most recent panic attack was triggered by the presence of dizziness, a sensation for which she was already vigilant. As this sensation has been associated with panic attacks in the past, Anna experienced fear and increased heart rate. She interpreted these sensations as signs that she was having a heart attack; this interpretation was likely strengthened by a core belief that she is highly vulnerable and a tendency to recall people she has known who had heart attacks. She responded by escaping from the situation and seeking reassurance, which brought some temporary relief of her fear but also left her continuing to fear her body sensations.

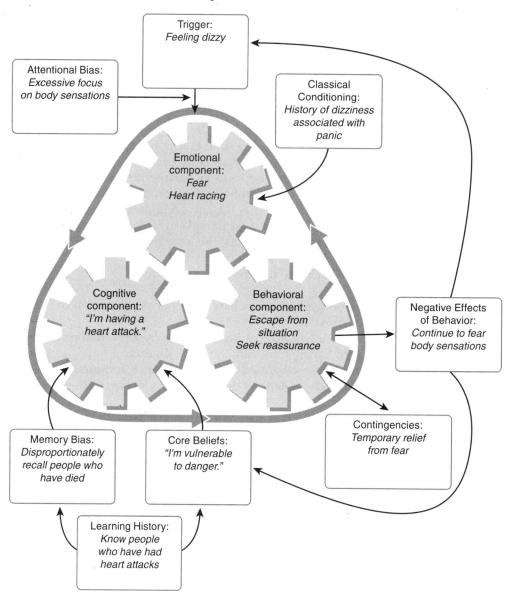

FIGURE 5.5. The full conceptual model for one of Anna's panic attacks.

Anna's conceptualization underscores the etiology-versus-maintenance issue we discussed in Chapter 1. We are most certainly interested in Anna's learning history. The past is important. However, we use historical information differently than do clinicians from some other theoretical orientations. We are interested in how Anna learned to view the world a certain way and how she came to acquire and rely upon certain behavioral responses. Some models of psychotherapy emphasize etiology of the problem—that is, the primary aim is to understand how Anna's panic attacks started. Such a conceptualization has relatively little meat on it—it doesn't show you what to work on. In our model, we emphasize maintenance of the problem—that is, the factors that cause her panic attacks to keep occurring, day in and day out. That meaty conceptualization leads directly to a solid, workable action plan.

Although the specifics will differ from client to client, we can ask similar questions about all our clients in order to understand "why." Let's try it again with our client Christina, who suffers from severe depression. Again, we want to build our meaty conceptualization on specific episodes of the problem, so we talk to Christina about the times when her depression is at its worst and ask her to describe a recent episode in which her mood really tanked.

Christina's Trigger

Christina tells us that she felt especially depressed a few days ago, when her friend, who has been calling to provide support and companionship through this depressive episode, failed to call at the agreed-upon time. This sent Christina into a tailspin. Through additional discussions, we learn that Christina is constantly looking for signs of distress in this (and other) relationships, so that's an *attentional bias* (see Chapter 3) that led her to detect the potential problem very rapidly. So this trigger came from outside of Christina (her friend failing to call), unlike Anna, whose trigger came from inside of her (a physical sensation).

Christina's Emotional System

Christina's emotional response consisted of the subjective feeling state of sadness, as well as a physiological sensation of heaviness. It turns out from our discussion that Christina also has an attentional bias toward her own feelings—she is constantly monitoring herself for sadness, so she picks up on this feeling rapidly as well. Her thoughts and behaviors (discussed below) probably fueled this feeling of sadness.

We also pick up on what appears to be some *classical conditioning* (see Chapter 4) for this emotional response. In this case, it's kind of subtle. We don't find any "smoking gun" experience, such as that the last time someone failed to call her it really did mean that the person hated her and the relationship was over. What we do find, however, is that sadness has been Christina's habitual reaction to this situation. Every time she's been stood up for a call, she has become increasingly depressed. So, if classical conditioning occurs when a person has learned that one thing is associated with another, we can hypothesize that Christina has learned that "being stood up means getting depressed." Perhaps she can articulate that connection, perhaps not; but given that history, it's no wonder that sadness became her reflexive emotional reaction. Situations become associated with feelings.

Christina's Cognitive System

Christina's mental reaction to her friend not calling was to think "I must have done something to upset her," followed quickly by the thought "What's wrong with me?" Those kinds of *interpretations* (see Chapter 3) would sadden just about anybody, so we can understand how her thoughts were intertwined with her emotions. It's important to note here as well that her thoughts are partly about the situation and partly about her own feelings. Thoughts about one's own emotions, and even thoughts about one's own thoughts, can be a big part of the problem.

There's another part of Christina's cognitive component that emerged as her depressive episode wore on. As she lay there in bed, feeling unhappy, she engaged in *rumination*.

She tried to think about all of the things she might have done wrong to upset her friend. She also devoted a lot of mental energy to wishing she could feel better, like everyone else seems to.

As we get to know Christina a little better over time, we start seeing a pattern in her thoughts that suggests that she has a *core belief* (see Chapter 3) in which she views herself, at a basic level, as being worthless and unlovable. Her *learning history* may have fed into that belief, as she was long considered an "outsider" among her peers, even when she was very young. That learning history might have also contributed to a *memory bias:* When she looks back on her own life, all she tends to remember are the times when she was isolated and lonely. To her, the past looks bleak. But it's a biased memory: She tends to forget or discount those times when she actually had friends and felt OK. Only the rotten stuff comes to mind.

Christina's Behavioral System

Feeling awful, Christina got in bed and remained there for most of the day, ruminating. There were some immediate *contingencies* (see Chapter 2) associated with that set of behaviors, however. Getting in bed and not having to deal with daily hassles and responsibilities did deliver some short-term relief. Ruminating didn't solve any of her problems, but engaging in that activity made her feel *as if* she was solving them. So, because those behaviors made her feel slightly less bad, the behaviors were *reinforced* and became her "go-to" moves. But there were also longer-term, unhealthy consequences of this behavioral pattern. She got in bed and didn't take the initiative to call her friend. That resulted in increased distance from the friend—the very thing she was concerned about—and means that her friend is less likely to call tomorrow as well. Being in bed and ruminating also meant that she wasn't doing anything else that would be good for her, such as engaging in activities that might give her a sense of pleasure or accomplishment.

Let's add another piece to this puzzle. Why didn't Christina just call her friend? Was it just because she was too depressed to do so, or because other behaviors had been so heavily reinforced that there was no room for anything else? That seems to be a big part of it, but with additional discussions, it also became clear that Christina had a *behavioral skill deficit* (see Chapter 2). Calling up a friend, asking that friend for support, and letting him or her know that you're not happy about being stood up, requires the skill of *assertion.* Christina has always had difficulty in the assertion department—some might even call her a "doormat." She doesn't know what to say, or how to say it, so she doesn't handle those complicated interactions smoothly. That's yet another reason why she didn't pick up the phone.

Christina's Full Conceptualization

How would you diagram this episode of Christina's depression? My diagram is shown in Figure 5.6. A verbal description of Christina's meaty conceptualization might go like this:

Christina experienced increased depression after her friend failed to call at the expected time. Because Christina was vigilant for signs of relationship distress, she quickly perceived a problem and assumed that she must have done something to upset her friend. As this has always been a trigger for sadness in the past, Christina once again felt increasing sadness and a sense of heaviness and focused on her unpleasant feelings. She wondered what was wrong with her. Her thoughts may relate to a core belief that she is basically worthless and unlovable; she has a history of feeling like an "outsider" and a tendency to selectively recall instances of loneliness; these processes likely contributed to her interpretation of the events. As her capacity for assertive behavior is limited, she responded by getting in bed and engaging in ruminative thinking; this brought some degree of short-term relief but also contributed to ongoing isolation and diminished positive activities, setting the stage for further depressive episodes.

I want to point out that Christina's diagram is constructed similarly to Anna's. We have a lot of the same basic underlying processes (e.g., a core pathological process of emotional, cognitive, and behavioral responses; attentional and memory biases; classical conditioning; contingencies; core beliefs), although the content and expression of the processes are different for these two clients.

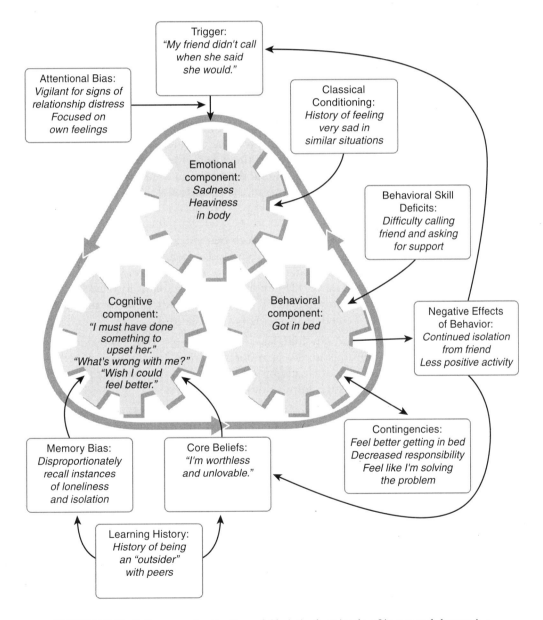

FIGURE 5.6. Full conceptualization of Christina's episode of increased depression.

But there are also some person-specific alterations here. For example, Christina has a noticeable behavioral skill deficit, whereas Anna does not. As you create meaty conceptualizations for your clients, you will probably find that not every element of the diagram will apply to every client. This is a representation of the elements of psychological problems that *could* be there; part of your task as the therapist is to determine whether they *are* there.

I also know that many clients have multiple problems. Anna and Christina are fairly straightforward cases (diagnostically speaking), so I chose them to illustrate the basic points. Your clients, on the other hand, might have all kinds of issues going on. Therefore, it's not assumed that one diagram will capture everything that's wrong. You're going to use this diagram to conceptualize various incidents of the client's problem(s) as they come up in therapy. For any given client, you might end up drawing 2, 3, or 10 of these conceptualizations throughout the course of treatment. Doing so is an integral part of therapy.

Turning Meaty Conceptualizations into Treatment Plans

Conceptualizing the case and making diagrams is not merely an intellectual exercise. It's our road map for treatment. For every client, we have to determine where the problem areas are and which ones seem to be "driving" the core pathological process. In theory, nearly all of the items in the model are potential targets for treatment (although some we can influence more than others). In terms of the core pathological process, we might choose any of the following interventions.

• If maladaptive behavioral responses seem to be central to the problem, we might provide direct behavioral instructions for more adaptive behaviors, perhaps practicing those behaviors in session. We might have the client practice a competing response that makes the maladaptive response more difficult for a time. We might instruct the client to engage in activities that have a high likelihood of being rewarding, or we might instruct the client to disrupt avoidant behaviors by facing scary situations.

• If unpleasant emotions and physiological sensations seem to be central to the problem, we might select interventions aimed at reducing physical arousal (e.g., relaxation, exercise, meditation, distraction), or we might select interventions that teach greater ability to tolerate distress (e.g., exposure, mindfulness, or acceptance).

• If maladaptive interpretations and beliefs seem to be central to the problem, we might select interventions aimed at correcting erroneous thoughts (e.g., challenging cognitive distortions, Socratic questioning, behavioral experiments). Alternatively, we might teach the person to notice and accept his or her thoughts without becoming bogged down in them.

In addition, we might select interventions for those elements that are outside of the core pathological process but are nevertheless still important to the maintenance of the problem:

• If the trigger is inherently toxic (i.e., it is not reasonable to expect that the person would be able to have an adaptive process), or the behavior is so strongly connected to the trigger that it's hard to break the association, we might consider altering the person's environment.

- If the person has an attentional bias for triggers (i.e., disproportionately allocating attention toward threatening stimuli), we might teach him or her how to redirect attention toward less evocative stimuli.

- If the person has a behavioral skill deficit (e.g., poor social skills), we might teach him or her a new skill and have him or her practice it.

- If the person's current contingencies lead him or her to select maladaptive behaviors (e.g., if he or she is being reinforced for unhealthy behaviors, or isn't being reinforced for healthy behaviors), we might alter the current system of rewards and punishers (either by working with the person or with others who interact with the person) so that adaptive behaviors are rewarded and maladaptive behaviors are not rewarded. We might also make use of systematic reinforcement for desired behaviors in the session.

- If the person has a memory bias that influences his or her interpretations (e.g., he or she disproportionately recalls negative information), we might cue him or her to remember other information that would change the interpretations.

- If the person's core beliefs have a negative influence on his or her thoughts in uncomfortable situations (e.g., he or she has basic, unhealthy beliefs about him- or herself), we might challenge those core beliefs using dialogue or by constructing new experiences that can alter his or her beliefs.

Note the key word *might* in all of the above. Selection of any given intervention is a matter of clinical skill, informed by the best available research data. For any given client, some things are more likely to work than others.

The core pathological process is a self-perpetuating cycle. This is bad news for the client (e.g., maladaptive thoughts lead to more negative emotions and to more unhelpful behaviors) but good news for the clinician (e.g., making thoughts more adaptive can lead to more positive emotions and more helpful behaviors). So successfully intervening in one part of the process has the potential to indirectly affect the other parts as well. In Part II, we talk about how to develop a treatment plan based on our meaty conceptualization.

THE ESSENTIALS

✱ A meaty conceptualization does not just tell a story about the client; it provides meaningful targets for intervention.

✱ For any given client, our targets might be the client's symptoms, the mechanisms that maintain those symptoms, or the functional outcomes of those symptoms.

✱ Meaty conceptualizations are often facilitated by dissecting specific episodes of the client's problem.

✱ Meaty conceptualizations form the basis of our treatment plan. We might decide to directly target elements of the core pathological process, such as maladaptive behaviors, thoughts, or emotions. We might also decide to directly target elements outside of the core pathological process, such as environmental factors, information-processing biases, skill deficits, unhelpful contingencies, or core beliefs.

KEY TERMS AND DEFINITIONS

Functional analysis: Understanding a behavior in relation to its antecedents (triggers) and consequences (contingencies).

Functional outcome: Impaired ability to function in one or more areas of life due to the symptom.

Learning history: The person's history of experiences that have shaped his or her way of thinking and perceiving the world.

Meaty conceptualization: A conceptual model that provides clear and actionable information about the processes by which the problem persists.

Mechanism: A psychological variable that contributes to the persistence of the symptom.

Symptom: The presenting behavioral, emotional, or cognitive complaint.

Target: The specific mechanism that we wish to address directly in treatment.

Trigger: The external or internal stimulus that begins an episode of the problem.

Making a Meaty Conceptualization

Identify a recent instance of your personal target. It's important that you have a specific instance in mind, not just a general impression. Fill in as many boxes in the figure below as you can. (Don't worry, you'll have lots of opportunities to refine this; we're just taking an initial crack at it.) Remember, not all components will apply to all people.

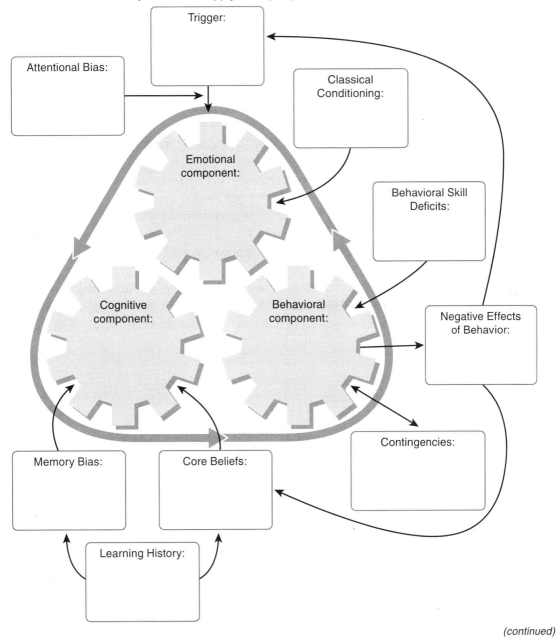

(continued)

From *Doing CBT* by David F. Tolin. Copyright © 2016 The Guilford Press. Permission to photocopy this worksheet is granted to purchasers of this book for personal use only (see copyright page for details). Purchasers can download enlarged versions of this worksheet (see the box at the end of the table of contents).

Think about all of these elements:

Trigger: What internal or external stimuli seem to be at the beginning of the personal target? Is there a particular place? Time of day? People? Weird sensation? Thought that pops into your head? Activity?

Attentional bias: What do you focus on? What do you fail to focus on?

Emotional component: What kind of feelings do you have? What does your body feel like?

Cognitive component: What thoughts go through your mind? How do you interpret the trigger?

Behavioral component: What do you do? What do you fail to do? How well do you do it?

Classical conditioning: Do you feel a certain way because the trigger reminds you of something else or has been associated with something else?

Behavioral skill deficit: Are there skills that seem to be lacking, things you can't do (or can't do very well)?

Contingencies: What do you get out of the behavior? Or, if there's a behavior you're not doing, has that behavior not led to good things in the past?

Negative effects of behavior: What happens in the longer term as a result of your behavior (or lack thereof)?

Core beliefs: What basic assumptions do you have about yourself, other people, or the world that influence how you interpret the trigger?

Learning history: What learning experiences have you had that have shaped your basic assumptions about yourself, other people, or the world?

Memory bias: What memories do you recall that add fuel to the personal target? What do you fail to recall?

PART II

How Do We Help?

The next several chapters describe ways that CBT therapists work with clients on psychological problems. Many of these interventions have been used as stand-alone procedures, whereas others are frequently combined into multi-intervention treatment "packages." Many CBT treatments, such as (to name just a few) cognitive therapy (A. T. Beck et al., 1979), emotion regulation training (Mennin, Heimberg, Turk, & Fresco, 2002), dialectical behavior therapy (Linehan, 1993), acceptance and commitment therapy (Hayes et al., 2012), functional analytic psychotherapy (Kohlenberg & Tsai, 1991), metacognitive therapy (Wells, 2009), and specific cognitive-behavioral therapies designed for a variety of disorders, are actually collections of multiple interventions. Some emphasize one specific kind of intervention over another; some were developed with different client populations in mind; some select certain targets over other ones. But the central point is this: There is a limited number of CBT interventions that exist. Selecting, combining, and adapting these interventions is the scientific artistry of CBT. In the coming chapters, I'll give some examples on adapting the process for different kinds of clients you might see. You might treat high-functioning people who have jobs and decent relationships but are struggling somehow. Or you might treat lower functioning people, such as those with severe psychiatric illness, chronic unemployment, poor interpersonal functioning, or intellectual disabilities. You might treat children, or you might treat clients in groups. Adaptation is a complex process, and there's no way we could cover every possible adaptation in one book. But I'll try to give you some preliminary ideas to get you on your way.

In Part II, we're going to focus on these specific CBT interventions, rather than the treatment packages—for example, we're not going to have a complete discussion of how to perform dialectical behavior therapy, but we will address its component interventions, such as *mindfulness* and *behavioral skill training*. Similarly, we're not going to discuss Beck's cognitive therapy for depression in great detail, although we will address its component interventions, such as *cognitive restructuring* and *activity scheduling*. For a more in-depth discussion of the treatment packages, I recommend consulting the source materials that are listed in Appendix A.

Where Do I Start?

Your first question might well be, "Given all of these different interventions that make up CBT, how do I decide which ones to use with my client?" As discussed in Chapter 5, our selection of specific interventions is based on several factors, including:

- Which intervention has the strongest research evidence for this client's presenting problem?
- Which aspect of the pathological process seems to be contributing most strongly to the problem (i.e., seems to be "driving")?
- Which aspect of the pathological process can I most strongly impact right now?
- Which aspect of the pathological process has the greatest likelihood of creating a positive "downstream" sequence of changes?
- Which changes will have the greatest impact on the person's quality of life?

Why I Lean Behavioral

It's important to note that even though many elements of CBT have been shown to be effective for many different problems, not all are created equal. Broadly speaking, in my own practice I tend to emphasize the behavior-level interventions over the cognitive-level and emotion-level interventions. So with most clients, I usually start with, and spend more time across the course of therapy focusing on, the behavior-level interventions. I think of it in the way I show in Figure II.1. Imagine that your entire course of CBT is a dinner. The behavior-level interventions are your main course, and the cognitive-level and emotion-level interventions are the side dishes.

And what about the therapeutic relationship? That's the plate that the meal is served on. It's how you deliver the interventions to the client. If the plate's broken, the meal can't be served, and the client goes hungry.

There are a lot of skilled and smart CBTers who will disagree with me on this point. Many CBTers base their work on a cognitive model of psychological disorders that posits:

$$\text{Thoughts} \rightarrow \text{Feelings} \rightarrow \text{Behaviors}$$

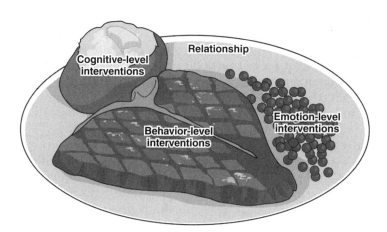

FIGURE II.1. If CBT were a dinner, behavior-level interventions would be the main course, and cognitive- and emotion-level interventions would be the side dishes.

That is, the way you think affects how you feel, and subsequently how you act. It would therefore follow from this model that:

Change in thoughts → Change in feelings → Change in behaviors

So the argument is that if you want to change the client's feelings and behaviors, you should target the way he or she thinks. This linear model was central to the cognitive therapy movement that gained steam in the 1970s (Bandura, 1977; A. T. Beck, 1976; Ellis, 1977; Mahoney, 1977; Meichenbaum, 1977) and remains highly prominent today. More recently, however, there has been renewed debate in the field (see the sidebar, "The Science behind It") about whether challenging cognitions is necessary or sufficient for changing emotions and behaviors. But there is *no* debate at all about whether you need to have your client change his or her behaviors. Even the most hardcore cognitive therapists (i.e., those who are really into challenging cognitions) agree that direct prescriptions for behavioral change are necessary. Ultimately, in order to get better, the client has to change what he or she is doing. Even Beck (Beck et al., 1979), considered by many to be the founder of cognitive therapy, starts his "cognitive therapy" for depression with a behavior-level intervention (activity scheduling) prior to doing cognitive-level interventions (cognitive restructuring).

The Science behind It

We know people often start therapy with distorted thoughts and leave therapy with more realistic thoughts. But there is conflicting evidence about whether cognitive change is a *causal* mechanism in recovery from psychological problems (e.g., Hofmann, 2008; Longmore & Worrell, 2007). That is, did the person feel better because he or she changed his or her thoughts? Or did his or her thoughts change because he or she was feeling better?

It has been noted, for example, that dismantling research (in which elements of a complex treatment are studied separately) has often failed to demonstrate that the addition of cognitive-level interventions to behavioral-level interventions adds to the outcome. In a meta-analysis of available CBT studies for anxiety, the addition of cognitive-level interventions did not appear to add appreciably to outcomes when compared with behavior-level interventions alone (Adams, Brady, Lohr, & Jacobs, 2015).

A classic example of dismantling research comes from research on depression. Beck and colleagues' (1979) cognitive therapy for depression consists of two major elements: *cognitive restructuring*, which involves identifying and disputing maladaptive thoughts and beliefs, and *behavioral activation*, which involves encouraging the client to engage in a greater range of activities that produce a sense of mastery or pleasure. The efficacy of this treatment for depression is well established (Dobson, 1989), but why does it work? There is a fair amount of evidence to suggest that the treatment works, in part, by means of changes in maladaptive thoughts and beliefs. As one example, DeRubeis et al. (1990) assigned clients to receive 12 weeks of either cognitive therapy or antidepressant medication. In addition to measuring depressive symptoms, the researchers also measured the presence of dysfunctional (depressive) thoughts. In the cognitive therapy group, early changes in thoughts predicted later changes in depression symptoms; this relationship was not observed among the medication clients. Thus, changes in thoughts preceded and predicted changes in depressive symptoms.

So we know that cognitive change is an important mechanism in recovering from depression. But are cognitive-level interventions the best way to get there? N. S. Jacobson et al. (1996) assigned depressed clients to receive a treatment focused primarily on activity scheduling (see Chapter 10), to a treatment that included both activity scheduling and modifying interpretations, or to the full treatment that included activity scheduling, modifying interpretations, and identifying and modifying core beliefs (see Chapters 14 and 16). There were no differences in short-term or long-term outcomes across any of the treatments. That is, clients receiving activity scheduling alone fared just as well as did clients who also received the cognitive elements of treatment. Interestingly, the "behavioral" treatment (activity scheduling) had just as strong an impact on maladaptive beliefs as did the "cognitive" treatments (modifying interpretations and core beliefs). In a later study, for clients with severe depression, activity scheduling proved even *more* effective than did cognitive restructuring (Dimidjian et al., 2006).

How much emphasis we should put on thoughts, and the rationality or irrationality of those thoughts, is a tricky issue. We know that thoughts change in CBT, and we know that the degree of cognitive change is significantly associated with the degree of emotional and behavioral change. But, on the other hand, a lot of studies have shown that CBT that *doesn't* target thoughts directly can be as effective as CBT that *does* target those thoughts. Remember our meaty conceptualization in Chapter 5. Yes, thoughts can influence feelings and behaviors. But feelings and behaviors influence thoughts just as much. It's a cycle, and there's no clear reason to believe thoughts are the *start* of the cycle; they are simply a *part* of the cycle.

However, I continue to think there is merit to learning about, and using, cognitive interventions. There are several reasons for this:

• Cognitive interventions, even without behavioral interventions, do have a demonstrated treatment effect on their own—although most "cognitive" treatments include some degree of behavioral intervention, including the "behavioral experiments" used to test the accuracy of beliefs (Longmore & Worrell, 2007). Some studies have suggested an incremental benefit of adding cognitive restructuring to behavioral interventions, although, as described above, the research on this is mixed.

• Often we confuse the *mechanism of treatment* (the means by which an intervention works) with *what the therapist does* (the specific interventions). It's easy to assume that the two are intertwined—that is, if you want to produce a cognitive change, you should use a cognitive treatment, and if you want to produce a behavioral change, you should use a behavioral treatment. Sometimes that's the case, but sometimes it isn't. In many cases, a behavioral intervention will produce a cognitive change, and a cognitive intervention will produce a behavioral change. Remember, the core pathological process is a cycle in which cognitive, emotional, and behavioral processes all influence each other. As one gets better, so do the others.

• The state of the dismantling research (see "The Science behind It") is muddy at best. In many cases, and for many disorders, we just don't know what the active ingredients of therapy are—even when our therapies are clearly shown to work.

• The dismantling research to date can tell us only about averages, but they don't tell us much about how a given client will respond. Yes, for depression it appears that the average client responds as well (or better) to behavioral interventions as he or she does to cognitive interventions—but that doesn't necessarily mean that *your* client will.

• In real practice, many clients do not respond to the first intervention you try (Westen, Novotny, & Thompson-Brenner, 2004). That doesn't mean, however, that they won't respond to the second or third intervention you try. So it's important to have room for flexibility.

We don't want to fall into the trap of thinking that there's a suitable "one size fits all" solution. Going back to our dinner plate analogy, we can easily think of lots of exceptions to the standard meal. There might be a vegetarian coming to dinner, who doesn't want the steak I prepared. Or maybe someone has a food allergy that makes it unwise for them to eat the shrimp scampi. I'm certainly not going to tell them, "Look, this is the dinner I've prepared, and that's what I'm going to give you." I have to be flexible in order to meet the specific needs and wants of my guests. Similarly, it might well be that one of my guests likes one of the side dishes so much that he or she wants to make a whole meal out of it. That's fine, too.

And so it is with CBT. When I'm treating a client with depression, I'm most likely going to emphasize the behavioral activation component of *activity scheduling* (see Chapter 10), and when I'm treating a client with an anxiety disorder, I'm likely to emphasize the behavior-level intervention of *exposure* (see Chapter 11). However, I also realize that there will be some clients for whom those "main course" interventions will be unnecessary, or not well tolerated at first. Alternatively, I could have a client who responds so beautifully to a "side dish" intervention, such as cognitive restructuring or relaxation, that it seems reasonable to make the whole CBT about that intervention. That's fine, as long as it's clearly working. So even though I'm probably going to offer behavior-level interventions such as activity scheduling and exposure as the first-line interventions, I'm also keeping cognitive-level and emotion-level interventions in my back pocket—and I pull those interventions out quite often. Remember, we always want to employ the best available research in our intervention plan, but that research might well be adapted to specific client characteristics, based on the clinician's judgment.

It's also quite possible, in our dinner, for a guest to have a great experience with only the main course; no side dishes required. That's also perfectly fine. I like to make my CBT as simple as possible, without sacrificing efficacy. So if my depressed client shows a complete recovery using activity scheduling, or my client with anxiety recovers using exposure therapy, I don't feel obligated to start introducing cognitive-level or emotional-level interventions. That would be fixing what ain't broke.

Picking Your Targets

Let's come back to our meaty conceptualization from Chapter 5, which suggests that any given clinical problem can be broken down into its component parts. We see in Figure II.2 that most components of the model can potentially be addressed using specific CBT interventions. I say "most" because there are some things we can affect more easily than others. We can't, for example, change whatever learning history the person had that shaped his or her core beliefs. However, we can work on those beliefs in order to help the person overcome the learning history.

You can see from Figure II.2 that different CBT interventions have different targets. As we discussed in Chapter 5, targets in CBT are the maintaining factors that we aim to modify directly (with the understanding that there are also lots of ways to modify those factors indirectly). For any given client, we must pick one or more targets and then identify interventions that are likely to affect that target. For example:

• If we choose to target triggers and external events, we might choose *situation selection* and *stimulus control*. These are interventions that address the circumstances under which the problem occurs and the relationship between the circumstances and the target behavior. We'll review these interventions in Chapter 8.

• If we choose to target the cognitive component of the core pathological process, we might consider *cognitive restructuring*. Cognitive restructuring, which we'll discuss in Chapters 12 and 13, addresses distorted patterns of thinking by having the person identify the mental error and practice a more realistic, adaptive way of thinking. Alternatively (or in addition), we might select *acceptance*, which refer to a process of giving up fruitless struggles against unpleasant thoughts. By redirecting clients away from internal struggles and avoidance and toward more meaningful and value-directed action, we may

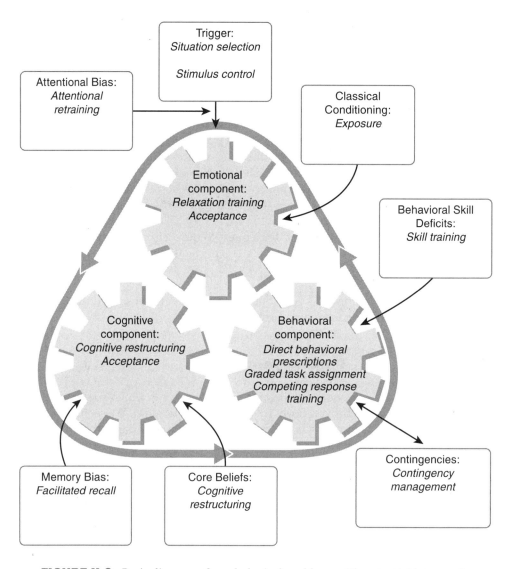

FIGURE II.2. Basic diagram of psychological problems with potential interventions.

be able to reduce much of their discomfort. We'll talk about acceptance of thoughts in Chapter 15.

- If we choose to target the emotional component of the core pathological process, we might try *relaxation training* and related interventions, which target physiological arousal (e.g., anxiety, anger, stress). As we'll discuss in Chapter 18, by reducing physical arousal levels, we can also (indirectly) affect related thoughts and behaviors. We could also employ *acceptance* for emotions (see Chapter 19) to steer clients away from struggling against their own feelings.

- If we choose to target the behavioral component of the core pathological process, we are likely to use *direct behavioral prescriptions*. Fundamentally, CBT asks clients to do something differently. In Chapter 10, we'll discuss how we use direct instructions for our clients to try new things or reduce maladaptive behaviors. One such prescription is *activity scheduling*, in which we get our clients with depression or anhedonia doing things so that they can obtain natural reinforcement from the environment. We might use *graded task assignments*, in which we break complex tasks down for clients into smaller, more manageable steps, so that they are less likely to become overwhelmed and demotivated. We could use *competing response training*, practicing the direct opposite of a maladaptive behavior. This is particularly useful for habitual, repetitive behaviors.

- To the extent that we wish to directly target information-processing biases, we could use *attentional retraining* and *facilitated recall*. We'll review these in Chapter 17.

- If we choose to target maladaptive contingencies that maintain behavior, we might opt to use *contingency management*. As its name implies, contingency management targets behavioral contingencies (reinforcement, escape, punishment, penalty). The general aim is to rearrange the contingencies so that the desired behaviors are being reinforced and maladaptive behaviors are not being reinforced. More on that in Chapter 9.

- *Exposure* could be used to address both classically conditioned emotional responses and avoidance behavior. When clients are unnecessarily fearful and avoidant of certain situations, activities, objects, or thoughts, we need to help them face those fears in a controlled manner. In Chapter 11 we'll review how to do this for a variety of psychological problems.

- If a behavioral skill deficit is our target, we would opt for *skill training*. In Chapter 12, we talk about how to assess, train, and practice behavioral skills so that the client can interact more effectively with his or her environment.

As you can see, the intervention for any particular disorder stems from our meaty conceptualization. Therefore, it is critical that you perform an accurate and thorough therapy assessment (see Chapter 6) before starting your intervention.

A Diagnosis Is Not a Target

As I discussed in Chapter 1, the DSM diagnosis is a blunt instrument. Selecting the right intervention(s) is often not as simple as "If diagnosis X, then treatment Y." The diagnosis, and the outcome research associated with that diagnosis, can give us important clues about what will be helpful—if the person has OCD, for example, I can make a pretty strong hypothesis that exposure and response prevention will be a successful treatment—but to really tailor the treatment effectively, we need to understand the client in front of us, not just know what diagnosis he or she has.

CBT Style

In addition to the specific interventions listed above, there are several elements of CBT style that will show up throughout this section. They show up in multiple places, permeating the therapy. They include:

- *Holding up a mirror.* Often, clients fail to see their own thoughts, feelings, or behaviors, or they fail to see the consequences of these processes. Part of the therapist's job is to increase the client's awareness, showing the client what is happening.

- *Bringing the problem into the room.* Talking about problems in the abstract often doesn't get you much traction in therapy. In many cases, the client needs to be fully in touch with the target problem in the session—meaning that he or she needs to feel some of the feelings, think some of the thoughts, and even enact some of the behaviors. That way, the problem is right in front of us so we can work on it.

- *Engaging the frontal lobes.* The frontal lobes are the "thinking" part of our brains. In many cases, maladaptive thoughts, feelings, and behaviors persist because we have mentally disengaged from them, or only think about them a certain way. By having clients analyze and even mentally "play with" the problem, we engage them in a new way of thinking and processing information.

- *Committing to change.* Because CBT is an active treatment with clearly defined goals and outcomes, the process relies on the client's willingness to engage in treatment and make changes. Of course, not all clients come in with that kind of motivation and commitment, so that becomes a big part of our job as therapists.

- *Doing better in order to feel better.* Many clients come to therapy with the belief that their first order of business is to feel better. Only then, their logic goes, can they start to live a better life. We turn that notion on its head, teaching clients that living a better life—doing better—is a good pathway to feeling better.

- *Acting the opposite.* Sometimes, when the client has maladaptive thoughts, emotions, or behaviors, it's helpful to prescribe behaviors that directly conflict with the pattern. By asking clients to do things that directly oppose their core pathological process, we can loosen up entrenched ways of thinking, improve emotional flexibility, and "try on" new behavioral patterns.

- *Devil's advocate.* Sometimes, it's helpful for the therapist to articulate the "sick" role so that the client can play the "healthy" role. By structuring the conversation in this way, the client will often come to realize that the "healthy" role is a bit closer to the truth, or that it is a more desirable way to be.

- *Metaphor.* Metaphors are often a helpful way to illustrate complex concepts. They require clients to think a bit more deeply about what you're trying to convey and provide a mental template that they can call up later in distressing situations.

- *Show me, don't tell me.* Often we get our point across most effectively be engaging the client in some kind of demonstration. An experiential exercise will often be much more memorable and meaningful than will a bunch of words.

HOW WE ENGAGE THE CLIENT

In the next two chapters, we review how we interact with the CBT client. Our interactions have several aims, over and above those of any specific CBT intervention. When we engage with the client, we want to:

- Determine whether the client is a good candidate for therapy.
- Know how to find the best scientific evidence about how to treat the client's presenting problem(s).
- Establish a strong and trusting collaborative relationship.
- Increase or maintain the client's motivation to change.
- Develop a shared understanding with the client about why the problem is persisting.
- Establish clear goals for treatment.
- Provide the client with a clear rationale for the treatment.
- Know whether our treatment is working.

In order to do this, we're going to incorporate several important elements into our interactions with the client, starting at the first session and continuing many of them until the end of treatment. Our interactions with the client will include:

- Assessing (and potentially correcting) expectations for improvement.
- Searching for the best scientific evidence of treatment efficacy.
- Collaborative model building.
- Repeated measurement.
- Expressing empathy, genuineness, and unconditional positive regard.
- Fostering a sense of collaborative empiricism.
- Using motivational interviewing strategies.
- Assuming roles of teacher, co-scientist, and scaffold as needed.

CHAPTER 6

Therapy Assessment and Case Formulation

Diagnostic Assessments

A therapy assessment is different from a diagnostic assessment, although some elements might be combined within visits. A diagnostic assessment should be done for all clients prior to intervention. Much of the time, we want to know the person's diagnosis according to the DSM or the *International Classification of Diseases* (ICD). To accomplish this, we might use diagnostic interviews such as the Structured Clinical Interview for DSM-IV Axis I Disorders (First, Spitzer, Gibbon, & Williams, 1995), the Mini-International Neuropsychiatric Interview (Sheehan et al., 1998), the Anxiety Disorders Interview Schedule (T. A. Brown, DiNardo, & Barlow, 1994), the Schedule for Affective Disorders and Schizophrenia for School-Age Children (Kaufman et al., 1997), or the Diagnostic Interview for Anxiety, Mood, and Obsessive-Compulsive and Related Disorders (Tolin et al., in press). Although I don't think the diagnosis necessarily serves as a very good guide for treatment, structured diagnostic interviews can be helpful in making sure you haven't missed anything.

We also want to have information about the severity of symptoms. Just knowing that a client meets DSM criteria for OCD, for example, doesn't tell us much about the type of OCD symptoms that person has or the severity of those symptoms. One way to get at that is with formal instruments—often paper-and-pencil self-report scales that clients can fill out quickly. This is an extremely abbreviated list, but some useful measures include: the Beck Depression Inventory (A. T. Beck, Steer, & Brown, 1996), the Beck Anxiety Inventory (A. T. Beck & Steer, 1993), the Depression Anxiety Stress Scales (Lovibond & Lovibond, 1995), the Yale–Brown Obsessive–Compulsive Scale (Goodman et al., 1989), the Liebowitz Social Anxiety Scale (Heimberg et al., 1999), the Panic Disorder Severity Scale (Shear et al., 1997), the Penn State Worry Questionnaire (Meyer, Miller, Metzger, & Borkovec, 1990), the PTSD Diagnostic Scale (Foa, Riggs, Dancu, & Rothbaum, 1993), the Eating Disorder Examination Questionnaire (Fairburn & Beglin, 2008), the Drug Abuse Screening Test (H. A. Skinner, 1982), the Alcohol Use Disorders Identification Test (Saunders, Aasland, Babor, de la Fuente, & Grant, 1993), and the Adult ADHD Investigator Symptom

Rating Scale (Spencer et al., 2010). Broad-based symptom severity measures, such as the Minnesota Multiphasic Personality Inventory (Ben-Porath & Tellegen, 2008), the Personality Assessment Inventory (Morey, 1991), the Millon Clinical Multiaxial Inventory (Millon, Millon, Davis, & Grossman, 2009), the Symptom Checklist–90 (Derogatis, 1992), or the Child Behavior Checklist (Achenbach, 1991) might be used as well.

We may also want to understand the impact that the person's condition has on his or her quality of life, using measures such as the Medical Outcomes Survey Short Form (Ware, 1993; Ware, Kosinski, & Keller, 1996), the Quality of Life Inventory (Frisch, Cornell, Villanueva, & Retzlaff, 1992), the Quality of Life Enjoyment and Satisfaction Questionnaire (Endicott, Nee, Harrison, & Blumenthal, 1993), the Satisfaction with Life Scale (Diener, Emmons, Larsen, & Griffin, 1985), or the Life Satisfaction Index (Wood, Wylie, & Sheafor, 1969), as well as the impact of the condition on daily functioning, using measures such as the Sheehan Disability Scale (Sheehan, 2008), the Liebowitz Self-Rating Disability Scale (Schneier et al., 1994), the Work and Social Adjustment Scale (Mundt, Marks, Shear, & Greist, 2002), or the Range of Impaired Functioning Tool (Leon et al., 1999).

The great thing is that a lot of measures are available at no cost. You can find a wealth of free measures online. Other measures are available for a fee, but are worth looking into.

A diagnostic assessment should also include a thorough history, including a history of psychiatric and medical problems and treatments, as well as behavioral observations of the client. In some cases, behavioral observations and self-reported concerns will be assessed in a formal manner, such as with the Mini-Mental State Examination (Folstein, Folstein, & McHugh, 1975), in which the interviewer records the client's subjective symptoms, overt behaviors, and responses to brief cognitive screening tests. A somewhat broader screen for cognitive impairment can be found in the Montreal Cognitive Assessment (Nasreddine et al., 2005), which is available for free (at *www.mocatest.org*).

Therapy Assessments

A **therapy assessment** has different aims. Although it may be combined with the diagnostic assessment, in the therapy assessment we are interested in determining suitability for therapy, understanding the factors that increase or decrease the client's chances for success, and beginning to develop a model of the illness or presenting problem. The therapy assessment might take one session or it might take more. In some ways, the therapy assessment never truly ends, as we'll see later.

Determining Suitability for Therapy

I have often been asked, "How should I determine whether this client should be treated with CBT versus another kind of psychotherapy?" Ultimately, this is an empirical question. Based on what you know about the client, what treatments have scientific support of efficacy?

I'm partial to doing my own literature searches. PubMed (*www.ncbi.nlm.nih.gov/pubmed*), for example, is a great place to find research articles, and it's free. But I also recognize that practitioners are busy, and it's not easy to carve out time to search the literature from scratch. There are some helpful sites out there that have condensed a great deal of the treatment outcome literature. These include the empirically supported treatments website managed by the Society of Clinical Psychology (Division 12 of the American Psychological Association; *www.psychologicaltreatments.org*) and a similar site managed by the Society of Clinical Child and Adolescent Psychology (Division 53 of the American Psychological Association; *www.effectivechildtherapy.org*).

So let's say I'm working with Lauren, who has schizophrenia. I go to the Society of Clinical Psychology website and select "schizophrenia," and I find the following treatment information:

- Social Skills Training (SST) (strong research support).
- Cognitive Behavioral Therapy (CBT) (strong research support).
- Assertive Community Treatment (ACT) (strong research support).
- Family Psychoeducation (strong research support).
- Supported Employment (strong research support).
- Social Learning/Token Economy Programs (strong research support).
- Cognitive Remediation (strong research support).
- Acceptance and Commitment Therapy (ACT) for Psychosis (modest research support).
- Cognitive Adaptation Training (CAT) (modest research support).
- Illness Management and Recovery (IMR) (modest research support).

This gives me a good starting point in knowing what kinds of interventions might be helpful. Many of the treatments with strong research support are within the broad scope of CBT.

Sometimes, of course, we find that both CBT and non-CBT treatments have documented efficacy. Let's say I'm working with Shari, who has bulimia nervosa. When I search *www.psychologicaltreatments.org*, I find the following:

- Cognitive Behavioral Therapy (strong research support).
- Interpersonal Psychotherapy (strong research support).
- Family-Based Treatment (modest research support).
- Healthy-Weight Program (controversial research support).

Here I have a bit of a conundrum. CBT has strong research support for bulimia, but so does interpersonal psychotherapy (IPT). Which one should I use?

We don't have a set of criteria that will reliably tell us whether a client is likely to respond to one kind of treatment versus another. That would require us to have a set of research studies in which we identified a set of variables that were negative predictors of outcome for one kind of therapy, but not for another kind of therapy. We have some isolated examples of that, but not enough to make broad decisions about treatment for a wide range of clients. So at this time, I don't have data that would tell me whether CBT or IPT would be the better choice for Shari. According to the literature, either would be a good option. So why do I pick CBT? For me, it comes down to this: When two different treatments seem equally appropriate, make the selection based on your expertise and the characteristics of the client. That filtering of information is central to the notion of *evidence-based practice* discussed in Chapter 1. In my case, I have expertise in CBT, and during my interview with Shari, I can see several aspects of her cognitive, emotional, and behavioral processes that make CBT look promising. There is, admittedly, a judgment call to be made.

And then we have the issue that many of our clients have multiple problems or don't fit neatly into the diagnostic categories that figure prominently in lists of empirically supported treatments. What then? My strategy is to start with an *anchor diagnosis*—a presenting problem that seems closest to what the person is describing and seems to account for a large proportion of his or her problems. William, for example, doesn't meet full diagnostic criteria for any specific DSM disorder. But that doesn't mean I'm out of luck. I know that he is highly dependent on others, so I could take a look at proven treatments for dependent personality disorder. That will likely get me in the right ballpark. I also know that he experiences chronic pain from fibromyalgia, so I could investigate studies of CBT for pain disorders. So I have selected two anchor diagnoses that don't fit William's situation exactly but will likely address some of the same underlying mechanisms that we'll have to deal with in this case.

Who Will Do Well in Therapy?

In the absence of research providing clear direction of who will respond best to what kind of treatment, my best guess is this: *If the client is an appropriate candidate for psychotherapy, he or she is an appropriate candidate for CBT.* Generally good signs (Castonguay & Beutler, 2006) for psychotherapy (including CBT) include:

- Less chronic and complex disorders.
- Ability to form a reasonable therapeutic alliance.
- Absence of ongoing severe stressors.
- Ability to identify thoughts and feelings.
- Good expectancy for improvement.
- Adequate motivation to change.
- Accepting the rationale for treatment.
- Clearly defined treatment goals.

There are relatively few straight-up contraindications for CBT, though it has been suggested (Wright, Basco, & Thase, 2006) that altered cognitive function (e.g., delirium, acute psychosis, intoxication) or antisocial personality disorder would preclude effective treatment. That's likely true of any psychotherapy. If the person can't focus on you and have a meaningful conversation, it's going to be hard to get anywhere. There may be contraindications for specific *procedures* within CBT—for example, I might not attempt to use cognitive restructuring (see Chapter 14) with a client who has severe developmental disability—but that doesn't rule out CBT as an overall approach. I would choose different targets and different interventions.

When we look at the global predictors of therapy success, you'll see that some of these are characteristics that the client brings to the session, but others are potentially modifiable, either during the therapy assessment or during the therapy itself.

GOOD EXPECTANCY FOR IMPROVEMENT

Part of the therapeutic assessment should include evaluating, and potentially modifying, the client's expectations. Of course, we want our clients' expectations to be realistic, first and foremost; we don't want to fool them into thinking that treatment will be more effective than it is likely to be. There are formal measures for this, such as the Expectancy Rating Form (Borkovec & Nau, 1972), although it's also fine to ask a simple question such as, "How much better do you expect to feel after treatment?" (Sotsky et al., 1991). Sometimes, we see that clients' expectations are too low—that is, they don't expect to feel much better when, in fact, the research literature tells us that they are likely to have a good response to treatment. Sometimes, the expectations are too high—for example, clients expect that their problems will go away completely and never come back, when the research literature tells us that partial recovery and relapse are common. Here, we can use psychoeducation (see Chapter 7) to correct their expectations. When more than one form of treatment has adequate scientific evidence to justify its use, client preference can come into play. So, for example, with Shari, it might be helpful to discuss CBT and IPT with her and see which treatment seems to be a better "fit" with her ideas (i.e., which treatment is associated with stronger expectations for improvement).

CLEARLY DEFINED TREATMENT GOALS

Sometimes, the client knows exactly what he or she wants from treatment. Other times, his or her goals are fuzzier. I've had lots of clients say, at the first session, "I just want to have someone to talk to." That's a pretty vague goal, which is a recipe for treatment failure. Other clients come to treatment with a semblance of a goal, such as: "I just want to feel less depressed." That's better, but still probably not sufficient to give us a strong sense of direction. So in either case, we have to help the client develop specific desired outcomes for the therapy.

Solution-focused therapy uses the **miracle question** (de Shazer, 1988), which asks clients to define their goals in more concrete, often behavioral, terms. An example of the miracle question might be: "If you woke up tomorrow, and a miracle happened so that you were no longer depressed, what would be different?"; "What would the first signs be that the miracle occurred?"; "What would someone else notice that would tell them that the miracle had occurred?" To answer this question, the client has to think not only about his or her overall goal of "feeling less depressed," but also to consider how he or she would act differently if he or she were less depressed. Perhaps he or she would spend less time in bed and more time with friends. Or perhaps he or she would perform better at work. Those concrete behavioral indicators are good potential goals of therapy:

> "It sounds like overall, you'd like to feel less depressed. And some ways that we might know that you're feeling less depressed are that you would be spending less time in bed, that you'd be doing more things with your friends, and that you'd be performing better at work. I wonder if we might include those activities in our immediate goals for treatment, and see what impact that has on your feelings of depression?"

Note as well that this kind of goal setting flips a common way of thinking on its ear. Clients frequently assume that they should feel better first, and then start living better—"Feel better in order to do better." CBT, particularly the more behavioral elements of CBT, puts forth the notion of "Do better in order to feel better": If you start *living* better, you will start to *feel* better.

ACCEPTING THE RATIONALE FOR TREATMENT

As part of the initial therapy assessment, we use **psychoeducation** to help the client understand why we want to use the treatments we do. As we'll see in Chapter 7, psychoeducation is more than just lecturing the client. It involves steering the dialogue, through judicious use of questions, to help the client arrive at the rationale. When the client figures out the rationale, even though you steered him or her in that direction, he or she tends to be more accepting of that rationale because it seems "intuitively obvious." And, often, it is.

As we go through the process of model building (see the next section), it's helpful to ask such questions as "Given the fact that avoiding social situations seems to be one of the factors causing your social anxiety to persist, what do you think we might do about that?" or "Since lying in bed during the day seems not to be helping you to feel much better, and may even be making you feel worse, what solutions do you think might be helpful to you?" Chances are, the client will come up with ideas similar to exposure therapy (for the former client) or behavioral activation (for the latter client), which then allows you to say, "That's a good idea. I think you're right on the money there. Let's talk about some ways we might be able to accomplish that."

Remember that there's a balance here. The therapist does need to be directive, and we are trying to lead the conversation in a particular direction. At the same time, your client may have his or her own ideas about what will be helpful and what won't. His or her ideas might be accurate or inaccurate, but in either case they should be discussed and entertained seriously.

ADEQUATE MOTIVATION TO CHANGE

Because CBT is an active and directive treatment, it assumes a certain level of **motivation** on the part of the client. We assume, correctly or incorrectly, that the client:

- Knows he or she has a problem.
- Fully appreciates the severity of that problem.
- Wants to do something about the problem.
- Is willing to initiate and maintain efforts to work on the problem.

Often, we get a client like this, especially if we work in a private outpatient setting. But quite often, the client:

- Doesn't seem to understand that he or she has a problem, placing blame on others or deflecting responsibility for the problem.
- Doesn't seem to appreciate the severity of that problem, minimizing the symptoms or their impact.
- Doesn't seem particularly interested in doing something about the problem.
- Shows low or inconsistent willingness to initiate and maintain efforts to work on the problem.

We can measure level of motivation formally with tools such as the University of Rhode Island Change Assessment Questionnaire (Greenstein, Franklin, & McGuffin, 1999) or Readiness Rulers (Biener & Abrams, 1991) in which the client is asked to rate, on a numeric scale, how ready he or she is to change. But we can often get a good sense of the client's level of motivation just by talking with him or her directly about it: "How much does this problem bother you?"; "How important is it for you to make a change now?"; "How do you feel about the idea of being in therapy for this problem?"

Miller and Rollnick (2002) suggest that motivation is best as something that one *does*, rather than something that one *has*. That is, they suggest that motivation is a set of behaviors a person might or might not do at any moment, rather than an overall personality characteristic. It follows, therefore, that there is no such thing as a globally "unmotivated client," nor is there such a thing as a globally "motivated client." Rather, motivation is a state that can fluctuate over time.

Many clinicians identify a client's motivational state according to his or her **stage of change** (Prochaska & DiClemente, 1982). These stages have been defined in various ways, but generally include:

- *Precontemplation.* This is the stage of the client who seems defensive, doesn't acknowledge the problem, or doesn't express interest in changing.
- *Contemplation.* This is the stage of the client who is "waffling." She or he may have acknowledged that a problem exists but isn't convinced that she or he needs or wants to do something about it.
- *Action.* This is the stage of the client who is ready to go and is working on the problem.
- *Maintenance.* This is the stage of the client who has already made a behavior change and is trying to keep the ball rolling.

Progression along these stages of change is not necessarily linear, nor is it unidirectional. Clients may increase or decrease their readiness to change over time based on several factors.

In Chapter 7, we'll talk about specific ways to incorporate stages of change into your conversations with the client and maximize motivation to change.

Collaborative Model Building

Collaborative model-building begins early in treatment, often during the therapeutic assessment, but will be an ongoing process throughout therapy. The basic aim of collaborative model building is to understand the client's presenting problem(s) from a cognitive-behavioral perspective.

As you may recall from Chapter 1, we are interested in the etiology of the problem (the factors that initially contributed to the development of the problem), but we place greater emphasis on the maintenance of the problem (those factors that cause the problem to persist in the present).

As we develop the conceptual model, some important points to keep in mind include:

- The model should be *collaborative.* That is, the therapist and client should develop the model together. Each person has something unique to contribute to the process. The therapist has the educational background and often will have experience assessing and treating these kinds of problems with other clients. The client, on the other hand, has direct experience with his or her problem and can provide the details about specific thoughts, feelings, behaviors, and so on.

- The model should be *clear* to the client. This model will form the basic framework for the CBT, so it is critical that the client understand it. Keep the language simple; avoid technical or jargon-ish terms like *codependency, transference, conditioned stimulus,* and so on. Use the simplest terms possible to describe what you mean.

- The model should *demystify* the problem. In many cases, clients don't have a good understanding of why they experience what they experience. They don't know why they feel the way they do, or why they act the way they act, or why the world responds to them as it does. Part of the aim of model building is to take the mystery out of it—to help the client understand that these things are usually not random and that they often happen for understandable reasons.

- The model should be *parsimonious*. This is good science and good practice. Remember Ockham's razor: "One should not increase, beyond what is necessary, the number of entities required to explain anything." In practical terms, this means that you should strive for the simplest explanation that will explain what's going on, making as few assumptions about things that can't be verified as possible. Generally speaking, this means that our model will stick to things that can be observed by the client or by others, such as behaviors, emotions, physiological sensations, and thoughts, as well as external events such as triggers, reinforcers, and learning history.

- The model should be *empirical*. In **empiricism,** all ideas are treated as hypotheses, rather than facts. (This will come up later as an important part of certain CBT interventions in Chapter 14.) Throughout the process of collaborative model building (and, indeed, throughout the process of CBT), we are taking educated guesses. We have to, because we will simply never have all of the facts at our disposal. So we take the best guess we can based on the science we know and what we learn from the client. Part of treating our ideas as hypotheses is the fact that we will be wrong some of the time. The CBT therapist, being a scientist at heart, is willing to be wrong and repeatedly checks whether his or her ideas are still holding up or whether they need to be revised.

- The model should be considered a *work in progress*. As you learn new things about the client over the course of CBT, you will want to revise your model accordingly. Perhaps the client comes up with a new insight or idea. Perhaps a homework assignment yields an unexpected result. Perhaps you make some new behavioral observations of the clients. The model is never set in stone, and as these things come up, the therapist and client together should revisit the model to ensure that it reflects the best understanding possible.

Here's just one example of a therapist (T) introducing collaborative model building to Anna (A), our client with panic attacks:

T: Now that you and I have talked a bit about your panic attacks, I think I have a pretty good understanding of the kind of things you experience when these attacks come on. They sound very scary, especially since they seem to just come from out of nowhere. I'd like to see whether you and I can begin to understand why you're having these panic attacks. Can you think of a recent panic attack that we could use as an example?

A: Sure, I had a panic attack just yesterday and it was really bad. I was just at the mall shopping, and all of a sudden boom, I started freaking out for no reason. My heart was pounding and I felt like I couldn't breathe.

T: Wow, that sounds frightening. Can you recall the first thing you noticed? What was the first sign that something was wrong?

A: I think the first sign was that I started feeling kind of dizzy, like I was lightheaded.

T: (*taking out a piece of paper*) OK, I'm going to write that down here at the top of the page: "Dizzy and lightheaded." Let's think of this as possibly being a trigger for the panic attack. When you noticed yourself feeling dizzy and lightheaded, what did you make of that? Did you think something was up?

A: Oh, yeah. I thought, "Oh no, here it comes again."

T: Can you elaborate on that a bit? Here what comes again?

A: I just thought I was going to have another one of my attacks.

T: OK, and if you did have an attack, did you predict what was going to happen?

A: Yeah, I thought maybe I was going to pass out, or throw up or something, and it would be really embarrassing in front of all those people.

T: (*writing on the paper*) OK, so I'll write that here as well. It sounds like when you noticed yourself feeling dizzy and lightheaded, you had some thoughts about it. Specifically, you thought you were going to have a panic attack, and that you'd pass out or throw up, and get embarrassed. Does that sound right?

A: Definitely.

T: OK, so here you are feeling dizzy and lightheaded, and thinking that you're going to panic, pass out, or throw up, and get embarrassed. What did you notice then?

A: My heart started pounding really hard. And I felt like it was getting harder to breathe. And I started feeling sweaty and clammy.

T: (*writing on the paper*) I'll write that here, that after thinking these bad things were going to happen, you started experiencing more physical sensations, like heart pounding, feeling like you can't breathe, and feeling sweaty and clammy. I wonder whether your thoughts about panicking, fainting, and throwing up had anything to do with that?

A: What do you mean?

T: Well, if I told you right now that you were going to panic, faint, or throw up, and you believed me, how do you think you would feel?

A: I'd probably feel pretty nervous and scared.

T: In your body, what does nervous and scared feel like?

A: Well, it feels like heart racing, and maybe being sweaty or tense.

T: Yeah. I think most people would feel that way, if they truly believed that something bad was going to happen. So perhaps we might take a guess that your thoughts about what was going to happen to you made your scared feelings get worse?

A: I guess that's possible.

T: OK, for now we'll just treat it as a hunch. So when these symptoms got bad, what did you do then?

A: Well, I started gasping for air, you know, like trying to breathe really deeply.

T: And did that make things better or worse?

A: Worse, I think. I just felt even dizzier.

T: So breathing hard just made the dizziness worse. Did you do anything else?

A: I walked really quickly out of the mall and went and sat in my car so no one could see me.

T: (*writing on the paper*) Ah, so let's write that response here, that you left the situation and sat in your car. How did that feel when you did that?

A: I felt better. I knew no one could see me so I wouldn't get embarrassed, and after a while my body started to go back to normal and so I just drove home.

T: Any idea about why your body started to go back to normal at that time?

A: I guess maybe because I got out of there in time?

T: (*writing on the paper*) OK, so what you got out of leaving the mall and going to your

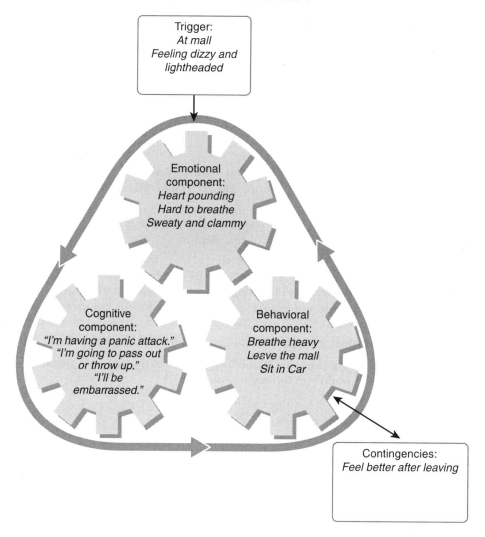

FIGURE 6.1. Initial model developed during Anna's therapy assessment.

car was that you started to feel less fearful, like you were safer. And your body did start to go back to normal, so that seemed like more evidence that you needed to get out of there. So we're starting to put together an understanding of how this might go [see Figure 6.1]. As you look at this, what comes to mind for you?

A: It looks exactly like what happens to me. Seeing it written down like this makes it really clear.

Note that in this example, the therapist hasn't yet developed a completed model of the problem. Rather, at this stage the therapist is just starting to generate ideas, collaboratively with the client, about how the problem unfolds. Later, other parts of the model will be added as the therapist learns more. But the therapist has started the process by generating hypotheses about triggers, cognitive processes, emotional processes, behavioral processes, and reinforcers. Specifically, we now know:

- The *trigger* for the episode was being at the mall and feeling dizzy and lightheaded (remember, triggers can be internal to the person).
- The *core pathological process* included *thoughts* of having a panic attack, passing out, throwing up, and being embarrassed; *physiological sensations* of heart pounding, feeling like it is hard to breathe, and feeling sweaty and clammy; and *behaviors* including breathing heavily, leaving the mall, and sitting in the car.
- The behavior was *negatively reinforced* (escape) because Anna felt better immediately after leaving the mall. She also *interpreted* her return to feeling normal to her escape behaviors.

As the conversation with Anna proceeds in this and subsequent sessions, the therapist and Anna will return to collaborative model building to flesh out the model. For example, here's a bit of a conversation that happened in the fourth therapy session:

A: I didn't do my homework this week. I know I was supposed to practice getting my heart rate up, but I just couldn't bring myself to do it.

T: That's interesting. Thank you for telling me that. Let's see if we can understand what was going on. What got in your way?

A: I guess I was starting to get my heart rate up and then I just started thinking about how my uncle had a heart attack. He didn't even see it coming. And I remembered that a friend of my mom's had a heart attack too and died.

T: And you thought that this would happen to you, too.

A: Yeah, I guess maybe.

T: OK, so let's see if we can add this new information to our understanding of what's happening. (*Takes out the model drawing.*) It seems like you have some learning history here. You know people who have had heart attacks. What would you say is the impact of that learning history on you?

A: It makes me think of them when I'm scared.

T: Right. Those are the people who come to mind for you when you're scared. Your memory focuses in on those people. What else is the effect on you?

A: I guess it just makes me feel more vulnerable.

T: Vulnerable sounds like a good word here. So you're kind of carrying that belief around with you, that you're vulnerable.

A: Yeah.

Here, the therapist has made lemonade out of lemons. Although the discussion began with the fact that Anna hadn't done her exposure homework (which we discuss in Chapter

---

Holding Up a Mirror

The act of collaborative model building is an early step in holding up a mirror to the client. By helping the client link thoughts, feelings, and behaviors, we're encouraging the client to look closely at his or her own reactions in a manner that he or she probably hasn't before.

Adapting the Process: *Collaborative Model Building . . .*

. . . with high-functioning clients. High-functioning adults will usually respond well to collaborative model building and can easily grasp the concepts. Where there are gaps in the available knowledge, you can assign them various kinds of homework to try to fill in more information.

. . . with low-functioning clients. For lower-functioning clients, collaborative model building is still important, although you will be using simpler terminology and a more limited range of concepts. It might be helpful to begin with simply having the client practice identifying thoughts, feelings, and behaviors and recognizing the differences among them.

. . . with children. A child's ability to engage in collaborative model building will depend very much on his or her developmental stage. Some older kids will take to the process as well as adults do (sometimes better). Younger kids, or those with limited attention or more concrete thinking, will require adaptation. At times, it can be helpful to externalize the presenting problem by giving it a name, like "OCD" or "Stinky Breath." We can then ask questions such as, "How did Stinky Breath make you feel inside? What words did Stinky Breath say to you in your head? How did you act when Stinky Breath showed up?"

. . . in groups. In groups, it's hard to do individualized model building. However, to the extent that there is homogeneity in the group (e.g., everyone is there for treatment of non-suicidal self-injury), you can make some reasonable generalizations based on the common presenting problem and ask the group members to come up with their own examples.

. . . on the inpatient unit. The biggest limitation to model building is time. In inpatient treatment, you will likely only have enough time to flesh out a few of the elements of the model. Try to focus on the ones that seem most critical or would give you the most traction— for example, specific maladaptive behaviors, contingencies, and skill deficits.

11), the therapist used this to gain valuable information about Anna's problem. We found out a bit about Anna's learning history and started to see evidence of a memory bias and a maladaptive core belief.

Repeated Measurement

Remember that CBT is inherently an empirical process. We formulate hypotheses (which may be wrong), generate a strategy to test those hypotheses, and then gather information to determine whether the hypothesis was accurate. For example, as a therapist, I might formulate a hypothesis that social skill training (see Chapter 12) will help Scott, our socially anxious client. The therapy then becomes an experiment, in which Scott and I try the intervention and then check to see whether his social anxiety is better, the same, or worse.

There are a number of nice, transdiagnostic computerized programs that will track clients' progress on a session-by-session basis, including the Partners for Change Outcome Management System (S. D. Miller, Duncan, Sorrell, & Brown, 2005) and the Outcome Questionnaire–45 (Lambert et al., 1996). If I wanted to go lower-tech, I could periodically administer one of several brief measures of social anxiety or social functioning (many of which are available for free on the Internet). Even lower-tech than that, I could simply ask Scott at each session to rate the severity of his social anxiety on a scale from 0 to 10. The latter strategy is less than ideal from a measurement perspective, but at the very least, from the perspective of the therapeutic relationship, I'm checking in with Scott, seeing whether what we're doing is working or not, and discussing the results openly with him.

The decision about what to measure is determined on a case-by-case basis, but repeated measurements for any given client could include:

- Standardized measures of the target symptoms.
- Standardized measures of functional impairment or quality of life.
- Numeric ratings (e.g., "On a scale from 0 to 10, how depressed have you felt this week?").
- Self-monitoring of the frequency of problem behaviors.

Some advantages of using standardized measures versus "homemade" measures are that standardized measures have known reliability and validity and that they usually are normed on both healthy and unhealthy populations so that you have a sense of what the "normal range" looks like.

Interpreting a reduction in a particular test score or other measure can be tricky. Let's say you're treating Christina, our depressed client, and are using the Depression Anxiety Stress Scales (DASS; Lovibond & Lovibond, 1995), a nice self-report measure that is well validated, applicable to a broad range of adult clients, easy to use, and free to download (at *www2.psy.unsw.edu.au/groups/dass/*), to measure her level of depression at each session. Christina begins treatment with a Depression subscale score of 25, in the Severe range. At today's session, the score is 19, in the Moderate range. Is that a meaningful reduction? Is Christina really getting better? Or is this just random fluctuation in how she answers the questions?

A really helpful strategy is to calculate the presence of *reliable change* and *clinically significant change* (N. S. Jacobson, Follette, & Revenstorf, 1984). If you're not into statistics, don't tune out on me just yet. This is easy. **Reliable change** tells you whether a reduction in test scores is statistically reliable—that is, that it's not just random fluctuation in test scores. From day to day, a person's test score will fluctuate, even if the problem being measured isn't really changing (e.g., Christina's DASS scores will change over time, whether or not she is truly becoming less depressed—on any given day, people respond to verbal and written questions slightly differently). So to determine reliable change, you have to first determine how much random fluctuation can be expected, taking into account the standard deviation of the measure (how much "scatter" there tends to be around the average) and the test–retest reliability of the measure (how strongly scores at two administrations correlate with each other). If your client's score has changed by more than that amount, you can conclude that the change is reliable—that is, that it's a real change, and not just random fluctuation.

Clinically significant change tells you, in various ways, whether the client's score reflects that she or he is doing well. Depending on what kind of data you have, this could mean that (1) the person's score is sufficiently far away from the clinical (unhealthy) mean that the person could be called "not unhealthy" on that measure; (2) the person's score is sufficiently close to the normative (healthy) mean that the person could be called "healthy" on that measure; or (3) the person's score is closer to the normative (healthy) mean than to the clinical (unhealthy) mean, so that the person could be called "closer to healthy than unhealthy" on that measure.

I mentioned that it's easy. You don't have to be a statistics whiz to do this. There's a handy website from Dr. Chris Evans at Nottingham University in the United Kingdom (*www.psyctc.org/stats/rcsc.htm*) that does the work for you. To calculate reliable change, you need to know:

- The clinical (unhealthy) standard deviation of your measure.
- The test–retest reliability of your measure.

To calculate clinically significant change, you need to know:

- The clinical (unhealthy) mean and standard deviation of your measure and/or
- the normative (healthy) mean and standard deviation of your measure.

As an example, Table 6.1 shows the normative data for the DASS. I obtained data from research on the DASS (T. A. Brown, Chorpita, Korotitsch, & Barlow, 1997; Lovibond & Lovibond, 1995) and used the free online calculator (at *www.psyctc.org/stats/rcsc.htm*). Note that in this example, I am defining clinically significant change as a score that is closer to the normative (healthy) mean than to the clinical (unhealthy) mean. That's the definition that works best for me in clinical practice.

So let's go back to Christina, whose DASS Depression score has decreased from 25 to 19. That's a decrease of 6 points. We see from Table 6.1 that the score has to decrease by 16 or more points in order for us to call the change reliable—that is, that it's definitely a real decrease in depression and not just random fluctuation on the measure. So Christina has not yet obtained reliable change. We also see that in order to achieve clinically significant change—that is, for us to call Christina closer to healthy than to unhealthy—we'd need to see a DASS Depression score of 14 or lower. So Christina is still in the unhealthy range and has not yet obtained clinically significant change.

What do we do with that information? In the spirit of collaborative empiricism, we talk to the client about it, of course! I like to do this at the beginning of each session, after the client has completed the measure in my waiting room. Here's an example of such a discussion with Christina (C):

T: Let's take a look at your test results today. When we started treatment, your Depression score was a 25, which is usually considered to be in the Severe range. Today, it's 19, which is usually considered to be in the Moderate range. That seems like a nice decrease; would I be correct in interpreting this to mean that you're seeing some improvement in your depression?

C: I guess. I still feel depressed a lot of the time, but I'm noticing that it doesn't feel quite as intense as it used to. It also seems like I'm not spending quite as much time in bed as I used to, and I'm starting to think that maybe I should try calling some friends to go out and do something fun one of these days.

T: Those seem like very good signs, and it really does sound like things are getting better. It sounds like your efforts are starting to pay off; congratulations! This also suggests to me that we're probably on the right track with our treatment; would you agree?

C: Yeah, I think that the things that we're working on really seem to be helping. That daily schedule of activities you gave me gives me a sense of structure for my day

TABLE 6.1. Determining Reliable and Clinically Significant Change for the Depression Anxiety Stress Scales

DASS scale	Clinical (unhealthy) mean	Clinical (unhealthy) SD	Normative (healthy) mean	Normative (healthy) SD	Test–retest reliability	For reliable change you need . . .	For clinically significant change (closer to the healthy mean than to the unhealthy mean) you need . . .
Depression	25.31	10.24	6.34	6.97	0.71	A decrease of 16 points or more	A score of 14 or lower
Anxiety	15.48	8.81	4.70	4.91	0.78	A decrease of 12 points or more	A score of 8 or lower
Stress	22.36	9.90	10.11	7.91	0.81	A decrease of 12 points or more	A score of 15 or lower

and it seems like I'm spending less time sitting around not knowing what to do with myself.

T: Great. Now let's look at the flip side of this issue, which is the fact that on this test, you still seem pretty depressed. Based on research with lots of people who do and don't have a depression problem, I would consider a score of 14 or lower to mean that you're answering these questions more like a nondepressed person than like a depressed person. So right now, someone just looking at this test result would still conclude that you have significant depression. Does that seem accurate to you?

C: Yeah. Things are better, but I wouldn't go so far as to say that my depression has gone away.

T: OK. So I'm thinking, then, that since we seem to be on the right track, but we haven't gotten you all the way there, it seems like we should continue with our treatment. Perhaps it would make sense for us to plan on reevaluating things after perhaps five more sessions, and see where we are?

C: That sounds like a good idea to me.

Note that with this dialogue, and with all of the other dialogues in this book, you may have clients who are more or less able to talk about things at this level of sophistication.

Holding Up a Mirror

Repeated measurement is a great way to hold up a mirror to the client. It's often hard to know exactly how we feel, and it's particularly hard to say with any certainty whether we feel better this week than we did 1 week ago. Try it yourself: Do you feel better or worse today than you did 1 week ago? It's a tough question to answer, and we usually end up guessing based on our immediate mood. Without capturing how you were feeling last week, and doing it again this week, it's hard to know.

That's OK. You may have to change the language—for example, when talking to people who are cognitively impaired, when talking to children, and so forth—but the basic point is the same, and you should still have the discussion.

What if the score was 9, instead of 19? According to the table, that would mean that the client has achieved both reliable change—that is, the decrease is definitely real—and clinically significant change, that is, the person is scoring closer to healthy than unhealthy. This might mean that it's time to talk about termination. We can't base our clinical decisions solely on a test score, but we should at least begin having the conversation. With Christina, it could go something like this:

> T: Let's take a look at your test results today. When we started treatment, your depression score was a 25, which is usually considered to be in the Severe range. Today, it's 9, which is usually considered to be in the Normal range. That seems like a very big decrease; would I be correct in interpreting this to mean that you're feeling much better?

> C: Definitely. I really feel like my depression is pretty well controlled. I still have occasional times when I feel down, but I'm not spending a lot of time in bed, I'm not avoiding my friends, and I feel like I'm keeping fairly active and doing things that make me feel good.

> T: Wow, I'm glad to hear that things are going so well! Your score here, in fact, is low enough that most people looking at it would conclude that even though you might feel down once in a while, you don't have a significant problem with depression. Does that seem accurate to you?

> C: Yeah. It really feels like I'm doing much better.

> T: When we started our treatment, we identified some goals for what we wanted to accomplish. I wonder whether it feels like you have met those goals?

> C: I think so. I'm feeling a lot better, and I'm living life much more the way I want to, rather than letting my depression boss me around and take control of my life.

> T: I wonder, then, whether it might be time for us to think about ending our treatment?

> C: Yeah, I was thinking the same thing. I worry a little that the depression might come back, though.

> T: That's a very natural worry. Your depression was pretty bad, and I don't blame you for not wanting to experience that again. It's also true that at least some of the time, people do experience a return of depression down the road. Let me make a suggestion here: How about we spend our time today making a plan for ways that you could help prevent the depression from coming back, and then perhaps we plan on one more meeting after a little bit of time has passed, say, a month or so from now? That way, we could check in and see whether you're continuing to feel better. We could have you fill out this measure again then, too, so that we can see if things are still looking good from that perspective. If so, then perhaps that would be a good time for us to wrap it up, although of course you're always welcome to call me to make another appointment in the future if it feels necessary. If you're not doing so well in a month, on the other hand, maybe that would be a signal to us that we still have some more work to do before stopping the treatment.

> C: That sounds like a good plan.

Of course, the termination discussion doesn't always go like this. Some clients want to hang on to the therapy much longer than is clinically necessary. Others seem to want to wrap things up prematurely, before the therapeutic goals have been met. The client's attitudes and feelings about treatment and about the therapist are always a worthy topic of discussion and can themselves be the targets of CBT conceptualizations and interventions.

Things That Might Bug You about This

You might be thinking that all of this repeated measurement seems a little technical, a bit wonky. You might even be thinking that it could get in the way of an effective therapeutic relationship. And it could, depending on how you handle it. Novice therapists can sometimes find themselves overrelying on measures, assuming that they are the final "truth," and spending way too much time talking about them. And certainly overemphasizing the measurement over the conversation can make the therapy session seem rather sterile and inhuman.

However, when one is being an artistic scientist (or is it a scientific artist? I forget), that measurement can be integrated fairly seamlessly into the discussion, and it fits with the general theme of trying to find the right answers together. The trick here is to introduce the concept of measurement early in the process, emphasize how it will help, and get the client's input. For example:

> As we go through this therapy, I'd like to be able to keep track of how you're doing. That way, when things are going better, we'll know right away, but if things aren't going better, we'll know that right away too so that we can reevaluate what we're doing. The idea is that I want you to get the very most out of this therapy that you can. So I'd like us to come up with something that we could check on every week, and we can use that as a source of information about your progress. In your opinion, what would be the most important thing for us to check repeatedly?

You might wonder whether clinical intuition is enough to get a sense of where the client is. Often, it's not. There's a wealth of research showing that clinician's judgments can be skewed by a number of logical fallacies (Garb, 2005). Just like our clients' brains, our brains take shortcuts that can distort our perceptions. So when we are faced with questions such as "How depressed is this client?" or "Is this client less angry than he or she was last week?" we are taking a guess that is subject to biases. We know that clinicians can make more accurate judgments when they use a standardized measure of some kind (Dawes, Faust, & Meehl, 1989). We preach to our clients that they should go get empirical data before making up their minds. Using a standardized measure—even a quick symptom checklist—helps model that approach.

I also can't stress enough the importance of taking measurements throughout therapy, not just at the beginning and end. Repeated measurements are often our best way of determining that the therapy is going off track. When we see that the client's depression, anxiety, drinking, quality of life, or whatever are not getting better, or perhaps are even getting worse, that's a strong signal that we need to stop what we're doing, return to our collaborative model, and try to identify what changes need to be made. And the client is doing that with us, every step of the way. I can't tell you how many times repeated measurement has helped me steer away from a potentially failed therapy.

THE ESSENTIALS

* The therapy assessment picks up where a sound diagnostic assessment leaves off.

* One aim of the therapy assessment is to determine the client's suitability for CBT.

* Collaborative model building, in which the therapist and client construct a shared understanding of why the problem persists, is critical and an ongoing part of therapy.

* Repeated measurement of the problem is an important part of CBT.

KEY TERMS AND DEFINITIONS

Clinically significant change: The extent to which scores on an outcome measure can be interpreted as being "healthy," "not ill," or "closer to healthy than ill," depending on which definition you use.

Collaborative model building: The process of developing a case conceptualization collaboratively with the client.

Empiricism: The notion that knowledge is best attained by forming testable hypotheses and observing outcomes.

Miracle question: A way of asking the client to identify specific, concrete indicators that the presenting problem has resolved.

Motivation: A fluctuating state that involves recognizing a problem, searching for a way to change, and then beginning and sticking with that change strategy.

Psychoeducation: A way of educating the client about his or her disorder, conceptualization of the disorder, or treatment of the disorder through dialogue, examples, metaphors, and other strategies.

Reliable change: The extent to which change on an outcome measure can be interpreted as "real," rather than as random fluctuation.

Stage of change: The client's level of readiness, at any given moment, to make a behavioral change.

Therapy assessment: A clinical assessment with the specific aims of determining suitability for therapy, understanding the factors that increase or decrease the client's chances for success, and beginning to develop a model of the illness or presenting problem.

Motivation to Change the Personal Target

Stage of Change: As you think about working on your personal target, what is your stage of change?

☐ *Precontemplation:* I'm not really interested in changing the personal target.

☐ *Contemplation:* I might be interested in changing the personal target, but I'm not really sure that I need to or want to.

☐ *Action:* I am sure that I want to change the personal target and want to get started.

☐ *Maintenance:* I have already been working on changing the personal target and have made a lot of progress so far.

Readiness Ruler: On the scale below, how ready are you to begin working on your personal target? (Circle the best number.)

0	1	2	3	4	5	6	7	8	9	10
Not at all ready		Not really ready			Kind of ready			Pretty darn ready		Extremely ready

Pros and Cons: What, in your opinion, are the pros and cons of changing the personal target? What are the pros and cons of leaving the personal target alone?

Pros of changing my personal target	Cons of changing my personal target
Pros of leaving my personal target alone	Cons of leaving my personal target alone

How, if at all, does listing the pros and cons impact your readiness to work on your personal target? Please write your answer here, and if your 0-to-10 number has changed, please indicate what the new number is.

From *Doing CBT* by David F. Tolin. Copyright © 2016 The Guilford Press. Permission to photocopy this worksheet is granted to purchasers of this book for personal use only (see copyright page for details). Purchasers can download enlarged versions of this worksheet (see the box at the end of the table of contents).

CHAPTER 7

CBT Finesse

Making a Relationship That Works

The therapeutic relationship is extremely important in CBT. As we discussed in Chapter 1, technique and relationship are both necessary components of effective therapy. The best therapists are those who select and implement the right techniques within the context of a solid therapeutic relationship.

Note that this view of the therapeutic relationship differs somewhat from those of our psychodynamic and humanistic colleagues. In some forms of psychotherapy, the therapeutic relationship is viewed as the causal mechanism of change—that is, the client gets better *because* of the relationship he or she formed with the therapist. That perspective assumes that the therapeutic relationship is *necessary* and *sufficient* to elicit clinical change. Our perspective is that the therapeutic relationship is *necessary* but not *sufficient*. That is, the relationship alone does not cause the clinical improvement. There are some possible exceptions to this, such as when the therapeutic relationship is used to deliver reinforcement (Kohlenberg & Tsai, 1991), but even then, there are some specific strategies (techniques) that the clinician must follow.

From our perspective, the therapeutic relationship forms a set of minimal conditions that must be present before any intervention will be effective. Going back to our discussion in Chapter 5, I think of the therapeutic relationship as the plate on which we serve our meal. It's not the meal itself, but it is nevertheless critical. If the plate is broken, or dirty, or simply nonexistent, the meal can't be served—at least not well.

Here's an example of how this can play out clinically. In a multisite trial of CBT for panic disorder, even though the treatment was highly structured, significant differences in treatment outcome were seen for different therapists—in some cases, the therapist accounted for as much as 18% of the variability in outcomes (Huppert et al., 2001). That's a lot. CBT seems to work very well in the hands of some people and less well in the hands of others. Why? It seems that even when the therapeutic techniques are held fairly constant, some therapists are better at managing the therapeutic relationship than others—that is, they interact with the client in a way that encourages more positive change and elicits fewer resistance behaviors.

The therapeutic relationship has been studied fairly extensively, and the results were summarized by an American Psychological Association task force on evidence-based relationships (Norcross & Wampold, 2011). Their main conclusions were:

- The therapeutic relationship contributes to outcomes, independent of the specific type of treatment. That is, regardless of whether you are doing CBT, psychodynamic therapy, pharmacotherapy, or whatever, the quality of the relationship affects the outcome of the treatment, over and above the effects of everything else you are doing.
- The therapeutic relationship can and should be tailored to specific client characteristics. That is, the therapist can control much of how the relationship goes and can modify that relationship depending on what the client needs. It's not simply a matter of whether the client and therapist like one another, nor is it simply a matter of whether the client happens to do well with a particular therapist's style.

The task force found that across studies, the following elements of the therapeutic relationship were demonstrably effective:

- *Therapeutic alliance.* The therapeutic alliance has been defined in many different ways, beginning with Freud's (1912/1958) concepts of transference and countertransference. The concept has now largely been stripped of its psychoanalytic underpinnings (e.g., we no longer believe that how a client feels about the therapist is based on how he or she unconsciously feels about his or her parents) and is usually defined as three closely related constructs in which collaboration is a central feature (Bordin, 1994):
    1. The therapist and client agree on the goals of therapy.
    2. The therapist and client agree on the tasks that will make up therapy.
    3. The therapist and client share an interpersonal bond.
- *Empathy.* Carl Rogers (1957) was among the first to emphasize that therapists should display empathy: acknowledging the client's frame of reference, trying to see things from the client's perspective, and striving to understand the emotions the client is feeling. We can express empathy in various ways, including making reflective statements about what the client is saying, as well as what the client seems to be feeling. This is not simply parroting back what the client is saying; rather, the empathic therapist paraphrases, summarizes, and highlights aspects of the client's statements, as well as the emotional state suggested by the client's statements and in-session behaviors.
- *Collecting client feedback.* We talked at length about the usefulness of repeated measurement in Chapter 6. Research tells us that repeated check-ins are not only good for determining the course of therapy and making corrections, but they are also good for the therapeutic relationship. They demonstrate to the client that you are interested in his or her progress, want to make sure therapy is going as well as it can, and are receptive to getting corrective feedback.
- *Cohesion.* In group therapy (including group CBT), group cohesion can predict both treatment outcome and treatment retention. Like many of the other constructs in this chapter, group cohesion has been defined in different ways but is generally considered to reflect the strength of the relationship between group members and the group as a whole (Yalom, 1995). A group is thought to have a high level of cohesion when its members have positive feelings about one another, feel a sense of belonging in the group, and feel that the group is working together toward a common goal (Burlingame, McClendon, & Alonso, 2011).

Does this seem like a tall order? It is. Recognize that some of this may be out of your control. For example, a client may simply hate your guts, and there might not be much you can do about that. And in such a case, we need to acknowledge that the therapy might be less effective as a result. Sometimes we transfer clients to another clinician when it seems appropriate.

But on the other hand, a lot of the relationship is very much under your control as a therapist. And it's really not terribly difficult once you get into the groove and this becomes your default way of talking to clients.

Take the time, at the outset of therapy, to discuss what the goals are. If the client doesn't have specific goals, take the time to help him or her formulate those goals (see later in the chapter). Try to come up with a goal or set of goals that seem reasonable, attainable, and appropriate. When it seems appropriate over the course of therapy, revisit those goals to make sure that they still apply and that you are moving toward them.

Take the time to discuss the procedures of CBT with the client. Don't just "do stuff" to the client; explain what you want to do and why you think that will be helpful. Allow the client to contribute his or her own ideas and modifications, if appropriate (and if the client's ideas are way off, explain why you think so—remember, you get to be genuine here).

Express empathy for the client. Yes, even the client who has behaved badly. Recognize, in your own mind, that this person is struggling. Convey to the client that you appreciate their difficulties, using your words, your facial expression, your body posture, and so on. Empathy refers to understanding and accepting the client's feelings and perspectives without judging him or her. We can express empathy by making good eye contact with the client, having a responsive facial expression (no blank slate or grumpy face here), maintaining an open body orientation (facing the client, often leaning forward, without crossing arms or legs), and using verbal encouragers ("Tell me more about that"; "Can you elaborate on that point?") as well as nonverbal encouragers (nodding, saying "uh-huh").

Display a basic liking for the client. Yes, even the client who makes it hard. You don't have to like everything the client does, nor do you have to agree with what he or she says. But acknowledge that this is a worthwhile human being who deserves better than his or her current situation. Convey, with your words and actions, that your liking of the client is a constant, not changing according to the choices he or she makes, the behaviors he or she exhibits, or the clinical progress he or she does or does not make.

Metaphor

Kozak and Foa (1997, p. 55) use a "coaching" metaphor to explain the process of therapy, expectations, and elements of the therapeutic relationship to clients:

> A useful analogy is that of an athlete who gets help from an expert coach. Suppose that a baseball player is in a batting slump and does not know how to get out of it. An expert coach will watch the batter and figure out what has to be done differently. Then practice exercises will be assigned to correct the problem. If the coach is not very knowledgeable and does not analyze the athlete's problem correctly or provide useful exercises, no amount of practicing the wrong exercises by the batter will correct the problem. On the other hand, if the coach prescribes just the right exercises, but the batter rejects the coach's instructions, the coaching won't be useful. Also, even if the batter agrees with what the coach says but doesn't practice or changes the exercises around to make them easier, the expert coaching will be useless.

Adapting the Process: *Relationship Building . . .*

. . . with high-functioning clients. Most high-functioning adults without significant personality pathology will come into therapy with a generally positive expectation for the therapeutic relationship. You can usually ask direct questions about their perceptions, expectations, and concerns.

. . . with low-functioning clients. Some lower-functioning clients will have had negative, even coercive, therapeutic relationships in the past, and building a sense of trust will be critical. It's important to take things slow and not rush into your interventions. Take the time to listen to them and show that you take them seriously. Spend extra time engaging them as cotherapists to the extent possible.

. . . with children. Kids often develop relationships in a way that differs from adults. Often, the initial one or two sessions with a child (particularly one who seems a bit shy or reluctant) might be spent building rapport by playing with a toy, playing a video game, or talking about the child's areas of interest. Even young kids, though, need to be shown that you're interested in what they have to say and value their opinions.

. . . in groups. Much of the relationship building in groups involves building a sense of cohesion among the group members. One way to do this, particularly in early group sessions, is to encourage the group members to get to know each other. In some cases, "ice breaker" games have been helpful. As group members share their experiences, build a sense of common concern and purpose by asking whether other group members have had similar experiences.

. . . on the inpatient unit. Many inpatients are not in the hospital voluntarily, and some will view you as an obstacle to their freedom. They may be hostile in some cases, or in other cases they might try to impress you with how mentally healthy they are. The relationship will develop best when the client can view the therapist as nonthreatening. Ask gentle, open-ended questions, and don't push. Remember that in inpatient treatment, you're unlikely to bond with the client with the same depth that might happen in outpatient treatment.

Alliance Ruptures

All relationships have their ups and downs, and a therapeutic relationship is no exception. **Alliance ruptures** are points at which the therapeutic relationship seems strained, or feels like it is breaking down (Safran & Muran, 2000). Sometimes, alliance ruptures are hard to notice; at other times, they're right in your face. Ruptures may take place:

- When the client and therapist disagree about treatment goals. For example, a client is seeking relief from depressed mood, but the therapist believes that she first needs to cut back on her drinking.
- When the client and therapist disagree about the tasks of therapy. For example, a client believes that an in-depth exploration of childhood experiences is necessary, whereas the therapist believes that a more present-oriented treatment would be more helpful.
- When the client–therapist bond is strained. For example, a client may feel patronized or misunderstood by the therapist (Bordin, 1979; Safran, Muran, & Eubanks-Carter, 2011).

Things That Might Bug You about This

Someone might say, "Hold on there a minute, pal. You said I should be genuine, but also that I should display a basic liking for the client. So what if I just detest the client? What then?" To which I reply: Either find something to like and respect in this client, or transfer the client to another clinician. Brutal, I know, but them's the facts. You're not going to form a successful therapeutic relationship with someone you can't like or respect, and your CBT will go nowhere. And, I would add, a failed CBT is potentially worse than no CBT at all. So don't set yourself and the client up for failure.

I've done plenty of on-the-fly CBT on myself for this issue, and you might find that helpful, too. If you start really having a lot of negative feelings about the client (which my psychodynamic friends would call *countertransference*), think of that as a personal target for yourself. You'll find that many of the CBT conceptualization strategies apply very well. Remember our basic conceptual questions, and think of how they might apply to your reactions to the client:

- What aspect of the client's behavior triggers your reaction?
- What emotions and physiological sensations do you experience with this client?
- What interpretations do you have about the client?
- How do you behave toward the client?
- To what extent do you have an attentional bias that makes you more likely to detect the client's aversive behaviors?
- What classical conditioning experiences have you had that influence your automatic emotional reactions to the client?
- What behavioral skill deficits might you have that contribute to how you respond?
- What current and past contingencies influence your behaviors toward the client?
- To what extent do you have a memory bias that influences your interpretation of the client's behavior?
- What core beliefs do you have that influence your thoughts toward the client?
- How does your own behavior contribute to the ongoing problem with the client?

As we go through the interventions in this book (which you will be practicing on yourself anyway), think about how you might apply them to a challenging therapeutic relationship.

You're going to have alliance ruptures in CBT. In some ways, these ruptures provide a unique opportunity for further exploration of the client's core beliefs and ways of relating to others (Safran & Segal, 1990). We'll discuss that process further in Chapter 16.

For now, we'll focus on repairing alliance ruptures when they come up. Sometimes therapists feel squeamish about talking about ruptures with clients. But it's important to address them, because unrepaired ruptures are significant predictors of poor outcome or treatment dropout (Muran et al., 2009). Some general principles to follow (Safran & Muran, 2000; Safran & Segal, 1990) include:

- *Encourage the client to express what he or she thinks and feels about the therapy or the therapist.* Sometimes, simple questions such as "How well do we seem to be working together?" or "What are your thoughts about how this therapy is going?" are sufficient. At other times, the therapist can point out the specific issue, using such questions as "It feels like we're struggling over what the goals of therapy will be. Does it seem that way to you, too? What's your sense of what's going on?" or "It seems like you and I are having some difficulty communicating. How are you feeling about what's going on right now?"

• *Respond in an open and nondefensive fashion, taking responsibility for your contribution to the rupture.* Notice that in the examples above, the therapist framed the questions as a problem of the dyad, rather than a problem of the client. Asking in that way invites open exploration rather than defensiveness. If your actions played some role in the rupture, acknowledge it openly, such as, "Yes, I can see that I responded a bit too bluntly to what you said. I apologize for that; I'll try to be more sensitive in what I say. Please let me know if you notice me doing it again."

• *Express empathy.* Show an effort to understand and resonate with how the client felt during the rupture, such as "I can certainly understand how that would have made you angry. I can imagine that I would be angry, too, if I were in that situation."

How to build a therapeutic relationship poorly	How to build a therapeutic relationship like a champ
Confront the client. The "tough love" or "get-in-their-face" approach, often shown on reality TV shows, used to be used widely in the field of addictions and flat out doesn't work (W. R. Miller, Wilbourne, & Hettema, 2003).	*Use motivational interviewing strategies.* Motivational interviewing appears to be much more effective in helping clients increase their motivation to change. The ultimate responsibility for change is left with the client, who is free to take our advice or not. The therapist does not assume an authoritarian role, but instead creates a positive atmosphere that is conducive to change. The therapist's tone elicits insight and ideas from the client.
Use negative processes. When the therapeutic relationship is hostile, pejorative, critical, rejecting, or blaming, it's unlikely to result in a good outcome.	*Separate the person from the problem.* We often need to call clients' attention to their maladaptive thoughts, as well as their unhealthy patterns of behavior. At times, we may engage them in exercises that dispute long-standing beliefs. The goal here is to make sure it's clear that you are disputing the person's thoughts and behaviors, not the person him- or herself. Make liberal use of empathy, genuineness, and unconditional positive regard.
Make assumptions. It turns out that therapists aren't always great at gauging clients' satisfaction with the therapeutic relationship or with treatment. It also turns out that many clients aren't going to bring up concerns about treatment spontaneously.	*Ask the client.* Therapists do best when they periodically inquire, "How are we doing?" "How are you feeling about this treatment?" "How well does it seem that we are working together?" "What aspects of our work together seem the most and least helpful to you?" There's an old saying in medicine: "When in doubt, ask the patient." Good advice for psychotherapists, too.
Be rigid. Often, in CBT, we have a treatment protocol that we are trying to follow. In some cases, this means the use of treatment manuals. At times, the client will experience concerns, emotions, or crises that necessitate a significant amount of flexibility in the treatment. Stick to the manual and don't acknowledge the client's concerns as they come up.	*Be moderately flexible.* Treatment manuals are great, in their own way. If you're learning how to treat a particular condition, a well-written treatment manual can be a helpful resource for both interventions and conceptualization. But adherence to a protocol only works up to a certain point. When a new concern or crisis comes up, you need to be flexible enough to address that issue in the therapy session, rather than blindly sticking to the manual.

Be overflexible. Don't worry about what the science says about treatments that work. Just listen to the client and discuss whatever comes up in the session.	*Be moderately structured.* Recognize that there are some treatments that have been proven to work. This body of research evidence should serve as the starting point for all of our clinical decisions. Although we may adapt and augment evidence-based treatments depending on our expertise and client characteristics, most of these adaptations and augmentations will not have been tested scientifically. Recognize that the farther we deviate from the treatment known to be effective, the more we are skating on the thinner ice of the empirical pond. So let me suggest a slight modification of Ockham's razor: *When in doubt, go with the intervention that has the strongest level of research support.*
Ignore alliance ruptures. The client will get over it, right?	*Address alliance ruptures immediately.* Encourage the client to express what he or she thinks and feels about the therapy or the therapist. Be empathic and nondefensive, validating the client's experience and taking responsibility for your contribution to the rupture.

Cultural Competency

Most of what we know about psychotherapy, including CBT, comes from the study of people who are in the ethnic and racial majority in Western societies. However, there is increasing recognition that cultural factors should be addressed in therapy (American Psychological Association, 2003; S. Sue, Zane, Nagayama Hall, & Berger, 2009; Whaley & Davis, 2007). Broadly speaking, CBT appears to be effective for members of ethnic minority groups (Miranda et al., 2005). However, several authors have suggested a need for improved **cultural competency**, defined as being aware of one's own values and cultural biases, having sufficient knowledge and appreciation of the client's culture and worldview, and intervening in a manner that is culturally sensitive and relevant (D. W. Sue, Ivey, & Pedersen, 1996). Many authors have suggested that specific cultural adaptations may improve outcomes (Gallagher-Thompson, Arean, Rivera, & Thompson, 2001; Hinton et al., 2005; Otto & Hinton, 2006; Rossello & Bernal, 1999; D. W. Sue, 2001; S. Sue, 1998). For example, in one study, CBT was adapted for use with depressed low-income African American women by changing the language used to describe CBT and including culturally specific content (e.g., African American family issues). Women receiving the culturally adapted CBT showed greater benefit than did women receiving nonadapted CBT (L. P. Kohn, Oden, Muñoz, Robinson, & Leavitt, 2002). Similarly, CBT was adapted for Hispanic clients by using bilingual and bicultural therapists, translating all materials into Spanish, training staff to exhibit the culturally valued traits of *respeto* (respect) and *simpatia* (sympathy) to patients, and allowing for warmer, more personalized interactions. Clients who received this culturally adapted CBT had lower dropout rates than did those who received nonadapted CBT (Miranda, Azocar, Organista, Dwyer, & Areane, 2003).

D. W. Sue (2001) suggests several characteristics of a culturally competent therapist. Specific culturally competent *beliefs and attitudes* include:

- Being aware of one's own heritage and valuing differences.
- Being aware of one's own background, experiences, and biases.
- Being aware of negative emotional reactions and stereotypes toward various cultural groups.

Specific culturally competent *knowledge* includes:

* Knowing how one's own heritage affects perceptions.
* Knowledge about the groups with whom one works.
* Understanding the effect of race and ethnicity in psychological problems.
* Understanding cultural aspects of family and community.

Specific culturally competent *skills* include:

* Seeking out multicultural consultation, education, and training.
* Reviewing research on racial/ethnic groups.
* Being able to engage in a range of verbal and nonverbal styles.
* Being able to seek consultation from traditional healers.
* Educating clients about the nature of one's own practice.

Motivate That Client

In Chapter 6, we discussed stages of change and the fact that motivation fluctuates over time. At any given moment, a client may be more or less ready to make the kind of behavioral changes we're looking for in CBT. But we know confronting the client isn't likely to be helpful. **Motivational interviewing** (MI) is a helpful way of speaking to clients, particularly so when the client is reluctant or ambivalent about treatment or about changing his or her behavior.

The overall aim of MI is to increase the client's readiness to make a behavioral change. Depending on the client's level of motivation at the time, that goal might be to help the client recognize the problem, to help the client accept a change plan, or to ensure homework compliance or continued attendance in treatment.

The general principles of MI include:

* The main task is to resolve ambivalence about changing or about treatment.
* The therapist does not take an authoritarian role in resolving ambivalence.
* It is understood that the client is ultimately responsible for changing.
* The therapist uses persuasion and support, not coercion or argument.
* The client, not the therapist, needs to be the one to articulate the arguments for change. It is well known that when we say something, we tend to believe it more and become more attached to that argument.

Adapting to the Client's Stage of Change

MI is all about meeting the client where he or she is, not where we want him or her to be. You can imagine that when you're talking to a client in the precontemplation stage, it would be rather pointless to start throwing a bunch of interventions at him or her—most likely, you would get a great deal of resistance.

Precontemplation and Contemplation

The philosopher Pascal (1623–1662) wrote, "People are better persuaded by the reasons they themselves discovered than those that come into the minds of others." So if we want to be persuasive, the best way to do that is to get the client to discover the reasons for changing, rather than simply handing those reasons to her or him. Therefore, a key goal of MI, particularly for clients in the precontemplation or contemplation stages, is to get the client to make *change talk:* to say things that suggest some increase in motivation to change.

For clients in the *precontemplation* stage—that is, clients who do not acknowledge that there is a problem or that they need treatment—it's important to discuss the client's feelings and experiences, trying to see the issue from his or her perspective. Don't assume the client is ready to change, and plan to start small. Our aim here is to try to increase the client's level of ambivalence and get her or him "waffling" a bit. Good change talk for a client in precontemplation would be, "Well, maybe I do have a problem" or "I just don't know whether I need treatment." It's movement in the right direction.

For clients in the *contemplation* stage, help the client weigh his or her options by talking about the pros and cons of changing, as well as any potential barriers to changing. Identify the client's personal reasons for wanting to make a change. Encourage short-term, achievable goal setting. Here, our aim is to decrease the client's ambivalence and help him or her decide what he or she wants to do. Good change talk for a client in contemplation would be, "I guess I need to do something" or "I know I don't want things to keep going the way they are." That sounds like a client in the process of making up his or her mind.

Action and Maintenance

When clients are in the action or maintenance stages of change, the principles of MI are emphasized less, although they never go away completely (remember, that action-stage client could be in contemplation next week). But here is where the client is no longer experiencing serious ambivalence and is ready to work. So we meet them there.

For clients in the *action* stage, provide continued encouragement and discuss ways for the client to slowly increase the frequency, intensity, and time spent on change strategies.

For clients in the *maintenance* stage, continue to provide praise and feedback for the client's efforts. Develop a plan for relapse, if one should occur.

Talking to Clients in a Way That Increases Motivation

A complete discussion of MI is beyond the scope of this book, but you can find more information in Miller and Rollnick (2002). Here, I discuss just a few elements of MI that are particularly helpful for the CBT practitioner.

The spirit of MI can be summarized by the acronym ACE:

- Autonomy: The ultimate responsibility for change is left with the client, who is free to take our advice or not. We want the client, not the therapist, to present the arguments for changing.
- Collaboration: The therapist does not assume an authoritarian role. Rather, the therapist seeks to create a positive atmosphere that is conducive to change.
- Evocation: The therapist's tone is not one of imparting wisdom, insight, or advice. Rather, the therapist elicits these things from the client.

Managing Resistance

The concept of **resistance** in psychotherapy has a long history in the psychoanalytic tradition (Freud, 1933/1965; Wachtel, 1982). Being late to appointments, failing to complete homework assignments, being unresponsive to conversation or suggestions by the therapist, acting in a hostile manner toward the therapist, denial of the problem, or engaging in excessive debate with the therapist are all possible examples of resistance. Psychoanalytic scholars argue that "Resistance defends the patient's illness. The patient's characteristic defense mechanisms designed to safeguard against unpleasant affects come to the fore during dynamic treatment. In fact, resistance may be defined as the patient's defenses as they manifest themselves in psychodynamic treatment" (Gabbard, 1994; p. 14). That is, they perceive resistance as being the result of largely unconscious defense mechanisms, which serve primarily to help the person avoid unpleasant feelings.

In CBT, we tend not to embrace theories based on nonfalsifiable constructs such as unconscious defense mechanisms; however, our thinking about resistance is otherwise not terribly far off from that of our psychoanalytic colleagues. Cognitive-behavioral theorists have defined it this way: "resistance entails those aspects of clients' functioning that seek to maintain the status quo in their psychological lives" (C. F. Newman, 2002, p. 166). Both the psychoanalytic and the cognitive-behavioral models perceive resistance as normal and perhaps unavoidable, as we encourage clients to make large, often frightening, changes to their behavior and their lives.

One of the critical issues in MI interactions is not to let resistance turn into an argument. You could respond to the client's resistance by stating your point more strongly or trying to convince the client you are right. And we could predict that if you chose that response, the client would become even more "stubborn," defending the status quo and dismissing what you have to say. You and the client would deadlock.

Just as one way of responding might *increase* the client's level of resistance, another way of responding might *decrease* it. That way of thinking about it suggests that resistance is not simply a characteristic of the client. It's an outcome of the interaction between therapist and client (Beutler, Moleiro, & Talebi, 2002). The therapist can increase or decrease the client's level of resistance by altering his or her style. In many cases, resistance is just the client's way of telling us, "You have misjudged my stage of change. Evidently you have mistaken me for someone in the action stage; however, in reality I am in the precontemplation stage."

When resistance shows up, we need to make sure that it doesn't lead to arguments and counterarguments, resulting in an entrenched "stuckness." The acronym OARS (W. R. Miller & Rollnick, 2013) provides some guidance for talking to the resistant client:

- Open-ended questions: Ask questions that are hard to answer with only one or two words. This encourages the client to open up more. Instead of asking our client Blaise, for example, "Do you think you use cocaine too much?" we could ask, "What concerns do you have about your cocaine use?" or "Tell me a bit about your cocaine use."

- Affirmations: Make positive statements about what the client is saying. As Shari objects to stopping her purging behavior because she's afraid of weight gain, instead of challenging her directly, we could say: "I can see how that would concern you," or "I can see what a struggle this decision is for you."

- Reflective listening: Use reflective statements to check whether you understand what the client meant. As we talk to William—who was dragged into therapy by his husband and is now grumbling about it in session—instead of pointing out all of the reasons he should be in therapy, we should say "It wasn't your idea to come see me today," "You feel pretty discouraged right now," or "You have mixed feelings about it." When you say these things as statements (meaning the vocal inflection goes down at the end of the sentence), the client can correct you if you're wrong—which leads to more conversation, which is good. But if you make them questions—"Was it your idea to come see me today?" "Do you feel discouraged right now?" "Do you mean that you have mixed feelings about it?"—you're getting into closed-ended questions, which tend to be conversation killers. Reflective statements can also help you to steer the conversation toward change talk (remember, getting the client to make change talk is one of our main goals in MI). So you can reflect back selected elements of what the client said to emphasize the point.

   • <u>S</u>ummarizing: Periodically summarize what you're hearing. Nick had expressed some reservations about coming to marital therapy with Johanna. Rather than siding with Johanna against Nick on this issue (which would likely have been a relationship killer), the therapist listened carefully and said, "Let me stop and summarize what we've just talked about. You're not sure that you want to work on the marriage and you really only came because Johanna insisted on it. At the same time, you've had some nagging thoughts of your own about what's been happening, the change in your marital satisfaction, the possible impact on your son, and the fact that you don't like the way you feel. Did I miss anything? I'm wondering what you make of all those things."

So we know that you want to avoid telling the client what he or she "should" do or lecturing him or her about why he or she needs treatment. But a tricky flip side of that principle is also not to agree too enthusiastically with the client's decisions. "I'm so glad you've decided to give therapy a try!" Now you've indicated to the client that you have a strong opinion about whether or not he or she should be in therapy. And because motivation fluctuates over time, when the client's motivation dips, he or she may be reluctant to discuss his or her ambivalence with you or may be inclined to turn that ambivalence into an argument with you. The client's choices need to belong to the client alone.

   Again, balance in all things. As CBT therapists, we are firmly on our client's side. We often cheerlead. We are genuine, and express our opinions when indicated. We make use of reinforcement strategies to promote change. So we are definitely not the neutral "blank slate" that characterizes some approaches to the therapeutic relationship. And yet, we can also see that when we push these elements too hard with a client who is in the precontemplation or contemplation stage of change, they can backfire. So there are times when it makes sense to temper our enthusiasm. If we want change more than the client does, it's going to get tricky.

Developing Discrepancy

When clients are in the precontemplation or contemplation stages of change, *developing discrepancy* is a critical maneuver to help move them closer to the action stage. For any given client, it's important to know what her or his long-term goals and values are. Does your client want to be successful in work? A good spouse or parent? A good friend? Where would she or he like to be in 5 years?

   Typically, we see that clients' behaviors do not fit well with those long-term goals and values. We reflect that discrepancy back to them:

"It sounds like you're in a tough spot right now. On the one hand, you're not sure you like the idea of being in therapy, and you really don't like the idea of being labeled as having an 'anger problem.' On the other hand, your family is very important to you, but you're noticing that lately the relationships with your spouse and kids have been strained, and that you're having a lot of arguments with them. I wonder how you reconcile that?"

Holding Up a Mirror

Developing discrepancy is a way of holding up a mirror to our clients. We are reflecting their own words back to them, but linking them in a way that shows them that their behavior is not in line with their stated goals or values. Now, it's worth noting that it can be uncomfortable to face the fact that your behavior is off track—that you are not acting like the person you want to be. For some clients, this awareness can have a temporary saddening effect. I don't think that's a bad thing. I think of this as *productive discomfort.* It's uncomfortable, yes, but you can do something about it. It's unlikely to cause a significant exacerbation or prolonging of depression, as long as the therapist follows up with a good plan to address the problem. So I don't hold back on this issue for fear of upsetting someone.

Committing to Change

MI is all about helping the client commit to changing his or her behavior. In that sense, it's very CBT. But first we have to identify how far away the client is from that commitment. Some clients (e.g., those in the precontemplative stage of change) are very far indeed, and so we need to loosen up their thinking and raise their level of ambivalence.

Sometimes we can get the client to agree to change some things, but not all things. For example, a client might be willing to commit to not drinking and driving but is not willing to commit to sobriety. Now, we could draw a hard line and say, "It's sobriety or nothing," but doing so would probably cause the client to retreat and become entrenched. It's probably more effective to accept this "micro-commitment" and meet the client where he or she is. The well-known "foot-in-the-door" phenomenon from social psychology (Freedman & Fraser, 1966) shows us that once someone has agreed to something small, he or she is much more likely to agree to something larger later on. So the client's willingness to make a small behavioral change might be a sign that larger commitments will follow.

Adapting the Process: *Motivational Interviewing . . .*

. . . with high-functioning clients. Even our highest-functioning clients will experience ambivalence. Recognize that it's perfectly normal. Because of their high level of functioning, these clients can probably tolerate a fairly straightforward discussion of the discrepancy between goals and behavior.

. . . with low-functioning clients. Lower-functioning clients may have less emotional capacity to cope with a direct discussion of discrepancies, so that aspect of MI should be broached delicately. However, these clients can usually identify some pros and cons of changing. For some, just generating insight into the problem will be helpful. Look for change talk that displays some degree of recognition that something is wrong.

. . . with children. Kids can often identify "hassles" associated with their problems. By asking the child questions such as how this problem affects their friendships, their family lives, their play time, and their school, the therapist may elicit some change talk. Sometimes,

"I just want my parents to get off my back" is enough of a goal that the therapist can start to elicit a plan.

...*in groups.* Pro and con lists adapt to the group setting well. It can be useful to have the group members identify the pros and cons of changing a particular behavior, while the therapist writes them on a dry-erase board. Be mindful, however, that the group members don't begin trying to convince each other to change. Remember that arguments will likely only lead to counterarguments.

...*on the inpatient unit.* Sometimes, the client's goals will be fairly modest. The client may simply wish to be discharged from the hospital, or may wish not to have to be readmitted, or may simply wish to have some private time or privileges on the unit without having to be checked and rechecked. That opens the door to a discussion of how the client might achieve those goals.

More CBTish Aspects of the Therapeutic Relationship

A CBT therapist has a tough job. You have to be empathic and show unconditional positive regard, and you have to match the client's stage of change and manage resistance. Those are the tasks of any good psychotherapist. In addition, you have some CBTish roles to play. As a CBT therapist, you are also a *co-scientist*, a *teacher*, and a *scaffold*.

The Therapist as Co-Scientist

A unique aspect of the CBT relationship is *collaborative empiricism. Collaborative* means that the client and therapist work together as a team to identify and change maintaining factors. The therapist serves in many respects as a coach. Part of the collaboration is the understanding that the therapist and client both bring unique ideas, perspectives, and knowledge to the table. You have the educational background and often will have experience assessing and treating these kinds of problems with other clients. The client has direct experience with his or her problem and can provide the details about specific thoughts, feelings, behaviors, and so on.

Empiricism means that the client and therapist work together to formulate hypotheses about the mechanisms of the pathology and what interventions will be effective. They then test these hypotheses through systematic collection of data. One really nice thing about empiricism is that you don't need to feel pressured to have all of the answers! Cherish your ignorance. It's one of your best tools. One of my favorite collaborative empiricism-style answers to client questions is "I don't know; how can we find out?" The *we* is collaborative; the *find out* is empiricism.

Another thing I like about collaborative empiricism is that the therapist and the client both have explicit permission to be wrong. Being wrong, at least some of the time, is just part of the scientific process. But the flip side, and one of the greatest strengths of the scientific method, is that if you are wrong, you will know—and you will have the opportunity to change course accordingly.

I like to set the tone for collaborative empiricism right off the bat, in the first session. Here's an example from our first session with Christina:

"Now that we've set some goals for the treatment of your depression, let's talk about how we can best work together. You and I both play important roles here. I know quite a bit about depression, and I've had the opportunity to treat a lot of people who were depressed. So I have a pretty good sense of what's likely to help. But only you know what it feels like to be in your shoes. You're the one who knows what this depression feels like, and how it's affecting your life. And you're probably going to notice when things are working, or when they're not, long before I do. So we each have an important job to do. My job is to listen to you very carefully, to try to understand why you're feeling depressed, and to come up with suggestions for what kinds of things we can do to help you reach your goals. Your job is to do your very best with the strategies we come up with, to pay very careful attention to how the treatment is working, and whether you're getting closer to those goals or not, and to give me feedback about that. It's entirely possible that some of the ideas we generate won't be the right answer for you. That's completely normal. What's important is that if it seems like we're on the wrong track, that we discuss it right away so that you can get the most out of our time together. If we both do our jobs to the very best of our abilities, I think you're likely to be satisfied with the results. How does that sound to you?"

The Therapist as Teacher

Psychoeducation is applied across the course of treatment but is particularly important in early stages. Clients need to be educated about their psychological problems, as well as the specific CBT understanding of those problems. They need to be educated about the specific kinds of treatment we'll be doing and what the expectations are of the client and the therapist. And they need to receive feedback about their own progress, which is facilitated by our use of repeated measurement (see Chapter 6).

Psychoeducation is more than education. The aim here is not just to lecture at the client. Rather, psychoeducation takes the form of a back-and-forth dialogue, in which the therapist teaches the important concepts by examining aspects from the client's experience. We often use **Socratic questioning,** a strategy that we discuss in detail later in this book, as an educational strategy. In brief, Socratic questioning means that we use questions, rather than statements, to help the client arrive at the conclusion. When we do it this way, the information tends to "stick" better. Here's an example of a therapist providing psychoeducation about the CBT model for Bethany [B], our teenage client with OCD, making heavy use of Socratic questioning:

> T: Let's talk a bit about OCD and see if we can understand a bit better why you are struggling with this. We know that a lot of the time, you'll have an intrusive thought, like that you might stab someone or otherwise hurt them.

> B: Right, but I really don't want to hurt someone. That's why it seems so strange.

> T: Understood. So here you have this thought come into your mind that just doesn't seem to make much sense. I wonder, how common do you think it is for people to have thoughts like that?

> B: You mean how often do people have thoughts that they want to stab someone?

> T: Yeah, or thoughts like that. Perhaps thoughts of doing something violent or uncontrolled like that.

> B: Wow, I just don't know. I hadn't really considered it.

> T: Well, let's think about that a bit now. If I conducted a survey on the street, and I stopped a hundred people, and I asked them all, "Have you ever had a thought about doing something violent or uncontrolled?" how many people do you think would say "yes"?

B: Hmm. Well, I guess a lot of them would probably say "yes," that they've had that thought at some point. Maybe 80 or 90%. But I bet they don't think about it all the time, like I do.

T: No, they probably don't get preoccupied the way you do; that's a good point. But let's go with this assumption that 80 to 90% of people will say that they've had that thought at some point. If I then asked them whether that thought scared them to the point where they felt like they had to do some kind of compulsion to make sure it didn't happen, how many do you think would say "yes" to that one?

B: I'd guess that would be pretty rare, maybe 10 people or something like that.

T: Leaving us with 70 or 80 people who had the thought, but they didn't feel scared about it. Why do you suppose that is? Why wouldn't those people be scared?

B: I guess because they would know that it was just a passing thought. They didn't think that it really meant something.

T: Exactly. So the difference here is not the presence or absence of the thought, but rather the fact that some people interpret that thought as being true or real, and the rest interpret it as just a thought?

B: Yeah, I guess so. But maybe the 70 or 80 people who aren't scared just don't appreciate the risks.

T: That's possible. Let's think about that one for a bit. If I say to you that I am a hamburger, would that make me a hamburger?

B: (Laughs.) No, it wouldn't.

T: No. But what if I really, really believed that I was a hamburger? Would I be a hamburger then?

B: (Laughs.) No, it would mean you needed to get your head examined.

T: (Laughs.) Exactly! So thinking it doesn't necessarily make it so, no matter how much I might believe it?

B: Right.

T: What if, instead, I told you that I was a violent person? Would that make me a violent person?

B: No. Just you saying it wouldn't make you a violent person.

T: And what if I really, really believed that I was a violent person?

B: No, that still wouldn't mean you were violent.

T: How would you know whether I was a violent person or not?

B: I guess I'd want to know whether you had actually done something violent.

T: Right. My actions, not my thoughts, would tell us the truth. People are violent when they do violent things, not when they think about doing violent things. Have you done violent things?

B: No, never. But then why do the thoughts keep coming up over and over?

T: I have a guess about that. It seems like at least part of the problem here is that when the thought comes up, instead of just dismissing it as a passing thought, you tend to believe it—you tend to think that it's true, and that thinking it means that you're a violent person.

B: Definitely.

T: So when that thought comes to mind, what do you tend to do about it?

B: I try not to think about it. I try to get my mind off it, or I try counting in my head to distract myself.

T: Do you think that's what the people in our imaginary survey would say they do?

B: I don't know. Maybe not.

T: Exactly right. What happens when we try not to think about something? For example, if I told you not to think about chocolate chip cookies right now, what would happen?

B: I'd probably think about chocolate chip cookies.

T: And if I told you not to think about stabbing someone?

B: I'd probably think about stabbing someone.

T: And if I told you to try for the whole day not to think about stabbing someone?

B: I'd probably think about stabbing someone the whole day.

T: So, then, one way we can think about this problem is that you have these thoughts, which probably lots of people have at some point. But unlike most people, you interpret these thoughts as being true, and you take their appearance in your mind as evidence that you are a violent and dangerous person. So you try, naturally, not to think those thoughts. But the more you try, the more the thoughts keep coming to mind.

Metaphor

Art Freeman (quoted in Seid & Yalom, 2009, pp. 31–32) uses a great metaphor to help his client Edward recognize that his thoughts can be distorted.

> Freeman: An awful lot of the way that we feel has to do with how we think and how we see things. For example, if I were to give you a pair of glasses with very, very, dark gray lenses, and you looked at the world, how would the world look?
>
> Edward: Dark and dreary.
>
> Freeman: Dark and dreary. If I gave you a pair of glasses with, say, pink lenses, and you looked at the world, how would the world then look?
>
> Edward: Pink, pink and rosy.
>
> Freeman: Pink and rosy. OK. Let's suppose I gave you a pair of glasses with blue lenses. And I showed you a lemon. What color would the lemon be?
>
> Edward: Green.
>
> Freeman: Listen again. If you're wearing blue lenses and I show you a lemon, what color would the lemon be?
>
> Edward: Well, green, because blue and yellow makes green.
>
> Freeman: That's true. But the fact that it looks green—what color is the lemon?
>
> Edward: Well, the lemon, still, is really yellow.
>
> Freeman: It's yellow. So the fact that it looks green doesn't make it green. It's still yellow. I think what I've seen over the years is that no matter how stressful a situation, how difficult a relationship, how problematic an interaction, that the way we see it is really important because we may in fact see it as far worse than it really is, far more serious than it is.

Note that in this example, the therapist used questions to lead Bethany to an understanding of a cognitive-behavioral model of obsessive thoughts. Bethany, not the therapist, was the one who came up with most of the important points. At the end, the therapist simply has to summarize what's been said and tie it up with a bow. Bethany is now likely to be in a much better position to understand and accept the rationale for treatment.

The therapist doesn't always have to know all of the answers in advance, before engaging in Socratic questioning. There are times that we know exactly where we want to lead the client. But sometimes, it's a bit less clear, and we can't accurately predict what the client will say. It's all good. You do not have to be a genius to do CBT, nor do you have to know everything up front. You just have to ask the right questions. Your conceptualization can emerge from the discussion.

The Importance of Homework in CBT

Homework is an integral part of CBT. Most sessions end with an assignment of some kind. Homework assignments may include targeted reading assignments, self-monitoring, rehearsing a prescribed behavior pattern, or practicing skills learned in the session in the natural environment.

TARGETED READING ASSIGNMENTS

There are a lot of good books and web pages out there that can help clients understand their problems or understand what kinds of treatments might be helpful. A couple of websites I like are the National Institute of Mental Health (*www.nimh.nih.gov/health/publications*) and the Association for Behavioral and Cognitive Therapies (*www.abct.org/Information/?m=mInformation&fa=FactSheets*). These sites provide solid information for clients about psychological problems and CBT.

SELF-MONITORING OF THE TARGET PROBLEM

Once we have identified a target problem, it's often helpful to have the client monitor that problem in his or her day-to-day life. In our intervention chapters later in this book, we review several examples of self-monitoring. Briefly, however, **self-monitoring** is extremely helpful. Self-monitoring over time helps us make more fine-tuned determinations of whether or not the treatment is working. In the case of Christina, for example, we could use a measure such as the DASS to see whether depression scores are decreasing over time. But because the DASS measures many different aspects of depression, we might not expect to see a whole lot of improvement right away. We might get more useful information if we use self-monitoring to determine whether Christina is spending less time in bed across successive weeks of therapy. Even if the DASS scores aren't changing, we might take decreased time in bed as preliminary evidence that our treatment is having the desired effect.

What should the client monitor? We have all kinds of potential targets for treatment: triggers, thoughts, emotions, behaviors, and more. There are a few things I tend to do:

- I tend to emphasize monitoring of maladaptive behaviors. Behavior is often the most straightforward and obvious thing to target in treatment (e.g., getting out of bed). So I want measurement reactivity to be aimed toward that behavior.

Holding Up a Mirror

Self-monitoring is a classic way to hold up a mirror to the client—to have him or her take a good, hard look at something he or she is thinking, feeling, or doing. Self-monitoring provides helpful information about how frequently a problem is occurring. As we discussed in Chapter 3, retrospective memory is pretty unreliable. Even a simple question such as "How much time did you spend in bed this week?" is likely to lead to an answer that somewhat over- or underestimates the amount of time Christina actually spent in bed. Her mood state at the time you ask the question plays a powerful role in influencing what she does and does not recall. When Christina actually tracks it over the week, you get a different (and usually more reliable) answer.

Self-monitoring also tends to elicit a phenomenon known as *measurement reactivity.* The mere act of measuring something tends to affect the thing you're measuring. If I ask Christina to monitor, on a daily basis, the amount of time spent in bed, she is probably going to start paying much more attention to how much time she spends in bed. This may lead her to start to make efforts to spend less time in bed. Basic scientists consider measurement reactivity a problem; I consider it a bonus. It's perhaps the easiest thing we can do to start to elicit a behavioral change: Identify a target, and have the person start monitoring it. I've had a few cases in which just self-monitoring led the person to get a lot better.

Could self-monitoring be demoralizing? For example, if Christina is depressed and sees how much time she's spending in bed, might that make her feel even worse? It could. But more often than not, it gives the client a clearer sense of what she's dealing with and what she needs to accomplish. If she has some negative interpretations about the results of her self-monitoring, a skillful CBT therapist will elicit them and address them (see Chapters 13 and 14).

- When a person is habitually having negative interpretations (see Chapter 3) that are potentially modifiable, I might have him or her monitor the thoughts he or she experiences in stressful situations.
- But . . . when the thoughts are *intrusions* (for example, in Bethany's obsessions, Melissa's intrusive memories of PTSD, or Lauren's auditory hallucinations) and the person is already way too focused on them, I might not opt to have her or him focus more on them with self-monitoring. Instead, I might use self-monitoring to redirect her or his focus to her or his behavioral responses.
- When the illness occurs in discrete episodes (e.g., Anna's panic attacks), I might use self-monitoring of an episode, in which I ask the client to record triggers, thoughts, feelings, and behaviors for each episode as it occurs.

REHEARSING A PRESCRIBED BEHAVIOR PATTERN

Often, part of our treatment involves a prescribed behavioral change. We ask the client to do something that he or she wouldn't normally do, or we ask him or her to do something in a different manner. In the case of Christina, for example, one of my direct behavioral prescriptions might be to spend more time interacting with friends. I may, therefore, assign a homework task to spend some time talking to a friend (in person, by phone, or online) at least once per day for the week.

CBT also includes skill training for many clients (see Chapter 12). I might have spent some time in session, for example, teaching my client how to act more assertively. I might then instruct the client to identify three assertiveness situations in the coming week and to practice the assertive behaviors with other people.

The Therapist as Scaffold

The therapist provides necessary structure to the therapy. This allows the client to feel less overwhelmed, stay on track, and maintain a clear sense of where we are headed. Generally speaking, structured therapy is more effective than unstructured therapy. But, as we've discussed, there are limits to this: Rigid adherence to a schedule, without being responsive to changing client experiences, needs, and feelings, is likely to be unhelpful.

Structuring applies to both the therapy as a whole and to the individual session. At the therapy level, the therapist provides structure in discussions of what the client's goals for the therapy are, how long the therapy is likely to be, what interventions we are likely to use, how we will determine whether the treatment is effective, and expectations of the client and the therapist.

An example of a therapy structuring, given in the first session, might be: "Let's talk about how this therapy will go, so that we both have a good idea of what we want to do, what we can expect, and what our respective roles will be." The therapist can then begin a dialogue about the topics listed above. This way, the client leaves that first session with a pretty good idea about what to expect from treatment.

At the individual-session level, the therapist provides structure in discussions of what the client wants to discuss during that session, what the therapist wants to discuss during that session, and what specific interventions will be used in that session.

An example of a session structuring, which is repeated near the beginning of each session, could go like this for Anna:

> "Let's set an agenda for our meeting today. I'd like to review the homework assign-ment from last week and get a sense of how things are going for you. I'd also like to continue our work using exposure therapy for your panic attacks. At the end of our session, I'll have some new things for you to try as homework. Does that sound good to you? Is there anything else you would like to add to that agenda?"

As you might imagine, the structuring sets the tone for the therapy and for the rest of the session. You can imagine that after that initial structuring conversation, the client and therapist are likely to work together toward a common goal. Imagine how different that is from some other ways of opening a session, such as "So, how was your week?" or a blank stare, waiting for the client to say something. The opening of the session sets the tone for the rest of the session.

Now, of course, there are always exceptions to the rule. Sometimes life throws a curve-ball at the client. People die. Marriages break up. Jobs are lost. When the client comes in to the session with a crisis or something that really seems pressing, it would be odd (and counterproductive) to adhere to a fixed agenda. Sometimes, the crisis is big enough that it should dominate the session. So the therapist might respond with "OK, that sounds like it's really important for us to discuss. Let's put the rest of our agenda on hold for now, so that we can talk about this." Sometimes, the crisis is not quite so big and doesn't require abandoning the rest of the agenda. So the therapist could say, "OK, let's add that to our agenda to make sure we get to it today. Can we reserve the last 10 minutes of our meeting to talk about that issue?"

And, of course, there are exceptions to the exceptions. Some clients seem to be in perpetual crisis, and there's always some disaster that comes up. In such cases, it can be hard to work on any goals productively because there's no continuity from session to session. This happened with Elizabeth, who kept bringing up crisis after crisis and seemed not to be moving forward. The therapist thought that Elizabeth might benefit from some increased structure:

"It sounds like you're going through a lot. I want to see if we can find a way to discuss and acknowledge what's going on, and also have time to keep working on the things we need to work on in order for you to get better. How about if we take some of our time today to review the events that are troubling you, and some of our time to keep working on the skills we've been discussing?"

Goal Setting

In order to set an effective agenda for the therapy, we need to agree on a set of *goals* for the therapy. This is usually done right after the initial assessment and before starting any active interventions. As we discussed in Chapter 6, the "miracle question" and other strategies are helpful to focus the client on identifiable behavioral goals. "I want to feel better" is a fine objective, but it's not terribly helpful for treatment planning. Better defined treatment goals might include (but are certainly not limited to):

- A decreased score on a particular measure of psychological distress.
- Decreased frequency of alcohol use.
- Decreased frequency of self-injurious behaviors.
- Decreased frequency of panic attacks.
- Increased time spent in social interaction.
- Resumption of responsibilities such as work or school.

Now, I'm aware that no client in history has ever come into a therapist's office saying "What I really want to get out of therapy is a decreased score on the Beck Depression Inventory." Much more likely, the client says "I want to feel less depressed." The therapist's question, however, is "How will we know you are less depressed?" The client might say "I don't know; I'll just feel better." But we know that it's often hard for depressed people (or anyone else, for that matter) to know when they are feeling better. And we also know, memory bias being what it is, that a depressed person will probably look back on his or her week in a rather bleak manner.

Remember that different clients have different ideas of what they want from therapy. Some know exactly what they want; others don't—they just know something is wrong and they need help. In either case (or everything in between), goal setting is important. It just takes more time with some clients than with others. But it is worth every minute you invest in it. Yogi Berra is (probably mis-) quoted as having said, "If you don't know where you're going, you'll probably end up somewhere else."

Goals are not set in stone; they can be changed as needed. But they should always be kept firmly in mind, and the client and therapist should always know and agree on what the specific goals are. If you find yourself confused about what the goals of treatment are, stop what you are doing and revisit the topic.

Treatment goals must be agreed on, but a suggested hierarchy of goals (based on Linehan, 1993) is:

- *Threats to safety of self or others.* Generally speaking, when someone is in danger, there's little sense working on anything other than directly trying to reduce the danger.

- *Therapy-interfering behaviors.* When clients engage in **therapy-interfering behaviors** (TIBs) such as failing to attend appointments, failing to do homework assignments, or derailing the discussion in session, it's hard to accomplish much of anything. So if TIBs are present, your therapy should be about TIBs. For example, missing therapy sessions becomes your target behavior, and you develop a CBT conceptualization about that behavior.

- *Problems that have an immediate negative impact on functioning or quality of life.* These are the things that most people come into treatment for: anxiety, depression, drinking, interpersonal conflict, and so on. Of course, as described above, when there's a safety risk present, or there are TIBs, then you're probably not going to be able to treat these problems successfully until the safety risk or TIB is reasonably resolved.

- *Problems that are likely to worsen and cause a negative impact on functioning or quality of life.* These are the issues that may not be of immediate concern but that could get worse and become a problem. Heavy drinking is one possible example. Some clients' alcohol use is not necessarily causing problems for them immediately, but it seems reasonable to expect that over time, the problem is likely to get worse. In such a case, the client's drinking might not be the immediate target of treatment (the client may, e.g., be here primarily to work on depression or anxiety attacks), but it may become a target once the more pressing issues are reasonably resolved.

On Boundaries and CBT

At times, a CBT session looks much like any other psychotherapy session: two people sitting in chairs talking to each other, or maybe a group of people sitting in chairs talking to each other. At other times, however, CBT looks different from other forms of psychotherapy.

- CBT may take place outside of the therapist's office. I have treated people with OCD in their homes. I have treated people with disturbed eating in a restaurant. I have treated people with agoraphobia in cars and shopping malls.
- CBT may involve people other than the client. I have had several cases, for example, in which it was very helpful for me to include the client's friends or family members in sessions (with the client's clear permission, of course). I've had some cases, in fact, in which I spent more time talking to family members than to the client.
- Good CBT therapists are genuine. In sessions, I'm not trying to be a blank slate. I'm a real person, who has opinions, emotions, and ideas that I share with the client. I demonstrate a genuine positive regard for the client (even clients whose actions I find objectionable, or whose behaviors in sessions are obnoxious).

So how do I know when I'm acting appropriately, and respecting appropriate therapeutic boundaries? The critical issue is always *whether the therapist's action will benefit the client.* Is it in the client's best interest for us to bring in a family member? To have a session at a shopping mall? Is there likely to be a demonstrable benefit that would not be obtained in a more traditional therapy setting? I respect the fine line between being friendly and being a friend. I am unfailingly friendly toward the client, but my role as the therapist is never in doubt. I don't, for example, meet clients out for a social lunch. I don't share my own personal problems with clients. And when in doubt, I seek consultation from a colleague or supervisor. A second pair of eyes or ears can help a lot.

THE ESSENTIALS

* The therapeutic relationship is essential to good CBT, as it is with any therapy.
* Elements of a good therapeutic relationship include building a strong therapeutic alliance, expressing empathy for the client, collecting client feedback, and (in group settings) fostering cohesion.
* At any given time, a client is in a particular stage of change (readiness to work on the problem and change behavior). The therapist must adapt his or her style and goals accordingly.
* Client resistance is a sign that the therapist has misjudged the client's stage of change and needs to adjust his or her approach.
* Motivation can be increased by highlighting the discrepancy between the client's behavior and his or her larger goals and values.
* The CBT therapist acts as a co-scientist (e.g., using collaborative empiricism), a teacher (e.g., providing psychoeducation, giving instructions, and assigning homework), and a scaffold (structuring the therapy and sessions, and helping the client identify treatment goals).

KEY TERMS AND DEFINITIONS

Alliance rupture: A tension or breakdown in the therapeutic relationship.

Cultural competency: The ability to intervene in a culturally sensitive manner, being aware of personal values and biases, and possessing knowledge of the client's culture and worldview.

Motivational interviewing: A way of interacting with the client that aims to increase the client's readiness to make a behavioral change.

Resistance: Client behaviors that maintain the status quo and impede progress in therapy.

Self-monitoring: The process of actively tracking and recording a target of treatment outside of the session.

Socratic questioning: A way of helping the client arrive at a conclusion by asking carefully worded questions.

Therapy-interfering behaviors: Behaviors that are likely, if left uncorrected, to reduce the efficacy of treatment.

Goal Setting

Set at least one goal for your personal target. Define your goal(s) in clear behavioral terms: What will you do and when? If a miracle occurred and your personal target were resolved, what would you be doing differently?

Goal(s):

1. _____
   _____
   _____

2. _____
   _____
   _____

3. _____
   _____
   _____

From *Doing CBT* by David F. Tolin. Copyright © 2016 The Guilford Press. Permission to photocopy this worksheet is granted to purchasers of this book for personal use only (see copyright page for details). Purchasers can download enlarged versions of this worksheet (see the box at the end of the table of contents).

BEHAVIOR-LEVEL INTERVENTIONS

In this section, we discuss the behavior-level interventions in CBT. As I mentioned in the introduction to Part II, on average (with many notable exceptions) you should strongly consider using these strategies as the "main course" in your CBT.

Figure IIB.1 shows the targets for our behavioral-level interventions. Your targets here are:

- Triggers for behaviors.
- The behaviors themselves.
- Contingencies for behaviors.
- Behavioral skill deficits.
- Negative effects of behavior.

To affect these targets, we can select from several interventions, including:

- Situation selection and stimulus control.
- Contingency management.
- Direct behavioral prescriptions.
- Activity scheduling.
- Graded task assignment.
- Exposure.
- Behavioral skill training.

And remember from our core pathological process that behavioral, cognitive, and emotional systems all influence each other. So a behavioral intervention can create cognitive and emotional change as well.

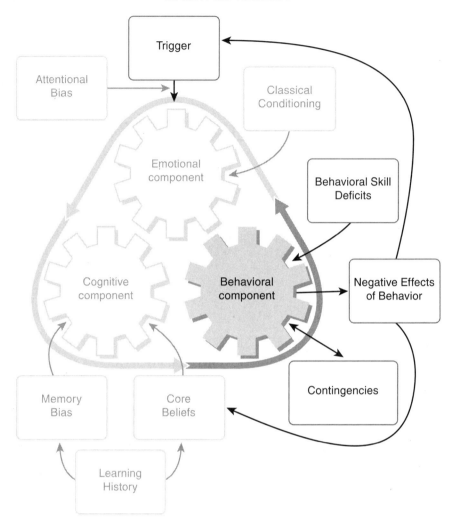

FIGURE IIB.1. The targets for behavioral-level interventions.

CHAPTER 8

Adjusting the Triggers

Situation Selection and Stimulus Control

In psychological therapy, we spend a lot of time thinking about ways to help the client to change. In CBT, for example, we might be interested in changing the client's emotions, cognitions, and behaviors. However, it often makes sense for us to think farther "upstream" and consider interventions that affect the triggers (also called **antecedents**) to the core pathological process.

Positive Cues, Negative Cues

How do you know when it's time to get up in the morning? If you're like me, you have an alarm clock that tells you. How do you know not to cross a city street at a particular moment? There's a sign in front of you that flashes the "don't walk" sign.

It's easy to overlook how strongly these **cues** affect our behavior. They don't completely control us—for example, I might hit the snooze button and keep sleeping, or I might jaywalk if no cars are coming—but there's no doubt that they influence us. The alarm clock in the morning is telling me to do something (get out of bed). Let's call that a *positive cue*. Conversely, the "don't walk" sign is telling me *not* to do something (cross the street). Let's call that a *negative cue*. Throughout the day, we see all kinds of positive and negative cues, and they guide our behaviors. The technical name for a positive or negative cue is a **discriminative stimulus.** Discriminative stimuli inform us about likely contingencies—for example, whether we will be reinforced or punished for a particular behavior in a particular context.

What if the cues were messed up, though? As just one example, what if my alarm clock was malfunctioning and went off at random times throughout the night? Most likely, it would no longer help me get up because I'd start ignoring it. Or what if the "don't walk" sign never came on at all? I might walk into traffic. So if the cues are messed up, the behavior can get messed up, too.

And so it is with many psychological problems. Many people engage in too much of the wrong behavior or not enough of the right behavior, or their behavior is "all over the place," in part because they are responding to messed-up cues in the environment.

In psychological problems, cues can be either internal to the person or external to the person. Internal cues may include over- or underarousal, physiological sensations, or negative cognitions. Each person's behavior is different and is controlled by a different set of cues. Our therapy assessment (see Chapter 6) helps us identify cues that are consistently associated with the problem behavior. If internal cues are identified, it may be useful to consider cognitive-level or emotion-level strategies, which will be discussed later in this book. In this chapter, we focus most of our attention on the management of *external* cues. We discuss two categories of cue-related interventions: *situation selection* and *stimulus control*.

Situation Selection: Choosing Your Environment

One cue-focused strategy is **situation selection.** By choosing to enter or avoid a specific situation, we increase or decrease the likelihood of the emotions and behaviors that follow from that situation. For example:

- For a client in a violent or abusive environment, we might encourage them to leave that situation (or, in the case of a minor, elder, or other vulnerable person, advocate for their removal from the environment).
- For a client with an alcohol use disorder, we might encourage him or her to stay away from bars, and we might also encourage him or her to remove alcohol from the home.
- For a child who is not complying with parental requests, we might alter which requests the parents make, or how they make them.

In this next dialogue, the therapist works with Blaise (B), our client who is struggling to recover from substance dependence. The therapist uses situation selection to help reduce Blaise's likelihood of using.

T: Let's talk a little bit about your pattern of using. In particular, I'm curious to know about the circumstances that have been associated with using in the past. For example, where, when, with whom, and so on.

B: Well, I would usually use with a certain group of friends. There were four of us, and we would just get together all the time and use together.

T: I see, so getting together with these other three people has been associated with using. Would you see them when you weren't using?

B: Not much. We didn't really hang out together unless we were using. Every once in a while we'd get together and not use, but mostly we were there to get high.

T: OK. When and where would it happen?

B: Usually at this one girl's house; her name is Kate. She was usually the host. And we would usually get together and use in the evening.

T: How much of your substance use would occur at Kate's house, compared to somewhere else?

B: I guess around 90% of the time I used, I would do it over there.

T: Not usually in other places like your apartment.

B: Not usually, no.

T: So if we're thinking about your substance use, we can think of some specific circumstances that are associated with using. It seems like when you're at Kate's house, or when you're with this group of three other people, you use. I wonder whether these people, and that setting, have started to serve as a cue for you?

B: What do you mean by a "cue"?

T: Well, I'm thinking that maybe when you see these people, or when you go to Kate's house, that's a signal tells you that it's time to use.

B: I guess that's possible. I do sometimes crave when I get a text from her, or when I think about going to her house.

T: So if your goal is not to use, what would make sense, from that perspective?

B: Maybe it would be better if I didn't see them so much. But they are my friends, after all.

T: Yes, they are. How much do you think you could see them, and still stay clean?

B: Umm. . . . I guess it's hard to do that.

T: So we have a dilemma here. On one hand, you like seeing your friends, and on the other hand, it's hard to stay clean when you do see them. So how do you resolve that?

B: Maybe just take a break from them or something?

T: Yeah, maybe at least for the time being, until you get clean.

B: I guess I could probably do that.

T: This doesn't necessarily mean that you should never see them again. But right now, you're having a hard time getting control of this problem. And part of getting control means putting yourself in situations that will help you, not hurt you.

In this example, the therapist hypothesized that this group of friends, and her friend Kate's house, were serving as *positive cues* for substance use. Several factors make this seem likely.

- Blaise's substance use usually occurred in the presence of this situation.
- Blaise was less likely to use substances outside of this situation.
- Blaise's contact with this situation was limited to times she was using substances.

Because it seemed that Blaise had limited capacity for self-control in the presence of those cues, the therapist encouraged her to temporarily avoid the situation.

Situation selection can be tricky business, however. Often, clients become overly rigid in their selection of situations, relying on maladaptive behavioral strategies such as chronic avoidance. For example:

- Anna, our client with panic disorder, avoids anything that might elevate her heart rate, for fear of having a panic attack.
- Melissa, who has PTSD, avoids anything that could remind her of her traumatic experiences, for fear of being plagued by painful memories.

- Christina, our depressed client, avoids anything that she predicts will be unfulfilling or disappointing, for fear of being dragged further into sadness.
- Shari, our client with bulimia, avoids desirable foods throughout the day for fear of gaining weight (though she later grazes and binge-eats in the evening).

As we discussed in Chapter 2, chronic avoidance behavior often does more harm than good. Not only does the person miss out on important activities or events, but the avoidance also contributes to the maintenance of the disorder by allowing maladaptive beliefs to persist.

Part of the reason that situation *mis-selection* comes up so frequently in mental disorders is that people tend to be bad at predicting how they are going to feel in a future situation. This may be particularly true in clients who are anxious (and overestimate how frightened they will feel) or depressed (who underestimate how much pleasure they will feel).

So how do you know whether avoidance is likely to help or harm? The best way is to go back to your meaty conceptualization. Based on the information in front of you, does avoidance behavior currently seem to be involved in the maintenance of the problem? For example, does avoidance contribute to the maintenance of maladaptive beliefs or get in the way of developing more adaptive coping strategies? If so, avoidance would seem to be part of the problem here, and you'd want the client to reduce that avoidance. Conversely, is the problem being driven more by the fact that the client keeps putting him- or herself into situations that are not functionally adaptive and diminish his or her capacity for self-control? That would suggest that some directed avoidance might be helpful.

Remember as well that any intervention you try doesn't have to be permanent. For example, we've encouraged Blaise to avoid certain friends and places, but that doesn't necessarily mean she can never see those friends or go to those places again. It just means that right now, Blaise can't handle it. So by prescribing situation selection, we get her a bit of breathing room that makes space for her to develop more adaptive coping strategies. Once she's stronger, we could test out her capacity to reenter those situations.

Stimulus Control: Manipulating Your Environment

Another cue-focused emotion regulation strategy is **stimulus control.** Through conditioning, emotional and behavioral responses can become associated over time with a variety of internal and external cues. Simply stated, if one engages in the behavior repeatedly in a certain context, over time that context begins to elicit the behavior. For example, if you frequently snack on potato chips while sitting on the couch and watching television, you

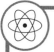

The Science behind It

Stimulus control has been used independently and as part of multicomponent behavioral interventions for such diverse problems as obesity (Hall & Hall, 1982; Stuart, 1971), study skills (Fox, 1962), and health maintenance (Mayer & Frederiksen, 1986; Meyers, Thackwray, Johnson, & Schleser, 1983). The incremental efficacy of stimulus control has been established in the treatment of obesity, in which the addition of stimulus control to other forms of behavior therapy significantly improved long-term outcome (Carroll & Yates, 1981).

Things That Might Bug You about This

This discussion about adjusting environmental cues might seem a bit simplistic. After all, many of our clients have severe and complex problems of behavior, emotion, and thought. So don't things like situation selection and stimulus control miss the boat?

First, let's recognize that these external interventions are, for most people, only part of the solution. Changing the client's external circumstances and experiences does not necessarily preclude the need to change the client's cognitive, emotional, and behavioral *reactions* to his or her circumstances or experiences.

Second, you might be surprised by how powerful these "simple" interventions can be, used alone or in conjunction with other strategies. They often get overlooked, to the client's detriment. For example, a therapist might spend session after session trying to build up the client's ability to resist urges to drink without addressing the fact that the client hangs out in a bar. Or a therapist might try to help an insomniac client relax and reduce bedtime anxiety without addressing the client's unhelpful bedtime routine. When the environment is exerting a powerful "pull" on the client, it's helpful and often necessary to adjust that environment.

might find that you become hungrier (physiological sensation) as soon as the TV is turned on (positive cue) and have the urge to start eating (behavior).

This means that some emotions and behaviors can become **habits,** partly dependent on their environmental context. They have become semi-automatic responses to a particular set of environmental cues. Controlling the habit, therefore, may depend partly on controlling the context in which it occurs. In other words, by placing oneself in a different situation or by changing the environment in some meaningful way, it becomes easier to control the problem behavior.

Using Stimulus Control for "All Over the Place" Behaviors

Sometimes, a particular behavior is considered OK or even desirable, but the problem is that the behavior doesn't happen when we want, where we want—instead, it's all over the place. The "all over the place" aspect of the behavior tells us that the behavior is under *poor stimulus control* (meaning it's not very responsive to any particular cues), and we want to get it under *good stimulus control* (meaning it gets clearly and consistently cued).

For illustrative purposes, let's take sleep as just one example of an "all over the place" behavior. Obviously, we need to sleep. But we need, for a variety of reasons, to sleep at some times and not others. When sleeping is all over the place—meaning it doesn't happen when and where you want it to happen—that's a problem. Maxmen and Ward (1995) wrote a great piece called "How to Become an Insomniac." Their advice is:

> Keep an unrealistic goal of the number of hours of sleep you should have. If you really only need 6 or 7 hours, make 8 or 9 the goal. If you are age 65 or over and once needed 8 hours but now need only 7 hours, ignore that and shoot for 8 hours.
>
> Catastrophize about not meeting this goal, especially in the middle of the night. For example, think, "I will never be able to function tomorrow unless I get more sleep. I probably will (fail, flunk, get fired—nonsleeper's choice) if I don't sleep enough."
>
> Remember, hours of insomnia expand proportionally to the number of hours spent in bed. If you need 7 hours of sleep in every 24 hours and spend 9 hours in bed, you can

guarantee at least 2 hours of insomnia. Taking a 1-hour nap during the day can help increase this to 3 hours of insomnia. Because you now have had 3 hours of insomnia, spend 10 hours in bed the next night trying to get enough sleep.

Spend all of the desperate hours fighting to get to sleep in bed. In Pavlovian fashion, this will make the bed a stimulus for profound upset.

Make the bed a center for many other daily activities—reading, writing, TV, etc. The bed then becomes a cue for many more things than sleep.

If you have the opportunity, start taking sleeping medications. Over-the-counter antihistaminic ones are best; they are relatively ineffectual, tolerance develops within days, and they suppress REM sleep. Consequently, if you try to stop taking them, you will have vicious REM rebound with many nightmares. Continue to increase the dosage to get enough sleep. The benzodiazepines aren't quite as effective at creating insomnia, but over weeks and months tolerance can develop, some REM rebound can occur, and variations on benzodiazepine withdrawal might also occur, worsening the insomnia (p. 369).

As you can see, some of the ways to become an insomniac are cognitive (e.g., catastrophizing), but many suggest that people with poor sleep have maladaptive cues (discriminative stimuli) for sleep. Their environment does not consistently tell them the right times and places for sleeping. To them, bed and nighttime do not mean "time to sleep." Instead, bed and nighttime mean other things like "time to worry," "time to watch TV," and so on.

Let's see what we can learn about our client Samuel (S), who came to a sleep clinic because of insomnia.

T: Let's take a look at your sleep routine. Where do you usually sleep?

S: In my bed.

T: Anywhere else?

S: Sometimes I'll take a nap on the couch if I'm really sleepy.

T: I see. When do you take those naps?

S: In the afternoon, usually. Sometimes when I get home from my shift I'm really wiped out and I'll fall asleep watching TV.

T: OK. Coming back up to your bed, what other kinds of things do you do there?

Try This

Do you consider yourself to be a *good sleeper* (meaning you fall asleep fairly quickly, remain asleep through the night, wake up at the right time, and feel rested in the morning), a *poor sleeper* (meaning it takes you a long time to fall asleep, or you wake up repeatedly during the night, or you wake up at the wrong time, or you don't feel rested in the morning), or somewhere in between? Now ask yourself the following questions:

- Under what circumstances are you more or less likely to sleep?
- Where do you sleep? And what else do you do in the place that you sleep?
- What time do you sleep? And what else do you do around that time?
- What other behaviors are associated with going to sleep for you?
- Why do that location, and that time, and those behaviors lead to sleep?

S: Um . . . sex? (*Laughs nervously.*)

T: (*Laughs.*) OK, seems reasonable. What else? For example, do you have a TV in your room?

S: Yeah. A lot of the time I'll watch TV in there if I can't sleep.

T: Anything else? Like eating, reading, stuff like that?

S: I don't eat in bed. But I do go in there to read.

T: Is that at bedtime, or at other times?

S: Sometimes I'll just go in there and lie down to read because it's a nice, quiet place.

T: And at bedtime, what other things do you tend to do?

S: You mean like besides brush my teeth and stuff?

T: Yeah, I mean are there things you do around bedtime that aren't related to your sleep routine?

S: A lot of the time my wife and I will talk. We talk about stuff that needs to get done, or problems that we've been having.

T: And when, in relationship to trying to sleep, do you have those conversations?

S: Usually like right when we get into bed.

T: I see. And those are relaxing conversations for you, or something different?

S: No, a lot of the time they're kind of stressful.

T: What time do you try to fall asleep?

S: It really varies. On some days I need to get up early for work, so I go to bed a lot earlier, like 9:00. But if I don't have to work the next day, and I know I can sleep in, I'll stay up until 1 in the morning or so because I know I can sleep until noon if I want to.

T: When you go to bed at 9, that's because you know you need to get up? Not because you feel sleepy?

S: Right. I just know that if I can't get 8 hours, I'm gonna be a mess.

T: And when you find yourself not able to sleep, what do you do?

S: I might watch TV or read.

T: Still in the bed?

S: Yeah. Or maybe if I don't want to disturb my wife, I'll just lie there and stare at the ceiling.

T: Checking the clock, too?

S: Oh, yeah. I keep looking at it, and only like 5 minutes will have gone by, and I just think "Man, if I can't get to sleep, I'm in big trouble tomorrow."

Good and bad sleepers tend to have very different bedtime routines, as shown in Table 8.1. For good sleepers, sleeping is clearly associated with certain cues: a particular place (bed), a particular time (night), and a specific set of behaviors (lights off, room quiet, perhaps a limited period of quiet activity). For these people, we would say sleep is under *good stimulus control*. For bad sleepers, on the other hand, sleeping is not clearly associated with any particular location or time. For these people, we would say sleep is under *poor stimulus control*.

TABLE 8.1. Common Cues for Good and Bad Sleepers

	Where?	When?	With what behaviors?
Good sleeper	• In bed • Bed is only (OK, mostly) used for sleeping	• At night, consistently around the same time (even on weekends)	• Lights off • Room quiet • After a period of quiet activity (e.g., reading)
Bad sleeper	• In bed, on couch, at desk, in class • Bed is also used for reading, doing homework, eating, talking on phone	• At night, late through the morning, in the afternoon	• TV on • After important work or discussions • Many nighttime activities besides sleep • Talking on the phone, using the laptop, or other nonsleeping behaviors in bed • Checking the clock

So, having determined that Samuel's sleep is under poor stimulus control, we can use stimulus control strategies to improve his sleep (Bootzin, 1979; Engle-Friedman, 1994; Jacobs et al., 1993; Morin & Espie, 2003).

T: Let's talk about some ways that you might be able to improve your sleep. At the end of our visit today, I'll write these down to make it easier to remember. The first one involves your bedtime. I'd like you to stay out of bed until you feel sleepy. That might mean that you don't get into bed until later.

S: But what about the days I have to get up early? If I don't get to bed early, I won't get enough sleep.

T: I can see why that would worry you. But I'd also like to point out that you're not getting enough sleep doing it this way, either. So when you go to bed earlier, it's not really having the desired effect. What it does instead is cause you to spend more time in bed not sleeping. The problem there is that your brain learns to associate bed with being awake, instead of associating it with being asleep. Does that make sense?

S: Yeah, I get it. It's not like I fall asleep at 9 anyway.

T: Right. The second thing is to cut down the activities that you do in bed. I'd like you to reserve the bed for sleeping and sex, and that's it. No reading, no TV, no stressful conversations. Again, we want your brain to learn that bed is where you sleep. Right now, when you get in bed, your brain is kind of asking, "Is it time to watch TV now? Is it time to read?" So we want to show it what bed is for.

S: OK, I can do that.

T: Now, since you're only using the bed for sleeping and sex, that means that if you find yourself not sleeping, you need to get out of the bed. So let's say that if you haven't fallen asleep after 10 minutes or so of lying there, get up and go into another room.

S: You mean get up in the middle of the night?

T: Exactly. Remember, the goal is to associate your bed with falling asleep quickly.

S: Well, what am I supposed to do in the middle of the night?

T: You could go into another room and watch TV if that helps, but be careful not to fall asleep on the couch. We want your brain to learn that bed, and only bed, is the place you sleep. Or you could do something productive, like a household chore. That way, it doesn't feel like the time is being wasted. And then, when you feel sleepy, go back to bed. But if you don't fall asleep after another 10 minutes or so, get back out of bed.

S: I could imagine that I could spend the whole night out of bed.

T: That could happen, at least at first. But look at it this way: You're already not sleeping. So lying in bed and waiting for sleep isn't doing the trick. So if you spend the whole night watching TV or doing chores or whatever, you're no worse off than you are now. But I'm guessing that after a bit of time, your brain and body are going to adjust to this new routine and you'll find that sleeps starts to come easier for you.

S: OK.

T: Now, this last part might not be much fun, but it's important. I want you to get up at the same time every day.

S: You mean, even on the days I don't have to work?

T: Yes. Let me explain why. Your brain and body have a natural rhythm of sleeping and being awake. But that rhythm is easily disrupted. When you get up at different times on different days, your cycle gets off, and then it becomes harder to fall asleep when you want to. It might seem tempting to try to "catch up" on your missed sleep on your days off, but that doesn't really work. You don't really end up feeling more rested, and the problem just gets worse.

S: That's true that I don't feel more rested.

T: And so related to that point, I bet you can guess what I'm going to say about naps.

S: Don't take them?

T: Perfect. Can you guess why?

S: Because they throw off my cycle.

T: Exactly.

You can see from this example that for Samuel, stimulus control involves modifying the *where* and *when* of sleeping, as well as the *behaviors that are associated* with sleeping.

Let's look at other clients who have "all over the place" behaviors that need to come under better stimulus control.

- Shari's eating pattern is all over the place. During the day, she eats little, avoiding desirable foods. When she gets home, she starts "grazing," including snacking in front of the TV. At some point in the evening, this escalates into an eating binge. We might consider having Shari eat at specified times and places (this procedure is sometimes called **narrowing**). We could, for example, instruct her to eat only at certain times of day, at the dinner table or in the cafeteria where she works, with the TV off. Over time, the aim is to weaken the associations between certain stimuli (e.g., the TV) and the desire to eat, making the behavior more controllable.

- Suzanne's worrying is also all over the place. We might consider having her designate a specific "worry time" at some point during the day. Each day at a certain time, her job is to go to a specific location and worry for 30 minutes. By associating her worrying behavior with a specific time and place, she may be better able to control the behavior at other times.
- Johanna and Nick, our distressed couple, tend to talk about their problems all the time. Although we don't want to discourage talking about marital problems, this behavior too seems to be all over the place. So perhaps we could get that behavior under better stimulus control by identifying a certain time of day that will be used for a "State of the Union" discussion. So, for example, every day after they put their son to bed, they have time to discuss their grievances.

Using Stimulus Control for Behaviors We Want to Decrease or Stop

Sometimes, the pattern we're trying to affect is different. It's not that we're trying to get the behavior to shape up in terms of time and location; rather, our aim is to decrease the behavior or stop it altogether. There's still a role for stimulus control interventions in such cases, but the emphasis is somewhat different. Sometimes, an unwanted behavior has become associated with a particular context, such as a place, time, or activity. One example would be smoking—the person wants to stop completely but habitually smokes after meals or during coffee breaks. For this person, we might hypothesize that mealtimes and coffee breaks are serving as *positive cues* for smoking.

When we're trying to eliminate a behavior, one kind of environmental intervention is to build *negative cues* into the environment. Specifically, we could try introducing stimuli into the environment that remind the person not to engage in the behavior. I've known smokers, for example, who have put pictures of their children on their cigarette packs because it discourages them from lighting up. If we determine that the smoking habitually occurs after meals or during coffee breaks, we might think of ways to build negative cues into the person's environment at those critical times. Concurrently, I would look to eliminate *positive cues* from the environment. What in this person's environment is inviting him or her to smoke? Ashtrays in the home, lighters, T-shirts with cigarette brand logos, and so on are potentially powerful smoking cues, so I would encourage the client to get rid of them.

Another behavior-reducing intervention would be to create *barriers* to the behavior—that is, to make it more difficult to engage in the behavior. In the case of a smoker, for example, I would think about taking steps that would limit the client's access to cigarettes, particularly during those high-risk times (e.g., leaving the pack at home or throwing it away). I might also use situation selection, such as encouraging the client not to be around others who are smoking.

Let's take a look at the use of *negative cues* and *barriers* when we want a behavior to stop. Here, the therapist is working with Samantha (S), our young client with trichotillomania. They're using stimulus control strategies (Franklin & Tolin, 2007) to try to alter the environment in a manner that will reduce the hair-pulling behavior.

T: OK, Samantha, you've told me a bunch about your hair pulling and how it usually goes. Let me see if I have it right. Usually, when you pull, you're studying at the desk in your room, with the door closed, and a lot of noise going on in the house.

S: Right.

T: Perhaps this would be a good place for us to start. It seems like what has happened is that you've pulled so often in that situation, that the situation itself can start to trigger urges to pull.

S: Maybe, but I don't always feel an urge to pull when I'm sitting there. The urge comes later.

T: You're right; you don't start to really feel the urge until you start stroking your hair and find a really good one, right?

S: Right.

T: So let's talk about that moment when you've found a good hair and have an urge to pull it. Once you start to really notice the urge, it's gotten really strong, and so it would be harder for you to do something about it then. Maybe, in this situation, your best strategy would be to act early, maybe even before you start to notice the urges. It's a little bit like when you play soccer. The goalie's job is to keep the ball out of the net, right?

S: Yeah, but she doesn't always succeed.

T: Exactly. So if you're the coach, what's the best way to make sure the other team doesn't score any points?

S: Well, I guess the best strategy is to make sure they don't get the ball anywhere near the net, so the other players can take care of it.

T: Right again! In fact, your team will probably do best if you don't let the other team even get onto your half of the field! Good defense takes place not just at the goal, when things are down to the wire, but earlier, before the other team has really started to advance. Fighting hair pulling is kind of like that. When you're really feeling the urge, and you have a good hair between your fingertips, the ball is already down by the net. At that point, it's going to be pretty hard to stop "trich" from doing what it wants to do.

S: So I need to stop it before it gets to that point.

T: Now you've got the idea. So let's think of some things that might help while you're studying. Anyone ever come into the room while you're studying at your desk, or stroking your hair, or even pulling?

S: Sometimes my mom or my little brother will come in to bug me. They've never come in while I was pulling, but they have come in while I was stroking my hair.

T: What happened when they came in?

S: I took my hand out of my hair right away. I didn't want them to see me doing it.

T: So when other people are around, you don't do it as much?

S: No, I don't. Are you saying that should invite everybody into my room while I'm studying? I wouldn't get anything done!

T: (*Laughs.*) No, I agree that it would be pretty tough to study with a bunch of people in your room. But what would happen if you left your bedroom door open?

S: Well, I guess I would worry that someone would see me pulling.

T: And what would be the result of that?

S: I probably wouldn't pull. But it's so noisy in the house, I need to keep the door closed.

T: What if there was another way? For example, what if we talked to your mom to see if there could be some special quiet time during the evening so you can study? For example, what if they sent your brother out to play in the yard for an hour, or kept him downstairs in the living room? Would that give you enough peace and quiet to study?

S: It might. I guess it's worth a try.

T: Great! We've got something we can try. Now the other part of this is that while you're studying, you sit like this. (*Rests head in hand, touching hair with fingertips.*) What do you think about that?

S: I suppose it makes it easier for me to start pulling.

T: Yes, and it also makes it more likely that you'll find a really good hair with your fingers, and then . . .

S: Whammo.

T: Right. So what would be a good solution?

S: I guess maybe I shouldn't sit like that.

T: Maybe not. How else could you sit?

S: I guess I could put my hands on the desk in front of me, or maybe hold onto my book. Maybe I could even sit on my hands, or put my hands in my pockets.

T: Great ideas! Now, how about something to help you remember not to pull?

S: You mean, like a sign or something?

T: Something like that. What do you think would work for you?

S: I guess I could make a big stop sign on my computer, you know, something in bright red, and tape it to the computer screen.

T: That sounds like a terrific idea.

S: You know, now that I'm thinking about it, maybe I could change my screensaver on my computer to say, "Don't pull."

T: Very creative! I think you're on your way.

We see here that the therapist is trying to enlist Samantha in a process of altering the environment by creating *negative cues* and *barriers* to the unwanted behavior. They've identified certain environmental stimuli that increase or decrease the likelihood of the behavior and are trying to rearrange Samantha's experience so that she gets fewer of the positive cues and more of the negative cues.

Let's look at other clients who have behaviors that we want to reduce or stop and how stimulus control interventions might help.

 Metaphor

Note that in the discussion with Samantha above, the therapist illustrates some of the stimulus control concepts by using a metaphor of a soccer game. Because Samantha is a soccer player, the example of "keeping the ball away from the net" was a concept to which Samantha could easily relate, and she could grasp the concept more easily than if the therapist had provided a dry and technical description of the methods of impulse control.

• Blaise engages in substance abuse that feels out of control. As part of helping her gain control over her drug use, we could consider building in barriers to drug use. Flushing her existing supply of cocaine down the toilet would be one obvious choice. Of course she can get more, but we're making it more difficult for her to use by building in the additional step of having to go get the drugs. We would also want to know whether she's keeping drug paraphernalia in her home. The existence of such paraphernalia not only makes it easy for her to use, but it probably also serves as a cue to use. So getting rid of that would likely help improve her ability to get control.

• Elizabeth, our client with borderline personality disorder, engages in several impulsive behaviors when she is distressed, including excessive shopping. (In fact, she's encountered a great deal of financial hardship because she has difficulty paying off her credit cards; this leads her to be even more distressed.) Although we can't reasonably stop her from buying things, we can use stimulus control to reduce the behavior. One step might be to create barriers to the behavior. Cutting up her credit cards, or at least putting them in a safe place in her home, might be one way to make excessive shopping more difficult. Rather than carrying credit cards, she could carry only a limited amount of cash with her. We could discourage wandering aimlessly through stores, where she's bound to encounter several buying cues. We could also use cues such as a written shopping list that she takes with her when she needs to go to a store—perhaps with a written reminder not to buy anything that's not on the list. Again, that doesn't necessarily eliminate the problem, but by making it a bit more difficult to engage in the behavior, we keep the ball downfield (to borrow the soccer analogy from Samantha's transcript) and may buy her a bit more time to regain control of herself. We could also consider posting, in a strategic location, a list of alternative coping behaviors that she could try when she is feeling distressed.

Using Stimulus Control for Behaviors We Want to Increase or Start

There are times when the desired behavior isn't happening at all, or isn't happening enough. In such cases, our environmental interventions involve *removing existing barriers* to the behavior and incorporating *positive cues*. I'm not very good about going to the gym. I know I should go, but frankly, I just don't seem to have enough control over that behavior to make it happen consistently. So my strategy was to pack a gym bag every evening and put it on the passenger seat of my car. That way, when I was driving to or from work, I had the gym bag right there. I had removed a potential barrier to the behavior (the need to go get my gym clothes) and had created a positive cue (the gym bag served as a reminder of what I was supposed to do). That's a stimulus control intervention.

Christina, our depressed client, isn't getting out of the house much. So that's a behavior we want to increase. How could stimulus control interventions help here? First, we could think about the *existing barriers* to the behavior, even small ones, and figure out ways to lessen or remove them. Second, we could think of ways to build *positive cues* into her environment. Here, the therapist is working with Christina (C) on those issues.

T: Let's think about what kinds of things get in the way of going out. I realize that your feelings of depression and low energy play a big role here, and we should discuss those. However, for the moment I'd like to discuss the environmental factors that get in the way, or make it more of a hassle to get out of the house.

C: Um . . . well, I guess one thing is that I don't have a bus pass.

T: I see. How does that interfere with going out?

C: Well, it means that if I do decide to go out, I have to go look for the right change, and if I don't have change, I have to go to the store downstairs and try to get change, and they don't always want to give me change unless I'm buying something, so sometimes I have to just buy something so I can get change for the bus.

T: I can see how that could be a hassle. Without a bus pass, it becomes a big headache to get the right change. So if we want to make it as easy as possible for you to go out, what could we do about that?

C: I guess I could get a bus pass.

T: Yes, you could. What do you think about that?

C: I guess it would make it easier. And I'd save money, too, because it's cheaper to use a pass than to pay every time.

T: Sounds like a win–win situation. Would you be willing to commit to getting a bus pass this week? You don't necessarily have to use it if you don't want to, but it seems like just having it would help.

C: I could do that.

T: Great. That's a very good step in the right direction. I think it might also be helpful if you had some kind of reminder to go out—something that tells you to try. What could you think of there?

C: A reminder? Like someone calls me and says "go out now"?

T: Well, if you had someone like that, sure. But do you have someone like that?

C: No.

T: So what else could you try?

C: I can't think of anything.

T: You have a smartphone, right?

C: Yeah. Oh, maybe I could do something with that.

T: You could. Do you know how to set appointments with alarms?

C: Yeah, I can just tell it every day at such-and-such o'clock to remind me to go outside.

T: Good idea.

The stimulus control intervention for Christina, for whom we want to increase a behavior, was the opposite of what we did for Samantha, for whom we want to decrease a behavior. We're trying to alter Christina's environment by creating *positive cues* for the desired behavior and by *removing existing barriers* to the behavior.

Adapting the Process: *Stimulus Control . . .*

. . . with high-functioning clients. We all respond to positive and negative cues for behavior. Posting an article about obesity on the refrigerator door, leaving your sneakers by the door to remind you to go jogging, or programming reminders into your smartphone are all examples of this. Smartphone users can use the standard reminder app, and there are many third-party apps that are designed for this purpose (Any.do, Wunderlist, and Remember the Milk are good examples).

... *with low-functioning clients.* Lower-functioning clients may, for a variety of reasons, have many barriers to the desired behaviors. Therefore, it's often not enough simply to instruct the client to engage in a certain behavior. A thorough discussion (perhaps including family members or other people who interact regularly with the client) about barriers and how to resolve them is often necessary. Prompts to engage in desired behaviors or not to engage in unwanted behaviors should be direct, clear, and frequent.

... *with children.* Kids tend to respond well to stimulus control interventions. Reminder notes for behaviors, posted in a conspicuous place, can be helpful. For kids who like technology, there are even fancy gizmos that clients can purchase, such as Fitbits or watches that will prompt the desired behaviors at random intervals or at scheduled times (e.g., *www. watchminder.com*).

... *on the inpatient unit.* Inpatient units are a great place for stimulus control interventions, because the clinician has a good deal of control over the client's environment. Staff can verbally remind the client to engage in the desired behaviors on a regular basis, or reminders can be posted in the client's room. Staff can place limits on behaviors such as sleeping and eating, so that they take place at certain times and not at others. These interventions may help the client gain greater control over the behaviors.

How to do situation selection and stimulus control poorly	How to do situation selection and stimulus control like a champ
Prescribe avoidance of things that aren't objectively dangerous. If the client is excessively fearful of something, tell him or her to avoid that situation altogether. That way, the client never gets distressed (and the problem won't get solved, either).	*Prescribe approach for fearful clients.* For clients with excessive fears, it is likely that approaching the feared situation will not cause anything bad to happen (other than transient feelings of anxiety). Therefore, other strategies such as *exposure* (see Chapter 11) are usually more appropriate.
Prescribe approach for a client with limited capacity for self-control. When clients have impulsive, aggressive, or addictive problems, send them back into situations with which they can't realistically cope. That sets the client up for failure.	*Prescribe judicious avoidance for clients with limited capacity for self-control.* Sending a person with poor self-management ability back into a difficult situation can set him or her up for failure. Some degree of avoidance may be useful, at least on a temporary basis, until the client has had the chance to build and strengthen his or her capacity for self-control in CBT.
Ignore the cues. If you're looking to decrease a behavior, go ahead and leave positive cues in place so the client will constantly be encouraged to engage in the behavior he or she hopes to decrease. If you're looking to increase a behavior, leave negative cues in place so the client will constantly be discouraged from doing the behavior you want him or her to do. That'll keep the client confused.	*Emphasize the addition or subtraction of cues.* If you're looking to decrease a behavior, get the positive cues out of there and add some negative cues. If you're looking to increase a behavior, get the negative cues out of there and add some positive cues.
Ignore the barriers. Leave barriers to the desired behavior in place, so that it's extra hard for the client to make progress.	*Emphasize the addition or subtraction of barriers.* Remove barriers to the desired behavior and add barriers to the unwanted behavior.

Let's look at other clients who have behaviors that we want to increase or start and how stimulus control interventions might help.

- Nick and Johanna don't have many positive interactions with each other. They don't compliment each other or show appreciation for each other much. They don't express affection toward each other. These are behaviors we'd like to increase. We've already talked about using stimulus control to contain their problem-focused interactions, so what if we also tried to increase the frequency of loving behaviors? A strong positive cue for those behaviors might be a weekly date night in which they are instructed *not* to talk about their problems but rather to engage in more pleasant conversation—art, sports, ideas, plans, whatever. They also might benefit from some time- or situation-based reminder, such as "Every day when you get home from work, go over to Johanna, give her a kiss, and ask her how her day was." This builds a routine that serves as a positive cue.

- William, our dependent client, isn't taking the initiative to do things for himself. As we learn more about William, we find that his husband serves (accidentally) as a *negative cue* for self-sufficient behavior, because he usually sees how helpless William seems and does things for him. Since he's part of William's environment, we might consider changing the husband's behavior so that he serves as a *positive cue:* Instead of taking over and doing things for him, he could gently remind William that he can do it for himself and provide some encouraging words.

- Lauren, our client with schizophrenia, doesn't take her medications reliably. That's a big problem, because when she goes off of her medications, she deteriorates rapidly and can end up in the hospital. So we want to increase her medication-taking behavior. We might first look to eliminate barriers. Perhaps we find that Lauren keeps her medications in the living room. Simply moving them to the bathroom, where she goes first thing every morning, would help reduce that barrier. The use of a pill box for each day might similarly reduce barriers to taking medications. What about a big sign on her bathroom mirror that says "Lauren, remember to take your meds"?

 TIB Alert!

In Chapter 7, we discussed a potential hierarchy of treatment goals. TIBs are right near the top of that list. Importantly, in that hierarchy, TIBs are a higher priority than are the symptoms for which the client is seeking treatment. After all, you're not going to make much progress with a client who is not fully participating in treatment.

Of all the TIBs clients engage in, homework noncompliance is one of the most common and damaging. Clients who don't complete their CBT homework assignments tend not to get much better. We have lots of ways of addressing this problem, but stimulus control can be an important part of the intervention. Think about homework completion as a behavior that we want to increase or start. We know that stimulus control for that kind of behavior change involves creating *positive cues* for the desired behavior and *removing existing barriers* to the behavior. There are lots of ways to create reminders to complete CBT homework and reduce barriers. Making sure that the homework paperwork is easily accessible, or even using a computer program or smartphone app (there are lots of them out there for various aspects of CBT) might make homework completion easier for the client. We can schedule homework for specific times of day or create reminders in calendars or on the phone. I've sent text messages to clients reminding them to do homework, and I've even programmed my e-mail account to send a reminder e-mail once per day. All of these are stimulus control procedures aimed at increasing the behavior.

To be clear, as is true with all of the stimulus control interventions discussed in this chapter, I don't necessarily believe that stimulus control will solve the entire problem (though sometimes it does). Behavior is complex and multidetermined. If a client isn't doing homework, I'm also going to want to know about motivation, interpretations, the therapeutic relationship, contingencies, emotional factors, and much more. But stimulus control can be an important element of your intervention. I find it helpful, when a client hasn't done his or her homework, to start by asking questions such as "What got in your way?" and "What could we do about that?" rather than immediately jumping to the (mind-reading) conclusion that this client just isn't motivated enough.

THE ESSENTIALS

* Behavior is influenced by the presence of positive and negative cues.

* Situation selection refers to choosing environments to enter versus those to avoid. When using situation selection, make sure that you are not starting or perpetuating a cycle of unnecessary or unhelpful avoidance.

* Stimulus control refers to changing aspects of the person's environment in order to influence behavior.

* When the target behavior is "all over the place," stimulus control involves modifying where and when the behavior takes place, as well as associated behaviors.

* When we are trying to stop or decrease a target behavior, stimulus control involves building negative cues into the environment, removing positive cues from the environment, and creating barriers to the behavior.

* When we are trying to start or increase a target behavior, stimulus control involves building positive cues into the environment, removing negative cues from the environment, and removing barriers to the behavior.

KEY TERMS AND DEFINITIONS

Antecedents: External or internal stimuli that precede a behavioral response.

Cues: Environmental signals that tell us to perform (or not to perform) a particular behavior.

Discriminative stimulus: A stimulus that serves as a cue or signal for a certain behavioral response.

Habits: Behaviors that are performed semi-automatically in response to environmental cues.

Narrowing: A form of stimulus control that involves restricting the range of stimuli associated with a behavior.

Situation selection: Entering or avoiding certain situations in order to alter emotional and behavioral response.

Stimulus control: Altering the environment in order to increase or decrease the likelihood of a behavioral response.

Situation Selection and Stimulus Control

Note: As we get into interventions, you may find that some of the interventions do not apply to your personal target. That's OK. Do your best.

How might you use *situation selection* (e.g., avoiding certain situations or cues) to modify the personal target?

What would be the pros and cons of using situation selection in this case?

Pros	Cons

Examining the behavioral aspect(s) of your personal target, would you say that the behavior is under good stimulus control, or under poor stimulus control? Explain.

(continued)

From *Doing CBT* by David F. Tolin. Copyright © 2016 The Guilford Press. Permission to photocopy this worksheet is granted to purchasers of this book for personal use only (see copyright page for details). Purchasers can download enlarged versions of this worksheet (see the box at the end of the table of contents).

How might you use *stimulus control interventions* to modify the personal target? For example, would you modify . . .

    Where the behavior occurs?

    When the behavior occurs?

    Associated behaviors?

    Cues for the behavior or to refrain from the behavior?

    Creating or removing barriers?

Try using a situation selection or stimulus control intervention, or both, for a period of at least 3 days consistently. Write down what you tried, what it was like to do it, and whether your efforts affected the personal target.

CHAPTER 9

Contingency Management in Therapy

Behavior and Its Contingencies in Therapy

Contingencies, which we discussed in Chapter 2, are all about making a behavior go up or down. So at the most basic level, before implementing a contingency with a client, we need to think about whether the client has a *behavioral excess* or a *behavioral deficit,* what kind of movement in behavior we're trying to achieve with operant conditioning.

Expanding on our discussion of behavioral excesses and behavioral deficits from Chapter 2, sometimes it's clear that the client has a behavioral deficit, and you therefore want a certain behavior to go *up.*

- Scott, the socially anxious client, doesn't go out with his coworkers, strike up conversations with others, or go to parties. We would therefore say that he *is not interacting enough with others* and *needs to do more of that.*
- Christina, our depressed client, stays home by herself all day watching TV rather than engaging in potentially more rewarding activities. We would therefore say that she is *not doing enough rewarding activities* and *needs to do more of that.*
- William, who is highly dependent on others, rarely makes decisions for himself or initiates activities. We would therefore say that he is *not engaging in self-sufficient behaviors enough* and *needs to do more of that.* Related to his chronic pain, we might also say that he is *not engaging in enough physically challenging activities* and *needs to do more of that.*

Note that I don't include Samuel's insomnia on this list. When we talk about operant therapy, we're targeting the person's volitional behaviors. Falling asleep is a biological reflex, not a volitional behavior. Therefore, if we tried to reward Samuel for falling asleep, that probably wouldn't work. We could, however, use stimulus control (see Chapter 8) to intervene in all of the volitional behaviors he does that are related to sleep, such as encouraging his going to bed and getting up on a regular schedule, avoiding TV in bed, and so on.

Sometimes, it's clear that the client has a behavioral excess, and you therefore want a certain behavior to go *down*.

- Samantha, our client with trichotillomania, pulls her hair out. We would therefore say that she is *pulling her hair too much* and *needs to do less of that*. We want certain behaviors to go *down*.
- Lauren, our client with schizophrenia, shouts at people whom she (incorrectly) believes are harassing or following her. We would therefore say that she is *shouting at others too much* and *needs to do less of that*.
- Blaise, our client struggling with substance use, feels unable to stop using. We would therefore say that she is *using substances too much* and *needs to do less of that*.
- Shari, our bulimic client, engages in bingeing and purging behaviors. We would therefore say that she is *bingeing and purging too much* and *needs to do less of that*.

I'm not including expression of emotions here. Christina cries a lot. Anna has panic attacks. Scott blushes and trembles. I think of those kinds of emotional expressions as largely biological reflexes and not good targets for operant therapy. The volitional behaviors that *accompany* those expressions, of course, are good targets. So I'm not going to target Christina's crying directly, although I might want to see that improve as we work on other behaviors that are more under her control, such as spending less time in bed. And I might not target Anna and Scott's physiological anxiety reactions directly, but I might target their escape and avoidance behaviors and see if they experience less physiological arousal as a result.

Much of the time, there's a mix in which we want some behaviors to go up, and we want others to come down. A client engages in too much of one kind of behavior and not enough of another kind of behavior.

- Elizabeth, our client with borderline personality disorder, cuts herself. We would therefore say that she is *cutting herself too much* and *needs to do less of that*. We want certain behaviors to go *down*. Elizabeth also doesn't use appropriate, assertive communication to express herself to others, which is part of why she feels a need to cut herself. We would therefore say that she is *not asserting herself enough* and *needs to do more of that*.
- Melissa, our client with complex PTSD, stays home at night because of her fears. We would therefore say that she is *not going outside enough* and *needs to do more of that*. She also lashes out at the people around her. We would therefore say that she is *lashing out too much* and *needs to do less of that*.
- Nick and Johanna, our distressed couple, argue and yell at each other frequently. We would therefore say that they are *arguing and yelling too frequently* and *need to do less of that*. At the same time, we see that they also don't express affection or speak kindly to each other very much. So they are *not expressing affection or speaking kindly enough* and *need to do more of that*.

We previously discussed how contingencies are implicated in the etiology and maintenance of maladaptive behaviors. We now turn our attention to how the CBT therapist can employ the same principles to promote positive behavior change (see Table 9.1).

TABLE 9.1. Potential operant Strategies to Increase or Decrease a Behavior

Desired Outcome	
To increase a behavior	To decrease a behavior
• Reinforcement • Escape • Premack principle	• Punishment • Penalty • Extinction • Differential reinforcement of other behavior • Differential reinforcement of lower rate of behavior (DRL) • Noncontingent (free) reinforcement

Do More of That: Increasing Desired Behavior

Let's start with getting a low-frequency behavior to occur more frequently. We know from operant conditioning that *reinforcement* of some kind will likely increase the desired behavior. We also know that there are two kinds of reinforcement: *positive reinforcement* (also called *reinforcement*) and *negative reinforcement* (also called *escape*).

Positive reinforcement (reinforcement) means that we will add something to the person's experience following the desired behavior, with the outcome being an increased likelihood that he or she will do it again (i.e., he or she is motivated to get that reinforcer again). Treats, extra privileges, attention, and praise are all examples of possible positive reinforcers (assuming, of course, that the person is motivated to obtain those things).

Negative reinforcement (escape) means that we will remove something from the person's experience following the desired behavior, with the outcome being an increased likelihood that he or she will do it again (i.e., he or she is motivated to get away from something). Negative reinforcement isn't used much in CBT, because it essentially means that you start with some kind of aversive circumstance that is alleviated when the person performs the desired behavior. In addition to having a potential for pretty negative side effects, one could certainly raise ethical questions about creating (or allowing) aversive conditions for the client.

We have another potential way to implement reinforcement, called the **Premack principle.** Simply put, the Premack principle (Premack, 1962) means that you can reinforce low-frequency behaviors (those things that the client isn't doing enough of) with higher-frequency behaviors (those things that the client is happy to do). Did your mom ever tell you that you couldn't have dessert until you ate your veggies? If so, she was using the Premack principle. Eating veggies was your low-frequency behavior (meaning if you had a choice, you'd do it at a low frequency), so she reinforced it by pairing it with the high-frequency behavior (meaning if you had a choice, you'd do it at a high frequency) of eating dessert. We use the Premack principle whenever we employ a "you get to do this after you do that" guideline. This principle can be self-directed, such as when we instruct a client to delay TV until after his or her CBT homework has been completed, or it can be directed by external parties, such as when parents require a child to do his or her chores before going out to play.

Do Less of That: Decreasing Undesired Behavior

Sometimes, we want a high-frequency behavior to become less frequent or to stop altogether. We know that *punishment* is one way to make a behavior go down, and that there are two kinds of punishment: *positive punishment* (also called *punishment*) and *negative punishment* (also called *penalty*).

Positive punishment (punishment) means that we will add something to the person's experience following the unwanted behavior, with the outcome being a decreased likelihood that he or she will do it again (i.e., he or she is motivated to avoid whatever we added). Spankings are one kind of punishment (note: don't spank your client). So are things like electric shocks or drugs like disulfiram (Antabuse), which causes vomiting when the person drinks alcohol. So are interventions in which the person has to correct, clean up, or "fix" the aftereffects of his or her undesired behavior.

Negative punishment (penalty) means that we will remove something from the person's experience following the unwanted behavior, with the outcome being a decreased likelihood that he or she will do it again (i.e., he or she is motivated to not have that taken away). Time-outs are one kind of penalty, because they involve a removal from desired social stimulation. Financial penalties, in which the person gives up an amount of money after performing the behavior, are another.

We also know from operant conditioning that *extinction* procedures will decrease behavior. We use extinction when we stop reinforcing the behavior. So, for example, if a client is engaging in an unwanted behavior in order to receive attention from others, cutting off attention for that behavior would be predicted to reduce the behavior over time. Of course, finding out what's been reinforcing the behavior is often tricky. In addition, when we use extinction we may have to contend with the short-term *extinction burst*, which can be a small problem or a big problem, depending on the person, the behavior, and the situation.

We can add a few more strategies for decreasing an undesired behavior that avoid a lot of the pitfalls of punishment and extinction. One is called **differential reinforcement of other behavior,** or DRO for short. If we find a behavior that naturally competes with the undesired behavior, we can reinforce that as a way of "crowding out" the undesired behavior. We could decrease screaming, for example, by positively reinforcing the client for speaking calmly. We could decrease time spent in front of the TV by reinforcing more productive activities. The trick is to find a behavior that is inherently incompatible with the undesired behavior (e.g., it is impossible to scream and speak calmly at the same time).

Similarly, **differential reinforcement of lower rates of behavior (DRL)** uses reinforcers for a *decrease* in, or absence of, the behavior. That is, we can provide reinforcers when the rate of behavior decreases to a certain cutoff. We could decrease screaming, for example, by providing a reinforcer for each day (or hour, or whatever) that the client doesn't scream. Or, if that's too difficult, we could set a threshold of screaming (say, 50% of the baseline rate or less) and provide reinforcement when the frequency of the behavior falls below that baseline level.

Finally, **noncontingent (free) reinforcement** can be used to "uncouple" the behavior from its reinforcer. Let's say, for example, that the client is screaming as a way of obtaining attention from others. In this case, attention is serving as the positive reinforcer for the behavior. If we make attention freely available—that is, you can have as much attention as you want, whenever you want—then there is less incentive to engage in the unwanted behavior.

Preparing for Contingency Management

Step 1: Pick Your Target

The first step in successful contingency management is to *identify and define the target behavior.* The aim here is usually not to try to change every behavior at once; rather, we want to pick a small number (perhaps one or two at first) of target behaviors that are really important and relevant to the client's presenting problem. Defining the behavior is often tricky, because we want to make sure that everyone (e.g., the therapist, the client, family members, or other involved people) can understand and agree on our definition. We know that Melissa, our client with PTSD, is lashing out at people, but what exactly do we mean by "lashing out"? Similarly, we know that William, our dependent client, is not engaging in enough self-sufficient behaviors, but what would such behaviors entail?

Often, it's not possible to come up with an exact behavior definition for everything we want to accomplish. We might not be able to define every aspect of Melissa's lashing out, nor will we be able to define every possible example of self-sufficient behavior we want William to do. But it's important to get as close as we can to a solid definition. In general, good definitions of behavior are *objective, clear,* and *complete* (Kazdin, 1989).

- *Objective* means that the definition should refer to the observable characteristics of the behavior. That is, we want to state specifically what the client does and does not do (e.g., "Melissa speaks in a loud tone to people"), rather than the presumed emotions or internal characteristics of the person (e.g., "Melissa gets angry" or "Melissa is aggressive").

- *Clear* means that the definition would make sense to anyone who reads or hears it. So we want to make sure that we use simple terms (e.g., "William will pay household bills, without asking his husband for assistance"), rather than ambiguous terms (e.g., "William will take more initiative to do things").

- *Complete* means that we have to agree on what does and does not constitute an instance of the target behavior. We've identified the fact that Melissa speaks in a loud tone to people, but how loud is loud? Similarly, we want William to pay household bills, but does that mean all of them, or just some of them? These details need to be discussed in advance so that everyone understands them. Note that "complete" doesn't necessarily mean "addressing the entire problem." Melissa and William certainly have problems that go well beyond the finite behaviors we've identified here. But we've identified these particular behaviors as being relevant to the presenting problem and good things to work on in the short term, so we want to make sure our definitions adequately capture those behaviors.

Step 2: Know the Base Rate

The second step is to *understand the base rate of the behavior.* That is, before intervening, we need to know how frequently the behavior is occurring. How many times per day does Samantha pull out her hair? How often does Christina leave her house and engage in rewarding activities?

There is always a judgment call about what kind of base rate is considered maladaptive and what kind of base rate would be considered adaptive or at least acceptable. How much social interaction *should* Scott be having? Should he be an extrovert, or just less isolated than he is now? How much hair pulling would we accept from Samantha? None at all, or just not enough to cause visible hair loss? Should Blaise aim for complete abstinence, or should we strive for moderation in her substance use?

There are few hard and fast answers here. Therefore, this needs to be addressed collaboratively with the client. What would the client find acceptable or desirable (e.g., how active a lifestyle would Christina ideally like to have?). Similarly, the therapist must use his or her knowledge about the target behaviors to make recommendations (e.g., is moderate substance use likely to be effective in the long term for Blaise?). In some cases, especially in institutional settings, other staff members may need to be involved in the discussion (e.g., what frequency of shouting would be acceptable in Lauren's case and make her a candidate for discharge?).

In many cases, the client can and should help with this. Self-monitoring is a great way to assess the frequency of a behavior. For example, we could give Samantha a self-monitoring form and ask her to record, for one full week, each time she pulls out a hair. Sometimes, we can enlist the aid of people who have the opportunity to observe the client in his or her environment. We could, for example, ask Christina's husband to record every time Christina goes out to do something. Our own observations during therapy can be helpful. For example, we can keep track of how many times a desired or unwanted behavior occurs during therapy sessions. In some therapeutic settings, we have the opportunity to engage in prolonged observations of the client. On an inpatient unit, for example, we might opt to watch the client for an extended period of time, noting how many times a desired or unwanted behavior occurs.

Defining the base rate requires some decision making. Some kinds of behaviors lend themselves more naturally to one kind of assessment over another.

- In some cases we might choose to attend to how *often* a behavior occurs. For example, Samantha's hair pulling might lend itself to this kind of measurement—in a given day, how many times does she do it?

- In other cases, we might choose to attend to how *long* the behavior continues. We want Scott to interact with people more, so rather than trying to count every social interaction he has (especially if Scott makes them very brief), it might be more productive for us to measure how much total time per day he spends interacting with people. A sample form for the measurement of frequency and duration of behavior is shown in Figure 9.1 and reprinted in Appendix B.

- In still others, we might want to know the *proportion of time* that is being spent performing desired and unwanted behaviors. This is particularly helpful when our ability to observe is limited. If Christina is on an inpatient unit, for example, we might not be able to watch her all day and add up how much time she spends in and out of bed. But we could check on her every 15 minutes and make a rating of whether she is in or out of bed at that moment. By calculating the proportion of total observations in which she was out of bed, we can get a rough idea of the proportion of the day she was out of bed. A sample form for this use is shown in Figure 9.2, and a blank version is provided in Appendix B.

Date and time	Antecedents: Describe what was happening right *before* the behavior.	How many times did the client do the behavior?	How long did the client do the behavior?	Consequences: Describe what happened right *after* the behavior.
10/23 4:00 pm	Watching TV and feeling stressed out	3 hairs pulled	10 minutes	Felt a sense of relief

FIGURE 9.1. Sample monitoring form for frequency, duration, antecedents, and consequences of behavior.

Observation	1	2	3	4	5	6	7	8	9
Behavior present?	(Y) N	(Y) N	Y (N)	(Y) N	Y (N)	Y (N)	(Y) N	Y (N)	(Y) N

FIGURE 9.2. Sample form for monitoring the proportion of observations in which a behavior is present.

Step 3: Functional Analysis: What Comes Before and After?

The third step is to develop a *functional analysis* of behavior. As described in Chapter 5, functional analysis is a means of understanding *why* a behavior does or does not occur by looking at the *antecedents* (what comes before the behavior) and the *consequences* (what comes after the behavior). Antecedents are our triggers (modified by internal factors such as attention, thoughts, and emotions), and consequences are our contingencies.

So, as one example, let's say we want to understand Elizabeth's self-injurious behaviors. We might find out that a common antecedent of these behaviors is an interpersonal conflict of some kind, especially when the other person seems to ignore or belittle her. And we might further learn that a common consequence of (reinforcer for) her behavior is attention from other people.

We can find out the antecedents and consequences of the behavior in the same ways that we find out the base rate of the behavior. So, in many cases, the client is a good source of information. Even clients who struggle to understand "why" they do something can tell us about what came before the behavior and what came after the behavior. Self-monitoring forms can be used for this. An example is shown in Figure 9.3, and a blank version is provided in Appendix B.

We can often observe these things ourselves. Whether in a therapy session or in a contained treatment setting, as we note the behavior's occurrence, we can track the antecedents and consequences of the behavior, as shown in Figure 9.1.

Step 4: Pick Your Contingencies

The fourth step is to *identify the contingencies to be used.* If reinforcement is to be used, we have to have an idea of what the client would find reinforcing. Everyone is different, so this has to be determined on a case-by-case basis.

Reinforcers may include (but are certainly not limited to):

- Interpersonal (e.g., attention, praise, extra time with a liked person).
- Food (e.g., special snacks or drinks).

Date and time	What was happening right *before* the behavior?	How many times did you do the behavior?	How long did you do the behavior?	What happened right *after* the behavior?
9/10 2:30 pm	With my friends who were drinking, felt left out	5 drinks	2 hours	I felt better, buzzed, like I was part of the group

FIGURE 9.3. Sample self-monitoring form for behavior.

- Material (e.g., magazines, toys).
- Desired activities (e.g., watching TV, playing games—this is the Premack principle).

Punishers (positive punishers) should be used with extreme caution, if at all, and, in general, reinforcement seems to be a better strategy. But I'll discuss punishment briefly here. For positive punishment, the idea is that the punisher should be strong enough that the person is highly motivated to avoid it and that therefore it won't have to be used much. Mild punishments are often not strong enough to deter the behavior—over time, the client can habituate to the mild punisher, and the clinician ends up overusing the punisher (indeed, the person administering the punishment can be negatively reinforced for doing so)—so mild punishment can actually pose a greater ethical problem than strong punishment. Whenever we're considering the use of punishment, we need to think clearly about whether the benefits of using punishment outweigh the costs. That is, are you doing the client a greater disservice by using punishment or by *not* using punishment and allowing a potentially dangerous behavior to persist? Or, alternatively, what are the pros and cons of using punishment versus other potential methods of behavior control, such as restraints or sedating medications? I can think of some cases in which one could make an ethical argument for the use of punishment. As one example, some researchers have used electrical shocks to stop dangerous head-banging behavior in people with autism (Linscheid, Iwata, Ricketts, Williams, & Griffin, 1990). One method involves a sensor, worn on the head, that detects potentially self-injurious blows to the head and transmits a signal to a module on the arm or leg that delivers an electric shock (roughly the pain equivalent of a rubber band snapped on the arm or leg) whenever the head is strongly hit or banged against a wall. Overall, these devices seem to dramatically reduce head banging, have fairly durable effects, and don't seem to have severe adverse effects (Lichstein & Schreibman, 1976). Now, I'm not necessarily endorsing this method, but it does raise a really challenging ethical question about which is the greater evil—using pain to decrease the behavior or allowing the client to continue behavior with a potential for serious injury.

I'm not going to talk much about the use of physically aversive punishment in this book. But if an aversive punishment is to be used, I would recommend you include the following steps (see Matson & Kazdin, 1981):

1. Determine first that punishment is absolutely necessary. That means, in most cases, that you have already tried other strategies and they have not been effective.
2. Do a careful cost–benefit analysis. What are the costs and benefits of using punishment in this case? What are the costs and benefits of *not* using punishment in this case?
3. Obtain consultation from at least one "neutral" party who can advise and monitor the ethical issues that come up. If you work for a hospital, for example, include someone from the administration or an in-house review committee who is tasked with overseeing the well-being of the client.
4. Make sure that you have obtained informed consent from the client or, if the client has been declared incompetent, from a legally appointed guardian.
5. Find the right level of punishment. As I mentioned previously, the punisher should be strong enough that you don't have to use it very much. At the same time, however, it should not be so strong that it harms the client.
6. Do it extremely carefully and deliberately. Don't get sloppy with punishment. Have one person, or a small team of people, whose job is to administer, monitor, and document the use of punishers.

7. Include a reinforcement arm (e.g., DRO) to the program. That is, whenever you try to stop one behavior, try to encourage a different one.
8. Make sure that the necessity of the punisher is decreasing over time. Theoretically, if the punisher is effective, then the behavior will decrease, and the punisher will not be needed as much. If you find that the behavior is *not* decreasing, then your punisher is not really serving as a punisher, technically speaking. That signals a need to reevaluate the plan quickly.

One alternative kind of punisher, which does not employ physically aversive stimulation, is **overcorrection.** In overcorrection, following the occurrence of an unwanted behavior, the client is instructed to engage in a more desirable behavior. Overcorrection includes two components: First, the client corrects the environmental consequences of the unwanted behavior (e.g., if the client made a mess during an outburst, the client is instructed to clean up the mess). This step is sometimes called *restitution.* Second, the client overrehearses the desirable behavior (e.g., the client is instructed to clean up messes made by other people as well). This step is sometimes called *positive practice.*

Penalty (negative punishment) is more commonly used and is generally fraught with fewer cost–benefit and ethical concerns than is positive punishment (though such concerns are by no means absent). Here, the idea is that something is taken away following an unwanted behavior.

Perhaps the most readily identifiable example of penalty is the **time-out.** In this strategy (which can range from being sent to one's room at home to being placed in a seclusion room on a hospital unit), the person is physically removed from the location where the unwanted behavior is taking place and brought to a location that is devoid of potential reinforcers (e.g., attention from other people).

Other penalty strategies include **response cost,** in which the client gives something up following an occurrence of the unwanted behavior. My administrative assistant has a "swear jar" on her desk, and every time I or one of my staff curses in her office, we have to put a quarter in the jar. That's response cost. It costs something to swear, so we reevaluate how much we want or need to swear. In clinical settings, clients have been "fined" tokens in a token economy (see later discussion), or clients have agreed to pay a certain amount to someone when they engage in an unwanted behavior. As one classic example, a man who drank excessively agreed to pay his wife $20 to spend as she wished every time he drank more than a specified amount in a day. His drinking behavior quickly came under control (P. M. Miller, 1972). My all-time favorite, though, is a case example of penalty for nail biting. The client, who was politically conservative, agreed to donate $10 to the American Communist Party (an organization she hated) if she did not exhibit evidence of nail growth. Nail biting stopped immediately, and the client remained free of nail biting 8 months after treatment ended (Ross, 1974).

Step 5: Get Buy-In from Everyone

The fifth step is to *get agreement from as many parties as possible.* Depending on the treatment setting, the client, and the nature of the problem, the parties involved in contingency management might include the therapist, the client, family members (e.g., parents, spouse), other treating clinicians, and unit staff. Contingency management requires consistency in order to be successful. Often, it takes just one person to be "not on board" with the program for it to fall apart.

Some clients in some treatment settings are unlikely to be invested in behavior change, at least at first. Some clients are being treated involuntarily, either through hospitalization or because of a court order. Some children might be in treatment primarily at the insistence of their parents. Cases such as these pose a special set of problems for contingency management (and for any other therapeutic intervention).

It's important to try to get some degree of buy-in from the client. Motivational interviewing strategies (see Chapter 7) can be a helpful way to get the client thinking about the pros and cons of behavior change. Less insightful clients might have a hard time identifying intrinsic benefits of changing behavior. Sometimes, however, they might be motivated by external goals such as "getting my parents off my back" or "getting released from the hospital sooner." It's not ideal, but it might be enough to work with.

Contingency management *can* work, at least to some extent, without the client's buy-in, so long as the selected contingencies are powerful enough to be motivating. But it will likely be much more effective if you can help the client find a reason to get involved with the process.

The agreement from all parties should include, at a minimum:

- A clear definition of the target behavior(s), either desired or unwanted.
- The specific, concrete aims of the contingency management plan.
- An objective description of what the behavioral contingencies will be, how they will be delivered, who will deliver them, and when they will be delivered.
- The duration of the contingency management plan.
- The frequency of check-ins to monitor progress, who will conduct the check-ins, and what information will be gathered.

Contingency Management in Action: Prompt–Praise–Ignore

A very straightforward program of contingency management that can be used in a variety of institutional settings is what I call the **prompt–praise–ignore plan.** This plan uses interpersonal contact in a variety of ways, without relying on tangible reinforcers. The steps are:

1. *Prompt:* The therapist or other staff member prompts the client to engage in the desired behavior when they see that it is not occurring when it should, or when identified antecedents of the behavior are present. So, for example, staff might use a prompt such as "This would be a good time to make eye contact," or "Remember to use your assertive speaking skills." This is an example of creating *positive cues* (see Chapter 8).
2. *Praise:* When the client engages in the desired behavior, staff praises the client with statements such as "Nice job!" or "Great!" In this way, praise is used as a *reinforcer.*
3. *Ignore:* When the client engages in an unwanted behavior, staff withdraws attention from the client. Usually this means something like abruptly walking away from the client and ignoring him or her for a specified period of time (e.g., 10 minutes). In this way, withdrawal of attention is used as a *penalty* (specifically, *response cost*). To the extent that attention was a desired reinforcer for the unwanted behavior, withdrawal of attention may also serve an *extinction* function.

Of course, the prompt–praise–ignore plan will only work under certain conditions. The client has to be able to attend to, and comprehend, the prompt. The client also has to find the praise reinforcing (meaning he or she will do more of the desired behavior in order to obtain it). Finally, the client has to find being ignored somewhat aversive. It goes back to your meaty conceptualization of this particular client. No two clients are exactly the same, and therefore you can't automatically assume that a reinforcer or punisher for one client will serve as a reinforcer or punisher for another client. It's only a reinforcer if the person will do more of the behavior to get it, and it's only a punisher if the person will do less of the behavior to avoid it.

A Note on Extinction

Whenever we talk about ignoring a problem behavior, such as in the prompt–praise–ignore plan, we have to think through a few potential pitfalls. Perhaps the biggest concern is the *extinction burst*. Sometimes, the client's initial reaction to the absence of reinforcement will be to increase, rather than decrease, the behavior in an attempt to get the reinforcer (attention). And sometimes unit staff will give in at that point and give the client the attention he or she seeks. Now we've just reinforced the escalation, and we're in trouble. So extinction plans need to be administered carefully and consistently. Another concern is that sometimes it's simply not safe to ignore an unwanted behavior altogether. For example, if a client is self-injuring, ignoring it just can't happen. But we can try, in such cases, to minimize the amount of attention the client receives. I have instructed medical staff, for example, to tend to a client's self-inflicted wounds but to not make small talk or eye contact with the client other than the minimal amount necessary to provide appropriate medical care.

Contingency Management in Action: The Token Economy

As you might imagine, it's often not feasible to hand out tangible reinforcers for every instance of a desired behavior. First, that can add up to an awful lot of reinforcers, which would become burdensome for clinical staff. Second, providing tangible reinforcers might interrupt the client, keeping him or her from doing the very thing we want him or her to do. Third, when we overreinforce, **satiation** kicks in, in which the reinforcer stops being reinforcing. As just one example, let's say we're using pieces of candy as a reinforcer. The client can only eat so much candy. After a while, he or she becomes full, and then candy loses its reinforcement value.

It's often helpful, therefore, to use smaller, symbolic reinforcers that can be cashed in later for the real reinforcer. Money is a great example of a symbolic reinforcer. You can't eat it, you can't wear it, you can't live in it—but after accumulating some of it, you can use it to buy the things you want.

Now, I'm not (necessarily) suggesting we start handing out cash when clients engage in the desired behavior. But we can do something analogous to this. Many behavioral plans involve a **token economy** (Ayllon & Azrin, 1968), in which clients earn some kind of symbolic reinforcer (a token, such as a poker chip or a star on a chart) and these tokens can later be cashed in to "purchase" a desired tangible reward, activity, privilege, and so forth.

I have a token economy going on in my house. My kids don't like to do their homework for school (chips off the old block, they are). So I have a chart on the refrigerator in which they get a star each day they do their homework. At the end of the week, an amount of money is given, which serves as their allowance. So the star serves as a token *reinforcer*, which is later cashed in for money (in itself a token reinforcer), which they then use to buy what they want (the actual reinforcer).

Let's look at a couple of clinical examples of token economies. Nick and Johanna, our distressed couple, are having a hard time controlling their son, James. In particular, they've been having trouble getting him to get ready for school and out the door on time. Every morning is a huge struggle between James and his parents. James argues about getting out of bed, getting dressed, eating breakfast, and getting out the door. Often, he misses the school bus, and Nick or Johanna has to drive him to school. That causes Nick and Johanna to be more rushed and cranky, and they end up even more frustrated and less willing to work together as partners. So let's help Nick and Johanna set up a token economy for James.

1. We want to *identify and define the target behavior* in a manner that is objective, clear, and complete. So rather than making it something vague like "James has a bad attitude in the morning," we'll identify it as: "James does not get out of bed on time, get dressed, eat breakfast, and get on the bus on time." We want him to do *more* of certain behaviors that are currently not happening enough, so we're probably going to want to use a reinforcement-based program.

2. We want to *understand the base rate of the behavior*. It's probably easiest for now to have Nick and Johanna monitor James's morning routine (although if we can get James to do it himself, so much the better—we want to include him and give him a sense of control over the process). So for a full week, let's ask Nick and Johanna to use a checklist indicating, for each day, whether or not James did the desired behaviors. We'll use the frequency of the behavior as our measure.

3. We want a *functional analysis* of James's morning behavior. From his parents' monitoring form, we find that the behavior can occur on any day but seems more likely to happen on Monday mornings after he's been home for the weekend. We find a potentially important *consequence* of the behavior, which is that Nick and Johanna let him be late (often he watches TV while they get ready to leave) and drive him to school.

4. We want to *identify the contingencies to be used*. We know that James likes to watch TV. Currently, he gets to watch just about as much TV as he wants—indeed, as mentioned above, TV is actually serving as a reinforcer for his disruptive school routine. We can turn that around and use TV as a reinforcer for the desired behaviors. We're not seeing an immediate need for punishers at this time. We could think of his arguing behavior as something to decrease, but let's see how reinforcement works first. We want to use the least aversive program possible.

5. We want to *get agreement from as many parties as possible*. We need to make sure that both Nick and Johanna are fully on board with the process, so that they don't end up sending him an inconsistent message. You can just imagine how disastrously this will turn out if Johanna enforces the rules and Nick doesn't.

For James's token economy, a star chart seems like a reasonable thing to try. We create a chart such as that shown in Figure 9.4 and provided as a blank form in Appendix B.

Note that we're not addressing all of James's behavior problems right now. He certainly has a bunch of them. But contingency management programs work best when you keep them simple. Once we have a sense that James can reliably go through the morning routine and go off to school on time, we may switch the program so that he will earn stars for other desired behaviors.

By the way, let me just make a side note that even though James is not our client, by working on James's behavior in this way, we're working toward our treatment goal of helping Nick and Johanna with their marriage. First, we hope that James will shape up a bit and therefore put less stress on our clients. Second, and perhaps this is even more important, we're giving Nick and Johanna an opportunity to work together on a common problem in a way that is productive and doesn't start arguments. We might even program in some shared pleasant activities by having Nick and Johanna go out for coffee together to review James's behavior plan.

Token economies can also be used in institutional settings. Lauren, our client with schizophrenia, is on an inpatient psychiatric unit. She has been screaming at people, which is highly disruptive to the other clients. Let's work through the steps of setting up a token economy for her.

1. *Identify and define the target behavior.* We want to define screaming as objectively as possible. Assuming we can't realistically follow her around with a decibel meter, we could come up with something like "speaking at a volume that could be heard down the hall."

2. *Understand the base rate of the behavior.* For this, we would probably want to have the unit staff complete a checklist of some kind so that we can track the behavior over time. Unit staff members are busy, so it might not be realistic to have them record every single instance of the behavior. Instead, we could use periodic observations with a check-list, such as that shown in Figure 9.2. The frequency of observations depends on a lot of feasibility factors; however, we know that there are shift changes at 7 A.M., 3 P.M., and 11 P.M. We could ask the outgoing charge nurse, at the end of each shift, to rate whether the unwanted behavior was observed during that shift. That would give us three observation periods per day.

The desired behavior is: _Go through the morning routine and get on bus on time._

Defined as: _Get out of bed by 7 am, get dressed, eat breakfast, and get on the bus when it arrives._

The reward for the desired behavior is: _James will earn 1 star for each weekday he does the above (maximum 5 per week), and will be allowed to watch 1 hour of TV per star he earns._

	Sun	Mon	Tues	Wed	Thurs	Fri	Sat	Total
Week 1			★					1
Week 2			★			★		2
Week 3			★		★	★		3
Week 4		★		★	★	★		4

FIGURE 9.4. Sample Behavior Star Chart.

3. *Conduct a functional analysis.* We want to know the antecedents and consequences of Lauren's screaming behavior. We might do some observation on the unit for this. We learn, in this case, that Lauren's screaming often follows some other kind of chaos on the unit, such as mealtime or large numbers of clients moving from one area to another. We also learn that Lauren's screaming is often followed by an increase in attention from staff, asking her what's wrong. We might hypothesize (though it is just a hypothesis at this point) that the extra staff attention is serving as a reinforcer for the unwanted behavior. But that also signals to us that Lauren finds attention to be reinforcing. We can use that information.

4. *Identify the contingencies to be used:* We want Lauren to do *less* screaming. We know that punishment, penalty, extinction, DRO, DRL, and noncontingent (free) reinforcement are the strategies that can decrease behavior. Let's take punishment off the table for the moment (see earlier discussion for the many reasons to do so). Extinction and DRO could come into play by using the *prompt–praise–ignore* plan. That is, if we identify a more desired behavior, such as speaking calmly to people in a normal tone of voice, we could (a) remind her to speak calmly when a social interaction is coming up, (b) reinforce her for that behavior when it occurs, and (c) ignore her when she screams. We may want to increase the reward value of the program for Lauren, so we talk to her and get a sense of what she likes and values. It turns out that she does like attention from people. She also likes certain magazines that they don't have on the unit, and she likes listening to music. All of these are potential reinforcers.

Note that I don't want to select reinforcers that Lauren naturally has a right to have. Nor do I want to select reinforcers that are already freely available on the unit (these would be ineffective). The idea is that Lauren should be able to earn something "extra."

5. *Get agreement from as many parties as possible.* This might be the hardest part of the program. With so many unit staff members over three shifts per day, we need to make sure that everyone understands the plan, knows exactly what they're supposed to do, and agrees to stick to the plan. Most likely, we're going to have to have a series of staff meetings in order to make this work. Remember, one person can wreck it. For example, if the night shift staff reinforces a behavior you've been trying to extinguish during the day, you're probably not going to get a good result.

For Lauren's token economy, we'll use a chart kept at the nurse's station, combined with poker chips to be given as tokens. We create a chart such as that shown in Figure 9.5 and provided as a blank form in Appendix B. Lauren will earn a token when she goes through a full shift without screaming, and she can later cash those tokens in for things she wants.

Note that, in this case, we are using DRL, in which we provide reinforcement when the rate of behavior decreases to a certain cutoff (in this case, zero per shift). Doing that by itself may not be terribly effective. But here we're combining it with the *prompt–praise–ignore* plan, so rather than just telling Lauren what not to do and hoping she can earn tokens for that, we're giving her clear instructions about desired, alternative behaviors.

We could opt to employ a punishment strategy, specifically *penalty,* in this case. That would mean that Lauren can *lose* tokens as well as gain them. If the reinforcement plan we have here doesn't seem to be sufficient, we could consider a penalty aspect in which Lauren loses a token, for example, whenever she screams at someone. But again, we always want to use the least aversive plan possible, so let's try reinforcement first.

The desired behavior is: _Decrease screaming._

Defined as: _Speak at a normal volume. Do not speak at a volume that can be heard down the hall._

The reward for the desired behavior is: _Lauren will earn 1 token for each shift she does the above, and will be allowed to purchase items from the list with her tokens._

Behavior (_screaming_) present? Y/N				Total "no"
	7 am–3 pm	3 pm–11 pm	11 pm–7 am	
Monday	(Y) N	(Y) N	Y (N)	1
Tuesday	Y (N)	(Y) N	Y (N)	2
Wednesday	Y (N)	Y (N)	Y (N)	3

List of items that can be purchased:

Magazine: 1 token

30 minutes of listening to music: 2 tokens

30 minutes of extra individual staff time: 3 tokens

FIGURE 9.5. Sample Token Economy Chart for Institutions.

The Science behind It

There are a multitude of variations of the token economy, and there's no way I could possibly do them all justice here. In brief, though, token economies have been used effectively for purposes as varied as decreasing aggressive behavior on inpatient psychiatric units (LePage, 1999; LePage et al., 2003), improving social functioning and decreasing disorganized behavior among psychotic clients (Maley, Feldman, & Ruskin, 1973; Schwartz & Bellack, 1975), improving treatment attendance and drug abstinence (negative urine screens) among substance-using outpatients (Ledgerwood, Arfken, Petry, & Alessi, 2014; Petry & Carroll, 2013; Petry et al., 2005), improving treatment compliance in medically ill children (Carton & Schweitzer, 1996; da Costa, Rapoff, Lemanek, & Goldstein, 1997), improving healthy eating habits among obese individuals (L. H. Epstein, Masek, & Marshall, 1978), and improving functional behavior in people with autism (Matson & Boisjoli, 2009). In one novel group therapy application, the tokens function like raffle tickets. All members of the group put their tokens in a bowl (and those performing more of the desired behaviors get more tokens to put in), and tokens are then drawn and prizes given out (Petry, DePhilippis, Rash, Drapkin, & McKay, 2014).

Contingency Management in Action: Self-Control Strategies

So far we've talked about operant interventions that are administered by another person or people. But operant strategies can be self-administered as well. **Self-control** is a broad term that refers to operant treatment that is largely directed by, and administered by, the client (with the therapist's guidance). The basic steps of self-control interventions (Kanfer, 1971) are:

1. Identifying and monitoring the target behavior.
2. Conducting a *functional analysis* of the antecedents and consequences of the behavior.
3. Intervening at the event level (see Chapter 8), such as situation selection or stimulus control.
4. Constructing a process of self-reinforcement for desired behaviors.

It's often helpful to use a **contingency contract,** which specifies the specific target behaviors and the contingencies to be used. The contract can be between two people (e.g., a parent and child, or between spouses), or the person can make it with him- or herself. In either case, we're formalizing the agreement and clearly identifying what will happen. A sample contingency contract for Blaise, our client struggling with a substance use relapse, is shown in Figure 9.6, and a blank contract is provided in Appendix B.

In this example, Blaise selected two different kinds of contingencies. The first was *reinforcement* for two specific behaviors (abstaining from substance use and attending support group meetings). She also opted to use *penalty* for substance use. Again, punishment strategies such as penalty may or may not be needed; you'll need to review this on a case-by-case basis, carefully weighing the pros and cons. Should the penalty arm of the contract prove financially burdensome or emotionally demoralizing to Blaise, the therapist might recommend dropping it and switching to a reinforcement-only plan.

I, *Blaise*_____, intend to make the following behavior change(s):

1. *I will not use drugs*

2. *I will attend all of my meetings*

3. _____

My reward system for making these change(s) will be:

1. When I *stay clean for 48 hours*_____, I will *go out for coffee and dessert*____ .

2. When I *attend 7 meetings in a row*____, I will *go to the movies*____ .

3. When I _____, I will _____ .

My penalty system (optional) for not making these change(s) will be:

1. When I *use drugs*_____, I will *give $10 to a charity I don't like*__ .

2. When I _____, I will _____ .

3. When I _____, I will _____ .

FIGURE 9.6. Sample Contingency Contract.

It can be helpful to identify *competing behaviors* as part of a self-control strategy. This relates to the principle of DRO. Ideally, we find a behavior that is fundamentally incompatible with the problem behavior. One example is the use of **competing response training.** Originally devised as part of a broader package called *habit reversal training* (Azrin & Nunn, 1973), competing response training involves identifying a behavior that competes with, or is otherwise incompatible with, the unwanted behavior.

Here, the therapist uses competing response training with Samantha (S), our young client with trichotillomania (adapted from Franklin & Tolin, 2007). The idea is to try to have Samantha practice some kind of competing behavior as an alternative to hair pulling. Initially, the aim is simply to get Samantha used to the exercise, rather than to prevent pulling.

T: Let's start to work on reducing your hair pulling. I'd like to see if we can identify something else you can do with your hands whenever you find yourself pulling. We want to make sure it's something that you can do easily, without needing a lot of preparation. It also has to be something that you can sustain for three minutes. It also has to be something that would physically prevent you from pulling—meaning you couldn't pull hair while doing it. Any ideas?

S: Hmm, that's hard. I've tried things like playing with a stress ball; that really didn't work for me.

T: When you tried using the stress ball before, how did you do it?

S: Well, I would just go get it when I felt like pulling, and then I'd just play around with it for a few seconds. But a lot of the time I found that I would start pulling while I was looking for the ball. And even if I could hold out until I found the ball, it seemed like I'd just start pulling again once I put it down.

T: So perhaps we could make that work better by changing a couple of things. First we have the fact that searching for the ball isn't helping. How could we fix that?

S: I guess I could keep the ball in my pocket. It's pretty small so I could do that.

T: Great idea. But I know that sometimes you pull in the bathroom, right when you get out of the shower. What would you do then?

S: Well, I have a couple of those stress balls—maybe I could just keep one on the bathroom counter?

T: That sounds like a good plan. And we have this other part—in your experience, you start pulling as soon as you put the stress ball down. There are a couple of things you told me about how you use the ball that give me some clues about how we could improve that. You said that you would just kind of play around with the ball—what would you do, exactly?

S: I'd just, you know, hold it, maybe give it a squeeze or two.

T: So perhaps we could change that up by having you squeeze the ball right from the start and hold onto it really tightly the whole time, like you're trying to fatigue the muscles of your hand. The other thing you said was that you would only play with the ball for a few seconds. How about if we increase that, and have you squeeze the ball for 3 whole minutes?

S: Well, I get the part about squeezing the ball; that makes sense. But why 3 minutes? That seems like a long time.

T: Yes, it is a long time. That's part of what may be helpful about it. You see, often, beating urges to pull doesn't necessarily mean that you have to be 100% free of the urges, 100% of the time. In many cases, all you really need is to be able to get through that immediate period when the urges are really strong. By squeezing the stress ball for 3 minutes, what you're doing is making sure that you're squeezing long enough for the urge to come down to a level where you can resist it.

S: But what happens if I get another urge after the 3 minutes?

T: My hope is that after 3 minutes, your urges will feel a lot more controllable. But if you get another urge, then you would just squeeze the ball again for another 3 minutes.

S: OK, I guess I can try it.

T: Great. Let me show you how it will go. (*Takes a stress ball from the desk drawer and places it on the desk.*) I have my stress ball here, on the bathroom counter, just like we agreed. Now I'll start brushing my teeth, just like you do. (*Mimics brushing teeth.*) Now, I start looking at my hair in the mirror, and my hand goes up to my head. (*Starts playing with hair.*) I find a hair that feels kind of coarse, one that I'd really like to pull. (*Removes hand from hair and picks up stress ball with the same hand.*) So now I drop what I'm doing, grab the stress ball, and squeeze. And I'll hold it that way for 3 minutes. Now you try it. (*Places the stress ball in front of Samantha.*)

S: OK. (*Mimics brushing teeth.*)

T: That's good. Now, look in the mirror and see that hair. Put your hand up there and feel around until you find a really good, coarse hair. (*Samantha does so.*) Very good. What are you experiencing right now?

S: I'd like to pull it.

T: Perfect. On a scale from 0 to 10, how strong is that urge to pull?

S: About an 8.

T: OK. Now, quickly, drop your hand away from your head and grab the stress ball. Squeeze it nice and hard—not so hard that you hurt your hand, but hard enough that it would make your hand muscles start to get tired. (*Samantha does so.*) Now let's look at the clock and wait for 3 minutes to go by. (*Both wait for 3 minutes.*) Excellent; you can put the ball down now. On a scale from 0 to 10, how strong is your urge to pull hair right now?

S: Maybe a 2.

T: So you see, your urge can come down even if you don't pull hair—you can wait it out and just stay on top of the urge, without giving in to it, and it will eventually decrease.

Samantha's self-monitoring sheets showed that her hair pulling frequency decreased over the next 2 weeks but was not completely eliminated. The therapist used this information as a starting point for a trouble-shooting discussion.

T: It looks like you're really doing a good job with the stress ball, and your records show me that you're pulling less hair. I also see that although you've been able to reduce the hair pulling, you're still pulling some of the time—it looks like more in the bathroom now than on the couch. Let's see if we can make this even more helpful for you. Tell me a little about the times that it's working.

S: Well, the times that it's working are when I notice that I have a hold of the hair on my head and I'm about to pull it, and I can get myself to put my hand down and pick up the stress ball. Usually, if I can do that, I'm OK.

T: And the times that it's not working?

S: Sometimes, when I have my hand up on my head, it seems like I just don't have enough willpower to put my hand down. It's like I'm out of control or something.

T: I think I understand. And I should tell you that in my opinion, it's not an issue of willpower—you have plenty of that. When this strategy isn't working, I think it's because there are some ways that it could be more effective, not because there's something wrong with you. Perhaps what's happening is that you pass a "point of no return" when your hand is up to your scalp, and at that point it's just really hard for you to stop yourself.

S: That's definitely what it feels like. It's just too hard to take my hand away from my head.

T: OK, so knowing that, what could we do differently?

S: I don't know. . . . I guess maybe if I didn't let myself get to that point. . . .

T: You're on to something there.

S: So are we talking about grabbing the squeeze ball before my hand gets up to my head?

T: I think that might be a very good solution for you. There's a chain of events that leads up to your pulling the hair. It probably starts when you enter the bathroom, maybe even earlier, and then gathers steam when you look in the mirror, gets even stronger when you start looking at your hair, and so on, so by the time you have that one hair between your fingertips, the train is going 100 miles an hour and it's hard to put on the brakes.

S: That really seems true. It does feel like a train picking up speed.

T: And so the best way to stop the train may be to catch it while it's still moving slow, just pulling out of the station. The question, then, is: When would be the best time for you to act to interrupt that chain of events?

S: What about right when I walk up to the mirror?

T: Good idea.

S: But should I do that even if I'm not having any urges to pull?

T: Yes, I think so. Because we know from your experience that, even if you aren't having an urge right then, the urge is likely to show up eventually. So let's try to nip it in the bud.

There are several elements to note in this transcript. First, the therapist corrects Samantha's inaccurate beliefs about her lack of "willpower." A lot of clients explain their behavior in these terms. However, in our model, Samantha's hair pulling is viewed as persisting not because she lacks willpower but because she doesn't have an effective plan of action. Unwanted behaviors are viewed as being elicited by certain antecedents and reinforced by certain consequences, rather than as signs of personal weakness.

Second, the therapist emphasizes that Samantha should continue the competing behavior for an extended period of time. In some respects, this follows the principle of *overcorrection* described earlier. Primarily, however, the recommended long duration is designed to allow Samantha's urge to pull to subside while she is doing the competing behavior; briefer durations may not be as successful (Twohig & Woods, 2001), as Samantha's prior experience with the stress ball suggests.

Third, the therapist pays attention to Samantha's **behavioral chain.** Samantha's hair pulling does not happen randomly. Rather, it's part of a "chain" of behaviors that occur in sequence. In the bathroom, for example, Samantha's behavioral chain is:

1. Step out of the shower.
2. Go to the mirror.
3. Look at hair.
4. Touch hair.
5. Find an abnormal hair.
6. Pull hair.

The therapist encourages Samantha to use her competing response progressively earlier in the chain. Masters, Burish, Hollon, and Rimm (1987) make this point nicely: "Self-control procedures are most easily implemented early in a response chain. . . . Certain people seem to believe that the mark of self-control is the ability to withstand any and all temptation. In fact, it is far more correct to say that the mark of self-control is the ability to minimize temptation by early interruption of such behavioral chains" (pp. 451–452).

Contingency Management in Action: Reinforcing Clinically Relevant Behavior in Session

Operant therapy shows up in the conversation between the therapist and client as well. *Functional analytic psychotherapy* (Kohlenberg & Tsai, 1991) is a form of CBT that is based on exactly this principle.

Clinically Relevant Behaviors

In psychotherapy sessions, many clients, particularly those with impairments in interpersonal functioning, will engage in **clinically relevant behaviors** (CRBs)—that is, behaviors that are related to the problem for which the client is being treated. These behaviors can be unhealthy, or they can be healthy. Examples of unhealthy CRBs (adapted from Kohlenberg & Tsai, 1994) include:

- Elizabeth, our client with borderline personality disorder who has a long pattern of impaired interpersonal relationships, avoids eye contact during the session, answers questions by talking at length in an unfocused manner, and presents with one "crisis" after another.
- Melissa, our client with complex PTSD, is reluctant to disclose personal information during the session. At times she seems suspicious and irritable; at other times, she seems inappropriately nonchalant, making jokes rather than discussing potentially painful topics.
- William, our dependent client, often waits for the therapist to bring up topics for discussion. He rarely comes up with his own ideas, seeming to want the therapist to solve his problems for him.
- Scott, our socially anxious client, "freezes up" and is hesitant to speak during the session.

In each of these cases, we can hypothesize that the client's behavior during the therapy session is the same kind of behavior that the client displays in day-to-day life. That is, the problem is not simply that Melissa acts suspicious of the therapist; it's that she acts suspicious of people in general, and she's displaying that behavior during the session. Part of the therapist's job is to watch for these unhealthy CRBs in session. Over the course of the conversation, the therapist notices how often the behaviors occur and when they tend to occur (antecedents).

Readers familiar with psychodynamic therapy might notice the overlap here with the concept of *transference*. In both psychodynamic therapy and CBT, we're interested in how the client behaves toward the therapist, and we intend to make therapy out of it. But we're interpreting the behavior in different ways and doing different things with it. In the classic psychodynamic perspective, we view transference behaviors as reflecting unconscious conflicts, often stemming from childhood. In the CBT perspective, we don't necessarily disagree that childhood can be a factor, but we're more interested in viewing unhealthy

---

Bringing the Problem into the Room

In order to use CRBs constructively in session, the therapist has to *evoke* both unhealthy and healthy CRBs during the session. Evoking unhealthy CRBs may seem a little counterintuitive at first, but remember that therapy is most effective when the client experiences at least some of the problem during the therapy session. That gives us the opportunity to use our session time working on it. Working on a problem behavior that is occurring *right now* is potentially far more powerful than discussing it in the abstract (Goldfried, 1982).

In most cases, unhealthy CRBs will be evoked naturally throughout the course of therapy. Starting therapy with a new person, completing paperwork, doing homework, having therapeutic conversations, and preparing to terminate therapy are all naturally evocative, and different people will respond to them in different ways. The therapist pays attention to the client's behavioral reactions to these different facets of therapy.

The therapist can also evoke CRBs by asking direct questions about the therapeutic relationship (Kanter et al., 2009). For example, when discussing a client's problems of interpersonal relationships, the therapist might ask questions such as "Does that ever happen in here?" or "Do I make you feel that way as well?" These are deliberately evocative questions that may lead to a discussion of how the client's in-session behavior parallels that in real life.

We can also evoke CRBs by asking the client to indicate how he or she is thinking and feeling at any given moment. Questions such as "What's your reaction to what I just said?"; "What were you thinking or feeling on the way to therapy today?"; and "What are your feelings about our session today?" are all ways to get the client to elicit either healthy or unhealthy CRBs.

Much of the time, all we need is to evoke a *flavor* of the CRB. We don't, for example, want Elizabeth to start cutting herself in the office; we don't want Melissa to storm out of the room; we don't want Scott to be paralyzed with fear; we don't want Nick and Johanna to get into a screaming match; and we certainly don't want Shari throwing up in our office. But most of the time, when the therapeutic relationship is handled sensitively and deliberately, that's not what will happen. By asking evocative questions, we can see the client's behavioral pattern becoming activated, even if the behaviors aren't at full force.

The bottom line is that we don't need to be afraid of unhealthy CRBs, nor do we need to take great pains to avoid them. If these behaviors are part of the client's problem, we want them in the room so that we can work on them.

CRBs as an important sample of the client's overall pattern of interpersonal functioning. We further hypothesize that working on those behaviors in the session can help the client change his or her behavior pattern outside of the session.

Applying Contingencies to CRBs

During sessions, the therapist watches for and reinforces healthy CRBs during the session. Examples of healthy clinically relevant in-session behaviors may include:

- Elizabeth makes appropriate eye contact, answers questions in a focused manner, and stays on topic rather than presenting in "crisis" mode.
- Melissa discloses personal information to the therapist and displays a friendly yet serious affect.
- William initiates topics of discussion, comes up with ideas, and works to solve his own problems.
- Scott speaks freely during the session.

Reinforcing healthy CRBs can take several forms, and the therapist has to develop an understanding of the kind of therapist behaviors that the client will find reinforcing. William, for example, might respond well to the therapist saying things like "I'm glad you were able to come up with that idea." Melissa, on the other hand, might find similar comments annoying but might be reinforced when the therapist responds to her self-disclosure warmly and without criticism. In either case, the therapist is reinforcing the healthy CRB. Remember, there's no predetermined rule about what people find reinforcing. Reinforcement is whatever makes the client more likely to do the behavior, and one person's reinforcement is another person's irritant.

Generally speaking, the most reliably reinforcing therapist behaviors are those that are consistent with what might happen in the real world (Ferster, 1972; Kohlenberg & Tsai, 1994). So, for example, if an unassertive client disagrees with the therapist, one potential response would be to say something like "Thank you for disagreeing with me! That's great!" However, such a response is probably not what the client will experience outside of therapy. Rather, the therapist will likely have greater impact by demonstrating that he or she takes the statement of disagreement seriously (e.g., does not dismiss it), acknowledges the validity of the point, invites further discussion, and so forth.

Reinforcing healthy CRBs requires a great deal of self-awareness and genuineness from the therapist. To provide accurate feedback to the client about his or her in-session behavior, the therapist must first be aware of his or her personal reactions to the client's behavior and then convey, while still maintaining professionalism and appropriate boundaries, the impact of the behaviors on the therapist.

- Elizabeth's poor eye contact, unfocused responses, and "crisis" presentations make it hard for the therapist to work with her—there's little continuity from one session to the next, and Elizabeth's behavior seems to thwart the therapist's efforts to empathize with her and feel a sense of connection to her. She has to have that feedback, because this is how she acts outside of the therapy as well. But, of course, the trick is giving her that feedback in a manner that is productive rather than destructive.
- Melissa's nondisclosure, suspiciousness, and irritability get in the way of building a collaborative working alliance. Her inappropriately timed jokes, which seem to be a way of avoiding intense discussions, make it hard to know when she's being serious and what she really needs. Again, because these behaviors are representative of her

larger pattern of interpersonal behavior, the therapist points out how her behaviors are affecting their discussion in order to allow Melissa to examine and reflect on these behaviors.

● William's passivity and overreliance on the therapist is frustrating and makes it hard for the therapist to see his strengths. And because that's how he behaves toward others in general, the therapy session provides a good place to notice and address the behavior.

Now, let me throw in a big caveat, to be clear about what I'm *not* talking about. I'm not suggesting you vent your frustration at the client. I'm not suggesting you drop your empathy and unconditional positive regard. I'm not suggesting you make globally negative statements toward or about the client. What I am suggesting, however, is that we gently challenge the client's *behavior* (not the client him- or herself) in the context of the therapy session. If the client is acting in a maladaptive fashion during the session, we do the client no favors by acting as if that behavior has no effect on other people. So we call the client's attention to the behavior, suggest an alternative behavior, and reinforce that more adaptive behavior (DRO).

It's also important to note that the idea is not to punish unhealthy CRBs. Punishment has nasty side effects that you probably don't want in your therapy. Rather, we simply want to call the client's attention to them and make him- or her aware of their impact. It is best to do so after we've established a reasonably solid therapeutic relationship. It's a good idea to start that process by describing it explicitly and obtaining the client's consent (e.g., "We've talked about how it's hard for people to follow what you're saying when you go off on tangents. Is it OK for me to interrupt you when you do that with me?"). If possible, when calling attention to an unhealthy CRB, it's helpful to refer back to a previous healthy CRB as a counterexample (e.g., "You know how sometimes you are really able to express yourself with me? What's stopping you from doing that right now?"; Tsai, Kohlenberg, Kanter, & Waltz, 2009).

Let's see an example of this. Here, the therapist reinforces Melissa's (M) healthy CRB and redirects her unhealthy CRB.

T: Tell me how you felt about coming in today.

M: I was a little nervous. I didn't really know what we were going to talk about, or if I was going to get upset. But I'm glad I'm here now.

T: I'm glad you're here, too. It's nice to talk to you.

M: Whatever. It's your job to say that. I mean, what are you gonna say, "I hate talking to you?"

T: Now you seem to be withdrawing from me and using sarcasm. That makes it hard for me to understand how you really feel about things, and it makes it hard for me to know what you really need. So what is it that you're really feeling?

There are some things to note about this conversation (Callaghan, Summers, & Weidman, 2003). First, the therapist addresses Melissa's *behavior*, not her character or personality. Second, the therapist reinforces Melissa's healthy CRB—when she discloses that she felt nervous but is glad to be there, the therapist responds warmly and affirmatively. Third, the therapist points out Melissa's unhealthy CRB—when she dismisses the therapist's comment in a sarcastic manner, the therapist points out the negative impact of that behavior and suggests Melissa try more self-disclosure (the healthy behavior).

Things That Might Bug You about This

It's natural for questions to come up when you're learning about operant therapy. I'll try to address some likely ones.

- **Is this just manipulating clients?** Any therapeutic intervention has, at its core, an aim of changing the client's behavior. Sometimes we do that by changing environmental antecedents, sometimes we do it by changing or accepting thoughts and beliefs, sometimes we do it by changing or accepting emotions, and sometimes we do it directly by working on the behavior itself. Behavioral interventions, therefore, are no more or less "manipulative" than any other aspect of psychological therapy.

Let me also offer some food for thought: There is no such thing as not doing operant therapy. Let's take, as an example, perhaps the most "nonbehavioral" therapist in history, Carl Rogers. Rogers firmly believed in unconditional positive regard and accepting the client no matter what, and his debates with the behaviorist B. F. Skinner were legendary at the time (Rogers & Skinner, 1956). Yet, when one of Rogers's own cases was examined systematically over time, it was determined that: (1) he demonstrated greater empathy and acceptance behaviors when the client talked about his own feelings or made insightful statements, (2) he demonstrated less empathy and acceptance behaviors when the client spoke in an ambiguous or unclear fashion, and (3) those client behaviors to which Rogers responded with increased empathy and acceptance behaviors increased significantly over the course of therapy (Truax, 1966). So Rogers was using systematic reinforcement, as do we all. We can choose to be good behavior therapists or bad behavior therapists, but we can't choose *not* to be behavior therapists.

One possible source of this concern is the fact that in many cases the contingencies are being managed by someone other than the client. In a token economy, for example, the therapist or other clinical staff are the ones prompting the behavior and providing the tokens. I think about it this way: If the client had control over his or her behavior, then none of this would be needed. We wouldn't establish an operant intervention for a behavior that the client can and does control reliably. Our job is to provide some external structure while the client builds up his or her own internal structure. This is a bit like putting a splint on a broken leg. The leg can't support itself right now, and therefore we have to add some external support. Over time, however, the leg heals, and it's not our aim to have the client wear the splint forever. The end goal of an operant therapy (and indeed any therapy) is for the client to have self-control over behavior and to be able to get natural reinforcement from the environment for desired behavior.

- **Is the use of reinforcement just a form of bribery, and, by extension, icky?** The term *bribery* implies that there is somehow a moral or ethical transgression taking place. But contingencies are part of everyday life. There's no such thing as *not* having contingencies on our behavior. I go to work because I get paid to do so. If my employer decides to stop paying (reinforcing) me, you can bet that I won't go in any more, and I'll seek another source of reinforcement. That doesn't imply, however, that I'm being "bribed" to go to work. It simply means that the behavior (working) and the reinforcer (my paycheck) have been effectively paired.

Sometimes, people use the term *bribery* to signal a discomfort with reinforcing someone for doing a behavior that they should already be doing (there's a nice "should" statement for you). A parent, for example, might object to paying a child to clean his or her room, because, after all, the child *should* be doing that anyway. Others have objected to paying drug addicts to stay clean because the addicts *should* stay clean anyway (Kirby, Benishek, Dugosh, & Kerwin, 2006) or have objected to reinforcing children in residential care for good behavior because that's what they *should* be doing (Bailey, Gross, & Cotton, 2011). Well, if shoulds were dollars, we'd all be rich. The fact is that clients' behavior gets out of control, in part, because the contingencies got messed up along the way. The wrong stuff got reinforced, and the right stuff either didn't get adequately reinforced or it got punished. We use operant interventions to correct a broken contingency system.

• ***Does the use of operant strategies infantilize the client?*** Operant therapy has its roots in the treatment of people with severe developmental disabilities, people with severe mental illness living in institutions, children, and other groups of people who are globally unable to take care of themselves or sometimes even to make their own decisions. And for that reason, there are times that operant therapies such as contingency management can seem paternalistic. But that need not mean that operant therapy is only for the grossly impaired, nor that using operant therapy implies that we think of the client that way.

It's worth noting that many clients, including high-functioning ones, like the idea of earning rewards for desired behaviors—as one example, medical clients with diabetes favor the idea of earning rewards for appropriate treatment adherence (Blondon, Klasnja, Coleman, & Pratt, 2014). So not everyone finds the idea infantilizing.

As with everything, there's an art to this. You can present operant interventions in an infantilizing way, or you can present them in a way that is appropriate to the client's age and level of intellectual functioning. Some of the operant strategies in this chapter, such as self-control and reinforcing healthy CRBs in session, are quite appropriate for moderate- to high-functioning clients. Even the strategies we've discussed that seem readily applicable to lower-functioning and institutional clients, such as token economies and chaining, have a potential role in therapy for a wide range of clients, regardless of age, diagnosis, functional status, intellectual capacity, and so forth. The principle can translate across clients and settings, although the style of delivery will likely change. Even that high-functioning client struggles with behavioral problems, and we're not doing him or her any favors by not addressing those problems directly. I've used operant strategies with people with significant developmental disabilities and people with severe mental illness. I've also used them with doctors and lawyers and people with low-grade depression and anxiety. I've used them with people with and without severe personality disorders. I've used them on my kids. I've used them on myself.

• ***Does the use of contingencies undermine intrinsic motivation?*** The concern here is that when we use external reinforcers for a behavior, we undermine the person's *intrinsic motivation*—that is, the person's innate liking of, and desire to perform, the behavior. This concern stems from early research that suggested that when we pay people to do a behavior that they already like doing, they report liking it less (see Deci, Koestner, & Ryan, 1999, for review). I like fishing, for example. So if you started paying me to go fishing, my liking of fishing would probably decrease over time because it would become my job, rather than my hobby. In clinical settings, however, it's a different story. We're not reinforcing clients for something that they already do and like. We're reinforcing those behaviors that are not currently being performed enough. If the client had sufficient intrinsic motivation, we wouldn't be doing this in the first place.

It's worth noting as well that when we use reinforcers for things that the person doesn't naturally do and enjoy, intrinsic motivation either doesn't change or increases. Using task-dependent positive reinforcement has, in many cases, been demonstrated to increase liking of the task being performed in samples as diverse as boys doing math problems (McGinnis, Friman, & Carlyon, 1999), college students building erector sets (Wimperis & Farr, 1979), and telephone operators performing their jobs (Lopez, 1981).

• ***Does changing a behavior in one situation generalize to other situations?*** *Generalization* of therapeutic change is always a concern. In most (though not all) cases, we want the client's behavior to change outside of the therapeutic setting. We can't automatically assume this will happen (Hersen, 1976), and assessing and promoting generalization of behavior is an important part of the therapist's job. Generally speaking, we will maximize generalization by including *self-control* procedures in the program. That is, at some point we want the client to be able to identify behavioral targets, to self-monitor, to make environmental adaptations, and to self-reinforce. This strategy, in addition to giving the greatest level of autonomy to the client, is also the most "portable," meaning the client can most easily use these strategies outside of the therapy session.

We can promote generalization by having multiple people, not just the therapist, involved in the contingency management program. So, for example, we might want to get the client's parents or spouse involved (assuming the therapist can train these people appropriately). In an inpatient or residential setting, we want to increase the number of staff members who are involved. These strategies decrease the likelihood that the therapist, or one staff member, will serve as the sole signal that the operant therapy program is in place.

We also increase the likelihood of generalization when we establish the new behavioral pattern very strongly. Behavior, both good and bad, tends to develop momentum (Nevin, 1992; Plaud & Gaither, 1996). It is important, therefore, to spend a lot of time engaging the client in interactions or situations that reinforce the desired behavior(s). We want to build up the strength of the desired behavior pattern and get it reinforced a lot.

We can also promote generalization by *changing the context* of the behavior. That is, once the client is able to perform a certain behavior or behaviors reliably in one setting, it is helpful to then change up the setting in one or more important ways. Ideally, these changes will approximate real-world settings that the client is likely to encounter. For example, let's say that Scott, our socially anxious client, has become reliably able to speak naturally with the therapist. The next step would be to bring in another person for Scott to speak to, perhaps about a different topic than what has been discussed before. In this way, we're asking Scott to practice the same behaviors in a new context.

- ***Does reinforcement just change what the client does, while ignoring what he or she thinks and feels?*** Remember that thoughts, feelings, and behaviors are linked in the *core pathological process*. They all mutually influence each other. So changing behaviors can and does lead to changes in thoughts and feelings. As one example, substance-abusing clients in a contingency management program not only showed better drug abstinence outcomes than did clients receiving standard treatment, but they also reported a greater satisfaction with life (Petry, Alessi, & Hanson, 2007) and reduced symptoms of psychiatric distress such as depression and anxiety (Petry, Alessi, & Rash, 2013).

Contingency Management in Action: Changing Aversive Contingency Patterns in Couples and Families

As we discussed in Chapter 2, couple and family distress is viewed, in part, as a mutual failure of reinforcement. Distressed couples primarily rely on escape (negative reinforcement) and punishment as a means of behavioral influence (N. S. Jacobson & Margolin, 1979), providing little positive reinforcement. Distressed families get into coercive processes, with harsh and inconsistent discipline and little positive interaction among family members (Patterson et al., 1989). People in these couples and family systems are inadvertently training each other to behave badly.

When treating distressed couples and families (or when using a couple or family intervention as a means of intervening with an individual's problem), the therapist should look for coercive processes. This can be done by carefully interviewing the couple or family (e.g., "When you see him acting like that, how do you respond?"; "How does your mom usually react when you do that?"; "When your wife talks to you calmly and directly, what do you do then?"), by using behavioral self-monitoring, or by asking the couple or family to role-play a typical problem scenario in the office while the therapist observes.

CBT for couples may be used when the relationship itself is the target problem (e.g., a couple isn't getting along well with each other) or as part of an intervention directed toward an individual (e.g., one member of the relationship is suffering from depression, substance abuse, or other problems). CBT for couples incorporates several behavioral interventions described in this book, adapted to address the reciprocal concerns of two people. Operant elements of CBT for couples (N. S. Jacobson & Margolin, 1979) include:

- Instructing each partner to track his or her own behavior, as well as relevant behaviors of the partner, to examine relationships among behaviors and to understand the reinforcement/punishment value of certain behaviors.
- Instructing each partner to increase the number of "pleasing" behaviors toward the other, in order to increase the likelihood of positive reinforcement.
- In some cases, using written contingency contracts between partners to specify desired behaviors (Baucom, 1982).

Here, the therapist is working with Nick (N) and Johanna (J) on their coercive processes. The aim is to pull them away from the use of escape and punishment strategies and toward the use of positive reinforcement. Remember that negative begets negative, and positive begets positive. So by having them deliberately start using positive behaviors toward each other, the therapist hopes to set a reciprocal cycle in motion.

T: It sounds like last night was another one of those times when each of you is trying to control the other using hostility of some kind.

J: I just felt like there was nothing I could do right. It seemed like whatever I did, I was going to get criticized. I felt like crap all night.

N: Well, what about me? It's not like you're treating me well at all, but as soon as I say one little thing about it, all of a sudden I'm the bad guy.

T: I'm hearing some defensiveness there, Nick. Hold up for just a second. Remember that defensiveness—that need to justify yourself—is one of our "four horsemen of the apocalypse." The fact that you feel a need to defend yourself is important, and we'll get to that, but in a way that's productive for both of you. Is that OK to hold off on the defense for now?

N: Yeah, that's OK.

T: I also just want to point out here that it seemed like you did a little bit of what I was talking about a minute ago. Johanna was saying something that didn't sit right with you, and you responded by trying to control her using a hostile statement. Can you see that you just did that?

N: (Sighs.) Yeah.

T: Let's be clear, that doesn't make you a bad guy or a bad husband. You're not driving this problem. You aren't either, Johanna. Neither of you is in control of this. Rather, the system that exists between the two of you has taken on a life of its own, and now it's got you both acting in ways that hurt the marriage and that you're not happy with. Does that make sense?

J: Yeah, I guess that makes sense.

T: Let's call these actions "displeases." It's a way of slapping someone on the wrist when they do something we don't like. Nick, when Johanna says something you don't like, you give her a "displease" as a way of shutting her down. And Johanna, when Nick doesn't do things the way you want them done, you give him a "displease" to try to get him in line. But the problem is that one "displease" seems to lead to another, and so it goes back and forth, becoming more and more unpleasant. Does that ring true to you?

N: It is a cycle. Once we start, it just keeps getting worse.

T: So let's take a look at the flip side of it—"pleases." When was the last time that you did something nice for each other? I don't mean like on a special occasion like a birthday; I mean just for no particular reason?

J: God, I can't even remember.

N: Months, maybe. I have no idea.

T: Seems like that's part of our problem. Nick, have you ever brought Johanna flowers just for the heck of it?

N: Not since we were dating, no.

T: Johanna, when you were dating, did you like it when Nick brought you flowers?

J: Yeah, I did.

T: So Nick, what do you think about that? What about bringing Johanna some flowers?

N: I'd feel silly doing it. I'm still pissed off at her and it would feel like I wasn't being genuine. And we both know that I'd only be doing it because you told me to.

T: So what? The bottom line is that Johanna likes it when you bring her flowers. Who cares why you're doing it? And who cares who gave you the idea?

N: I guess that doesn't really matter.

T: It doesn't. What's most important to the marriage is what you do for Johanna. Now Johanna, how about you? What kind of a "please" can you think of for Nick?

J: Um . . . I know he likes steak. I haven't made that in quite a while.

T: And so what would happen if you cooked him a really great steak, just the way he likes it? Would that be a silly thing to do?

J: I guess not.

T: Nick, would you enjoy the steak less because I suggested she cook it for you?

N: (*Laughs.*) No. I'd like it no matter what.

T: Right. These things like steaks and flowers are pleasing and helpful, no matter their reason. So here's what I'd like you to try this week. Nick, I'd like you to surprise Johanna with flowers. And Johanna, I'd like you to surprise Nick by cooking his favorite kind of steak for him. And I want you to do this whether or not you feel like it. That's important. Even if you're pissed off at each other, I still want you to do it. But I want you both to pay attention to some things. I want you to notice how your partner reacts when you do the "please," and I also want you to notice your own reactions, how you feel and how the marriage feels.

N: But even if she cooks me a steak, it's not like that solves anything. Sure, I'll enjoy the steak, but we still have serious issues between us.

T: Indeed you do. And we will work on those issues. But for right now, I'd like to see if we can experiment with breaking you out of this nasty cycle you're in, even temporarily. If it seems promising, we can experiment with increasing the number of "pleases" in the relationship.

In family CBT, we will often employ **parent management training** (Barkley, 1997; Kazdin, 2008; Patterson, 1982), which relies heavily on operant strategies to disrupt coercive processes. Aspects of parent management training include:

- *Teaching parents to identify and track the problem behaviors.* This part is easy to take for granted, but it's important. Many distressed parents, especially those of kids who are behaving badly, tend to describe their children's problems in vague terms, such as "He has a bad attitude" or "He just doesn't listen." Those descriptions don't give us much to work with. The therapist should help the parents identify the specific behaviors involved with having a "bad attitude" or "not listening"; for example, muttering nasty comments under his breath or rolling his eyes. Then, parents should identify the positive opposite of the problem behaviors, such as speaking clearly with polite language and making direct eye contact (Kazdin, 2008). These positive opposites will become the targets for positive reinforcement.

- *Teaching parents to give clear directions.* Parents of well-adjusted children have been demonstrated to use primarily what have been called *alpha commands* (McMahon & Forehand, 2003), which are clear, specific, and direct, given one at a time, with about a 5-second wait for compliance. "James, please turn off the TV and start doing your homework" is an alpha command. In contrast, parents of conduct-disordered children frequently use *beta commands*, which are vaguely phrased, often worded as a question, and followed by excessive rationalization. "How many times have I told you that you watch too much TV? You're going to rot your brain, and besides, don't you have homework to do? How are you going to get your grades up if you don't finish your homework? What am I

The Science behind It

Across studies, behavioral interventions with couples have a significant positive effect on marital satisfaction (Baucom, Shoham, Mueser, Daiuto, & Stickle, 1998; Shadish & Baldwin, 2005; Shadish et al., 1993). Parent management training has been shown extensively to reduce children's externalizing problems, improve social competence, and decrease familial stress (Kazdin, 1997; Kazdin, Siegel, & Bass, 1992; C. R. Martinez & Eddy, 2005; Ogden & Hagen, 2008; Webster-Stratton & Hammond, 1997), with evidence of generalization to the classroom setting (McNeil, Eyberg, Eisenstadt, Newcomb, & Funderburk, 1991), of long-term maintenance of gains (Long, Forehand, Wierson, & Morgan, 1994), and of applicability even in the presence of co-occurring child psychopathology (Costin & Chambers, 2007; Sukhodolsky, Gorman, Scahill, Findley, & McGuire, 2013).

supposed to do with you? Answer me!" is a beta command. Even "It's time for homework" is a beta command, because it doesn't contain an explicit instruction for the child.

• *Teaching parents to use positive reinforcement for desired behavior.* As noted above, in distressed families, positive reinforcement often goes out the window. So when the child acts in a desirable manner, the parent ignores it, only responding to the child when he or she acts inappropriately. Or the parent tries to use reinforcement but messes it up by throwing an aversive "zinger" in there: "I like the way you cleaned up your room. Why can't you do this every day?" (Kazdin, 2008). Verbal praise is perhaps the most straightforward way of introducing positive reinforcement: "James, I really like the way you started your homework on time. Nice job!" Star charts and other token economies, as described previously in this chapter, are a good way to employ tangible reinforcers. Over time, as with any other operant strategy, this intervention should be faded gradually so that the child assumes increasing control over his or her own behavior.

Using a positive reinforcement strategy also has the important side benefit of combating the parents' likely attentional bias toward negative behavior from the child (Barkley, 1997). Now, we're making the parents look for and "catch" desirable behavior. In many cases, the parent would like the child to do *less* of something, and so they rely exclusively on punishment strategies. Extinction, DRO, DRL, and noncontingent (free) reinforcement are not on their radar screens, and so it becomes the therapist's job to teach them these alternative strategies for reducing behavior and guide them through daily practice.

• *Teaching parents to use a mild penalty for inappropriate behavior.* Because distressed families frequently overuse punishment, the therapist's job is often to get them to tone this way down and use appropriate punishers. Positive punishment (punishment) should be deemphasized, and parents can instead be coached about the appropriate use of negative punishment (penalty). So, when little Johnny is rotten (or little Sid is vicious), brief time-outs (e.g., 1–2 minutes for each year of the child's age [Barkley, 1997]) and time-limited loss of privileges can be effective negative punishers, particularly if they are paired with prompts to engage in appropriate behaviors and subsequent reinforcement of those behaviors. In general, instances of praise should greatly outnumber instances of punishment (Kazdin, 2008), and we should emphasize reinforcing desired behaviors more than punishing unwanted behaviors.

• *Teaching parents to be consistent.* Both kids and adults find uncertainty and unpredictability to be aversive and will engage in behaviors that try to increase the predictability of the environment (Staub, Tursky, & Schwartz, 1971). As parental inconsistency increases, so do coercive behaviors from the child (Wahler, Williams, & Cerezo, 1990). This occurs even when the parents attempt to punish the child for unwanted behaviors; all things considered, the child will select negative adult attention over unpredictability (Strand, 2000). This is a critical issue: Although a parental response (e.g., yelling at the child) might be expected to be punishing, and might indeed be punishing in some situations, within the overall context of the family system the parental response can actually be reinforcing (Herrnstein, 1970). Contingencies only work when we create a *family culture* of consistent expectations, prompts, rewards, and punishments.

• *Programming in some child-centered activity each day.* Frequently, the family system becomes all about the child's problem behavior. That becomes all the family talks about. In such cases, the child's only substantial interactions with his or her parents revolve around the problem. That's discouraging to the child and demoralizing for the whole family. So it's helpful to instruct the family to have some positive activities—perhaps just playing a game for as little as 5 minutes—each day.

Using Schedules of Reinforcement in Therapy

Remember from Chapter 2 that reinforcement can be *continuous*, meaning it always follows the behavior, or it can be *intermittent*, meaning it sometimes follows the behavior. Continuous and intermittent reinforcement have somewhat different effects on behavior and can be used for different aims. Continuous reinforcement tends to make a behavior increase rapidly. So, if the desired behavior doesn't occur very much, and you want it to occur more often, continuous reinforcement is the way to go. Intermittent reinforcement tends to make a behavior "stick," even in the absence of reinforcement (the person knows the reinforcer is coming eventually, so keeps at it). So once the behavior is occurring at the desired frequency, we shift to an intermittent schedule of reinforcement to make the behavior less dependent on the reinforcers.

As an example, we've been trying to get Christina to get out of bed and engage in potentially rewarding activities. So to start, we would use a continuous schedule of reinforcement to get the frequency up. Every time she gets out of bed, she earns a token. Once she's doing that reliably, we switch to an intermittent schedule of reinforcement, giving her a token only every once in a while when she gets out of bed. Of course, if Christina's behavior starts to slip, we could always switch back to continuous reinforcement to get it back up again.

Sticky Points in Reinforcement

What If the Person Never Does the Desired Behavior, So There's Nothing to Reinforce?

When the person never performs the desired behavior, we're a little bit stuck because the person never has the opportunity to obtain a reinforcer.

In such cases, we use **shaping** to try to create the behavior where it doesn't exist. Shaping requires that we reinforce **successive approximations** to the behavior. Successive approximations are behaviors that are progressively closer and closer to the desired behavior. A classic example of shaping is seen in the case of a teenage girl with developmental disabilities who spoke so quietly as to be inaudible. The desired behavior was speaking in a normal volume. The therapist first reinforced her, using tokens, for speaking at any volume above a whisper. Then, when she could do that reliably, the therapist shifted the reinforcement so that the client would be reinforced for speaking a bit louder than that, and so on until she was speaking at a normal volume (Jackson & Wallace, 1974).

Our client William usually waits for the therapist to bring up topics for discussion, doesn't come up with his own ideas, and seems to wait for the therapist to solve his problems for him. If we were to use a straightforward reinforcement plan, we might wait a long time before William gave us a behavior we could reinforce. So, instead, let's try shaping using the reinforcement of successive approximations. If the desired behavior is for William to generate substantive topics for discussion in therapy and to assist with solving his own problems, we could think about a number of successive approximations to that behavior:

- William brings up a new topic in the conversation, even if it's irrelevant.
- William brings up a new topic in the conversation that is relevant to the problem being treated.
- William brings up a new topic in the conversation that is relevant to the problem being treated and generates at least one potential solution, even if the solution is not feasible.
- William brings up a new topic in the conversation that is relevant to the problem being treated and generates at least one feasible potential solution.
- William brings up a new topic in the conversation that is relevant to the problem being treated and generates at least two feasible potential solutions.
- William brings up a new topic in the conversation that is relevant to the problem being treated, generates at least two feasible potential solutions, and initiates a discussion about the pros and cons of each one.
- William brings up a new topic in the conversation that is relevant to the problem being treated, generates at least two feasible potential solutions, initiates a discussion about the pros and cons of each one, and selects one solution to try.

So if the therapist is reinforcing healthy CRBs, in one session he or she might reinforce William for bringing up any new topic. In keeping with the idea of using reinforcers that have some real-world validity, the therapist might attend closely to whatever new topic William brings up, even if it's irrelevant, leaning forward, responding warmly, and encouraging William to elaborate. Once William gets to that level of behavior, the therapist would then switch the reinforcement to the next successive approximation. Now, when William brings up an irrelevant topic, the therapist might simply prompt William gently to bring up a topic that is more relevant to the therapeutic discussion. When William does so, the therapist attends closely, leans forward, responds warmly, and encourages William to elaborate. The therapist follows this pattern of switching reinforcement to each successive approximation until William can eventually perform the desired behavior in session.

What If the Desired Behavior Is Really Complex?

Many desired behaviors are actually a complex chain of smaller behaviors. Part of the problem is that the client may not know, or be able to perform, all of the smaller behaviors that make up the desired behaviors, in the required sequence, in order to obtain reinforcement. This is where **chaining** comes in. Chaining refers to breaking a complex behavior down into a series of smaller behaviors (called a **task analysis**), and then reinforcing those smaller behaviors in sequence.

For example, let's take the example of making a bed (W. L. Williams & Burkholder, 2003). This behavior is actually made up of a number of smaller behaviors, including putting on the bottom sheet, tucking in the bottom sheet, putting on the top sheet, tucking in the top sheet, putting on the bedspread, putting pillowcases on the pillows, and placing the pillows at the head of the bed. And these smaller behaviors have to occur in a specific sequence in order for the bed to be made (you can't put the bedspread on first, for example). If we were trying to increase bed-making behavior in someone who couldn't do it, we might use chaining to reinforce the smaller behaviors.

Because chaining often is used in teaching a new skill of some kind, chaining strategies often employ *modeling*, in which the therapist first demonstrates the skill or otherwise has the client watch the behavior being performed (more on this strategy in Chapter 12). Chaining can take several forms:

- *Forward chaining* means that we start at the first smaller behavior and work our way forward. So, in the bed-making example described above, we would first reinforce the client for putting on the bottom sheet and only move to the next step when the client can do that reliably. The benefit of forward chaining is that each step of the process is reinforced. It's also an intuitive sequence, making it easier for staff to remember and use.

- *Backward chaining* means that we start at the last smaller behavior and work our way backward. So, in the bed-making example, we would first reinforce the client for placing the pillows at the head of an otherwise already-made bed and only move to the previous step when the client can do that reliably. The benefit of backward chaining is that the entire program started off with the desired reinforcer—having a finished bed. Thus clients might be more eager to go through the steps.

- *Total task presentation* means that we go through every step of the sequence, in order, on every trial, assisting whenever the client has difficulty. So, in the bed-making example, we would prompt the client to put on the bottom sheet, then tuck in the bottom sheet, then put on the top sheet, and so on until the entire task was completed. The benefit of total task presentation is that the chain of behaviors can be learned fairly quickly and efficiently.

There are no consistent findings to tell us whether forward chaining, backward chaining, or total task presentation is the best strategy overall (e.g., Slocum & Tiger, 2011). However, some research suggests that total task presentation might be more effective in at least some cases, depending on many factors, such as client characteristics, the length and complexity of the behavior being taught, and how many of the smaller steps the client can already complete (Davis & Rehfeldt, 2007).

How Do We Make Sure the Person Doesn't Just Become Dependent on the Reinforcers?

One concern with any operant intervention is that the client will simply engage in the desired behaviors in order to obtain reinforcement but will not engage in the behaviors otherwise. In some settings, that's fine, but most of the time we want the client to engage in the desired behaviors independently. We have several strategies that can help.

- **Fading** refers to gradually decreasing prompts for the behavior and/or gradually reducing the reinforcement. Once the client can perform the desired behavior reliably, the therapist provides fewer prompts or waits progressively longer before making a prompt. The use of reinforcement can be faded as well; for example, in a token economy the number of tokens given out can be gradually decreased.

- As token reinforcement is decreased, it's often a good idea to make the desired reinforcers more freely available so they become "uncoupled" from the program. So, for example, if the person was earning tokens that could be exchanged for TV time, we might now allow free access to the TV.

- Relatedly, remember that *intermittent reinforcement* helps make a behavior more "extinction-proof." So when we want to decrease the client's reliance on the reinforcers, it's helpful to switch from continuous to intermittent reinforcement to make the behavior less reward-dependent. Eventually, the reinforcers can be faded out altogether.

- Teaching *self-control* strategies is a helpful transition from clinician-directed to self-directed reinforcement. In particular, we can teach the client to reinforce him- or herself over time. Tangible self-administered reinforcers are often fine, although in many cases it's good just to get the client to pat him- or herself on the back for successfully completing the desired behavior.

- Behaviors will be most durable when they can be accompanied by *natural reinforcement*. In many cases, the environment will naturally reward the desired behavior once the client can do it reliably. As we get Christina to get out of bed and do more positive activities, for example, the satisfaction of those activities starts to take over, making our involvement less necessary. As Scott engages in more social activities, he develops friendships that become more naturally reinforcing. As Samantha learns to stop pulling her hair, the growth of new hair and an improved appearance become rewarding in themselves. As we develop behavioral interventions, we should be thinking up front about how we can make the best use of natural reinforcers for the behavior so that we don't have to reinforce it indefinitely.

How to do contingency management poorly	How to do contingency management like a champ
Be confusing. Use vague terms like "acting out," "isolating," or "being sullen" instead of clearly defined behaviors. Don't explain the rationale for changing the behavior to the client.	*Be clear.* Remember that operant therapy works when we identify the target behavior(s) in a way that is objective, clear, and complete. At any given time, the client, the therapist, and any other staff members involved should be able to identify exactly what the target behavior is and why they are working on it.
Overrely on aversive techniques. Make use of punishment, penalty, and escape strategies when you want a behavior to decrease. Scold or criticize the client as a form of punishment, or take away privileges when the client does the undesired behavior. Nag the client until he or she either does the desired behavior to get you to shut up or lashes out at you in order to regain a sense of control.	*Make positive reinforcement the cornerstone of your program.* Before employing any aversive techniques, even mild ones such as criticism, it's important to ensure that there isn't a less aversive way to get at the behavior. Remember that if our aim is to decrease an unwanted behavior, we can use punishment and penalty, but we can also use extinction and DRO, which are far less aversive than punishment strategies, may work better in the long run, and are more humane.
Be inconsistent. One person can derail an operant therapy program. If you're in a therapeutic setting with lots of staff members, don't discuss the plan with the whole staff. That way, one or more staff members can fail to adhere to the plan and wreck it (Bailey et al., 2011). For example, some staff members may not administer reinforcers as agreed or may administer the reinforcers in a manner that is not contingent on behavior. Staff may even start to make up their own rules, such as withdrawing tokens (penalty) in a program based solely on reinforcement.	*Consistency, consistency, consistency.* The plan will work only when everyone follows the same rules. The amount of staff education and training required to pull this off is often quite substantial, and it is likely that multiple staff members will have to keep careful records and communicate with each other frequently throughout the process.
Fail to respect the client's autonomy. This relates to the issue of paternalism discussed above. A contingency management program almost always requires some degree of "buy-in" from the client. Even in an institutional setting such as an inpatient unit, clients can cooperate with the plan to a greater or lesser extent, and the results will vary accordingly.	*Make the client part of the treatment team.* Certainly, there are some clients who require that others make all of their decisions for them. However, that doesn't apply to most clients, whether in outpatient or inpatient settings. The determination of how to implement operant therapy requires a good understanding of the client's capacity to make decisions about behavior, his or her ability

and willingness to get involved in deciding what contingencies to use, and his or her ability and willingness to employ self-control strategies. As I mentioned earlier, I have used operant therapy with (to use just two examples) developmentally disabled children in a contained environment and with professionals seeking outpatient therapy for depression and anxiety. The underlying principles are the same (e.g., reinforcement does what it does), but the selection and implementation are different. I can't approach these two different kinds of clients in the same way and expect a good result.

Reinforce the wrong behaviors. It's easy to reinforce the wrong thing. For example, let's say I want William, our client with depression and dependency, to initiate topics of discussion, come up with ideas, and work to solve his own problems. Let's further say that today I'm tired and hassled, and we're running out of time in the session, and I really, really want to get to activity scheduling (see Chapter 10) today. And now William brings up a topic that is relevant to his therapy, yet not what I wanted to talk about today. If I want to do contingency management poorly, I should fail to reinforce William's healthy CRB, dismiss the topic he brings up, say what *I* want to say, and then, through words or actions, reinforce him for keeping his mouth shut and going with my agenda. William has now taken a step backward.

Reinforce the right behaviors. The therapist needs to watch constantly for the presence of desired and undesired behaviors, unfailingly reinforcing the desired behaviors and not reinforcing the undesired behaviors. In the case of William, who brings up a topic that is relevant to his therapy, yet not what I wanted to talk about today, I need to take the time to reinforce his healthy CRB (e.g., listening carefully and validating what he is saying) even if that takes the session in a slightly different direction. You have to be on top of your game with this stuff.

Expect the contingency management to solve everything. And, on the flip side, get frustrated and give up on it when it doesn't make everything better.

Recognize that contingency management is usually part of a larger whole. Although contingency management is great (and an important part of CBT), it is not a panacea. Nothing is. It's important to recognize that successful therapy usually requires a variety of tactics, including operant therapy but also such things as cognitive restructuring, skill training, environmental adaptations, and direct behavioral prescriptions, which we discuss in other chapters.

THE ESSENTIALS

❋ To increase a desired behavior, we can use reinforcement strategies.

❋ To decrease an undesired behavior, punishment strategies may be used but require additional consideration of costs and benefits.

❋ Less aversive methods of decreasing undesired behavior include penalty, extinction, differential reinforcement of other behavior (DRO), differential reinforcement of lower rates of behavior (DRL), and noncontingent (free) reinforcement.

❋ Steps in contingency management include picking your target behavior, knowing the base rate of the target behavior, conducting a functional analysis of the target behavior, picking the contingencies, and getting buy-in from all parties.

❋ Examples of contingency management include the prompt–praise–ignore plan, token economies, self-control strategies and reinforcing CRBs in session, and changing aversive contingency patterns in couples and families.

❋ Shaping can be used to reinforce successive approximations to the desired behavior.

❋ Chaining can be used to reinforce a complex set of behaviors.

❋ To reduce dependence on the reinforcers, we can use strategies such as fading, self-control strategies, and utilizing naturalistic reinforcement.

KEY TERMS AND DEFINITIONS

Behavioral chain: A sequence of behaviors that leads up to the target behavior.

Chaining: Teaching a set of smaller behaviors in a specific sequence to create the larger, desired behavior.

Clinically relevant behaviors (CRBs): Healthy or unhealthy behaviors, exhibited in the therapy session, that are related to the problem for which the client is being treated.

Competing response training: Practicing a behavior that competes with, or is incompatible with, an unwanted behavior.

Contingency contract: An agreement that specifies the contingencies to be used in a behavior change program.

Differential reinforcement of lower rates of behavior (DRL): Providing reinforcement when the frequency of a behavior is less than or equal to a prescribed limit.

Differential reinforcement of other behavior (DRO): Decreasing an unwanted behavior by reinforcing a competing, more desirable, behavior.

Fading: Gradually removing prompts to engage in a desired behavior and/or gradually decreasing reinforcement for the desired behavior.

Noncontingent (free) reinforcement: Decreasing a reinforced behavior by making the reinforcer freely available.

Overcorrection: Positive punishment by the repetition of appropriate behavior after the occurrence of an unwanted behavior.

Parent management training: A strategy for teaching parents to use appropriate contingency management with children.

Premack principle: The reinforcement of a low-frequency behavior by using a high-frequency behavior as a contingency.

Prompt–praise–ignore plan: A contingency management plan that relies on behavioral prompting, praise as a reinforcer, and ignoring as a negative punisher or extinction.

Response cost: Negative punishment by giving up something desirable following an occurrence of an unwanted behavior.

Satiation: Providing so much of a reinforcer that it loses its reinforcement value.

Self-control: Self-directed operant intervention that involves modifying antecedents and consequences of one's own behavior.

Shaping: Helping the client develop a new behavior by reinforcing successive approximations to the behavior.

Successive approximations: Behaviors that more and more closely resemble the desired behavior that is being shaped.

Task analysis: Identification of the smaller behaviors that must be performed to make up the larger behavior.

Time-out: Negative punishment by temporary removal from potential reinforcers.

Token economy: A contingency management system in which clients earn token reinforcers that can later be cashed in for tangible reinforcers, activities, or privileges.

Behavioral Self-Monitoring

Choose one or two target behaviors to monitor. These can be either: (1) a desired behavior that doesn't happen enough or (2) an unwanted behavior that happens too much.

The behavior to monitor is: _____

Each time the behavior occurs, complete a row of the form. You can use more copies if needed.

Date and time	What was happening right *before* the behavior?	How many times did you do the behavior?	How long did you do the behavior?	What happened right *after* the behavior?

Functional analysis: The antecedents for my target behavior are: _____

The consequences (reinforcers) for my target behavior are: _____

From *Doing CBT* by David F. Tolin. Copyright © 2016 The Guilford Press. Permission to photocopy this worksheet is granted to purchasers of this book for personal use only (see copyright page for details). Purchasers can download enlarged versions of this worksheet (see the box at the end of the table of contents).

Behavioral Charting

Track the one or two target behavior(s) you identified on the previous page. Because everyone's behavior is different, you'll have to come up with the right parameters for tracking, including: (1) whether to count the frequency of the behavior, the duration of the behavior, the proportion of time spent doing the behavior, or some other measure (e.g., number of cigarettes smoked, amount of food eaten, time at which you went to bed, etc.); (2) whether to measure it daily, hourly, in increments of a day, or other; and (3) how m⚫ny observations you need to make in order to get a good idea of the base rate of the behavior. Have no less than three, but it can be more if that's what's needed. Depending on your personal target, you may be looking for an increase or decrease in behavior.

On the left (white) side of the chart below, track your behavior over time. You want something that looks more or less like the left side of the chart below:

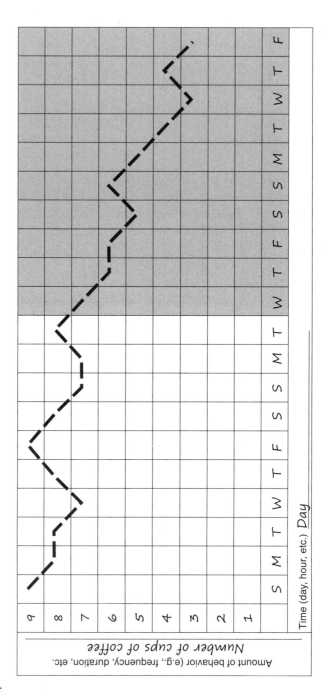

(continued)

From *Doing CBT* by David F. Tolin. Copyright © 2016 The Guilford Press. Permission to photocopy this worksheet is granted to purchasers of this book for personal use only (see copyright page for details). Purchasers can download enlarged versions of this worksheet (see the box at the end of the table of contents).

Now you try it.

Amount of behavior (e.g., frequency, duration, etc.)

Time (day, hour, etc.)

Contingency Contracting

If you feel ready to do so, complete and sign a contingency contract with yourself. If you find it helpful to have another person work with you on your contingency management, you can have that person co-sign the contract. Once the contract is signed, put a copy where you'll be able to see it regularly, and follow it.

Date: _____

I, _____, intend to make the following behavior change(s):

1.

2.

3.

Required: My reward system for making these change(s) will be:

1. When I _____, I will _____.

2. When I _____, I will _____.

3. When I _____, I will _____.

Optional: My penalty system for not making these change(s) will be:

1. When I _____, I will _____.

2. When I _____, I will _____.

3. When I _____, I will _____.

This system will remain in place until _____.

_____   _____
Signature   Co-signature (if applicable)

Now go back to the previous page and continue tracking your target behavior on the right (gray) side of the chart.

What did you notice?

From *Doing CBT* by David F. Tolin. Copyright © 2016 The Guilford Press. Permission to photocopy this worksheet is granted to purchasers of this book for personal use only (see copyright page for details). Purchasers can download enlarged versions of this worksheet (see the box at the end of the table of contents).

CHAPTER 10

Direct Behavioral Prescriptions and Graded Task Assignment

Much of the behavioral side of CBT comes down to **direct behavioral prescriptions.** Specifically, the therapist makes direct recommendations for the client to do something different. Sometimes this means we direct the client to do *more* of a certain behavior. Sometimes it means we direct the client to do *less* of a certain behavior. Sometimes it means we direct the client to do something *in a specific way*. But regardless of the specifics, the CBT therapist provides direct instruction to the client on what to do outside of the session.

As with anything else, we make certain assumptions when we make direct behavioral prescriptions to the client. We assume the client has been involved with the development of the prescriptions in a collaborative manner and is in agreement with the prescriptions. If you haven't reached that stage, review Chapter 7. We also assume the client possesses adequate skill to carry out the instructions. When this is not the case, we would likely use *skill training* (see Chapter 12) to build the requisite skills first.

Things That Might Bug You about This

The use of direct behavioral prescriptions does not mean that we're uninterested in the reasons why the behavior is the way it is. So I don't want you to get the idea that we're making simplistic behavioral recommendations that ignore bigger problems. We're interested in understanding what's wrong with Nick and Johanna's marriage; we're interested in understanding what's keeping Samuel up at night; we're interested in understanding how Blaise's life came to revolve around substances; we're interested in why Elizabeth has inconsistent interest in her therapy; and we're interested in why Shari feels a need to restrict her food intake. The direct behavioral prescriptions are a necessary part of the intervention, but they're not necessarily the whole intervention.

There are any number of direct behavioral prescriptions a therapist might make. For example:

- Nick and Johanna, our distressed couple, are locked in a cycle of negative interaction. The therapist might make a direct behavioral prescription by encouraging them to spend at least 15 minutes per day talking to each other about their days and schedule a weekly "date night" together.
- Samuel, our client with insomnia, engages in a number of behaviors at night that are incompatible with sleep. The therapist might make a direct behavioral prescription for him to change his nighttime routine, for example, to engage in quieter activities, to stop work earlier in the evening, to reduce food and alcohol intake late in the evening, and so forth.
- Blaise, the young woman recovering from cocaine dependence, has relatively few social or recreational outlets that don't involve using substances. The therapist might make a direct behavioral prescription for her to seek out new sources of enjoyment and companionship.
- Elizabeth, our client with borderline personality disorder and a long history of self-injurious behaviors, has been inconsistent in her willingness to stick with outpatient treatment. The therapist might make a direct behavioral prescription for her to attend a certain number of group therapy sessions before making up her mind about whether to continue or not.
- Shari, our bulimic client, restricts her food intake during the day, trying to avoid high-calorie foods. By evening, she is hungry and more likely to binge. The therapist might make a direct behavioral prescription for her to adhere to a regular meal schedule throughout the day.

These direct behavioral prescriptions might be paired with operant strategies such as *self-control* and *contingency contracting* (see Chapter 9).

Activity Scheduling

As we discussed in Chapter 2, clients' behaviors have consequences and feed into the core pathological process. Certain clients, particularly those suffering from depression, might be characterized as having a general *lack* of behavior—at least, a lack of behavior that would likely be pleasurable, that would lead to a sense of accomplishment, that is consistent with the client's longer-term goals and values, or that provides a sense of meaning and purpose. Christina, for example, spends most of her time at home by herself, and much of that time is spent either in bed or sitting on the couch. She watches a lot of TV, not because she's interested in the show but because she can't come up with anything better to do. She doesn't cook for herself or do many chores. On some days, she doesn't even get dressed or groom herself. In short, she acts like a depressed person.

As we discussed in Chapter 2, Christina's behavior has some serious consequences for her. Because of her inactivity, she feels even sadder, continues to believe that no one likes her, deprives herself of the opportunity for positive reinforcement, and has an ever-shrinking support network. We're going to have a hard time getting Christina out of this rut without having her do something different.

Christina seems like an excellent candidate for **activity scheduling.** Activity scheduling is a core component of a larger package of CBT strategies called *behavioral activation*

(Lejuez, Hopko, & Hopko, 2001; Lewinsohn, Biglan, & Zeiss, 1976; Martell, Addis, & Jacobson, 2001). You might hear these terms used interchangeably, although behavioral activation packages also include strategies such as stimulus control (see Chapter 8), contingency management (see Chapter 9) and skill training (see Chapter 12; Kanter et al., 2010). Activity scheduling results in large and durable treatment effects for clients with depression (Cuijpers, van Straten, & Warmerdam, 2007a). As we discussed in the introduction to Part II, it's entirely possible that activity scheduling accounts for most of the effects of CBT for depression, even changes in maladaptive beliefs (Dimidjian et al., 2006; N. S. Jacobson et al., 1996).

Self-Monitoring of Activities

As with many interventions, successful activity scheduling begins with *self-monitoring*. In this case, we want the client to keep track of his or her daily activities. I like to ask the client to track what he or she is doing on an hourly basis. It's important to note that there is no such thing as "doing nothing," and therefore there shouldn't be any blank areas on the self-monitoring form. Even sitting and staring blankly at a wall is doing *something*.

I also find it helpful, for each hour's activities, to ask the client to rate the degree of *mastery* and *pleasure* he or she derives from the activities. *Mastery* refers to a sense of accomplishment, whereas *pleasure* refers to enjoyment or happiness. It's great when an activity can deliver both mastery and pleasure, but in many cases it's fine when the activity delivers just one. Watching a great movie might give you a sense of pleasure, but not much of a sense of mastery. Finishing a paper for school might give you a sense of mastery, but not much pleasure. That's fine, as long as the day has an adequate amount of both.

Christina was instructed to complete a self-monitoring form every day over the course of a week. Her form is partly shown in Figure 10.1, and the entire form is reprinted in Appendix B. We can see some important patterns in Christina's self-monitoring that will be useful for our treatment planning.

- She spends an excessive amount of time sitting on the couch watching TV, as well as an excessive amount of time in bed.
- Overall, she has low levels of mastery and pleasure in her day.
- She does get a bit of mastery and/or pleasure from doing household chores and talking to her mom on the phone.

Of course, we can predict that Christina will view this exercise through depression-colored glasses, and we should be prepared to discuss with her what the information

Holding Up a Mirror

As with all self-monitoring, tracking one's behaviors can be an intervention in itself. *Measurement reactivity* occurs when the act of monitoring something changes what you're monitoring. In Christina's case, self-monitoring is a good way to increase her awareness. She might not have been aware of just how much time she was spending on the couch, or how little mastery and pleasure she was experiencing throughout the day. Just making her aware of these facts might stimulate her to change things.

Time	Activity	Mastery (0–10)	Pleasure (0–10)
6–7	Sleeping	0	0
7–8	Lying in bed, thinking	0	1
8–9	Lying in bed, looking at a magazine	0	2
9–10	Eating breakfast (cereal and coffee)	1	2
10–11	Sitting on couch and watching TV	0	2
11–12	Sitting on couch and watching TV	0	2
12–1	Sitting on couch and watching TV	0	2
1–2	Eating lunch (leftover cold pizza from last night)	1	1
2–3	Trying to do a little cleaning up around the house	4	3
3–4	Doing some organizing in the garage	5	4
4–5	Sitting on couch and watching TV	0	2
5–6	Calling my mom and talking about her new job	2	4
6–7	Ate dinner (more leftover pizza)	1	0
7–8	Went to bed early and read a book	2	2

FIGURE 10.1. Christina's self-monitoring form of daily activities.

means and what it does not mean. It means that her activities are part of the problem and that we should consider changing them. It doesn't mean that the situation is hopeless, that she is useless, or that she is to blame for everything that's going on.

Prescribing Activities

Next, we need to understand *what behaviors should be added*. It can be tempting at this point to toss out some behaviors that we think ought to be reinforcing, such as "go for a walk in the park." But we can never assume that what's reinforcing for us will be reinforcing for the client. So we have to figure out what kinds of behaviors would give Christina a sense of mastery and/or pleasure.

Sometimes, it can be helpful to have the client review a list of potentially rewarding activities and indicate which ones might be rewarding for him or her. A Mastery and Pleasure Checklist is provided in Appendix B.

Of course, we have to use our clinical judgment when selecting rewarding activities. We probably don't want our client with compulsive gambling to select going to the casino as a rewarding activity, and we might not want some of our clients with OCD to select cleaning up the house.

Here, the therapist reviews Christina's (C) self-monitoring form and identifies potentially rewarding activities.

T: Christina, as you look at these forms from the past week, what comes to mind for you?

C: Um . . . I see that I'm spending a lot of time in front of the TV.

T: Yeah, it looks like it's several hours a day. I also notice that you're not getting much of a sense of mastery or pleasure from that activity.

C: No. Mostly I just sit there flipping through channels. Or I just sit there like a zombie.

T: I see. I'm also noticing quite a bit of time spent in bed.

C: Yeah, sometimes I just lie in bed because I don't see much reason to do anything else.

T: And again, not much mastery or pleasure in that for you.

C: No.

T: I do see little bits of mastery and pleasure in there, though.

C: When I was doing some stuff around the house I felt kind of productive. But I didn't really get anything finished or accomplished, so it's not like I did anything useful.

T: Well, that might be something we need to address, but for now what I'd like us to notice is just the fact that doing it made you feel a little bit better.

C: OK.

T: And talking to your mom seemed to be a good thing.

C: Kind of. I mean, it wasn't great.

T: No, but it's something. I guess my overall question, looking at your forms, is whether you think your daily activities are making your feelings of depression better or worse?

C: Worse, I think.

T: I suspect so. And so if sitting around and being pretty inactive seems to be part of the problem, then what's a good solution?

C: Doing more?

T: Perhaps. Although I'd put some qualifications on that. Just "doing more" for the sake of being active probably isn't going to help much. The key for us would be to try to get you to have more experiences of mastery and pleasure in your day. So what kind of activities can you think of that would give you a sense of mastery or pleasure?

C: I don't know. Nothing really seems like it would be fun.

T: That's not surprising. Depression kind of sucks the fun out of things. It makes it hard for you to even imagine enjoying anything. Let me try asking it a different way. Before you felt this depressed, what kind of things used to give you a sense of mastery or pleasure?

C: Hmm. Well . . . I guess I used to like going out with my friends.

T: Ah. What kind of things did you like doing?

C: We'd go out and have lunch sometimes, or sometimes we'd just get some coffee and walk around downtown for a while.

T: Sounds nice.

C: It was. But I haven't talked to them in a while, so I don't know how I would even start that up again.

T: Let's worry about that in a bit. For now, we're just thinking of ideas. What else used to give you a sense of mastery or pleasure?

C: This is going to sound stupid, but I used to like just driving by myself through the country and blasting the stereo and singing.

T: That doesn't sound stupid to me. It sounds like something you enjoyed.

C: Yeah.

T: Let's keep thinking of ideas.

The therapist and Christina continue with this discussion until they have identified a large number of potentially rewarding activities. A couple of stylistic notes:

• The therapist keeps Christina focused on the task. In some cases, she throws up some potential roadblocks, such as not knowing how to get together with her friends. This is an important issue to problem-solve, but for now the therapist chooses not to allow the discussion to derail. In doing so, the therapist is modeling appropriate problem solving (see Chapter 12).

• The therapist makes a mental note of Christina's self-deprecating remarks, such as prefacing her idea with the statement "this is going to sound stupid." Statements like this can be conceptualized as unhealthy CRBs (see Chapter 9), as well as the cognitive distortion of *mind reading* (see Chapter 3). The therapist may come back around and address these remarks but for now chooses to stay focused on the task. Later, the therapist might opt to use a cognitive-level intervention (see Chapter 14) to address the distorted thought pattern.

• The therapist balances the reward potential of the activities against Christina's lack of enthusiasm. Depression makes it hard for an individual to accurately predict how enjoyable an activity will be. But the therapist uses cues from Christina's life before depression to generate hypotheses about what Christina might find pleasurable.

Activities will often be most rewarding if they are consistent with the client's longer-term *goals* and *values* (Hayes et al., 2012; Lejuez et al., 2001). The person's goals and values are what make something rewarding or reinforcing in the first place. I personally would find a chocolate chip cookie very rewarding. However, if you are the sort who really enjoys eating healthy, you might not find a cookie rewarding at all. So it's helpful to understand what the client's goals and values are—not just his or her goals for treatment but also in a broader sense of "What kind of life do you want to live?" and "What kind of person do you want to be?"

Orienting the client toward value-based action is not just for depressed clients. We often see that as clients struggle with various psychological problems, they focus more and more on trying to cope with their problems and less and less on acting in a value-based manner. So we go back to what's really important to the person—not just "being happy," but actually having a life that is consistent with long-term goals and values.

Here, the therapist is working with Suzanne (S), our client with GAD and benzodiazepine abuse, to help her identify the extent to which her behavior is consistent or inconsistent with her values.

T: We've been talking a lot about your actions to try to keep yourself from getting too anxious. In the last few sessions, you've told me about how you avoid doing things that would stress you out too much, and you've told me about how you use worrying as a way of trying to stay prepared for anything that might happen.

S: Right, that's pretty much what I do.

T: I'm wondering how much of your time and energy those activities take.

S: A lot. It seems sometimes like it just consumes my day, and I spend all of my energy fighting off the anxiety.

T: So fighting off the anxiety must be something very important to you.

S: Well, it is, because I just worry that I'm going to get overwhelmed.

T: You've got to wonder where that time and energy is coming from. I mean, if you're spending all of that time and energy fighting off anxiety, what aren't you doing instead?

S: Hmm . . . I guess I'm really not spending time with my friends and my family the way I used to. And if I do spend time with them, I'm not really focusing on them, because I'm so busy worrying.

T: So we have a question of what's really most important to you. It seems that you value your friends and family a lot, but in the moment you take your time and energy away from them and put it toward trying to fight anxiety.

S: I do.

T: So in the big picture, what do you really want your life to be about?

S: I'm not sure I understand.

T: Well, for example, you could have your life be all about fighting anxiety. You could put all of your time and effort into that. And maybe you would succeed at that, and then you would be the world champion anxiety fighter. Is that what you would really want for yourself?

S: No. Because I wouldn't have my friends and family.

T: Right, so even becoming the world champion anxiety fighter wouldn't really lead you toward a fulfilling life, because there are things that are more important to you than that. So if you don't want your life to be about fighting anxiety, what do you want it to be about?

S: Well, I want it to be about being a good friend and a good mother and a good wife. You know, having a life.

T: Yes. And somewhere along the way you jumped off of that track and it became all about trying not to feel anxious. So let's see if we can get you back on track. That's not to say that we don't want to help you feel better—we definitely do—but let's have you start working your way back to the person you want to be. What kinds of activities can you think of that would put you back on that track?

Finally, we need to *schedule the desired activities*. There are several important aspects of activity scheduling. First, we need to recognize that some activities are likely more difficult than others. For example, our client might be interested in climbing a mountain, but if he or she is out of shape, we might not want to schedule that immediately. Instead, we often recommend *successive approximations* toward the larger goal. Going for walks or hikes, for example, might be a useful first step.

We also need to specify the what, when, where, and how of the scheduled behavior (Kanter et al., 2010). Ideally, we come up with a concrete plan such as "play basketball at 2 P.M. on Saturday in the park with friends for 1 hour." That's much more likely to succeed than a vague instruction like "play basketball sometime this week." Of course, such clear specifications aren't always possible during the therapy session. In the case above, for example, the client might not know if his or her friends will be available on Saturday. But we want to push for concrete scheduling as much as possible. We can write the desired activities onto the client's daily activity form as a reminder. Alternatively, I've asked several clients to program the scheduled activity as an appointment (with alarm) on their smartphones (Boschen & Casey, 2008).

Here, the therapist works with Christina (C) to schedule potentially rewarding activities into the upcoming week.

> T: We've identified two activities that seem promising: getting together with friends and driving in the country and singing with the stereo blasting. What would it be like to try these activities this week?
>
> C: I don't know if I would enjoy them anymore.
>
> T: I don't, either. You might not enjoy them. But I do know that the old you used to like those things. So if we had to take a guess, would these be reasonable things to try?
>
> C: Yeah, I guess they could be reasonable.
>
> T: I would also suggest that if you don't enjoy them, that's not necessarily the end of the world. The aim here is not just to get happy by doing these things. Happiness would be a nice by-product of these activities, but perhaps what's more important is that you're taking some steps toward rebuilding a life. What would stop you from doing these things?
>
> C: Well, I don't think anything would really stop me from taking a drive. But if my friends weren't available, that could stop me from getting together with them.
>
> T: Yes. So maybe we need a backup plan. That is, if it turns out that none of your friends can get together with you, we should have something else for you to do rather than stay home on the couch.
>
> C: OK, that makes sense.
>
> T: What else could stop you?
>
> C: I guess if I felt too depressed?
>
> T: That would stop you? How would it stop you?
>
> C: If I were really depressed I just wouldn't want to go do anything.
>
> T: Let's rephrase that a little. If you felt really depressed, you might choose not to go out. You might choose to sit on the couch. That would be your choice, and of course you have every right to make that choice. But would that mean that your feelings had really stopped you?
>
> C: No, I guess it wouldn't mean that they stopped me. It's a choice I make.

T: Yes. And, by that logic, could you choose to do something different?

C: I don't know. A lot of the time I'd like to go out, but I feel depressed.

T: How about we say it this way: I want to go out, *and* I feel depressed. Do you see the difference there? You could have both things. One doesn't prevent the other.

C: So you're saying I should just suck it up?

T: Not necessarily. What I am saying is that you can choose what to do with your time. Your feelings might be one thing to take into consideration when you make that choice, but your feelings don't have to be the boss. You can be the boss. You could be a person who feels depressed and chooses to take her depression for a drive.

C: OK, I get it.

T: So let's figure out when you will take your depression for a drive. What day do you want to do this?

C: Saturday would be pretty good.

T: OK, Saturday it is. What time?

C: Maybe some time in the afternoon.

T: Can we get more specific? I suspect this will be easier if you know exactly what time you plan to do it, so that you don't sit around on Saturday saying "I'll do it later."

C: OK, let's say 3 P.M.

T: Perfect. And how long will this drive be?

C: I could probably do an hour.

T: OK. Shall we formalize that? You'll take your depression for a drive on Saturday at 3 P.M. for one hour?

C: Yeah, I can do that.

T: Great. Let's schedule that on your activity sheet.

Some stylistic points to note here:

• The therapist again sidesteps Christina's prediction that she won't enjoy the activities. This is not to say the therapist just chooses activities at random that seem pleasant; rather, Christina's history suggests a high likelihood that these activities will be rewarding.

• The therapist downplays the immediate need to feel good during the scheduled activities. Happiness is reframed as a "nice by-product" of the activities, but the therapist opts to emphasize the functional nature of the activities ("rebuilding a life"). If Christina is constantly judging these activities by whether she feels better in the moment ("Do I feel better now? How about now?"), she could easily become discouraged.

• The therapist asks Christina to anticipate potential problems in the plan by asking, "What would stop you?" This creates an opportunity to model and practice effective problem solving.

• The therapist challenges Christina's belief about her emotions being in charge of her behavior. The therapist makes a subtle change in wording, changing Christina's "but" to an "and" ("I want to go out, *but* I feel depressed" vs. "I want to go out, *and* I feel depressed"). By doing so, the therapist is emphasizing that Christina can act one way *and* feel another way and that these two things need not negate each other (Hayes et al., 2012).

- Toward this end, the therapist introduces the metaphor of "taking your depression for a drive." In so doing, it is emphasized that Christina does not have to feel better before acting better. This shift in perspective emphasizes redirecting her effort from emotional control to value-based actions. More on that topic in Chapter 19.

- The therapist takes it slow at first. Whenever we assign homework, we want to make sure that it's appropriate for the client's capacity. As Christina becomes a bit stronger (as evidenced by her ability to do these activities), we can increase the frequency of activities, the amount of time spent in activities, and the variety of activities assigned.

Graded Task Assignment

Breaking It Down

Often, the desired activities are too ambitious or overwhelming for the client. Lauren, our client with schizophrenia, for example, might have "get a job" as her desired activity. But it would probably not work very well for us to just assign that as next week's homework.

Graded task assignment (A. T. Beck et al., 1979) includes breaking a complex task (e.g., getting a job) into more manageable "bite-sized" components. The act of getting a job, for example, might include:

- Deciding what kind of job to seek.
- Looking at print and online want ads.
- Obtaining a job application.
- Completing the job application.
- Submitting the job application.
- Attending a job interview.

The first step in graded task assignment is to identify all of the smaller steps needed to accomplish the target and to put them in logical order. Once the smaller steps have been identified and put into order, the therapist schedules the first step with the client. The next steps are assigned in sequence.

Here, the therapist and Lauren (L) use graded task assignment to plan her strategy for getting a job.

T: Let's break this down into manageable chunks. If your aim is to get a job, what's the first thing you'd need to do?

L: Um . . . I guess I'd have to figure out what kind of job I want.

T: Yes, that sounds like a good idea. And what then?

L: I guess fill out the application.

T: Hold on, I think you might have skipped a step. Fill out the application for where?

L: For the job?

T: How do you know who's hiring?

L: Oh, I see. Yeah, I mean I guess I need to look at some websites and see who's hiring.

T: OK, so you find someone who's hiring. And then what?

L: Then I fill out the application.

T: If the application is online.

L: Right. And if it's not, get it and then fill it out and then hand it in.

T: Yes. That seems like a logical sequence to me. Getting a job might seem overwhelming, but if we look at it as one step at a time, maybe it's more manageable?

L: Yeah, maybe.

T: OK, so let's look at that first step: Deciding what kind of job you want. What could you do this week to accomplish that?

L: Um . . . I could think about it some.

T: You could. How about something more active?

L: I guess I could call my friends and see how they like the jobs that they have?

T: That could be a step in the right direction. Let's schedule that.

The alert reader might note that this form of graded task assignment parallels the *chaining* strategies discussed in Chapter 9.

Working Up to It

The term "graded task assignment" can also be used to describe a series of assignments that are progressively more difficult. This is a little bit like exercise (which is a great antidepressant in itself, by the way). You start off running around the block, then a mile, then 2 miles, and so on. Like exercise, the activity becomes progressively easier over time.

Here, the therapist has been working with Lauren (L) on searching online classified ads for jobs. But Lauren gets fatigued and distracted and has been unable to do it for very long. She's getting discouraged.

L: I just feel like when I start looking online, I just get tired and I get so frustrated with the process that I just give up and go watch TV.

T: OK, so you're having trouble sticking with it for a long period of time. How long can you go before you feel like you have to stop?

L: I think maybe 10 minutes. And then I just start thinking about other stuff and I don't want to do it anymore.

T: Let's see if we can find a solution here. This is a little like building up your muscles. If you try to bench press 300 pounds on your first day at the gym, it's probably not going to go so well.

L: No, it won't. And I guess that's kind of how I feel when I try to do this, like I'm just trying to do too much.

T: Well, at the gym, let's say it's your first day and you go over to the exercise machine. What's the best strategy?

L: I guess just lift what I can.

T: Right. So how would you know what you can realistically lift?

L: I'd lift a light weight and if it's too easy, then add a little weight and keep going like that until it gets hard.

T: Exactly. And that's the point where you want to be working—right when it gets hard. Too light and you're not really getting any exercise; too heavy and you're squashed. So what would be the equivalent of that strategy when it comes to looking at online ads?

L: I guess just see how much I can do until it gets hard, and then just do that much.

T: Yes. So if it feels like you can reliably do 10 minutes with no trouble, maybe we add just a little bit of weight to that? Could you do 15?

L: Yeah, I think I could probably do 15.

T: So let's make that the plan for this week. Now, thinking back to our bench press example, should you stay at the same weight forever?

L: No. Once you can do a certain weight you should add some more so you're challenging yourself.

T: Right. So if you can do 15 minutes this week . . .

L: . . . I should do 20 minutes next week.

T: Yes. We're building your stamina.

If you've snuck a peek at Chapter 11, you may have noted that this gradual "building up" to a behavior resembles the process of *exposure*.

THE ESSENTIALS

* CBT frequently involves making direct behavioral prescriptions to the client.

* Activity scheduling, commonly used for depressed clients, involves self-monitoring of activity, including examining the level of mastery and pleasure obtained from those activities. The therapist helps the client identify and schedule specific activities to add.

* Graded task assignment can be used to break down a complex task into its component parts. Graded task assignment can also be used to help the client perform successive approximations to an activity.

KEY TERMS AND DEFINITIONS

Activity scheduling: Increasing client activities that have a high likelihood of being naturally positively reinforced.

Direct behavioral prescriptions: Therapist instructions to the client to engage in some form of behavioral change.

Graded task assignment: Breaking down complex tasks into manageable components, or doing progressively more challenging activities.

Activity Scheduling

Part 1: For one full day, write down everything you do, and rate each hour's activity on a scale of 0–10 for mastery (the extent to which you felt a sense of accomplishment) and pleasure (the extent to which you enjoyed yourself).

Time	Activity	Mastery (0–10)	Pleasure (0–10)
6–7			
7–8			
8–9			
9–10			
10–11			
11–12			
12–1			
1–2			
2–3			
3–4			
4–5			
5–6			
6–7			
7–8			
8–9			
9–10			
10–11			
11–12			
12–1			
1–2			

(continued)

From *Doing CBT* by David F. Tolin. Copyright © 2016 The Guilford Press. Permission to photocopy this worksheet is granted to purchasers of this book for personal use only (see copyright page for details). Purchasers can download enlarged versions of this worksheet (see the box at the end of the table of contents).

Part 2: Make one behavioral change that is relevant to your personal target. You could use *activity scheduling, graded task assignment*, or *another direct behavioral prescription.*

What was the behavioral change you made?
What is your reaction to this exercise?

CHAPTER 11

Exposure

Many problems are associated with some form of *avoidance*. This is particularly true of clients who suffer from fear-related problems such as phobias, panic disorder, PTSD, GAD, and OCD. But avoidance is common in lots of forms of psychopathology, not just those classified in DSM as anxiety disorders. And identifying and reversing the pattern of avoidance is important for a broad range of clients.

Exposure is the process of confronting previously avoided stimuli. These stimuli might be external to the person, or they might be internal to the person.

Avoidance in Its Many Forms

Avoidance of *external* stimuli is quite common. For example:

- Scott, our socially anxious client, avoids parties, public speaking, and talking to people he doesn't know well.
- Melissa, our client with complex PTSD secondary to childhood abuse, avoids seeing movies on TV that remind her of her traumatic experiences and avoids close relationships with men.
- Christina, our client with depression, avoids activities that involve sustained effort.
- Anna, who has panic disorder and agoraphobic avoidance, avoids crowded places such as shopping malls or theaters.
- Suzanne, our client with GAD and benzodiazepine abuse, avoids air travel due to fears of a plane crash.
- Bethany, our client with OCD, avoids being around sharp objects due to a fear that she might use them to harm someone. She also avoids things that she thinks might be "contaminated" or "dirty," for fear that she will contract a disease.
- Lauren, our client with schizophrenia, avoids being out in public due to fears of being persecuted.

Avoidance of *internal* stimuli is often more difficult to detect but is equally important. For example:

- Suzanne avoids thinking about certain feared disasters, worrying instead about more minor things or taking pills to "quiet her mind."
- Melissa avoids thinking about her childhood abuse experiences, often drinking as a way to try to "numb" herself.
- Elizabeth, our client with borderline personality and self-injurious behavior, tries to avoid feeling angry, for fear she will lose control of herself.
- Anna tries not to allow herself to become physiologically aroused, which she fears might trigger a panic attack.
- Bethany avoids thoughts that she might hurt someone or that she might be contaminated, telling herself over and over again that she is safe or that she is clean.

Understanding Exposure

Through exposure, we confront these patterns of fear and avoidance. The overall strategy is a direct behavioral prescription to face the feared and avoided stimulus until the client's distress subsides or a sense of mastery has been achieved.

In most cases, exposure is conducted gradually, in the same fashion as the *graded task assignment* described in Chapter 10. The client is instructed to perform moderately challenging exposures at first and then, once those exposures become easier, more difficult exposures are assigned. In contrast, some clinicians have used a strategy called **flooding,** in which exposure begins with the most challenging exercises. In practice, graded exposure and flooding appear equally effective in the long run. Therefore, selection of graded exposure versus flooding is largely a matter of personal preference and comfort level. Some people like to tiptoe into the cold swimming pool, whereas other people like to do a cannonball off the side. Speaking for myself, I like to tiptoe in. But I understand why some other people prefer the cannonball. The choice is based on a trade-off of comfort versus efficiency: How much discomfort is the client willing to tolerate in order to speed up the process? One option is generally easier for most people to tolerate, but the other option will often get the job done more quickly. In the end, everyone ends up in the pool, and things tend to work out. Most clinicians and clients tend to prefer the graded approach (Moulds & Nixon, 2006; Öst, Alm, Brandberg, & Breitholtz, 2001), so that's what we'll emphasize here.

In Vivo Exposure

Whenever possible (and safe), the most effective and efficient way to perform exposure is to confront avoided situations in real life. This is called *in vivo* **exposure.** Examples of *in vivo* exposure might include:

- Scott goes to a party, speaks in public, and talks to people he doesn't know well.
- Melissa watches movies that remind her of her traumatic experiences and interacts socially with men.
- Suzanne flies on an airplane.
- Christina engages in progressively greater sustained effort.

- Anna goes to shopping malls and theaters.
- Bethany handles sharp objects and touches things that she thinks might be "contaminated" or "dirty."
- Lauren goes out in public.

Imaginal Exposure

Sometimes *in vivo* exposure is just not possible. Suzanne, for example, might find it financially prohibitive to fly repeatedly on an airplane. In such cases, **imaginal exposure** might be used to envision the avoided activity. So the therapist might instruct Suzanne to envision, in great detail, the act of getting on the plane, buckling in, taking off, and even experiencing scary turbulence. Imaginal exposure often makes use of audio recordings so that the exposure can be repeated. During an imaginal exposure session, the client's narrative might be recorded (e.g., on a smartphone app), with the instruction to listen to the recording repeatedly for homework.

In recent years, **virtual reality exposure therapy** (in which clients are immersed in a "virtual" world that allows them to confront their fears) has been examined as an alternative means of imaginal exposure, and preliminary data suggest that it can be quite effective (Meyerbroker & Emmelkamp, 2010; Michaliszyn, Marchand, Bouchard, Martel, & Poirier-Bisson, 2010).

Exposure to Thoughts

As I mentioned earlier, sometimes the feared and avoided stimuli are internal to the person. In many cases, the feared and avoided stimulus is mental, such as a thought or a memory. We might use **exposure to thoughts** as a way of confronting and reducing distress about these mental "triggers." Sometimes, these exposures are to intrusive, scary thoughts, such as the obsessions experienced by someone with OCD. In other cases, the exposures are to worst-case scenarios, such as the catastrophes imagined by someone with GAD. Examples of exposure to thoughts might include:

- Suzanne imagines the worst-case scenarios.
- Melissa deliberately recalls her childhood abuse experiences.
- Bethany deliberately thinks about harming someone, or that she is contaminated.

Exposure to Feelings

In other cases, the feared and avoided stimulus is physiological or emotional. We might use **exposure to emotions and physiological sensations,** sometimes called *interoceptive exposure,* to reduce distress toward those internal stimuli. Examples of exposure to emotions and physiological sensations might include:

- Anna deliberately engages in activities that cause her heart rate to increase or that cause her to feel dizzy.
- Elizabeth deliberately induces feelings of anger.
- When Christina experiences sadness in the session, the therapist points it out and asks her to sit with it, experiencing it fully.

Things That Might Bug You about This

A lot of therapists seem reluctant to use exposure therapy (Becker, Zayfert, & Anderson, 2004), often because they fear upsetting the client or damaging the therapeutic relationship. There are a lot of myths about exposure therapy that make some therapists squeamish (Feeny, Hembree, & Zoellner, 2003). However, when we look at the facts, it seems that fears about exposure are greatly overblown. I don't think I'm exaggerating when I say that one of the most common blunders therapists make is underutilizing exposure. Here are the most common myths out there:

- *Exposure will cause intolerable anxiety.* Exposure therapy does not routinely worsen anxiety. That is, although exposure is temporarily anxiety-producing, the evidence does not suggest that it causes a sustained increase in anxiety. In a large study of clients with PTSD (female assault survivors seen in a community clinic), imaginal exposure was used in which the clients deliberately and vividly recalled and described their traumatic experiences. Approximately a quarter of these clients reported a temporary increase in feelings of anxiety in the days following exposure, and about 1 in 10 reported a temporary increase in feelings of depression. Those who reported an exacerbation of anxiety or depression were no more likely to drop out than were those who did not report an exacerbation, and they benefited just as much from the treatment in the long run (Foa, Zoellner, Feeny, Hembree, & Alvarez-Conrad, 2002). Among 361 female assault survivors with PTSD, none showed a reliable worsening of PTSD symptoms, whereas 93% showed a reliable improvement in PTSD symptoms, when receiving exposure therapy (Jayawickreme et al., 2014).

- *Exposure will increase co-occurring problems, such as substance abuse, self-destructive behaviors, or psychosis and can't be effective with complex cases.* Exposure therapy does not routinely cause substance use to worsen in dually diagnosed clients. Several studies of clients with co-occurring PTSD and substance use disorders show that those receiving exposure-based PTSD treatment showed reductions in substance use, as well as reductions in their PTSD symptoms, with gains maintained over an extended follow-up period (Berenz, Rowe, Schumacher, Stasiewicz, & Coffey, 2012; Brady, Dansky, Back, Foa, & Carroll, 2001; Mills et al., 2012). In clinical practice, it's worth noting that we would usually be providing a substance-abuse-specific intervention concurrently with (or, in many cases, preceding) the exposure.

The available data suggest that clients with dissociative disorder also benefit from exposure. In trials of clients with PTSD, clients with significant dissociative symptoms did not drop out more frequently and showed equivalent improvement compared with clients without significant dissociation (Hagenaars, van Minnen, & Hoogduin, 2010; Halvorsen, Stenmark, Neuner, & Nordahl, 2014).

The available data do not suggest that exposure therapy exacerbates self-injurious behaviors. Exposure is an element of dialectical behavior therapy for clients with borderline personality disorder and self-injurious behavior (Linehan, 1993). In a trial of clients with co-occurring PTSD and borderline personality disorder with a history of nonsuicidal self-injury who were receiving dialectical behavior therapy that included exposure, rates of self-injury decreased significantly over the course of the program, and the rate of self-injury was not higher in weeks that included exposure than in weeks that did not include exposure (Krüger et al., 2014). When a similar group of clients was randomly assigned to receive DBT or DBT plus exposure to trauma memories and cues, those receiving exposure had double the remission rate of those receiving DBT without exposure and were 2.4 times less likely to attempt suicide and 1.5 times less likely to self-injure than were those in DBT without exposure (Harned, Korslund, & Linehan, 2014). Again, it's worth noting that in clinical practice clients usually receive some training in emotion regulation strategies (see Chapters 18 and 19) prior to exposure. In the Harned et al. (2014) study, clients did not begin exposure until they were judged to be not at imminent risk of suicide, had not self-injured in the previous 2 months, were able to control intentional self-injury when in the presence of cues for those behaviors, did not exhibit serious TIBs, and were able and willing to experience intense emotions without escaping.

The available data do not suggest that exposure therapy exacerbates psychotic symptoms. In an open trial of clients with co-occurring PTSD and schizophrenia, a PTSD treatment that included exposure (along with skill training, cognitive restructuring, and relaxation) resulted in significant improvements in PTSD symptoms, with no reported adverse events (Frueh et al., 2009). Similar results have been reported in a case of co-occurring OCD and schizophrenia treated with exposure therapy (Ekers, Carman, & Schlich, 2004).

- *Exposure can't be used for people with PTSD, childhood sexual abuse, or complex PTSD.* The U.S. Agency for Healthcare Research and Quality (Jonas et al., 2013) and the Institute of Medicine (2008) both identified exposure therapy as the *only* psychological intervention with high strength of evidence for PTSD. Extensive evidence demonstrates that exposure-based treatment for PTSD is effective in a wide range of clients, from motor vehicle accident survivors to combat veterans to rape victims (Powers, Halpern, Ferenschak, Gilihan, & Foa, 2010).Across studies, exposure appears to work just as well for people with childhood sexual trauma as it does for people with PTSD resulting from other forms of trauma (Powers et al., 2010). Adult survivors of childhood sexual abuse were more likely to respond favorably to exposure therapy than to a problem-solving therapy that did not include exposure (McDonagh et al., 2005), and across studies clients with childhood sexual trauma respond more favorably to interventions that directly involve discussing the trauma than to interventions that do not address the trauma directly (Ehring et al., 2014). A combined treatment of skill building and exposure proved more effective than exposure alone or skill building alone for survivors of childhood abuse, though all three were fairly effective in reducing PTSD symptoms (Cloitre et al., 2010).

A panel of trauma experts identified exposure as the first-line treatment for clients with complex PTSD (Cloitre et al., 2011), defined as a history of complex, extreme, and/or recurrent trauma and associated with emotion regulation difficulties, disturbances in relational capacities, alterations in attention and consciousness (e.g., dissociation), adversely affected belief systems, and somatic distress or disorganization. Exposure therapy proved effective in a sample of clients with complex PTSD resulting from childhood sexual abuse, not only in PTSD symptoms but also in related concerns such as dissociation, dysfunctional sexual behavior, and other maladaptive behaviors (Resick, Nishith, & Griffin, 2003).

- *Children can't tolerate exposure therapy.* Children actually do great with exposure therapy (Kendall et al., 2006; Tolin & Franklin, 2002). In one trial of exposure and response prevention (more on response prevention later) in children ages 3–8 with OCD, 65% were considered treatment responders, with no dropouts and high levels of client and parent satisfaction with the treatment (Lewin et al., 2014). Other studies with children and adolescents demonstrate the effectiveness of exposure for phobias (Ollendick et al., 2009), panic disorder (Pincus, May, Whitton, Mattis, & Barlow, 2010), and PTSD (Gilboa-Schechtman et al., 2010). Exposure therapy for children is often modified to incorporate the parents as co-therapists (Piacentini et al., 2011), and some have framed exposures as "show-that-I-can" (STIC) tasks (Kendall & Hedtke, 2006). Long-term beneficial effects of exposure therapy for children have been demonstrated as long as 13 years after treatment ended (Saavedra, Silverman, Morgan-Lopez, & Kurtines, 2010).

- *Exposure therapy can only work when you also provide extensive coping skill training.* There are certainly some clients for whom this is likely the case. Dialectical behavioral therapy for borderline personality disorder and self-injurious behavior, as one example, uses exposure for PTSD symptoms but also incorporates emotion regulation skills such as cognitive restructuring, mindfulness, and direct behavioral prescriptions. Some studies of PTSD have suggested that emotion regulation training (see Chapters 18 and 19) prior to exposure therapy may decrease dropout rates and improve efficacy (Bryant et al., 2013; Cloitre et al., 2010). Across studies, however, the incremental benefit of adding just about anything to exposure is fairly small (e.g., Kehle-Forbes et al., 2013; Meuret, Wolitzky-Taylor, Twohig, & Craske, 2012).

- *Clients don't want exposure therapy.* The available data suggest that clients generally find exposure acceptable, even preferable to many alternative forms of treatment. When women with PTSD were asked to choose between exposure therapy and the antidepressant sertraline, three times as many chose to receive exposure therapy (Zoellner, Feeny, Cochran, & Pruitt, 2003). Similarly, college students who experienced trauma were over four times more likely to select exposure over sertraline, and over three times more likely to select exposure over psychodynamic therapy; none selected eye movement desensitization and reprocessing, a variation of exposure therapy with questionable scientific support (Becker, Darius, & Schaumberg, 2007). Veterans receiving exposure therapy for PTSD report high levels of satisfaction with the program and state that they would recommend the treatment to a friend with similar problems (Mott et al., 2013). Similarly, clients with agoraphobia rate exposure therapy as more acceptable, and more likely to be effective, than drug therapy, cognitive therapy, and relationship-oriented therapy (G. R. Norton, Allen, & Hilton, 1983).

In my clinical experience, many clients report that they find the idea of exposure naturally intuitive. It makes sense to them. Most of us can recall being afraid of something, like swimming or the dark, when we were kids. How did we overcome those childhood fears? By avoiding swimming or the dark forever? No, in most cases we overcame them by gradually getting used to the thing we were afraid of. Maybe we took it slowly, maybe we had help from someone else, but at the end of the day, most people recognize that you beat fears by facing them.

- *Clients will drop out of exposure therapy.* The data do not suggest that exposure is associated with increased dropout rates. Across studies of PTSD, clients are no more likely to drop out of exposure therapy than they are to drop out of other psychological treatments (Hembree et al., 2003). When exposure has been compared directly with pharmacotherapy for anxiety-related disorders, exposure usually shows an equivalent dropout rate (Barlow, Gorman, Shear, & Woods, 2000; Foa et al., 2005; Heimberg et al., 1998).

These myths are not only erroneous, they are also harmful. First, believing in these myths makes clinicians much less likely to use exposure therapy with their clients (van Minnen, Hendriks, & Olff, 2010)—a problem that has been labeled *exposophobia:* "The extreme fear (and associated avoidance) of using exposure therapy procedures occurring in trained mental health professionals" (Schare & Wyatt, 2013, p. 252). That's a real shame, because exposure is one of the most well-validated psychotherapy procedures in existence. Its efficacy cannot be disputed across the anxiety, trauma- and stressor-related, and obsessive-compulsive and related disorders (Cox, Endler, Lee, & Swinson, 1992; Jonsson & Hougaard, 2009; P. J. Norton & Price, 2007; Powers et al., 2010; N. P. Roberts, Kitchiner, Kenardy, & Bisson, 2009; Tolin, 2010).

How Does Exposure Work?

Although it's abundantly clear that exposure works, there are competing theories about how it works (Barlow & Allen, 2004; Craske et al., 2008). Some have suggested that exposure causes **habituation,** which is decreased responding over time to any stimulus that is presented over and over (Groves & Thompson, 1970). For example, initial exposure to ocean water can be cold. However, over time and with continued exposure, the water feels less cold as the person acclimates. Similarly, when repeatedly facing a fear-provoking stimulus in exposure therapy, the client experiences habituation, or a natural reduction in fear response.

Much of what we know about how exposure therapy works is from studies of **extinction.** We previously discussed extinction in the context of operant conditioning (see Chapter 2), although the variation of extinction we're talking about now is based on a classical conditioning model of fear (see Chapter 4). According to this model, the feared object, activity, situation, and so forth serves as a *conditioned stimulus.* By repeated presentation of the conditioned stimulus (e.g., a dog) without an unconditioned stimulus (e.g., pain, harm), the conditioned response (fear) is weakened.

Essentially, extinction of emotional responses (such as fear) is a form of learning. Specifically, extinction seems to rely on **inhibitory learning:** One learning experience interferes with, or inhibits, another (Bouton, 1993). So, for example, if we have learned to fear a dog, through exposure we learn new information about dogs that inhibits our learned fear. The implication is that the old learning is not erased—we don't "unlearn" our fear—but rather we learn new things through experience that can override that fear.

We can see this inhibitory learning process in the brain when people receive exposure. During exposure, the "fear centers" of the brain, such as the amygdala, become active (Sehlmeyer et al., 2009; Sotres-Bayon, Cain, & LeDoux, 2006). Over the course of exposure, the frontal cortex of the brain becomes active (Sotres-Bayon et al., 2006) and overrides the activity of the fear centers (Delgado, Nearing, Ledoux, & Phelps, 2008).

Craske et al. (2008) have suggested that exposure may work by promoting fear *toleration* rather than fear *reduction.* That is, a central aim of exposure may be to help clients learn to tolerate feelings of fear rather than engage in desperate attempts to feel better. This principle relates closely to the idea of *distress tolerance*, which we discuss at length in Chapter 19. For practical purposes in therapy, the idea of fear toleration means that we aren't necessarily trying to help clients feel better, at least not in the moment. Rather, we are trying to change how they think about fear itself—for example, helping them discover that it doesn't last forever and is manageable. Supporting this idea is the fact that when exposure is combined with drugs that increase sympathetic nervous system activity (i.e., create more feelings of anxiety and tension), it actually seems to work better than when exposure is combined with placebo or with drugs that decrease sympathetic nervous system activity (Berman & Dudai, 2001; Cain, Blouin, & Barad, 2004).

There are likely other factors at work in exposure as well. Some have argued for a role for **emotional processing** (Lang, 1971), which suggests that exposure to fear-provoking stimuli results in a new way of processing information that corrects faulty representations of fear in long-term memory (Foa & Kozak, 1986). For example, social interactions in clients with social phobia can be perceived as rewarding, despite their having sweaty palms and feeling some anxiety.

Still others have suggested that exposure works by improving the client's **self-efficacy**. The idea here is that rather than simply reducing a fear response, exposure increases the client's sense of mastery over a situation or performance (Bandura, 1977), changing "I can'ts" to "I cans." Persons with anxiety disorders tend to underestimate their capabilities to cope with fear. Therefore, if a client is able to face his or her fear and successfully tolerate it without avoiding it or withdrawing from it, he or she begins to realize that he or she is more capable and resilient than he or she had imagined. Thus the person becomes more willing to face his or her fears in different contexts, generalizing treatment effects.

"Pitching" Exposure

Despite the fact that clients intuitively "get" the idea of exposure, it's natural to expect a certain degree of ambivalence (although many clients are gung-ho from the start). After all, exposure is inherently scary, and the client has usually taken great pains to develop an avoidant coping style. Whenever we're faced with client ambivalence, we rely on the basic principles of motivational interviewing (MI; W. R. Miller & Rollnick, 2013), as discussed in Chapter 7. The spirit of MI can be summarized by the acronym ACE: Autonomy, Collaboration, and Evocation. That is, the therapist neither shoves exposure down the client's throat nor abandons the idea just because the client is ambivalent. Rather, the therapist respects the client's choices and collaborates with the client to generate an understanding of the problem, rationale for treatment, and ideas for interventions, often using questioning to evoke these ideas from the client.

Muller and Schultz (2012) provide several considerations for effectively pitching exposure therapy to clients, including:

- *Be on board with exposure yourself.* In order to present the facts accurately and persuasively, you have to know what you're talking about and believe what you're talking about. If you're still hanging on to negative myths about exposure therapy, you're unlikely to get a client on board. If that's the case, go back in this chapter and reread the facts.

- *Assess the client's expectations.* Before even discussing the rationale for exposure therapy, it can be helpful to ask the client whether he or she has heard of it and what he or she thinks of it. Is the client imagining some nightmarish scenario of being strapped to a chair and having spiders and snakes dumped on him or her? If so, discuss the issue of gradual exposure rather than flooding. Does the client believe that it's not likely to help? If so, look up the facts and share them with the client. Does the client believe it will be a piece of cake? If so, caution the client that exposure is often difficult work.

- *Emphasize the rationale.* As you work on your CBT case conceptualization, help the client to understand the role that avoidance (be it behavioral or mental) plays in the maintenance of the problem. Explain the mechanisms of habituation, extinction, cognitive processing, and self-efficacy. Help the client to understand that although facing fears might be uncomfortable at first, exposure will help break him or her out of a persistent cycle of unhappiness.

- *Provide real-life examples of habituation.* Most of us understand the basic idea of habituation once it's explained to us. And we can all probably think of things we've habituated to. A cold swimming pool, a smelly locker room, or traffic noise outside our apartment are all things that might be aversive at first, but we quickly adjust to them.

- *Step outside of the client's fear.* Often it's easier for the client to understand the rationale for exposure when it's discussed outside of the context of his or her own specific fear. So, for example, if I'm treating someone with panic disorder, I might ask him or her to imagine how we might treat someone with a completely different fear, such as a dog phobia.

Here, the therapist pitches exposure therapy to Scott (S), our socially anxious client.

T: We've spent quite a bit of time discussing your social anxiety, and I think we have a pretty good idea of where it's coming from.

S: Yeah, I think so. It's helpful for me to see that my anxious thoughts are part of what's keeping me anxious.

T: Right. I want to focus in a bit on the avoidance part of the puzzle. You've told me quite a bit about how you avoid social and performance situations that feel scary to you. For example, you don't go to parties, you don't speak up in meetings, you don't approach people to talk to them, and so on. My question to you is: Do you think that this avoidance is helping you? Or hurting you?

S: Well, I feel a lot better when I can avoid something.

T: Understood, although I had a slightly different question in mind. We know that avoidance feels better than doing these things. But my question is, is that really helping you? That is, is avoidance making your life better?

S: Well, no, in the long term it's not.

T: OK. It's not helping. On the flip side, what could some of the negative consequences of avoidance be?

S: Negative consequences? Well, I mean, I guess I don't go to the party, so I don't make as many friends?

T: Yes, that's one possibility. Avoidance does mean that you miss out on some things.

S: But I don't really want to go to the party anyway.

T: That's true. You don't want to go, because it would be scary and uncomfortable.

S: Right.

T: Perhaps more to the point, let me ask it this way: In the long run, do you think avoidance makes you less anxious, or more anxious?

S: I don't know. Less anxious I guess? Because I'm not going to parties and stuff?

T: Let's think of it this way. Say I have a terrible fear of dogs. And you're my therapist. And I come to you and I say "Doc, I have this fear of dogs. I think they're all going to rip my face off. What should I do?"

S: (*Laughs.*) I don't know.

T: Perhaps I should just make sure I never see a dog again. So maybe I should just stay inside whenever there's a dog around. And for that matter, I won't even watch Animal Planet, just in case a dog comes on TV. Over time, what would happen to my fear of dogs?

S: I guess it wouldn't go away.

T: Why not?

S: Well, because you're not seeing any dogs, so how do you know that they're not dangerous?

T: Exactly. If I avoid dogs, I just keep on thinking that they're all dangerous. I don't learn the truth, which is . . . what?

S: That some dogs might be dangerous, but most of them aren't.

T: Right. My fear is overblown, but if I keep avoiding I don't get to learn that for myself. So Doc, should I avoid dogs as a way of controlling my fear?

S: No.

T: What should I do instead?

S: You should get used to dogs.

T: Ah, interesting idea. I should get used to dogs. You mean I should throw myself into a kennel filled with really vicious, mean-looking dogs?

S: (*Laughs.*) No. You should probably start small. Like with a little puppy or something.

T: I see. What should I do with the puppy? Stay on the other side of the room from it? Or wave a big stick at it so it leaves me alone?

S: No, you should go pet it. Or at least, you know, get closer and closer to it until you can pet it.

T: Yeah, but isn't that just going to make me anxious? I mean, won't I just get so anxious that my head will explode?

S: It'll probably be scary at first.

T: And then?

S: You'll probably feel better once you see that the puppy isn't hurting you.

T: OK, so I pet the puppy. Now I'm done, right? You cured my dog phobia!

S: Not yet, no. Once you pet the puppy and you see it's OK, then you work your way up to something a little bigger.

T: Gotcha. So let me see if I'm hearing you, Doc: Avoidance is part of my problem, and to beat the problem I should probably do what I'm afraid of, starting small and then working my way up, so that I can learn it's OK?

S: Right.

T: Perfect. I couldn't have said it better myself. Now let's talk about you again. Does it make sense for you to keep avoiding scary social situations?

S: (*Pauses.*) No, I guess not. It keeps me anxious.

T: It keeps you from learning the truth, which is . . .

S: . . . that these things probably aren't as bad as I think they will be.

T: And so to beat that fear you should . . .

S: . . . start small and do things that are scary.

Developing an Exposure Hierarchy

The first step in graded exposure therapy is to develop an **exposure hierarchy:** a list of exposure activities to be performed. Items are developed collaboratively with the client by identifying activities that are not objectively dangerous but would nevertheless elicit fear and a desire to avoid.

For each item, we assign a **fear level,** sometimes referred to as the *subjective units of discomfort scale,* or SUDS (Wolpe, 1990), a numeric rating of how scary each activity would be. I usually use a scale from 0 to 100, although the exact scale is not critical (I had one child client who preferred to use the terms *rare, medium rare, medium, medium well,* and *well done.* Good enough). The fear level is assessed by asking how afraid or distressed the client would be conducting each activity.

The exposure hierarchy is then ordered according to fear level. A sample fear hierarchy for a client with a fear of dogs is shown in Figure 11.1, and you can find a blank

Activity	Fear Level (0–100)
1. Letting a large dog lick my face	90
2. Petting a large dog	85
3. Being in a room with a large dog off leash	80
4. Being in a room with a large dog on leash	75
5. Letting a small dog lick my face	70
6. Petting a small dog	65
7. Being in a room with a small dog off leash	60
8. Being in a room with a small dog on leash	55
9. Visiting a pet shop and looking at dogs in cages	40
10. Watching movies of dogs	35
11. Looking at pictures of dogs	30

FIGURE 11.1. Sample Exposure Hierarchy. From Tolin (2012). Copyright © 2012 Turner Publishing. Reprinted by permission.

version in Appendix B. As you can see, we broke the fear down into several concrete steps and ranked the steps according to their predicted fear level. In this case, we'll start near the bottom, with something that's not too scary (looking at pictures of dogs). Once that step has been mastered, it's time to move up to the next step (watching movies of dogs). Once that step has been mastered, we move up to the next step, and the next one, and so on, until the client is able to do the most difficult exposure (letting a large dog lick his or her face).

Notice that the exposure hierarchy doesn't shy away from high-fear exposures. The client might say something like, "No way would I ever let a large dog lick my face! I'd freak out!" But that is exactly why it's important to include that item in the hierarchy. Remember, the client will be working his or her way up the hierarchy gradually, so that by the time he or she gets to that step, it won't seem nearly as scary as it does during the initial planning. Therefore, an important rule of the exposure hierarchy is that you should include the scariest exposures, even if the client doesn't feel able to do them right now.

There is no hard and fast rule about how many items to include on an exposure hierarchy. The idea is that you want enough steps to help the client work his or her way up gradually, but not so many that it takes forever to complete the hierarchy. Ten items, give or take a couple, might be a good place to start, but that's a rough estimate. I've had clients who did quite well with only four or five items, and I've had other clients who needed 50 items or more for fears that were more complex. You want to make sure that you have adequate representation of low-fear, moderate-fear, and high-fear situations or activities, so that the client can progress gradually up the hierarchy.

What kind of activities should go on the exposure hierarchy? Everyone's fear is a little different. What's scary for one person might not be scary for another. Table 11.1 shows some examples of exposure activities (adapted from Tolin, 2012) that people in my clinic have completed. As you can see, it's quite a long list, and successful exposure therapy requires a lot of creativity from the therapist.

TABLE 11.1. Sample Exposure Exercises

Specific phobias

Animal-related exposures
- Holding snakes, spiders, or other animals.
- Visiting a pet store.
- Reading about, looking at pictures of, or watching movies about the feared animal.
- Drawing pictures of or singing songs about the feared animal.

Situational exposures
- Going to tall buildings and looking down over the balcony.
- Taking commercial flights.
- Spending time in confined spaces like closets.
- Going outside during storms.
- Being in the dark.
- Going swimming.
- Watching or listening to people vomit or pretend to vomit.
- Reading about, looking at pictures of, or watching movies about the feared situation.
- Drawing pictures of, or singing songs about, the feared situation.

Blood, injection, or injury-related exposures
- Watching others get injections or blood draws.
- Donating blood.
- Visiting a dentist.
- Watching surgeries on television.
- Reading about, looking at pictures of, or watching movies about blood, injections, or injuries.
- Drawing pictures of or singing songs about blood, injections, or injuries.

Panic disorder, agoraphobia, or fears of panic-like body sensations

Exercises to induce dizziness, lightheadedness, or faintness
- Hyperventilating.
- Spinning in a chair.
- Shaking the head back and forth rapidly.
- Lowering the head between the knees for 30 seconds, then raising the head quickly to induce a "draining" sensation.
- Going on rides at an amusement park.

Exercises to raise heart rate
- Running up and down stairs.
- Watching scary movies.
- Drinking caffeinated beverages.

Exercises to create a smothering feeling
- Breathing through a straw.
- Holding one's breath as long as possible.
- Lying with a heavy stack of books on one's chest.
- Wearing a tight scarf or tie.

Exercises to induce muscle tension or soreness
- Tensing all of the muscles of the body.

Exercises to induce uncomfortable digestive system feelings
- Smelling spoiled food or cigar butts to induce nausea.
- Eating to the point of feeling stuffed.
- Keeping cotton balls in one's mouth to make the mouth and throat feel dry.
- Swallowing rapidly again and again.

(continued)

TABLE 11.1. *(continued)*

Exercises to induce hot or cold sensations
- Sitting in a steamy bathroom or in a car with the heat cranked up.
- Going outside in cold weather with no coat on.

Exercises to induce feelings of unreality
- Staring at a spot on the wall, or one's hand, or a mirror for several minutes.

Exposures to situations that are difficult to escape from
- Sitting in crowded places such as theaters or church, away from aisles and exits.
- Going to busy places such as supermarkets or museums.
- Driving through tunnels or over bridges.
- Driving on busy highways.
- Riding buses or subways.
- Driving in heavy traffic during rush hour.
- Using elevators or escalators.

Exposures to being away from sources of help
- Being home alone.
- Going far away from one's home or car.
- Going to unfamiliar places and deliberately getting lost.

Social phobia or other social and performance fears

Exposure to social interactions
- Attending parties or other social gatherings.
- Introducing oneself to strangers.
- Initiating and maintaining conversations.

Exposure to being the center of attention
- Giving speeches.
- Speaking up in classes or meetings.
- Performing music, sports, or other activities in front of others.
- Inviting others to watch one work.
- Doing things while being photographed or filmed.

Exposure to assertive situations
- Returning items to a store.
- Asking people to quiet down in a movie theater.

Exposure to having others see embarrassing behavior or signs of anxiety
- Sprinkling water on the face, hands, or armpits in order to appear sweaty, then interacting with others.
- Jogging in place to appear flushed, then interacting with others.
- Deliberately falling down in front of people.
- Deliberately making mistakes in front of people.
- Deliberately stammering while talking.

OCD and obsessive fears

Exposure to contamination
- Touching a doorknob.
- Touching a newspaper.
- Touching someone's sweaty shirt.
- Touching toilet seats in public bathrooms.

(continued)

TABLE 11.1. (continued)

- Touching money.
- Touching a dead animal.
- Touching household chemicals.
- Making food for others with dirty hands.
- Touching one's own children with dirty hands.
- Touching someone else's saliva.
- Visiting an AIDS clinic and touching things.
- Touching gas pumps.

Exposure to fears of harming others
- Holding a knife while around people.
- Reading books or watching movies about serial killers.
- Bumping into people.
- Throwing thumbtacks onto the street.
- Driving through a crowded pedestrian area.

Exposure to making errors
- Leaving the house after turning the stove (or other appliance) on and off.
- Lighting candles and leaving the house.
- Going to bed with the door unlocked.
- Making a deliberate mistake with paperwork.

Exposure to things being "not right"
- Messing up the clothes in one's own closet.
- Putting things in the "wrong" order (e.g., putting magazines out of chronological order).
- Sprinkling dirt on the kitchen floor.
- Walking through doorways or up stairs in the "wrong" way.
- Eating, grooming, or brushing teeth "wrong."

Exposure to fears of being immoral or blasphemous
- Deliberately making small "sins" such as littering or cursing.
- Saying or writing blasphemous things like "I hate God" or "I like the Devil."

Exposure to superstitious or magical fears
- Doing things a "bad" number of times.
- Stepping on sidewalk cracks.
- Praying for disasters, such as a plane crash or a tornado.
- Saying or writing "forbidden" or "bad luck" words.

GAD and excessive worries

"Worst case scenario" exposures
- Writing down a detailed story about the worst thing happening (e.g., a story in which loved ones die or the house burns down).
- Making a recording of the story and listening to it over and over.
- Holding a mental image of the worst thing happening (e.g., a mental image of loved ones lying dead, or the house on fire).
- Drawing pictures of the worst thing happening.

"Risk" exposures
- Leaving the house with the door or window unlocked.
- Sleeping with the door unlocked.
- Deliberately making small errors.
- Deliberately being late for an event.

(continued)

TABLE 11.1. *(continued)*

PTSD

Traumatic-event exposures
- Writing down a detailed story about the traumatic event.
- Making a recording of the story and listening to it over and over.
- Holding a mental image of the traumatic event.
- Drawing pictures of the traumatic event.
- Reading about, looking at pictures of, or watching movies about events that resemble the traumatic event.

Situational exposures
- Driving or riding in a car.
- Going outside alone at night.
- Talking to people who resemble an assailant but are objectively not dangerous.

It's important that the exposure hierarchy list actual activities that the client can do. It's less helpful to include things like:

- *Feared consequences.* Listing feared consequences doesn't provide the client with a clear exposure exercise to do. So, for example, it is not helpful to write things like "I'll get sick and die"; "The plane will crash"; or "Everyone will think I'm a big loser." Instead, try turning those fears into exposure items that the client can actually do. For example, instead of "I'll get sick and die," try "Touch some Lysol and then make a sandwich and eat it." Instead of "The plane will crash," try "Fly in turbulent weather on a small plane." Instead of "Everyone will think I'm a big loser," try "Deliberately fall down in a public place and scatter an armload of books."

- *Items that are too vague.* The exposure hierarchy is intended to be a list of specific exercises for the client to do. It is important, therefore, that the items on the list give the client concrete, clear instructions. So, for example, it is not helpful to write things like "Touch things that are dirty"; "Feel uncomfortable physical sensations"; or "Think of disaster scenarios." Instead, try to be clear about what it is the client will actually do. Instead of "Touch things that are dirty," try "Touch a public toilet seat." Instead of "Feel uncomfortable physical sensations," try "Hyperventilate until I feel lightheaded." Instead of "Think of disaster scenarios," try "Record a story about my family getting into a serious car accident, and listen to the recording over and over."

Here, the therapist is working with Bethany (B), the teenage girl with OCD, to develop an exposure hierarchy related to her fear of contamination (a similar process would be followed for her fear of harming others).

T: What I'd like to do now is start to brainstorm a list of the things that would be frightening to you; things that you'd rather avoid and that seem to set off your contamination fears. What's something you can think of?

B: Well, I'm afraid to touch a doorknob outside of my house. I usually use my sleeve to open the door, or else I have to wash my hands afterwards.

T: OK, so touching a public doorknob would be one activity that you find scary. Can you help me understand how scary that would be? Let's imagine a scale that goes from 0 to 100, where 0 is not scary at all and 100 is the scariest thing you've ever done, or could even imagine doing. Where would touching a public doorknob rank on this scale?

B: About a 50.

T: OK. Let's call that your fear level. So your fear level for touching a doorknob would be 50. What else can you think of?

B: I don't like touching the floor.

T: And what would your fear level be for that?

B: Maybe 40.

T: OK, 40. What else?

B: Well, I don't like using public bathrooms.

T: And that's because of fears of getting contaminated?

B: Right.

T: OK, so what if you went into a public bathroom and touched the doorknob in there?

B: That would be scary. Like a 60.

T: I see. And what about if you actually touched the toilet seat in the public bathroom?

B: Eww, why would I do that?

T: Just as an exposure exercise, to help you overcome your fear.

B: I think that would be really scary, like a 90. I don't think I can do that.

T: Understood. For now, we're just coming up with ideas.

Note that the therapist does not get bogged down at this stage with a discussion of whether or not Bethany actually intends to do the exposure. That discussion will happen, but the task here is simply to generate potential exposure activities. As Bethany works her way up the exposure hierarchy, the most strongly feared activities will likely seem less threatening.

Yeah, I Go There

When I talk to some of my friends about exposure therapy, I get comments like "Gross!" "That's so weird!" "But that's not *normal*!" When exposure therapy is done well, it's not normal at all. I don't make a habit of hyperventilating and touching toilet seats for fun. But if I were treating someone with panic disorder or OCD, those are exactly the kinds of things we might do.

Good exposure is not just mimicking "normal" behavior—rather, it is a series of exercises that are specifically designed to help the client overcome fear.

Why do you have to push the exposures beyond normal? There are two main reasons. First, life has a way of throwing curveballs at the client. We cannot possibly predict everything that will happen to the client in the future, and sometimes the client will be caught off guard by something that is scarier than usual.

The second reason is that low-grade exposures that don't address the really scary items risk teaching the client *conditional safety* (Otto, Simon, Olatunji, Sung, & Pollack,

2011). Conditional safety is a belief that a situation is safe only under certain conditions. Conditional safety beliefs often have a "yes–but" quality: "*Yes*, I drove on the highway, *but* I only survived because it wasn't rush-hour traffic"; "*Yes*, I went into the restroom, *but* I only survived because I didn't touch the toilet"; "*Yes*, I touched a snake, *but* I only survived because I didn't let it crawl on me"; "*Yes*, I went to a party, *but* I only escaped humiliation because I didn't go out on the dance floor." In exposure therapy, we want the client to learn *unconditional safety:* The situation is safe, period. So you have to eliminate the "buts."

Eliminating Safety Behaviors

Related to the need to teach unconditional safety, rather than conditional safety, is the importance of eliminating **safety behaviors.** In Chapter 2 we reviewed how avoidance behavior can serve to maintain erroneous beliefs about threat and can even increase fears over time. One of the main problems is that when avoidance behavior is present, the *absence* of disaster is interpreted as confirmation of the necessity of the avoidance behavior (Lohr, Olatunji, & Sawchuk, 2007).

In many cases, the avoidance behavior is blatant and easy to detect. A client with a fear of dogs, for example, might opt not to go anywhere near dogs. Safety behaviors, on the other hand, are often more subtle. They represent behaviors that help the client to feel safer (though not necessarily to *be* safer). So an individual with a fear of dogs might not blatantly avoid dogs but instead would carry a bottle of pepper spray with him or her, with the knowledge that he or she could use it to repel an attacking dog if needed. The pepper spray makes the client feel safer, though its actual safety value is questionable at best (note that most of us walk around without pepper spray and survive).

Perhaps the most obvious example of the safety behavior is the compulsions exhibited by clients with OCD. These behaviors (e.g., hand washing, ordering, checking) are "aimed at preventing or reducing distress or preventing some dreaded event or situation; however, these behaviors or mental acts either are not connected in a realistic way with what they are designed to neutralize or prevent or are clearly excessive" (American Psychiatric Association, 2013, p. 237).

Safety behaviors are not limited to OCD, however. Indeed, many problems, from anxiety disorders (Kamphuis & Telch, 2000; Wells et al., 1995) to psychosis (Freeman et al., 2007), are associated with subtle behavioral adjustments that serve to make the person feel safer yet do not actually improve safety to a degree that would make it helpful—and therefore the cons of avoidance outweigh the pros of feeling safer. Some examples are shown in Table 11.2.

It's quite understandable that anxious clients would want to try to feel better when faced with frightening external or internal stimuli. But it is important to recognize that safety behaviors can create the same kind of problems that blatant avoidance does. Though they feel better in the short term, they have the potential to allow maladaptive beliefs to persist and for fear to increase or remain "stuck." I think of safety behaviors as similar to crutches. If the client has a broken leg, he or she might well need to use crutches. But what would happen if the client continued to use crutches, even without a broken leg, indefinitely? Over time, his or her leg muscles would start to waste away from disuse. Eventually, the client's natural ability to walk without crutches would become less and less. And there isn't a physical therapist around who isn't going to recommend that the client practice walking without the crutches. That's how the client gets stronger.

TABLE 11.2. Examples of Blatant Avoidance and Safety Behaviors

Fear	Blatant avoidance	Safety behavior
Doctors, dentists, injections, or blood draws	• Do not go to the doctor or donate blood.	• Distract yourself and do not look at the needle. • Request extra anesthetic.
Physical symptoms such as racing heart or dizziness	• Do not exert yourself. • Do not drink caffeine.	• Keep checking your pulse. • Have a "safe person" with you. • Do relaxation or breathing exercises to stay calm.
Situations in which it would be dangerous to lose control of yourself in the event of panic sensations, like driving a car	• Do not drive.	• Stay in the right lane in case you need to pull over. • Only drive when you feel good.
Thoughts of catastrophes	• Never think about bad things.	• Check to make sure everything is safe and okay. • Ask others to reassure you. • Worry about something else.
Having repulsive, horrible, or immoral thoughts or mental images	• Try not to think about the thoughts or images.	• Say prayers or do rituals after the images to feel better. • Remind yourself that you don't really mean it.
Memories of unpleasant, stressful, or traumatic life experiences	• Try not to think about the memories.	• Distract yourself with music or TV. • Use alcohol or drugs to clear your mind.
Being near certain animals	• Do not go near animals.	• Only go near animals if you have something to protect you. • Only go near animals that are leashed or caged.
Interacting with people	• Avoid social interaction.	• Keep the conversation limited to "easy" topics like the weather. • Have something in your hands so you don't have to shake hands.
Flying in an airplane	• Do not fly.	• Use alcohol or tranquilizers when flying. • Grip the armrest tightly so the plane doesn't crash.
Touching things that seem dirty or contaminated	• Do not touch dirty things.	• Wash hands repeatedly or use hand sanitizer after touching dirty things. • Use paper towels or your sleeve to minimize contact.
Public speaking	• Do not give speeches.	• Only speak about familiar topics. • Stay behind the podium. • Stick to topics you're very familiar with. • Don't make eye contact with the audience.

Note. Adapted from Tolin (2012). Copyright © 2012 Turner Publishing. Adapted by permission.

The Science behind It

Several studies demonstrate that anxious clients do much better with exposure when they are encouraged not to engage in or have access to safety behaviors (Kim, 2005; Morgan & Raffle, 1999; Powers, Smits, & Telch, 2004; Salkovskis, 1999; Sloan & Telch, 2002; Wells et al., 1995); safety behaviors also appear to decrease objective performance during public speaking for socially anxious clients (Rowa et al., 2015). The deleterious effects of safety behavior during exposure have been demonstrated in children as well (Hedtke, Kendall, & Tiwari, 2009).

There is controversy (surprise, surprise) about how important it is to eliminate safety behaviors, and some (e.g., Rachman, Radomsky, & Shafran, 2008) have suggested that a little bit might not be so bad. Not everyone has found that safety behaviors detract significantly from the effects of exposure, at least in fearful college students (Deacon, Sy, Lickel, & Nelson, 2010; Hood, Antony, Koerner, & Monson, 2010; Milosevic & Radomsky, 2008; Rachman, Shafran, Radomsky, & Zysk, 2011; Sy, Dixon, Lickel, Nelson, & Deacon, 2011). Asymptomatic college students report that they find exposure more acceptable when they are allowed to use safety behaviors (Levy & Radomsky, 2014), although students with claustrophobic fears do not find exposure with safety behavior to be more acceptable than exposure alone (Deacon et al., 2010).

So, the bottom line on safety behaviors, based on the available research, is:

- Safety behaviors often do more harm than good.
- Sometimes they don't.
- But there's not much evidence to suggest that they help.

Safety behaviors, and the conditional safety lessons they teach, play right into the "yes–buts" of fearful thinking: "*Yes*, I went to the mall, *but* I only coped because my spouse was with me"; "*Yes*, I went to a party, *but* I only escaped humiliation because I kept a drink in my hand at all times so people wouldn't see me trembling"; "*Yes*, I used a public bathroom, *but* I only survived because I used my sleeve to open the door"; "*Yes*, I thought about a disaster, *but* I only managed because I got reassurance from my spouse."

Here's a joke I like. A guy is standing on a street corner in New York City. He's stomping his feet, clapping his hands, yelling, whistling, making a lot of noise. Another man walks up to him and asks, "Why are you making all this racket?" "I'm doing it to keep the alligators away," the guy replies. "Huh? There are no alligators here." The guy says, "See? It's working." This fellow has clearly learned a conditional safety message that is completely erroneous. He's safe from alligators, whether he makes noise or not. The fact that he's not being attacked by alligators only serves to strengthen his belief in conditional safety.

So all other things being equal, I consider it important to eliminate safety behaviors as part of the exposure program. When we generate an exposure hierarchy, I will often create a safety behavior list (which I'll call a "Don't list") to go along with it. An example for Anna, our client with panic disorder and agoraphobia, is shown in Figure 11.2, and a blank form is provided in Appendix B.

As you can see in the figure, the therapist and Anna identified examples of safety behaviors in four categories:

1. *Distraction.* Trying to think about something else, or deliberately allocating attention toward distracting stimuli, is a common safety behavior. Research generally suggests that this is less effective during exposure than is focusing on the exercise, including the feared stimulus and the feeling of fear (Grayson, Foa, & Steketee, 1982; Kamphuis & Telch, 2000; M. J. Telch et al., 2004).

2. *Increasing a sense of safety.* As described previously, many safety behaviors are performed in order to provide an erroneous sense of safety (e.g., "If I stay close to the exit or keep checking my pulse, I'll be safer").

3. *Relaxing and "feeling better."* Relaxation as a general principle seems fine. However, when people get hung up on trying to feel better during an exposure exercise, it seems to detract from the lesson of unconditional safety. (You can imagine the shaky ground we're on when we teach an anxious client "I'll be OK, as long as I can relax.") Relaxation and related "feel-better" strategies also interfere with the natural habituation process: Over time, the client's fear is likely to come down on its own, without doing anything. Relaxation has the potential to short-cut that process by imposing immediate relief, thus depriving the client of the ability to learn that fear habituates on its own.

During and after exposure, I will not do the following things that distract me:

1. Try to focus on the dresses in the window at the mall

2.

3.

4.

During and after exposure, I will not do the following things that increase my sense of safety:

1. Stay close to the exit

2. Check my pulse

3.

4.

During and after exposure, I will not do the following things to relax or feel better:

1. Take a tranquilizer

2.

3.

4.

During and after exposure, I will not bring the following things or people with me:

1. My cell phone

2. My husband

3. Bottle of water

4.

FIGURE 11.2. Sample "don't" list of safety behaviors. Adapted from Tolin (2012). Copyright © 2012 Turner Publishing. Adapted by permission.

I'll point out here that we used to think that relaxing during exposure was a good thing. The original form of exposure, called *systematic desensitization,* paired imaginal exposure with relaxation training (Wolpe, 1961). The theory was that by pairing these two the feared stimulus would be associated with the more pleasant feelings of relaxation and that this association would offset the fear. Subsequent dismantling studies showed that relaxation didn't add anything to the exposure (e.g., Agras et al., 1971). That is, imaginal exposure worked equally well with or without relaxation training.

The astute reader might be wondering about as-needed benzodiazepine medications. And you may be on to something there. Clients with panic disorder taking as-needed (or *prn*) benzodiazepines with CBT seem to do less well than do clients receiving CBT alone, or CBT with fixed-dose benzodiazepines (Westra, Stewart, & Conrad, 2002). Again, you can imagine the conditional safety lesson being learned: "I'm OK as long as I have my pills." In an illustrative study, individuals with claustrophobia received exposure therapy along with a placebo pill. They were told that the placebo pill (1) was a sedating drug that would make exposure easier, (2) was a stimulating drug that would make exposure harder, or (3) would have no effect on exposure. All three groups showed an equivalent reduction in fear during exposure; however, at a 1-week follow-up, 39% of the group that had believed they were taking a drug that would make exposure easier showed a return of their fear, compared with 0% of the other two groups. Those believing that they were taking a drug that would make exposure easier reported lower levels of self-efficacy, which in turn predicted the return of fear (Powers, Smits, Whitley, Bystritsky, & Telch, 2008). So when we use medications as an adjunct to exposure therapy, we risk teaching a conditional safety lesson that undermines the client's self-efficacy to handle the situation and reduces the long-term effectiveness of the treatment.

4. *Bringing things or people.* People with agoraphobia commonly rely on the presence of a "safe person" who, they presume, will help them escape the feared situation (Barlow, 2002; Rachman, 1984). Similar findings have been reported among individuals with social anxiety (Darcy, Davila, & Beck, 2005). As a result, some clinicians use a couples-based CBT approach to help "wean" the client from the presence of his or her partner and to teach the partner how to encourage and reinforce more adaptive behaviors (Byrne, Carr, & Clark, 2004; Daiuto, Baucom, Epstein, & Dutton, 1998; N. S. Jacobson, Holtzworth-Munroe, & Schmaling, 1989). Bringing things such as cell phones, bottles of water, and medications can equally impede the outcome of exposure, as they too teach a message of conditional safety.

Is It Safe?

Your client might ask (and you might ask as well), "Couldn't some of these things be dangerous? Wouldn't ordinary people be reluctant to do some of these things?" It's perfectly natural to wonder about safety. It's also important, however, to recognize that no exposure is 100% safe. Life, in fact, is not 100% safe. We take risks all the time; that's part of living a happy and productive life. People with anxiety-related problems often think that their job is to minimize all risk. The aim of our treatment is to demonstrate to the client that tolerating, even embracing, risk is one of the key ingredients of living a happy life. Therefore, rather than asking whether an exposure exercise is "safe," I encourage the client to consider whether it is *safe enough*. Part of our goal in exposure therapy is to help clients reappraise *safe enough* situations and to approach them without undue anxiety. Exposure may seem a little odd, but it all lies in the realm of *safe enough*.

How do you know when something is *safe enough?* Every situation might be a little different, but here are some good questions to ask:

- *Does this activity kill or injure people in large numbers? Is it a common cause of death?* The leading causes of death in the United States, by a large margin, are cancer and heart disease (as well as other complications of obesity and smoking). Airplanes? Dog attacks? Sharks? Touching toilets? Not even in the top 100.

- *Do other people do these activities and survive?* Think about janitors who touch toilets, dog trainers who handle dogs, flight attendants who take multiple flights every day, and so on. They seem to survive just fine.

- *Does the client have a known medical condition that would make this exposure risky?* Some people have medical conditions that make certain exposures more risky than they would be for the average person. People with known heart disease, for example, should talk to a physician before doing exposures like running up and down stairs. People with known deficiencies of the immune system should talk to a physician before doing exposures to dirty or contaminated objects. If you're not sure whether the client has a medical condition that would change the risks, consult with the client's treating physician.

- *Do the benefits outweigh the risks?* This is perhaps the most important question. Treatments, whether medical or behavioral, carry some risk. Here's an example from medicine. One could certainly argue that sticking a needle into your own body is risky: You could get an infection or bleed to death, or you could overdose on, or have an allergic reaction to, the medication in the syringe. Would ordinary people go around sticking needles and injecting chemicals into themselves? Certainly not, nor would I advise them to. That would be highly irrational. But what if the person had a serious bacterial infection? And what if that syringe contained penicillin that could save the person's life? That certainly changes the risk–benefit ratio. In this case, I wouldn't hesitate to recommend the shot. In fact, you could make the argument that it would be highly irrational *not* to get the shot. Exposure therapy is beneficial enough that it is worth taking some calculated risks.

So the aim here is not to come up with things that are objectively dangerous. I wouldn't, for example, do an exposure exercise that involved pointing a gun at someone, crossing a street against fast oncoming traffic, or dangling from a balcony. We're also not being outrageous for the sake of being outrageous—this isn't *Fear Factor.* But what we are trying to do is to determine what kinds of situations are safe enough though still feared and avoided, the confrontation of which would help the client feel less fearful.

How Long Should Exposures Be?

Many clinical researchers have argued that exposures should be long. This is based, in part, on early research with nonclients suggesting that brief exposures (e.g., 15–25 minutes) were less effective than were longer exposures (e.g., 45–50 minutes); some were also concerned that short exposures could actually make the problem worse by *sensitizing* the client to the feared situation or object (Chaplin & Levine, 1981; Stone & Borkovec, 1975).

Clinical research with clients, however, raises questions about the necessity of long exposures and within-session habituation for fear reduction (Craske et al., 2008). Some older research shows that long (e.g., 2 hours) exposures were more effective than briefer exposures for clients with agoraphobia (R. Stern & Marks, 1973) and OCD (Rabavilas,

Boulougouris, & Stefanis, 1976). However, more recent research suggests that exposure therapy might be just as effective when exposures are short and there is not sufficient time for within-session habituation (e.g., Nacasch et al., 2015). As one example, phobic clients have responded well to repeated exposures as brief as 2 minutes each (Seim & Spates, 2008). The degree of **between-session habituation** appears to be much more predictive of outcome than the degree of **within-session habituation** (Craske et al., 2008; Kozak, Foa, & Steketee, 1998; van Minnen & Foa, 2006). That is, it doesn't seem to really matter much whether, in any given session, the client experiences a decrease in fear. What matters more is whether the feared object, activity, or situation is less scary the next time the client approaches it.

Generally speaking, I don't worry much about the duration of any given exposure exercise. As a rough guide, I look for some decrease in reported fear, or I hear the client making new self-efficacy statements (e.g., "Hey, I can do this!") before moving on to the next exercise.

Variety and Repetition Are Critical

It's important that exposure not be to just one thing. Instead, exposures should be varied and conducted in multiple contexts. Some examples include:

- Scott, our socially anxious client, should make a point of interacting with as many different people, in as many different contexts, as possible. He might make a point of interacting not only with his coworkers but also with store cashiers, the mail carrier, and strangers on a bus. Every person he sees represents a potential opportunity to face his fear.
- Suzanne, who is afraid to fly, should take several different kinds of flights. She should plan on taking short flights and long flights, fly on small airplanes and large airplanes, and fly in good weather and bad. She needs to demonstrate to herself that she can handle a wide range of flying experiences, not just certain ones.
- Bethany, who has a fear of dirt and germs, should touch as many "dirty" things as she can. She should, for example, touch doorknobs, handrails, floors, and bathrooms at home, at school, and all over town. She should visit places that seem slightly dirty and places that seem very dirty.

We also know that once is usually not enough; therefore, exposures should be repeated. A lot. Here are some examples:

- For Scott's fear of public speaking, it's probably not enough for him to just to give one speech—that probably won't beat his fear for good. Instead, he should sign up to give a series of presentations at work. Or he might consider joining an organization such as Toastmasters, in which he'll have the opportunity to give multiple speeches at regular intervals.
- Anna, who has panic attacks in response to increased heart rate, should try to get her heart rate elevated on a regular basis, preferably daily. Her therapist might encourage her to join a gym and commit to going every day and really working up a sweat.
- Melissa, who is disturbed by intrusive, traumatic memories, should do lots of imaginal exposure. She should plan daily exposure sessions, preferably for an hour per

exposure. She will need to prioritize her exposures by setting aside enough time and making sure family members understand that she will be busy during these periods.

Getting in the Right Zone

There is no hard and fast rule about how much fear the client should experience during exposure exercises. The rule of thumb, however, is that we should try to have the client experience as much fear as he or she can reasonably tolerate at that moment, no more, no less. That is, it should not feel like torture, but it should not be tedious, either. Numerically, a fear level somewhere between 20 and 80 might be a reasonable rule of thumb, but of course these are just subjective numbers, and one person's 80 might be entirely different from another person's 80. Generally speaking, though, if the client's fear level is quite low (i.e., the client is not reporting much fear), that's a sign that you have started too low on the exposure hierarchy and you need to try something a little tougher. If the client's fear level is extremely high, that's a sign that you may have started too high and you need to start with something easier. This way, the client's fear level will serve as a constant guide, showing you how strong the exposures need to be.

Exposure Troubleshooting

Sometimes you try an exposure exercise and, for some reason, the client just doesn't feel scared at all. Sometimes that means that your exposure didn't quite hit the mark, and you need to rethink it. Ask yourself: Does this exposure really target what the client is afraid of? Am I leaving out (or avoiding) some critical detail that would make it scary? Because everyone's fear is a little bit different, it's sometimes necessary to get creative in order to access the fear. Here are a couple of examples:

Scott is afraid of public speaking. So the therapist arranges to have Scott give a speech in front of some colleagues in the clinic, and Scott just doesn't get anxious. Closer examination of Scott's fear, however, reveals that Scott is afraid not of the act of public speaking itself but rather that he might show signs of anxiety while giving a speech. The therapist therefore instructed Scott to dab water on his forehead to make it look like he was sweating, to deliberately stammer, and to drop his papers while giving the speech.

Anna is afraid of driving. But when the therapist went driving with her, she was not anxious. Upon further discussion, it became evident that Anna was primarily afraid not of driving but of what she feared would happen if she felt panicky sensations while driving. The therapist therefore had Anna practice driving while engaging in mild hyperventilation to bring on sensations of lightheadedness.

Bethany, who has OCD, is afraid that she might be seized with an irresistible urge to hurt someone. The therapist handed Bethany a sharp knife and had her hold the knife in the therapist's presence. When Bethany did not become anxious, the therapist asked what was impeding her fear. Bethany stated that she felt that the therapist was probably strong enough and quick enough to get away from the knife if she decided to attack. The therapist therefore recruited a coworker, who was much smaller, to sit in the room with Bethany while the therapist left the room, locking the door on the way out.

What about if the client's fear doesn't come down? Remember that within-session habituation appears not to be a critical factor in the success of exposure therapy. Therefore, if the client's fear does not come down during the session, that's not the end of the world.

That having been said, when fear does not come down during exposure, it makes sense to check for some likely culprits that could impede the process. These include:

- *Being outside of the therapeutic zone.* When fear doesn't come down, one possibility is that the fear was too low to begin with, and therefore there's not much room for it to decrease. Alternatively, it could mean that the fear was too high, and the client simply feels overwhelmed. Try changing the exposure to something challenging, yet manageable.
- *Safety behaviors.* Subtle safety behaviors could get in the way of exposure. It's often helpful to ask the client questions such as, "Are you doing anything, with your body or with your thoughts, to try to feel better?" "Are you trying to make this exercise safer in any way?" Watch the client's behavior: Is he or she trying to breathe a certain way? White-knuckling the chair? Bracing for impact? Chatting about other things? Doing subtle forms of avoidance? Point these behaviors out to the client and encourage him or her to try going without them.

In Vivo Exposure

Here is an example of *in vivo* exposure. Bethany (B) has developed a fear hierarchy for her excessive fear of contamination. In this initial session, the therapist starts fairly low on her *exposure hierarchy*.

T: Bethany, let's do an exposure exercise together to see if we can help reduce some of your fears. We've generated this hierarchy, and as you can see, I've ordered the items according to your fear level, ranging from low to high. What I'd like to do is start with something that's pretty challenging but not too much for you to handle. As you look at this list, what seems like a good starting point?

B: I guess I could probably handle something that's like a 50. Like maybe touching doorknobs.

T: That sounds fine. Ready to start?

B: I guess so. I'm nervous, though.

T: Yes, I imagine so. It is scary right now, because this is really new for you and I'm sure your OCD is fired up about it.

B: Yeah, it is.

T: But I'll be here with you during this exercise, and I'll do it along with you. And I bet that over time it won't seem so scary.

B: OK.

T: Now, let's review a couple of things before we start. The first thing is that I'm going to want to check in with you as we're going along, so I'll ask you what your fear level is every few minutes. That will help me pace things and will give us a shorthand way of communicating.

B: OK.

T: Another part of this is that we need to make sure that you don't undo our exposure by doing compulsions, during or after our meeting. That is, it's important that you don't try to make things easier or safer.

B: You mean you don't want me to wash my hands after?

T: That's exactly right. Whatever contamination we get on us, I want us to let it sink in, so if it's going to kill us, I want to give it a chance to do that. Of course, I'm pretty sure it's not going to kill us, so I'm not worried about that. But I know that your brain isn't so sure of that. So I want to make sure that we can demonstrate that to your brain.

B: Well, how long will that be?

T: I'd recommend you go 24 hours without washing.

B: Twenty-four hours without washing my hands? Doesn't that seem a little extreme?

T: It might seem that way, yes. But let's think it through a bit. When people go camping, how long do they go without washing their hands?

B: A long time, I think. Maybe a couple of days sometimes.

T: Yes. And does that kill them?

B: I guess not.

T: So going 24 hours won't kill you?

B: Probably not.

T: Probably not. Let's flip the scenario, and imagine that you go home after our meeting and wash your hands. And you live. What's the lesson your brain's going to come away with?

B: That I needed to wash.

T: Right. Your brain will just assume it was right all along and that the only reason you didn't die is because you washed. So it seems like not washing for 24 hours is unlikely to harm you, but washing could harm you by undoing your progress. So is that something you can agree to?

B: Yeah, I can agree to it.

T: OK. Let's start right here, with the doorknob in my office. I'll go first. (*Does so.*) I'm putting my hand all over the doorknob here. Before you do it, what's your level, just thinking about it?

B: It's about a 40.

T: So kind of moderate. OK. Now you try it.

B: OK. (*Does so.*)

T: I noticed that you only touched the doorknob with two fingers, and the other three fingers and the palm of your hand didn't touch it. Is that making it feel safer?

B: Yeah, it is.

T: So let's try it differently. Try putting your whole hand on it. (*Bethany does so.*) What's your level right now?

B: About a 60.

T: OK, so it went up, but still kind of moderate. Now I want us to try adding something.

This contamination is on our hands, but I want to make sure we really get the full effect of the contamination. So watch what I do here. First I rub my palms together (*does so*), then I touch my hands to my clothes (*does so*), then my hair (*does so*), then my face (*does so*), even my mouth (*does so*).

B: Eww, that's gross. Aren't you worried about touching your mouth?

T: I agree it's gross, but no, I'm not worried. I think the odds of this killing me are reasonably low. So it's safe enough, and I think I can tolerate whatever uncertainty there is around this. Now, can you do that?

B: OK, I can try. (*Does so.*)

T: And what's your level now?

B: Maybe a 70.

T: OK, it went up some more. Too much for you?

B: No. It's scary, but it's not too much for me.

T: Great. Let's do it again.

The therapist and Bethany did several repetitions of this exposure over the next hour, and Bethany's fear level decreased from a peak of 70 to 30. The therapist then brought Bethany to a number of other doorknobs in the building, doing the same touching exposure at each one. At the end of the session, the therapist assigned homework.

T: Wow, you did really well with that exercise. What was your experience?

B: Well, I definitely feel gross. But it did seem to get easier as we went.

T: Yeah, I noticed that your fear level came down as we did it. So now let's talk about homework. We've already talked about the no-washing rule, so I'd like to make sure we stick to that. The other part of the homework is that I'd like to have you keep practicing what we worked on today. You're now a pro at touching doorknobs in my building, so what do you think about doing some doorknob-touching outside of this building, on your own?

B: That's a scary idea but I think I could do it.

T: Terrific. Let's make a schedule of when and where you'll do it.

Imaginal Exposure

Melissa, our client with complex PTSD secondary to childhood abuse, has been trying to avoid thinking about her traumatic experiences. Over the past several sessions, the therapist and Melissa have worked on more general strategies for emotion regulation, careful evaluation of suicide risk and development of a safety plan, and reducing Melissa's alcohol use. In this session, the therapist introduces imaginal exposure for Melissa (M).

T: You've been trying for a long time to avoid thinking about your abuse experience. And the avoidance seems to have done more harm than good, do you agree?

M: Yes. I know I need to stop avoiding.

T: Shall we start now?

M: I'm scared to.

T: I know. These are scary, awful memories. But they are just memories, you know. They can't hurt you.

M: I know. (*Sighs.*) OK, I guess it's time.

T: OK. But if it gets to be too much for you, just let me know. You're in control of this process.

M: OK.

T: Here's how I'd like to proceed. I'm going to ask you to close your eyes, if you feel comfortable doing so.

M: I'm not sure I feel comfortable doing that. It feels out of control.

T: OK, that's fine. We'll have the opportunity to work on that too as we go. But for now, how about if you just look at the blank wall across from you so you won't be distracted?

M: I can do that.

T: Fine. I'm going to ask you to tell me a story about the abuse. I'd like you to walk me through the whole thing, from beginning to end, step by step.

M: God, that's just painful. (*Cries.*) I hate thinking about it.

T: Yes. It is painful, and you have every right to feel pain about it.

M: OK. There were a lot of incidents. Which one should I pick?

T: Is there one that stands out that's particularly bothersome to you?

M: Yeah, I can think of a couple.

T: So how about if you pick one of those?

M: OK.

T: When you tell me this story, I'm going to ask that you use present-tense language. For example, instead of saying "I was," say "I am." We want to try to bring it to life here. I also want you to give me as much detail as you can, detail about what you're seeing, hearing, smelling, and so on, as well as detail about what you're thinking and feeling.

M: OK.

T: Would it be OK with you if I recorded what you say, so that you can take it with you later?

M: Ugh, I really don't like the idea of taking it with me. I want to get rid of it.

T: Yes, that's understandable. I think, though, that you're going to find that over time, this awful story is just a bad memory, just words, and that they don't have to have any power over you.

M: OK.

T: (*Turns recorder on.*) OK, when you're ready, start the story. Perhaps you could start by telling me where you are and when this is.

M: (*Takes a deep breath.*) I was in my bedroom, sleeping.

T: Try, "I am in my bedroom, sleeping."

M: I am in my bedroom, sleeping. I'm 8 years old. And I wake up because I hear a noise. (*Pauses.*)

T: What's your level right now?

M: Maybe a 75. I feel kind of sick.

T: Yes. Is 75 too high for you, or are you OK to go on?

M: I'm OK. It's dark in my room but I can see that someone's in there with me. At first I don't know who it is.

T: And how are you feeling, what are you thinking?

M: I'm thinking it's probably my stepdad again and I'm scared. I'm thinking he's going to do it again.

T: OK. Go on.

M: And he gets closer and I see it is my stepdad, and I just have a sinking feeling in my stomach. And he comes right up to the side of the bed and puts his face really close to mine. And I pretend to be asleep. And he smells like cigarettes and beer. And I just pray to God that he'll leave me alone, and I hope that he thinks I'm asleep. Or maybe that I'll just die right there and I won't have to go through this again. And now he's putting his hand under the sheet.

T: And what's your level now?

M: Like an 85.

T: Too much?

M: Maybe a little.

T: OK, take a break if you need to. Want to talk about something else for a minute?

M: Yeah, I think so. (*Crying.*)

T: That's fine. Let's take some time and just talk about what you're experiencing so far during this exercise.

M: It's just really painful. It just feels like it's happening all over again.

T: Yes, that memory is very vivid and very painful for you. And I guess it's not surprising that you'd feel pretty overwhelmed by it. But at the same time, can you see how you are in control now? You're choosing to remember, and you're in control of how it goes. No one else.

M: Yeah, I do see that. (*Pauses.*) I think I can start again.

T: OK, when you feel ready, tell me what happens next.

Melissa continues with her narrative, describing the entire incident of abuse. Because Melissa has difficulty with *emotion regulation*, and because of the deeply painful nature of the memories being discussed, the therapist recommended she take a few short breaks during the process but always returned to the exposure. (Had the therapist stopped the exposure altogether, Melissa might have come away with the impression that she is not strong enough to tolerate the memories of her experience.) Over the course of this session, which lasted 90 minutes, her fear level fluctuated but decreased from a peak of 90 to 40. By the end of the exposure session, she reported that she was feeling calmer and stronger. The therapist gave Melissa the audio recording with an instruction to listen to it each day until the next session.

Interoceptive Exposure

Anna has been avoiding certain physiological sensations due to fear that they will trigger a panic attack or worse. Here, the therapist uses interoceptive exposure to help reduce Anna's (A) fear of her own body.

T: So we've come up with a lot of different physical sensations that bother you—dizziness, lightheadedness, feeling hot, having your heart race—and that you have been trying to avoid. Today I'd like to try experiencing some of those physical sensations so that you don't have such a strong fear reaction to them. Where do you think we should start?

A: I think dizziness. I get pretty scared whenever I feel dizzy.

T: Yes. What do you fear will happen when you get dizzy?

A: I just think I'm going to pass out. Or puke.

T: I see. And has that actually happened?

A: No. But it feels like it's going to.

T: So even though your experience tells you it's unlikely, you still feel the fear and so you avoid it.

A: Yeah.

T: Was it always like that? Were you always afraid of dizziness? Or was there a time when you didn't mind it so much?

A: I guess when I was a kid I didn't mind.

T: Can you recall that even being fun, when you were a kid? Like, did you ever like going on rides or playground toys that made you dizzy? Or would you ever just go out in the yard and spin around?

A: Yeah, I used to like that.

T: So what's changed?

A: I don't know. Somewhere it just got scary.

T: I suspect that what changed is that somewhere along the line you got the idea that this sensation was dangerous; that it meant something bad. Now, I don't know whether we'll make dizziness fun again, but maybe we can make it not so scary. Let's try something just initially. Do this with me: Let's roll our heads around slowly, down, and left, and up, and right. (*Does so.*) What sensation does this give you?

A: I feel a little dizzy from that.

T: Panicking over it?

A: No.

T: Puking? Passing out?

A: (*Laughs.*) No.

T: What's your level?

A: 20.

T: Not too high.

A: No, not too high.

T: Let's try something a little more challenging. Let's have you come over to my desk chair here. It swivels, so we can have you experience a little more dizziness. (*Anna sits in the chair and the therapist spins her around slowly.*) Feeling some dizziness?

A: Oh yeah.

T: (*Still spinning the chair slowly.*) What's your level now?

A: It's a 50.

T: Quite a bit higher. But you can handle it?

A: Yeah, I can handle it.

T: (*Still spinning the chair.*) Is this like the kind of dizziness you get when you're panicky?

A: Yeah, it's similar. I feel kind of sick to my stomach.

T: Like you want to puke?

A: Yeah.

T: Well, I tell you what, I have a trash can right here, so if you need to puke, you can puke right there. But let's see if you actually do puke, or whether this is just an idea in your head. What's your level?

A: A 40.

T: Going down. Puking yet?

A: (*Laughs.*) No. It just feels that way.

T: (*Stops spinning the chair.*) OK, let's just let you feel dizzy for a while. Is your mind still telling you you're going to puke?

A: Not as much.

T: How about telling you that you're going to have a panic attack?

A: Yeah, that's definitely on my mind.

T: And is that actually happening?

A: No.

T: And if you did have a panic attack, would that be a disaster?

A: I guess not. But I don't want to have a panic attack in your office.

T: I can appreciate that. But if it did happen, could you stand it?

A: I could stand it.

Over the course of the exercise, Anna's fear decreased from a peak of 50 to 20, and she reported being able to experience dizziness without also experiencing significant fear. The therapist gave Anna a homework assignment to practice getting dizzy every day.

Note that in this example the therapist includes some "on the fly" *cognitive restructuring* (see Chapter 14) to address Anna's *probability overestimation* and *catastrophizing*. Here, the cognitive intervention is included not as a formal exercise but is rather woven into the exposure.

Adapting the Process: *Exposure . . .*

. . . with low-functioning clients. Our lower-functioning clients can benefit from exposure therapy. We have to pay careful attention to the presence of co-occurring psychological problems such as self-injurious behavior, substance abuse, and psychosis. None of these is a good reason not to use exposure, but when problems such as these are present, we should take care to monitor the severity of those problems before and after an exposure session. If we see those problems increasing from the beginning to the end of a session (or, perhaps more importantly, across multiple sessions), we should pause and assess the situation carefully before proceeding.

With lower-functioning clients, it may be particularly important to pay attention to the presence of behavioral skill deficits (see Chapter 2); when they are present, behavioral skill training (see Chapter 12) should be used prior to exposure. So, for example, I'm not going to assign a social contact exposure until I know that the client possesses sufficient social skills to pull it off.

. . . with children. Kids usually do great with exposure therapy, especially if it has a play-like feel. Kendall and Hedtke (2006) describe exposure exercises to younger children as "Show-That-I-Can (STIC)" tasks; for adolescents, Albano (2003) assigns "Mission Is Possible" exposure tasks in sealed envelopes. In many cases, exposure exercises can be framed as a kind of game, and the therapist must get creative to come up with play-like tasks that involve touching contamination, interacting with others, experiencing feared bodily sensations, or whatever the feared object or situation is (e.g., Treadwell & Tolin, 2007).

Usually, exposure therapy with children is most effective when parents are included (P. M. Barrett, Dadds, & Rapee, 1996). I encourage parents not to provide excessive reassurance or reinforce the use of safety behaviors, although, as we saw in Chapter 9, whenever we use *extinction* such as this, we have to make sure that the parents are prepared for the *extinction burst*. The success of parent-driven extinction will depend on the parents' ability to apply the procedure consistently and to tolerate the temporary (but often intense) increase in their child's anxiety. Parents can also use reinforcement strategies such as a *token economy* or *star charts* to encourage kids to do exposure homework. Adolescents may prefer to take greater responsibility for their treatment, in which case less parental involvement may be required. The ideal amount of parental involvement is determined on a case-by-case basis: Parents who are underinvolved need to be instructed in more active ways to manage the child's behavior; parents who are overinvolved often need to be instructed to back off (Tolin & Franklin, 2002).

. . . in groups. The application of exposure to groups will depend largely on the degree to which group members have the same fears. Most therapy groups, even those for anxious clients, will have a mix of different disorders. Even if you are running a group for patients with a single disorder, there's likely to be substantial variation among the group members. For example, if you're running a group for clients with panic and agoraphobia, you might find that one group member is afraid of dizziness and driving over bridges, whereas another is afraid of racing heart and being in crowds. That makes it tough to do meaningful exposures as a group. I've had success with a group model in which we spend the first part of the group reviewing homework and discussing common themes such as cognitive distortions and then split off into smaller groups for the actual exposure—so we leave my office and one person goes to drive over a bridge, two clients practice hyperventilating, and three go down to the crowded cafeteria. In other cases, however, I have found that there are some things that virtually everyone in the group fears, and therefore doing it together can be highly productive. I had a memorable session with a group of six socially phobic clients in which we went to a place with a lot of foot traffic and, one by one, walked out and dropped an armload of books in a noisy, attention-getting fashion. After the exercise, the client would rejoin the group, there would be high-fives all around, and then the next client would go out.

. . . on the inpatient unit. The inpatient unit limits the amount of exposure stimuli available for use. We can't, for example, do an *in vivo* driving exposure with a client who is on a locked unit. We're probably not going to use much exposure with clients who will be discharged soon (e.g., a client on a 72-hour hold), because we want to make sure we have adequate capacity for follow-up. We don't want to get the client wound up and then discharge him or her. But if we have adequate time and access to feared stimuli, exposure can be a useful part of inpatient treatment. We do need to assess the presence of behavioral skill deficits, as described above. For acutely ill clients, it's also important to pay close attention to the client's capacity for emotion regulation. An acutely suicidal or self-injurious client, or a client who is overwhelmed with seemingly uncontrollable emotion, may require alternative strategies for regulating emotion prior to starting exposure.

. . . with medical patients. Exposure therapy can be useful for clients with illness anxiety (previously called *hypochondriasis*). These clients often use excessive amounts of health care, searching for a medical explanation for their unexplained symptoms. Recent conceptualizations have likened illness anxiety to panic disorder, in which clients react to bodily sensations with catastrophic interpretations. Interoceptive exposure to feared physical sensations has been helpful in such cases (e.g., Visser & Bouman, 2001).

Exposure therapy has also been used for clients with maladaptive reactions to chronic pain. Clearly, we don't want to create excessive or uncontrollable pain for our clients. But many clients with chronic pain have become trapped in a cycle of avoidance, in which they use excessive measures to try to prevent the flareup of pain. We might encourage such clients to engage in carefully paced exposures to situations that they view as risky and encourage them to remain in situations even when pain flares up (Allen, Tsao, Seidman, & Ehrenreich-May, 2012).

What If It Goes Wrong?

Exposophobia is often related to the therapist's fear that somehow the process will go horribly wrong and there will be a bad outcome. We might have such questions as:

"What if I assign a driving exposure and the person gets in an accident?"
"What if we're doing imaginal exposure and the person becomes so overwhelmed he or she can't function?"
"What if I'm doing interoceptive exposure and the client really does throw up?"

Let me share a story from my own practice. I was treating a teenage girl with OCD who had the obsession that she could harm people with her thoughts. She was afraid to think bad things about people for fear that it would cause some tragedy to occur. She was also afraid to step on cracks, for fear that it would not only break her mother's back (as the childhood rhyme goes) but would also cause other disasters to occur. So we constructed an exposure hierarchy in which we would do progressively more "dangerous" activities, while also refraining from her usual safety behaviors. We had a really good session outside my office. We were stomping on sidewalk cracks, trying to make airplanes overhead crash by using our thoughts, and wishing out loud for people to die.

And a couple of days later, her boyfriend was killed in an automobile accident.

Now, that's most certainly a setback. Here's how I handled it.

1. We took a break from exposure. It's always fine to pause and reassess when something goes wrong. You can take a break for a few minutes or a few sessions, whatever is needed.

2. I attended to the immediate situation. In my client's case, it was important to address her feelings and thoughts about her boyfriend's death. Quite understandably, she was grieving, and it would have been unresponsive to just stay the course. You can do likewise with your clients. Remember, there's an optimal balance between structure and flexibility. You always have a basic structure in mind for the treatment, but as new issues arise, you make time to address them.

3. The client and I looked carefully at the facts. I asked her whether she thought our exposures had caused her boyfriend's death. She said she didn't think so and then reviewed with me several facts she had learned: Her boyfriend had been under the influence of alcohol and cocaine and was driving at a very high speed on a dark rural road without his headlights on and without wearing a seatbelt. Identifying those factors had helped her to recognize that there were other reasons for his death.

I bring up this case to illustrate the fact that, every so often, something might go wrong. But I don't have exposophobia. Why? Because I examine the evidence. I know that the rate of adverse events across studies of exposure therapy is extremely small (much smaller than the rate of adverse events for such things as psychiatric medications, which we often prescribe without hesitation). Although I remember this case well (memory bias, anyone?), I am also aware that, in my own clinical practice, hundreds of other clients did just fine and nothing bad happened (in fact, even this client eventually restarted exposure therapy and had a good outcome).

I also take comfort in knowing that the most common adverse effects of exposure therapy are not catastrophic. If a client throws up in my office (which has never happened), that's regrettable, but it's not the end of the world. If a client has a full-blown panic attack (which has happened rarely), I know it's just anxiety and will pass. If a client feels emotionally overwhelmed, I know that we can always take a break and do something to help regulate the emotion if needed.

In short, it's "safe enough."

How to do exposure therapy poorly	How to do exposure therapy like a champ
Be squeamish. Allow your own exposophobia to come into the therapy. Don't allow the client to get anxious or upset. Try to minimize risk at all times. Don't encourage activities that would make you personally feel anxious.	*Model appropriate coping.* You don't have to be fearless to be an effective exposure therapist. In fact, if something makes you nervous during an exposure exercise, the client might actually benefit from your sharing your experience and then modeling appropriate coping strategies. But if your fear level is going to affect your behavior in session, that's not going to help the client. I will confess that I am no fan of snakes. So when I knew I was going to have to conduct *in vivo* exposure for a client with a snake phobia, I did some self-directed exposure

beforehand: looking at the snake, touching the cage, and eventually holding the snake. I made sure that I wasn't going to freak out when it came time to do the actual therapy.

I think that the squeamishness issue can be particularly important when you are treating clients with PTSD or other concerns related to traumatic experiences. Some of the stories you'll hear during imaginal exposure are god-awful, and they can leave you feeling really lousy. It can be hard to listen to the details of clients' traumas. Here, too, if you have an emotional reaction to a trauma story, that's fine—and it's fine to say that to the client. I've told clients when I felt sad, frightened, or angry when listening to their stories. I've cried with clients. But, importantly, I take care not to join the client in the avoidance. I try to convey the message that this is a really unpleasant and upsetting process, but it's necessary, and we'll go through it together.

Create an unambitious exposure hierarchy. Construct an exposure hierarchy that mimics "normal" behavior, rather than doing specific exercises that target the person's fear.	*Include high-fear exposure items.* As discussed previously, good exposure therapy means going after the client's strongest fears. We don't have to get there immediately, but we do want to get there. Remember that we have to prepare the client for unexpected events, and we also want to make sure that we teach the client *unconditional safety.* If I'm treating snake phobia, "Go outside and walk around" might be good "normal" behavior, but it's not at the top of an exposure hierarchy. The top is probably going to be more along the lines of "Hold a snake and drape it around your neck" or "Let a snake lick your face." As long as it's safe enough, go for it.
Try to minimize the client's anxiety during exposure. Go overboard to help the client feel better in the moment, thus joining the client in the cycle of *experiential avoidance.* Communicate through your actions that the client *shouldn't* feel this way and that we need to do something right now in order to feel better.	*Encourage the client to tolerate distress.* Part of the whole point of exposure is teaching the client that he or she is capable of tolerating distress and that distress, once elicited, tends to fade away on its own. So when I'm doing an exposure therapy exercise with a client, we don't chat about the weather or last night's ball game. I usually don't try to get the client to relax or do fancy breathing exercises. I want the client to focus on what we're doing and see for him- or herself that the fear will subside over time, even when we don't try to make it go away.
Be lenient with safety behaviors. Let the client do whatever he or she feels will help him or her get through the exposures. Let him or her take benzodiazepine medications, carry cell phones, or bring his or her spouse along on exposures, thus teaching a lesson of conditional safety.	*Eliminate safety behaviors as much as possible, as quickly as possible.* The bulk of the evidence tells us that exposure therapy works best when we get rid of the safety behaviors. There is just no need for them, and more often than not, they defeat the purpose of the exercise (or, worse, reinforce a lesson of conditional safety). When I'm doing exposure therapy, I aim to get rid of all safety behaviors as rapidly as possible—I don't taper them off gradually. I'd rather start with milder exposures, done properly without

safety behaviors, than work up the hierarchy using safety behaviors and only then try to wean the client off them. So when we go driving or hyperventilating or touching toilets together, we're leaving the benzodiazepines, cell phone, hand sanitizer, or whatever the crutch is behind.

THE ESSENTIALS

* Exposure refers to the process of confronting previously avoided stimuli.
* Avoidance may be of external or internal (e.g., thoughts, feelings, body sensations) stimuli.
* Exposure is usually done in a gradual manner.
* *In vivo* exposure is used to expose clients to real-life objects, situations, or activities.
* Imaginal exposure is used when *in vivo* exposure is not realistic or to expose clients to feared outcomes in imagination.
* Exposure may be to avoided thoughts, feelings, or body sensations.
* Exposure begins by constructing an exposure hierarchy, ranking each activity according to its fear level.
* Safety behaviors should be eliminated to the extent possible during exposure therapy.
* Variety, repetition, and keeping the client in a zone of productive fear are all important.
* Therapists must identify and conquer their own exposophobia.

KEY TERMS AND DEFINITIONS

Between-session habituation: The degree to which fear decreases from one exposure treatment session to the next.

Emotional processing: The development of new ways of processing information and correcting faulty representations of fear in long-term memory.

Exposure: Confronting previously avoided stimuli.

Exposure hierarchy: A list of exposure activities to be performed, ranked according to fear level.

Exposure to emotions and physiological sensations: Exposure to avoided emotional states or physical sensations.

Exposure to thoughts: Exposure to avoided thoughts, images, or memories.

Extinction (classical conditioning): Decrease of a conditioned response when a conditioned stimulus is presented in the absence of an unconditioned stimulus.

Fear level: A numeric rating of predicted fear toward each exposure activity.

Flooding: Exposure that begins with the most challenging exercise.

Habituation: Decreased responding to repeated presentations of a stimulus.

Imaginal exposure: Vividly imagining feared objects, situations, or activities.

In vivo **exposure:** Exposure to real-life objects, situations, or activities.

Inhibitory learning: When one learned association interferes with or inhibits another.

Safety behaviors: Behavioral adaptations that serve an avoidance function.

Self-efficacy: One's belief or confidence in one's ability to complete a task.

Virtual reality exposure therapy: Imaginal exposure that uses virtual reality technology.

Exposure

If it seems applicable to your personal target, identify some potential exposure exercises you could do. If it is not applicable, identify some potential exposure exercises for a client or other person you know.

Activity	Fear Level (0–100)
1.	
2.	
3.	
4.	
5.	

If it seems applicable to your personal target, identify some safety behaviors you could eliminate. If it is not applicable, identify some safety behaviors for a client or other person you know.

During and after exposure, I will not do the following things that distract me:

1.

2.

During and after exposure, I will not do the following things that increase my sense of safety:

1.

2.

During and after exposure, I will not do the following things to relax or feel better:

1.

2.

During and after exposure, I will not bring the following things or people with me:

1.

2.

If it is applicable to your personal target, and you feel ready to do so, try one exposure exercise.

What was your starting fear level? _____   What was your final fear level? _____

What is your reaction to this exercise?

From *Doing CBT* by David F. Tolin. Copyright © 2016 The Guilford Press. Permission to photocopy this worksheet is granted to purchasers of this book for personal use only (see copyright page for details). Purchasers can download enlarged versions of this worksheet (see the box at the end of the table of contents).

CHAPTER 12

Behavioral Skill Training

In Chapter 2 we discussed how *behavioral skill deficits* can play a major role in the etiology and maintenance of psychopathology. Sometimes people engage in a maladaptive behavior (e.g., screaming at someone) in part because they don't know how to engage in a more adaptive behavior (e.g., speaking calmly yet assertively). Sometimes people avoid engaging in an adaptive behavior (e.g., public speaking) in part because they're not good at it.

Here are some examples from our clients:

- Melissa, our client with complex PTSD, "blows up" at her roommate in part because she is not skilled at asserting her needs in a calm manner.
- Scott, our socially anxious client, avoids parties in part because he is not skilled at making "small talk" and is concerned that he appears "weird" to others.
- Christina, who suffers from depression, engages in depressive rumination in part because she is not skilled at solving problems. She also isolates from others because she is not skilled at meeting people and making friends.
- Blaise, who is struggling with substance dependence, consistently caves in to her friends' invitations to use, in part because she has difficulty saying "no."
- Elizabeth, who has borderline personality disorder and a long history of self-injurious behaviors, cuts herself in part as a way of expressing her despair to others, because she is unskilled at expressing herself verbally.
- Nick and Johanna, our distressed couple, are unhappy in their marriage, in part because they are unskilled at having rewarding interactions with each other. They also seem to have difficulty communicating effectively with their son James, relying excessively on punitive strategies.
- Lauren, who has schizophrenia, feels like an "outsider" around people, in part because she is unskilled at reading social cues, making appropriate conversation with others, and using nonverbal cues that foster a productive interaction.

I want to note that behavioral skill deficits are likely not the *only* reasons these clients engage in maladaptive behaviors. Research on nonsuicidal self-injury, for example, suggests that self-injurious behavior largely serves an emotion-regulation function, although interpersonal communication can be an important secondary function (M. Z. Brown, Comtois, & Linehan, 2002; Klonsky, 2007; Nock, 2009). It would be a mistake, therefore, to assume that Elizabeth's sole reason for self-injury is to communicate to others. It would also be a mistake, however, to overlook that function of the behavior.

Behavioral skill training, therefore, is an important part of CBT. The aim here is to train the client in behavior skills needed to engage effectively with the environment. Linehan (1993) outlines three important steps that are broadly applicable to behavioral skill training. They include:

1. *Assessment of the skill.* The therapist creates circumstances conducive to the performance of the client's skill, observes the client's behavior in sessions, asks the client how he or she would ideally handle a situation or problem, asks the client to try new behaviors during session, and role-plays with the client.
2. *Instruction of the skill.* The therapist describes the desired behavior and behavior sequence, breaks the instructions down into easy steps, begins with simple tasks and then proceeds to more difficult aspects of the skill, provides the client with examples of the skill to be learned, and provides handouts describing the skill.
3. *Modeling of the skill.* The therapist role-plays with the client, uses the appropriate skill when interacting with the client, thinks out loud (using self-talk to model adaptive thinking), discloses his or her own use of the skill in everyday life, tells stories illustrating the skill, and points to models in the environment (e.g., people the client knows, public figures, characters from books or movies) for the client to observe.

To these, I would add:

4. *Practice and feedback.* The therapist instructs the client to practice the skill in an artificial setting, provides direct feedback about the successful and unsuccessful aspects of the skill application, instructs the client to try again with particular attention to the aspects of the skill most in need of improvement, gradually widens the scope of practice with increasing challenge, and prescribes homework to practice the skill outside of the therapy session.

Two domains of behavioral skill training that come up a lot are *social skill training* and *problem-solving training.* These interventions can be implemented in many different ways, depending on the needs of the client.

It's also worth noting that all of these clients might be conceptualized as having a skill deficit in the area of *emotion regulation.* As we'll discuss later, emotion regulation is a broad term for strategies aimed at reducing maladaptive emotions and/or increasing adaptive emotions. So we could use an emotion regulation skill deficit formulation as follows:

- Melissa and Elizabeth have difficulty regulating the emotions of *anger and fear.*
- Scott, Anna, and Lauren have difficulty regulating the emotion of *fear.*
- Christina and William have difficulty regulating the emotion of *sadness.*
- Blaise has difficulty regulating the arousal she experiences as *urges.*

In Chapters 18 and 19 we discuss emotion regulation training as an intervention for negative emotions. For now, I note briefly that various *emotion regulation training* programs, in which clients learn and practice applying strategies to either downregulate or tolerate negative emotions, have proven effective for a wide range of concerns, including borderline personality disorder (Gratz, Tull, & Levy, 2013), depression (Berking, Ebert, Cuijpers, & Hofmann, 2013), substance use (Stasiewicz et al., 2013), and PTSD (Bryant et al., 2013).

Behavioral skill training is often overlooked, yet it can be a critical part of CBT. For some clients, you might find it beneficial to dedicate most or even all of the therapy to skill training. For others, you might opt to make skill training the focus for only one or two sessions. It depends entirely on your meaty conceptualization: how strongly you think skill deficits are implicated in maintenance of the problem, how severe the skill deficits are, and how rapidly the client is able to acquire new skills.

Social Skill Training

Defining Social Skill

There is no universally accepted definition of *social skill*, most likely because the range of behaviors required to navigate social encounters is so broad. Generally speaking, however, social skills may be thought of as "the ability to elicit social reinforcement from others" (Doty, 1975, p. 679). That is, a person is exhibiting good social skills when he or she behaves in a way that is both healthy and elicits positive responses from other people.

Naturally, how we define good social skills will vary depending on a multitude of factors, including age, gender, culture, race, local norms, and so on. Think about something as simple as a handshake or eye contact. There is no such thing as one "skilled" handshake, or one "skilled" way of making eye contact, because how we are expected to shake hands or look at someone varies depending on who the person is, what our relationship with that person is, the environmental context of the interaction, and so on.

We can divide social skills into a couple of broad categories: *content of speech, paralinguistic features,* and *nonverbal elements.*

- *Content of speech* refers to what is being said. For example, are the client's statements "off topic" or relevant to the conversation? Does the client ask appropriate questions, or engage in a monologue? Does the client self-disclose in an appropriate manner?
- *Paralinguistic* features of speech refer to *how* things are being said. For example, is the client speaking too loudly or too softly? Is the tone of voice appropriate to the situation? Is the timing of speech appropriate?
- *Nonverbal behavior* reflects what the person is doing with his or her body during a social interaction. These factors include *proxemics* (how close the person is to the other person), *kinesics* (how the person moves and gestures), eye contact, and facial expression.

A partial list of paralinguistic and nonverbal aspects of social skill is shown in Table 12.1. Remember, though, that what is considered "skilled" will vary according to the situational and person factors described above. Greater eye contact is *generally* considered to be a good thing, but there are certainly circumstances in which it's not. So identification of skill deficits and targets will necessarily be an idiosyncratic process for each client.

A subcategory of social skill is **assertion** (the term *assertiveness* is often used to describe a characteristic of the person's personality, whereas the term *assertion* simply describes behavior). Just as with social skill more broadly, there is no universal definition

TABLE 12.1. Paralinguistic and Nonverbal Elements of Social Skill

Nonverbal elements	Potential problems
Duration of speech	Too short or too long
Latency (hesitation) of speech	Too short or too long
Fluency of speech	Too few or too many pauses
Facial expression	Too serious or too light for context
Volume of speech	Too quiet or too loud
Intonation of speech	Too flat or too variable
Eye contact	Too little or too much
Posture	Too rigid or closed off
Hand gestures	Too few or too many, awkward

Note. Based on Liberman (1982).

of assertion. However, definitions usually focus on two major domains of behavior: (1) making requests of others and refusing unreasonable requests, and (2) communicating strong opinions and feelings (Duckworth, 2003). Linehan and Egan (1979, pp. 245–246) described it this way:

- Assertion generally involves self-expressiveness, standing up for one's rights, or other more general interpersonal verbal responses to assertive situations.
- The style of an assertive response is usually direct and open.
- The person behaving assertively does not exhibit undue or excessive anxiety or fear. Thus, the style is verbally fluent, well timed, with appropriate response latency, speech volume, and eye contact.
- Assertive responses are socially acceptable and appropriate for a given situation.
- An assertive response is not coercive or aggressive.
- Assertive responses are generally chosen to maximize effectiveness, although, according to some, a response could be assertive but not effective.
- Assertive responses often occur in situations where someone is trying to get a person to give in to a demand or do a favor at the person's own expense, is insulting or inconsiderate, or where someone could do something the person would like, but only at the person's initiation.

Using ratings of videotaped interpersonal behavior, psychiatric clients rated as assertive were differentiated from those rated as unassertive by a more rapid verbal response, louder voice, marked inflection of speech, less compliance with requests, and more behavioral requests of others (Eisler, Miller, & Hersen, 1973).

The Process of Social Skill Training

Social skill training can be used to add new skills (in the case of an acquisition deficit) to the client's repertoire, or it can be used to strengthen the client's self-efficacy and use of a given skill under stressful circumstances (in the case of a performance or fluency deficit). Table 12.2 shows basic steps that are common to social skill training programs.

The Science behind It

In actual practice, social skill training is frequently combined with other interventions (Heimberg, Montgomery, Madsen, & Heimberg, 1977), so information about the efficacy of "pure" social skill training is sparse. However, as an element of CBT, it's been studied repeatedly and in multiple contexts.

• Social skill training has been shown to improve social functioning in adults, adolescents, and children with autism spectrum disorders (Lopata et al., 2010; Mandelberg et al., 2014; Walton & Ingersoll, 2013). Impressively, the benefits of social skill training remain evident 1–5 years after treatment (Mandelberg et al., 2014).

• Among clients with schizophrenia, social skill training significantly improves social and daily living skills, negative symptoms, and community functioning (Granholm, Holden, Link, & McQuaid, 2014; Kurtz & Mueser, 2008; Smith, Bellack, & Liberman, 1996). Social skill training for the individual has proven particularly helpful for clients who live in families that display high rates of expressed emotion (Wallace & Liberman, 1985), and families with high expressed emotion appear to benefit from family-oriented skill training (Berglund, Vahlne, & Edman, 2003).

• Although there is little evidence to suggest that social skill training by itself is effective for social anxiety (Ponniah & Hollon, 2008) or avoidant personality (Alden, 1989), CBT plus social skill training appears more effective than CBT without social skill training (Herbert et al., 2005). A behavioral intervention emphasizing social skill training resulted in significant improvements in socially anxious children (Beidel, Turner, & Morris, 2000; Spence, Donovan, & Brechman-Toussaint, 2000), and gains were maintained 5 years later (Beidel, Turner, & Young, 2006).

• Data are mixed regarding the efficacy of social skill training for children with ADHD. In one study, children did not appear to benefit from the training (Storebo, Gluud, Winkel, & Simonsen, 2012); in another, children's assertive behavior improved, although beneficial effects were not seen in other domains of behavior (Antshel & Remer, 2003). However, among children and adolescents with aggressive behaviors and poor peer relationships, social skill training decreases aggression, improves self-concept and social self-efficacy, and decreases internalizing problems (Harrell, Mercer, & DeRosier, 2009; Ison, 2001; J. B. Stern & Fodor, 1989).

• Among women at risk for HIV, training in partner-directed assertion about sexual topics was shown to increase condom use and sexual communication. In addition, sexual partners of women who received assertion training were more likely to adopt norms for condom use in the relationship (DiClemente & Wingood, 1995).

TABLE 12.2. Steps in Social Skill Training

Step	Description
Assessment	Determine the specific social skill deficit(s) using self-reports, behavioral observations, and/or third-party assessments.
Direct instruction or coaching	Teach and explain the rationale for the desired social behavior, with specific suggestions for how to enact the behaviors.
Modeling	Perform the desired social behavior for the client. Alternatively, have a helper display the behavior or use a videotaped example of the behavior.
Role playing	Encourage the client to role-play the desired behavior with the therapist or with a helper.
Feedback	Provide feedback to the client immediately after the role play, calling attention to strengths and weaknesses.
Homework assignments	Instruct the client to perform the desired social behaviors in the real world. Start with easy behaviors and progress to more complex ones.
Follow-up	Debrief about homework assignments, reassessing and calibrating as needed.

Note. Based on Segrin (2008).

Assessment

The first step is to determine what the skill deficit(s) is or are. There are many self-report measures of social skill and assertiveness out there (J. G. Beck & Heimberg, 1983; Glass & Arnkoff, 1989), although a client's self-report of his or her own social skill may or may not reflect the actual skill. It is often helpful to obtain reports from third parties, such as parents and teachers in the case of children (Crowe, Beauchamp, Catroppa, & Anderson, 2011; Matson & Wilkins, 2009). More frequently, however, we tend to assess social skill by observing the behavior. Sometimes, it's quite obvious, such as when you have a CRB in the session (see Chapter 9). The other day, I came out to my clinic's waiting room to greet a new client who was seeking treatment for social anxiety. She made little eye contact, mumbled a barely audible "hello," and had a handshake like a wet noodle. Easy to spot the social skill deficits there. In other cases, however, the deficits might be a bit more subtle, or they might not show up in a therapy session. For example, some clients might have a skill deficit only when interacting with members of the opposite sex, with authority figures, and so forth. In such cases, role plays can be helpful as a means of observing social skills, although sometimes the client's performance during role play will be more skilled than in real life (P. J. Norton & Hope, 2001)—possibly suggesting a performance deficit, rather than an acquisition deficit.

Depending on what I'm trying to assess, I might instruct the client to "do as you normally do," or I might instruct the client to "act as you think the most skilled person would act." The latter strategy might help me to understand whether we're looking at an acquisition deficit (the person never learned the skill) or a performance deficit (the person knows the skill but has trouble performing it).

When possible, it can be useful to get a helper for these kinds of role plays. That way, the helper can engage in the role play while the therapist observes the client, looking for strengths and weaknesses in social performance. Helpers also are useful when the character-istics of the person matter. For example, I can't pull off a convincing performance of a young woman being asked out on a date (though I have tried), but some of my coworkers can.

Direct Instruction or Coaching

The therapist provides a rationale for the social skill in question. Note that this can tie in nicely with *holding up a mirror* when we provide feedback such as "When you don't look at me I get the sense that you're not interested in what I have to say." The therapist explains what the social skill is, as concretely as possible, and explains why this skill is important (e.g., telling Lauren, "When you make eye contact with people, it shows to them that you're listen-ing and interested in them, which makes them more likely to want to keep talking to you").

In the case of people with schizophrenia or autism spectrum disorders, we often see that part of their social skill deficit is an inability to read others' facial expressions accurately, leading to inappropriate selection of behaviors (one would not speak to a sad person, an angry person, and a happy person in exactly the same way, for example). We might, therefore, start by having Lauren practice interpreting facial expressions (either on the therapist's face, a helper's face, or in photographs) as part of social skill training (Har-rell et al., 2009; Lopata et al., 2010; D. L. Roberts et al., 2014).

Modeling

The therapist then performs the desired social skill while the client observes. The thera-pist might then call the client's attention to specific aspects of the therapist's performance (e.g., "Did you notice how I was looking you in the eyes just then?").

One interesting variation on this theme for children is having them engage in struc-tured activities (e.g., games in an office or on a playground) with healthy children. That strategy appears promising for socially anxious children (Beidel et al., 2000) and children with autism spectrum disorders (Flynn & Healy, 2012).

Role Playing

The therapist then encourages the client to try the skill in a role play. As was the case with assessing social skills, a helper can be useful for this. Often, in the role play the therapist will take the role of another person in the client's life (a spouse, a stranger, a boss, etc.). Some have even used virtual reality as a means of role-playing interpersonal situations (Park et al., 2011). In general, the role play should be as close as possible to real-world situ-ations to maximize generalization (Goldstein & Kanfer, 1979). The role plays should be fairly brief (often less than 2 minutes and sometimes as brief as 10 seconds), so that the therapist can provide immediate feedback.

Feedback

Immediately after the role play, the therapist provides feedback to the client about his or her performance. The feedback should be highly specific, reinforcing any improvement noted in the target social skill (e.g., "I noticed that you made much more eye contact that time"). That reinforcement has been demonstrated to be a particularly important part of skill training (S. N. Elliott & Gresham, 1993), so don't skip it. Some clinicians working with children have used tangible rewards for skilled behavior (Rinn & Markle, 1979). On the flip side, the therapist should also provide constructive feedback about weaknesses in the skill (e.g., telling Scott, "It seemed like you were speaking very softly, so it was hard to hear what you were saying").

I often like to videotape these role plays using a webcam connected to the computer in my office (deleting the recordings immediately afterward, of course). After the role play, we play back the recording so that the client can see his or her performance directly. Clients are often quite surprised, for better or for worse, when they get a good look at themselves.

Yes, this can be anxiety-provoking. For most clients, that's not only OK, it's an important part of *bringing the problem into the room,* and it can serve a dual purpose as an exposure exercise (see Chapter 11).

In the specific case of CBT for couples or families, the therapist watches for the presence of unhelpful interpersonal behaviors, stopping the process, labeling the problem, and providing a rationale for changing it. Some examples of therapist interventions in problem behaviors with our distressed couple Nick and Johanna (based on Lester, Beckham, & Baucom, 1980) include:

- *Deciding who is at fault.* "Hang on, Johanna. You seem to be trying to decide who is at fault. When you try to place blame, it takes you away from actually solving the problem, and just makes Nick angrier. Can you see how his facial expression changed when you did that? So rather than arguing about whose fault it is, let's look for a reasonable way to handle the situation."
- *Getting sidetracked.* "Nick, you seem to be changing the subject. Even though these things might seem related, they get you off track. Instead, try to stay on one topic at a time."
- *Labeling.* "Let's avoid name calling here, Nick. When you label Johanna, it just serves to make her angrier, and by using such a broad label you seem to be implying that she can't change. Instead, be specific about exactly what behavior you dislike."
- *Verbal and nonverbal mismatch.* "Johanna, you just agreed with what Nick said verbally, but then you rolled your eyes and sighed. That seems to imply that you don't really agree, so you send a mixed message. Try saying what you really mean."

In couple and family CBT, we also want to be sure to encourage members to engage in more positive interpersonal behaviors and verbally reinforce them when they occur. During the therapy session, the therapist encourages members to:

- *Talk directly to each other.* Nick and Johanna should spend much, perhaps even most, of the session communicating directly with each other, rather than having each person talk to the therapist.
- *Make eye contact with each other.* Eye contact is a critical social skill that conveys warmth and interest.
- *Make "I" statements.* As we saw with assertion training, when Nick and Johanna use statements such as "I feel . . ." or "I think . . ." it reduces the likelihood that they will fall back into their cycle of blaming and coercive processes. It also encourages Nick and Johanna to take responsibility for their own emotions and behaviors.
- *Practice reflective listening.* Reflective listening (e.g., repeating or paraphrasing what another member has said) slows down the process, decreasing the likelihood of escalation. It also communicates that the member has heard what the person said, thus combating the process of stonewalling.

- *Give praise.* This relates to the operant aspects of couple and family CBT discussed in Chapter 2. Because Nick and Johanna are trapped in coercive contingency patterns, they should be encouraged to praise each other for desired behaviors.
- *Use nonverbal encouragers.* Nonverbal behaviors such as head nodding or sounds such as "uh-huh" are another way to communicate that the person is listening attentively. Of course, these behaviors can also be done in a sarcastic or snarky way, so the therapist must watch for mismatch or overuse.
- *Stating wants and likes directly.* Encouraging Nick and Johanna to state openly what they like and dislike and what they want and don't want helps facilitate direct and open communication. It also encourages a healthy vulnerability among them, which is a line to increased intimacy and connection.

Homework Assignments

As with anything else we practice within a therapy session, generalization is a major concern. It's not very useful for the client to master a skill in the therapist's office and then not apply it in the real world. That's where homework comes in. The therapist and the client collaboratively develop a "to-do" list of real-world opportunities for the client to practice the target social skill. Just as we discussed with exposure (see Chapter 11), repetition and variety are critical. We want the client to practice the behavior a lot, and in a range of situations.

Homework assignments should start off fairly easy. We don't want to set the client up for failure. As the client's skill level and self-efficacy improve, we can move on to more challenging situations.

Follow-Up

The therapist should follow up at the next session by reviewing the homework, identifying what went well and what went not so well. The follow-up also provides an opportunity to challenge any negative beliefs that the client had—for example, unassertive individuals frequently believe that assertive behaviors are undesirable and will lead to negative reactions from others (Eisler, Frederiksen, & Peterson, 1978). We can target *probability estimation* (e.g., "Did the clerk act negatively when you asserted yourself? What does that say about your predictions?") or, if there was a negative reaction, *catastrophizing* (e.g., "When the clerk scowled at you, was it an intolerable disaster, or were you able to cope?"). We also want to make sure that we reinforce the use of appropriate social skills outside of the therapy session—in inpatient or residential settings, this means that all staff members should be on board, watching for and praising the target social skill throughout the day. Remember, it only takes one person to screw it up.

In the specific case of assertion training, we follow the same basic model of assessment, direct instruction or coaching, modeling, role playing, feedback, homework assignments, and follow-up, with a couple of additional considerations:

- When we provide direct instruction or coaching, it's important to clarify the difference between aggressive, passive, and assertive behavior (Duckworth, 2003). Clients often confuse these; I've had angry clients who think that I'm trying to get them to be passive, and I've had anxious clients who think that I'm trying to get them to be aggressive. *Aggressive* behaviors are those that unnecessarily infringe on the rights or well-being of others. *Passive* behaviors are those which respect the rights and well-being of others at the expense of the individual. *Assertive* behaviors, as described above, are those which allow the individual to stand up for his or her rights and well-being without infringing on the rights and well-being of others.

- Clients with substance use disorders often benefit from specific assertion training in the area of substance refusal (Monti, Kadden, Rohsenow, Cooney, & Abrams, 2002). Many clients relapse because they cave in to pressure from peers. Therefore, practicing assertive substance-refusal behavior is a standard part of relapse prevention (Marlatt & Gordon, 1985).

- Clients with anger management problems often require specific practicing in making their facial expressions match their internal feelings (Kassinove & Tafrate, 2002). I've seen some clients whose facial expressions just appear angry, regardless of whether they are actually angry or not—and this leads others to treat the individual as if he or she were angry. I've seen other cases in which the person reports that he or she is highly angry, yet his or her facial expression appears calm—and this leads others to underestimate the person's anger. In either case, you can imagine how others' misreadings of the client's emotion could cause problems. I've spoken about *holding up a mirror* to the client; in this case, I do it literally and have the client actually look at his or her facial expression.

- People with anger issues also benefit from emphasizing the use of "I" language when making assertive statements. "I don't like it when you come home late" is assertive; "you're so inconsiderate for coming home late" is aggressive.

- Because conflicts and disagreements are often the trigger for excessive anger, that's a good situation in which to do role plays. I'll often start with role-playing a disagreement about something silly (e.g., "I think the sky is green"), allowing the client to practice an assertive response (e.g., "I disagree; I think the sky is blue") and gradually work up to more realistic disagreements.

Here, the therapist (T) is working with Scott (S), our socially anxious client who is afraid to start conversations with people. The therapist has already made some informal behavioral observations during sessions, noticing that Scott often makes poor eye contact and speaks in a quiet, mumbling voice. First, the therapist wants to assess the problem.

T: We've been talking about how hard it is for you to strike up a conversation and make small talk with people. How well do you think you do that?

S: I don't think I can do it at all. It's just too scary.

T: Yes, it is scary. What I'm getting at, though, is something a little bit different. I'm wondering whether you actually know how to do it, and whether you could do it well if you had to.

 Metaphor

For kids (and some adults), I use a metaphor of sharks, mice, and bears (Polischuk & Collins, 1991) to illustrate aggressive, passive, and assertive behavior, respectively. Sharks (aggressive) go on the attack against others. Mice (passive) don't speak up for themselves, often out of fear. Bears (assertive) don't attack others unnecessarily but don't get pushed around, either.

S: Oh. I'm not sure.

T: Can we try something for a bit? I'd like to have you strike up a conversation with me so that I can see what you do. I know it seems a bit artificial, but could we try this just so I can take a look?

S: I guess so.

T: OK. So set up the scene for me. Let's think about a situation in which it might make sense for you to start a conversation with someone. What might that be?

S: Umm . . . I guess if I were at a party.

T: That sounds good. So let's pretend to be at a party, and you don't know me. Where should I be?

S: I guess over there, maybe by the food or something.

T: OK, I'm here at the food. (*Stands up and walks to the other side of the room.*) And so you'd like to start a conversation with me. Let's see how you do. (*Turns away from Scott, pretending to sample food.*)

S: (*Long pause.*) Um . . . I don't know what I'm supposed to do.

T: (*Turning toward Scott,*) OK, let's start with that then. I'm over here, you're over there.

S: I guess I should walk over and say something.

T: Good idea. Let's try that. (*Turns away from Scott.*)

S: (*Walks up behind therapist.*) Hi (*mumbling*).

T: (*Turns to face Scott, smiling.*) Hi.

S: Um . . . So. . . . How's it going?

T: Fine, thank you. And you?

S: Fine. Um . . . so . . . um . . . how's this party? I mean, do you like this party?

T: (*breaking character*) OK, let's stop there. How would you say you did?

S: Not very well, I think.

T: What can you identify as being good or bad about it?

S: I guess I just didn't know what to say.

T: Yes, it seemed like you were struggling with that. Anything else?

S: I don't know what else.

T: Well, let me start by telling you some things that you seemed to do very well. Your volume sounded just fine, and starting off by saying "Hi" seemed very appropriate. So that was good.

S: OK.

T: There's also a couple of things that I noticed that perhaps we'd want to work on. First, it seemed like much of the time you weren't looking directly at me. In fact, when you first came up to me, you were talking to the back of my head. And then when I turned around, it seemed like you looked at the floor a lot. Did you notice that?

S: Yeah, I wasn't really making eye contact.

T: Right. Another thing I noticed was that you seemed to be sort of mumbling, so that it was hard for me to hear what you were saying.

S: I didn't know I was doing that. God, I just suck at this.

T: I'm not sure I would label it that way. We all have our strengths and weaknesses when it comes to socializing. And I certainly could see some strengths in this exercise. But since we can see some areas that probably make it harder for you, now we have an opportunity to work on those things.

In this example, the therapist used a role play to gather more information about Scott's social skill. Note as well that the therapist challenges Scott's tendency to overgeneralize (see Chapter 3) and put himself down. Scott's skill deficits are reframed as something to work on, rather than as a global failure. Next, the therapist begins to help Scott work on the desired social skills using coaching and modeling.

T: So let's practice doing this differently. We've identified three important things for you to work on here. The first is knowing what to say, the second is eye contact, and the third is enunciation. Let's start with the first one, knowing what to say. What's a good way to start this conversation?

S: Um . . . I guess maybe talk about something interesting.

T: Yes, talking about something interesting would be a good thing to do. But how do you know what I would find interesting?

S: I don't.

T: So maybe we start off with something that's a fairly safe bet. What do you know about me so far? You know I'm here at the party, and you know I'm eating the food. So might that be something to talk about?

S: I could ask you how the food is?

T: You could. What else?

S: Well, I guess since you're at the party I could find out how you know the host.

T: Yes, you could. So maybe that's piece number one for you to focus on: Have an opening line about something of potential common interest. Even things like the news, or sports, or the weather, might be good things to talk about. How about the next thing, the eye contact? What makes sense for you to do there?

S: Look you in the eye?

T: Yes, looking me in the eye sounds good. But my back is to you, so what can you do about that?

S: I guess I could say something to get you to turn around or look up.

T: Yes. Or you could just position yourself closer to my field of vision, rather than right behind me.

S: Yeah.

T: OK, so piece number two is eye contact. And how about the enunciation?

S: Speak more clearly.

T: Perfect. Let's try it, but this time I'll be you and you be me. So you go over there and have some food. I'll come up and start the conversation. I'd like you to pay careful attention to what I say, my eye contact, and my enunciation.

S: OK. (*Goes to other side of room.*)

T: (*Walks up to Scott's side.*) Hey.

S: (*Looks up.*) Hey.

T: How's that spinach dip?

S: Not bad. I think it's homemade.

T: I tried making something like that once. It turned out terrible. It's harder than it looks to make it.

S: (*Laughs.*) Yeah, me too.

T: (*Extends his hand.*) I'm Dave, by the way.

S: Scott.

T: Nice to meet you, Scott. How do you know the host?

S: Oh, we work together.

T: Oh, what do you do?

S: We both work at an insurance company. I process claims.

T: Is that here in town?

S: No, I have about a 45-minute commute to work.

T: Wow, that's a lot of driving. Does that bug you?

S: No, it's all right. I listen to these books on tape so it doesn't seem that long.

T: (*Breaking character.*) OK, let's stop here. What did you notice about what I was saying?

S: You started by just asking me about the food and how I know the host.

T: Right. You might have also noticed that I used a fair amount of open-ended questions. Those are questions that are hard to answer with just one word. So I could get you talking a bit more. So if I just asked you, "Do you like the spinach dip?" You could have just said "yes" or "no," and then I'd be stuck having to come up with something. But by changing the words to "How's the spinach dip?" I invite you to say a bit more to me.

S: It also seemed like the conversation kind of flowed naturally.

T: Yes. That's because I would follow up on something you said. So when you said you work with the host, it was a fairly natural follow-up question to ask you where you work. Anything else about what I said?

S: You introduced yourself.

T: Yes. I told you my name and I extended my hand. I also told you that I can't make spinach dip. That's part of having a relaxed conversation—I tell you a little something about myself, even if it doesn't seem terribly important. How was my eye contact?

S: You looked me in the eye.

T: Yes. And how was my enunciation?

S: Good. I could understand you just fine.

Next, the therapist continues the work by using role play and feedback.

T: OK. So I'd like to try this again, and this time let's switch back to our original roles. This time, remember: common interest, eye contact, enunciation. So I'll go back over here to the food, and you start the conversation.

S: (*Walks up to the therapist's side.*) Hey.

T: (*Facing Scott.*) Hi.

S: Um . . . how's the spinach dip?

T: It's pretty good, actually. I don't usually like it but this is good.

S: I tried to make some once. It didn't turn out all that well.

T: Yeah, I can't cook at all.

S: (*Extending hand.*) I'm Scott.

T: Dave.

S: So . . . um . . . do you work with the host?

T: Yes.

S: (*Pause.*) Oh. Where is that?

T: At an insurance company. I process claims there.

S: Oh, is that here in town?

T: (*Breaking character.*) OK, let's stop there. How do you think that one went?

S: It seemed better.

T: Yes, it sure did. I noticed that you seemed to have more to say. You asked me about the food, and how I know the host. It seemed particularly effective that you introduced yourself to me. Were there any places where you felt stuck?

S: I think there was an awkward pause after you told me you work with the host.

T: Yeah, I noticed that. You had just asked, "Do you work with the host?" and I said "Yes." Perhaps you could have phrased the question differently?

S: I could have done open-ended.

T: Right. If you had asked, "How do you know the host?" I would have had to say more.

S: OK.

T: What about eye contact?

S: Better?

T: Better, yes. There were definitely some points where you were looking right at me and it felt like you were interested in what I had to say. I also noticed that there were other times when you were looking at your shoes. So let's try it again, and this time let's shoot for a little more eye contact.

Adapting the Process: *Social Skill Training . . .*

   . . . with high-functioning clients. The social skill deficits with higher-functioning clients are likely to be subtle. You might not see them immediately during your first visit, and the client might not be aware of them. But over the course of your meetings with the client, you might notice that the client talks too loudly or too quietly when feeling distressed or reports day-to-day encounters that suggest the presence of poor assertion. Asking about, or pointing

out, these problems in a straightforward yet empathic manner may help the client recognize the presence of a deficit that is affecting his or her experiences with others.

With higher-functioning clients, you're less likely to see *acquisition deficits* (in which the person simply does not know the appropriate social skill) than you are to see *performance deficits* (in which the person knows the appropriate social skill but is inhibited from enacting the skill due to cognitive or emotional factors) or *fluency deficits* (in which the person knows the appropriate social skill, but has difficulty performing it smoothly and naturally). Because the person likely knows the appropriate skill, the training can focus less on instruction and modeling and more on rehearsal and feedback.

. . . with low-functioning clients. Lower-functioning clients, including those with psychotic or autism spectrum disorders, may have acquisition deficits in addition to performance and fluency deficits. That means that they are likely to need significantly more instruction and modeling than are higher-functioning clients. Social skill deficits with this population are often immediately evident during sessions and provide an excellent example of CRBs (see Chapter 9) to work on. The ability to recognize and interpret others' facial expressions is commonly impaired in such clients, and that might be an excellent place to start (e.g., having them label emotions in pictures or on the therapist's face).

When the behaviors are complex, *chaining* strategies (see Chapter 9) might be used to help the client string together smaller microbehaviors: for example, looking at the person, saying hello, extending a hand for a handshake, and starting a topic of conversation. When the desired social skills are very difficult for the client, *shaping* (see Chapter 9) can be used to prompt and reinforce *successive approximations:* for example, in some cases, we might simply reinforce the client for sustaining eye contact for 5 seconds, then 10, and so on.

. . . with children. With kids, it's important to recognize that good social skills at one developmental level might not be good at another developmental level. How a 6-year-old approaches and interacts with peers is different from how a 16-year-old does those things. Many kids have a problem handling teasing. Sometimes, teasing from peers is the relatively good-natured "ripping on each other," known in some communities as "the dozens," that constitutes how some peer groups interact. In other cases, teasing is a form of outright bullying. In either case, children with poor social and assertiveness skills are likely to freeze up in these situations and not know what to do. Role plays that specifically address these situations can be useful. I've taught kids how to deliver comic insults when the situation called for it.

. . . in groups. What better place to practice social skills than in a group setting? In group CBT, we can have clients role-play with each other, taking turns being the focus of the exercise. Groups also allow us to role-play not only two-person interactions but also other situations, such as small parties or meetings.

. . . with medical patients. Assertion problems are surprisingly common among patients with complicated psychological-medical problems such as chronic pain, migraine, nonepileptic seizures, and irritable bowel syndrome. It may be that somatic symptoms can have a communicative function for some, or it may be that lack of assertive behavior is a marker for overall miserableness. But in either case, such patients will often benefit from learning and practicing assertive behavior. In many cases, the person can be taught a more assertive means of communicating with medical professionals, such as asking direct questions, requesting specific treatments, and so forth.

Problem-Solving Training

As noted in Chapter 2, many psychological problems are associated with poor *problem solving*. By extension, many of the maladaptive behaviors and volitional mental acts we see in psychological disorders represent either efforts to avoid the problem altogether or an ineffective way of trying to address the problem.

Defining Problem Solving

Effective problem solving generally involves several steps (D'Zurilla & Goldfried, 1971): adopting a positive problem orientation, defining the problem and attempting to understand its cause, generating multiple possible solutions to the problem, deciding on a particular solution, and determining whether the solution was effective.

Adopting a Positive Problem Orientation

Successful problem solvers are characterized by a general tendency to (1) appraise problems as "challenges," (2) believe that problems are usually solvable, (3) believe in their personal ability to solve problems successfully, (4) believe that successful problem solving takes time, effort, and persistence, and (5) commit to solving problems rather than avoiding them (Maydeu-Olivares & D'Zurilla, 1996).

By contrast, some people have a *negative problem orientation*. These people show a general tendency to (1) view problems as a significant threat to psychological, social, behavioral, or health well-being, (2) doubt their personal ability to solve problems successfully, and (3) become emotionally upset when confronted with problems (i.e., low tolerance of frustration and uncertainty).

Others have an *impulsive/careless problem-solving style*. These people have a problem-solving process that is careless, hurried, or incomplete. They usually consider only a few solution alternatives, often going with first idea that comes to mind.

Still others have an *avoidant problem-solving style*. These individuals habitually engage in procrastination, passivity, or inaction. They put off problem solving as long as possible and often attempt to shift responsibility for problem solving to other people.

Defining the Problem and Attempting to Understand Its Cause

Emotionally distressed people often are not very good at specifying the exact problems they are facing. They often describe their problems in overly broad terms, such as "Life sucks," or "My marriage is a wreck," or "I'm just overwhelmed." Good problem solvers identify, in concrete terms, exactly what is wrong, such as "I don't do enough enjoyable activities," "My wife and I argue too frequently," or "I have more responsibilities than I can manage." They then try, as best they can, to pinpoint some of the reasons that these problems are occurring. So the first step in effective problem solving is to have a well-defined problem. A well-defined problem is one that gives a clear description of exactly what is happening, whereas a poorly defined problem is vague or refers to how the person feels about the problem, rather than saying what the problem is.

Generating Multiple Possible Solutions to the Problem

Effective problem solvers consider multiple options. They will reserve judgment on the options until they have identified several. Poor problem solvers, by contrast, often have difficulty generating potential solutions, or, in the case of the impulsive/careless problem-solving style, they accept the first solution that comes to mind before they have a chance to think of alternatives.

Deciding on a Particular Solution

Good problem solvers weigh the costs and benefits of the various options they have generated. They think both in terms of short-term and long-term costs and benefits. They consider the feasibility of each one, ultimately deciding on a solution to try. Poor problem solvers often fail to consider one or more of these elements—for example, they fail to consider long-term outcomes, or they don't think about the feasibility of each solution.

Implementing the Solution and Determining Whether the Solution Was Effective

Good problem solvers try a solution and then check to see whether they have actually solved the problem. If the problem wasn't solved, they go back to the drawing board. Poor problem solvers, by contrast, don't check their work, so they don't have a good way of knowing whether the selected solution was actually effective. They just move on to the next problem.

A subcategory of problem solving that overlaps with social skill is *social problem solving*. Social problem solving incorporates the basic elements of problem solving described

The Science behind It

The efficacy of problem-solving training is well established for clients with depression (Bell & D'Zurilla, 2009; Cuijpers, van Straten, & Warmerdam, 2007b), including with depressed older adults (Areán et al., 1993; Areán et al., 2010). It's proven particularly helpful for suicidal or self-injurious clients, who report decreased depression, hopelessness, and suicidal ideation following problem-solving interventions (Eskin, Ertekin, & Demir, 2008; Hatcher, Sharon, Parag, & Collins, 2011; Husain et al., 2014; Joiner, Voelz, & Rudd, 2001; Salkovskis, Atha, & Storer, 1990). Promotion of positive problem orientation has been included in a successful CBT program for clients with GAD (Ladouceur et al., 2000), who tend to use worry as a replacement for effective problem solving. Problem solving has been used to decrease child aggression and externalizing behavior (van Manen, Prins, & Emmelkamp, 2004), and to reduce risk of substance use relapse (Platt & Hermalin, 1989).

Social problem solving has been emphasized in CBT for couples and families. Training in effective problem solving appears to be a helpful way to reduce harmful expressed emotion in families of clients with severe mental illness (Liberman, Wallace, Falloon, & Vaughn, 1981), and it plays a key role in successful treatment of distressed couples (N. B. Epstein & Baucom, 2002; Hahlweg & Markman, 1988; N. S. Jacobson & Margolin, 1979; Lester et al., 1980; Schmaling, Fruzzetti, & Jacobson, 1989) and families of children with disordered behavior (Kazdin, Esveldt-Dawson, French, & Unis, 1987; Kazdin et al., 1992).

above, with the additional challenges of detecting an interpersonal conflict, estimating the perceptions of others, and identifying solutions within the context of an interpersonal conversation (McFall, 1982; Platt & Metzger, 1978).

The Process of Problem-Solving Training

Problem-solving training follows the basic steps of defining problem solving outlined above, as applied to clients, and includes *promoting a positive problem orientation,* followed by four practical steps: *problem definition/formulation, generation of alternatives, decision making,* and *solution implementation/verification* (D'Zurilla & Nezu, 1999; Nezu, Nezu, & D'Zurilla, 2013). Research shows that problem-solving training is most effective when all of these elements are included (Bell & D'Zurilla, 2009).

Promoting a Positive Problem Orientation

As discussed above, many clients have a negative problem orientation, in which they tend to view problems as threatening and insurmountable. We need to help the client start to shift his or her perspective toward the idea that problems are normal, tolerable, and (often) solvable. There are several ways we can do this.

- *Frame problems in living as part of normal life.* Clients often come to therapy thinking that their problems are unique to them or that they are much worse than everyone else's. Sometimes they are, but often they're not. Problems at work or school, troubles in marriage, strained social or family relationships, health concerns, and financial stress are pretty widespread. We don't want to minimize the client's distress about these problems ("Oh come on now, everyone's got problems; buck up!"), but we do want to help the client recognize that many people experience these kinds of problems and that many have found decent solutions. A checklist, such as that shown in Table 12.3, can help "normalize" common problems in living for the client.

TABLE 12.3. A Checklist of Potential Problem Areas

1. Problems with marriage or intimate relationships
2. Problems with relationships with children, parents, siblings, or other family members
3. Problems with work
4. Problems with school
5. Problems with money
6. Problems with home or apartment
7. Legal problems
8. Problems with friends
9. Problems related to alcohol or drugs
10. Problems related to mental health
11. Problems related to sex or sexuality
12. Problems related to past or anticipated loss of someone or something

---

Note. Based on Hawton and Kirk (1989).

- *Help the client understand that his or her problem-solving ability has been compromised.* It's well known that depression, anxiety, substance use, and a wide range of other psychological problems have an adverse effect on one's problem-solving ability. Even extremely intelligent and capable people can, when experiencing a significant emotional overload, have difficulty thinking about and addressing problems adequately. Even routine life stress can diminish problem-solving capacity. So we let the client know that it's quite understandable that he or she would have difficulty solving his or her problems in living under the circumstances. That rationale by itself seems to have a beneficial effect for clients experiencing acute crises such as suicidality, providing hope and making the problem seem more manageable (Bilsker & Forster, 2003).

- *Discuss and normalize the limits of the human brain.* Many clients overestimate what they "should" be able to do cognitively. Perhaps one of the biggest myths is that people should be able to "multitask," or attend to multiple issues at the same time. Other clients believe that they should be able to remember everything or that they should be able to solve a big, thorny problem all at once. No wonder they end up feeling disappointed in themselves. It can be helpful, therefore, to discuss the fact that no one's brain is efficient enough to do all of that. Instead, we all tend to do best when we break larger problems down into smaller ones, take one thing at a time, and use external aids such as notebooks, calendars, or smartphones as needed.

- *Challenge maladaptive beliefs.* Challenging maladaptive beliefs about problem solving is, of course, a cognitive intervention, although it serves a distinctly behavioral aim: to help the client adopt a more positive problem orientation in advance of problem-solving training.

- *Train a basic strategy for emotion regulation and problem solving under stress.* Nezu et al. (2013) use the abbreviation SSTA, which stands for:

  - Stop. The client is taught that strong feelings, ineffective behaviors, and unpleasant thoughts are signals that a problem exists. That means it's time to use problem-solving skills.
  - Slow down. As discussed previously, it's hard to solve problems effectively under conditions of acute stress. The client therefore should be taught to slow down once a problem has been identified. Counting, deep breathing, and taking a brief time-out are all ways to slow things down enough to allow the person to think more clearly.
  - Think. Having slowed down, the client then goes through the specific problem-solving steps described below, thinking clearly about what to do.
  - Act. Once a solution has been identified, the client implements that solution in a manner that aims for effective coping.

Devil's Advocate

The *reverse-advocacy role play* (Nezu et al., 2013) is one interesting way to get the client to identify alternative ways of thinking. In this strategy, the therapist role-plays the maladaptive belief, for example, "Most people don't have problems, so if I have a problem, it means I'm crazy," "My problems are all my fault," or "I must find an absolutely perfect solution to this problem." The client then responds to the therapist by contradicting the belief.

Problem Definition/Formulation

Critical aspects of problem definition/formulation include:

- *Gathering information about the problem.* Clients are instructed to ask questions such as *who, what, when, where,* and *how* about a problem. At times, it can be helpful to encourage the client to "act like a detective" in order to obtain the relevant facts. To quote Detective Joe Friday from *Dragnet,* "Just the facts, ma'am."

- *Defining the problem objectively and concisely.* When we're under emotional strain, our language about problems can get pretty dramatic: "I'm so mad at my wife I think my head's going to explode!" or, "Being alone is a nightmare; it's like I'm going to go crazy!" So we want the client to describe the problem using objective language: "My wife and I have arguments about twice per week in which I feel very angry. My heart starts racing, and my fists clench up. I don't know what to do except leave." "My fear is at its worst when I'm alone. I worry that no one will be able to help me, and I start feeling dizzy and worrying that I'm going to faint."

- *Separating facts from assumptions.* This relates in many ways to the cognitive distortions we discussed in Chapter 3. People often react to what they *think* or *assume* is happening, rather than what actually *is* happening. So we often need to look at the evidence and consider alternatives (see Chapter 14) in order to see things as clearly as possible.

- *Identifying what makes this situation a problem.* In order to understand why a certain situation is a problem, we want to understand the obstacles to reaching the goal. Is there someone or something in the way? Does the person have conflicting goals? Does the client lack the necessary skills or resources? Is this a new and confusing situation? Is the problem particularly complicated and overwhelming? Is the person's emotional reaction serving as a barrier to effective resolution?

- *Setting realistic goals.* In Chapter 7, we discussed the importance of setting clear, measurable, attainable treatment goals. Although we don't want to discourage lofty goals such as "be completely financially independent by this time next year," it's usually most productive to identify manageable subgoals such as "decrease my overall expenses by 5% this month in order to build up my savings."

Generation of Alternatives

We emphasize to the client that there is often more than one solution to a problem, that often a problem will have no single "perfect" solution, and that often the first solution that comes to mind is not the best one. We therefore encourage *brainstorming* as a way to generate multiple potential solutions to the problem. Critical aspects of brainstorming include:

- *Quantity leads to quality.* In general, the more potential solutions one comes up with, the more likely it is that one or more of those solutions will be a good one.
- *Defer judgment.* During brainstorming, we want to keep the creative juices flowing. We don't want the client to get bogged down just yet in deciding whether or not something is reasonable, feasible, or sensible. That will come later. For now, we want to simply encourage as many alternatives possible, even "silly" ones.
- *Variety enhances creativity.* Potential solutions can be either *strategies* or *tactics.* Strategies are general courses of action, whereas tactics are specific steps needed to enact

a strategy. A client might, when generating alternatives, come up with 10 different tactics that all serve the same strategy. Encourage the client to come up with multiple strategies as well as tactics.

Decision Making

Having generated a variety of potential solutions, it's time to start evaluating each one in order to narrow down the list. Steps in decision making include:

- *Getting rid of the obviously ineffective ones.* In the spirit of brainstorming, the client probably came up with some potential solutions that were clearly not feasible, excessively risky, or extremely unlikely to be effective. We can cross those off the list without too much discussion. That leaves us with a smaller list of potentially more viable solutions.
- *Predicting a range of consequences.* Here, the client considers each potential solution in turn and evaluates (1) the likelihood that the solution is doable and would actually work and (2) the potential positive and negative consequences of the solution.
- *Evaluating the predicted outcomes.* For each potential solution, the client asks: (1) will this solution solve the problem? (2) Can I really carry this solution out? (3) What are the likely overall effects on me, both short term and long term? (4) What are the likely overall effects on others, both short term and long term? Here, we're doing a cost–benefit analysis. Do the pros outweigh the cons? It's often helpful to write out the pros and cons of the various options, as shown in Figure 12.1; a blank form is provided in Appendix B.
- *Identifying effective solutions and developing an action plan.* The first question to ask, having evaluated the potential solutions, is: Is this problem solvable? There's often no "perfect" solution to a problem. Sometimes, there isn't even a decent one. That's an important fact to recognize. Although identifying a problem as unsolvable might be frustrating, it can also be liberating. If a problem is deemed to be unsolvable, it frees up the client from feeling compelled to keep trying to fix it. Identification of unsolvable problems, in fact, is a key element of the social problem-solving aspects of some behavioral therapies for couples (e.g., N. B. Epstein & Baucom, 2002; Gottman, 1999), as couples tend to keep bringing up unsolvable issues, hashing them out over and over, with no good resolution. Sometimes, it's more effective just to recognize that there isn't a good solution here and find a way to cope with and work around the problem, rather than addressing it directly. Assuming that we determine that the problem is indeed solvable, the next question is whether we need more information before we can select a solution. If so, we need to make a plan for how to get that information. Finally, we identify which solution, or combination of solutions, the client will choose to implement. Often, it's helpful to identify both the preferred solution and a "back-up" solution in case the first one fails.

Solution Implementation/Verification

Once the client has selected a solution or combination of solutions, the next step is to actually try it out. But the process doesn't end there. We need to then check and see whether the solution was effective. Sometimes, this requires a bit of cognitive challenging, such as when a client has unrealistically high expectations for how well the solution

My problem is: *I'm too busy at work and am having a hard time finishing tasks on time.*

This is a problem because: *I'm not enjoying work and my performance is starting to decline.*

My goal for this problem is: *To not be behind on tasks and stressed out.*

Potential Solution	Pros	Cons
Quit my job	I wouldn't have to deal with the stress anymore	I would financially be much worse off and that would lead to other problems
Delegate tasks to more junior staff	I would lighten my workload	They may resent me for it
Talk to boss about expectations	She might learn that I have too much to do	She might think I can't do my job
Monitor workload and discuss with boss	She might learn that I have too much to do	She might think I can't do my job
Work longer hours	I would get more done	I won't have time to do other pleasant things
Find ways to be more efficient	I would get more done	It may cost a lot of money and take more time in the short term
Prioritize tasks and do most pressing tasks first	No one will know that I'm behind	It doesn't solve the problem that I can't do it all
Ask other people how long it takes them to do things	It will help me find out if I'm too slow or am just doing too many things	They may think I can't handle my job and tell my boss
Do extra training	May help me to do my tasks faster	Will take time to organize and get benefits from it

FIGURE 12.1. Sample problem-solving worksheet for evaluating potential solutions.

will work out. A satisfactory solution need not be perfect. Important questions to ask at this stage are:

"How well did this solution or combination of solutions solve the problem?"
"How satisfied are you with the effects of the solution on you?"
"How satisfied are you with the effects of the solution on others?"
"How well do the results match the predicted outcomes, both positive and negative?"
"Overall, how satisfied are you with the results?"

In the case of social problem solving in distressed couples, the same problem-solving steps are followed; however, this time each step is done jointly by both partners (N. B.

Epstein & Baucom, 2002; N. S. Jacobson & Margolin, 1979). Successful implementation of joint problem solving therefore requires that the partners have developed a reasonable degree of skill in their ability to communicate with one another. When treating couples, it can be informative to have the couple discuss problems, both large and small, in the office. The therapist observes both members, watching for instances of skill deficit (Datillo, 2010; N. B. Epstein & Baucom, 2002; Gottman, 1999; N. S. Jacobson & Margolin, 1979). Distressed families might be instructed to work on a project together in the office, such as making a craft (Friedberg, 2006).

When collaborative problem-solving skills are lacking in a couple or family, we would probably start with some of the basic conversational and listening skills described above before attempting to solve problems. And, of course, even when the basic interactional skills have been mastered, the therapist may still need to intervene during problem solving, interrupting the discussion and prompting the partners to use the appropriate skills.

Here, the therapist is working with Christina (C), our depressed client. As we've discussed, Christina tends to engage in depressive rumination, in part because she's not very skilled at solving problems. And, most likely, her depressive rumination, in turn, further worsens her problem-solving ability (Lyubomirsky & Nolen-Hoeksema, 1995). First, the therapist works on problem definition/formulation.

Adapting the Process: *Problem-Solving Training...*

. . . with high-functioning clients. With our higher-functioning clients, we often find that the person has intact problem-solving capacity in some areas and poor problem-solving in others. That suggests that problem solving is not foreign to the person; rather, the skill is breaking down, often being overwhelmed by strong emotion. In the case of depression or anxiety, the person may engage in rumination or worry as a form of pseudo–problem solving. So the depressed or anxious mood can serve as a cue for practicing what the person probably already knows how to do.

. . . with low-functioning clients. With lower-functioning clients, the problem-solving deficits are likely to be evident across a broader range of situations, and the person might not have acquired basic problem-solving skills at all. Training, therefore, may need to begin with simple situations, such as how to get across town or how to buy groceries in a store. It's different from the operant strategies described in Chapter 9 (e.g., chaining), in which we tell the client the desired behavior and then teach him or her how to do it and reinforce him or her for doing it. Here, we're teaching the client the process of how to come up with the answers by him- or herself.

. . . with children. The principles of problem-solving training can be explained to kids in a developmentally appropriate way. For example, we could train a kid to ask him- or herself a series of questions, such as: (1) What's the problem? (2) What are three things I could do? (3) What's the best solution?

. . . in groups. Groups are a great place in which to brainstorm possible solutions and evaluate the pros and cons of the different solutions. The group leader may opt to write the problem and brainstorming ideas on a dry-erase board and have the group discuss the likelihood that each idea would lead to a positive outcome.

T: We've been talking about your friend, and how she always seems to be taking advantage of you. And it seems like this really bothers you.

C: It does.

T: So let's start by defining this problem a little more precisely. (*Takes out the Problem-Solving Worksheet from Appendix B.*) You'll see here that I have a worksheet that might help us. The first question here is "My problem is:" So what can we say the problem is?

C: My friend's a jerk.

T: Well, that might be true, although I think here we'll find it most helpful to use objective language. What exactly is it that bothers you?

C: She just keeps taking advantage of me.

T: We're getting closer. Can you say it more exactly?

C: She keeps asking to borrow money. And she asks me to give her rides all over the place, and she doesn't even give me money for gas.

T: I see. And this happens how often?

C: At least a couple times a week.

T: So part of what we can write (*writing on the worksheet*) is "At least twice a week, my friend asks me for money or she asks for a ride, without offering to give me money for gas." And how do you respond to these requests?

C: I do it.

T: And that's a problem?

C: Well yeah, I don't want to do it.

T: So why do you, then?

C: Because I just can't say no to her.

T: And you're unhappy about that.

C: Yeah, I just feel resentful.

T: So perhaps that's the second part of our problem? "I don't feel like I can say no to her, so I do what she asks, and then I end up feeling resentful"?

C: That sounds right.

T: So what would your goal be? That is, how would you like things to be?

C: Well, I guess I just need to be able to say no to her when she asks for things.

T: That's a possibility. But let's keep our options open for the moment. You just told me about a possible solution, but what's the actual goal? What do you want the situation to be?

C: I want her to stop asking me for stuff and never paying me back and me always being resentful of her.

T: Ah. So that's the real goal.

Note that the therapist encourages Christina to use objective language and to pay attention to the facts. The therapist also redirects Christina when she confuses a solution with a goal (Nezu et al., 2013). Saying no to her friend is one potential solution, but the therapist focuses Christina on the resolution that she actually wants rather than the strategies she might use to get there. Next, the therapist helps Christina generate alternatives, using the worksheet.

T: Let's start thinking of possible solutions to this problem. You've already mentioned one, which is that you could say no to your friend when she asks for things. But let's see if we can think of some more.

C: Well, I guess I could just make an excuse, like I'm busy or I don't have any money. But I don't like the idea of lying.

T: For now, let's hold off on judging these solutions. They might be good ones, or they might be bad ones, or they might be somewhere in the middle. But at this stage, let's go for quantity. So anything we can think of is OK. So I'll write here "Make an excuse." What else?

C: Um . . . I could just not answer her calls any more or not answer the door when she comes over.

T: Yes! You could avoid her completely. What else?

C: Um . . . I could move?

T: Love it! You could move away so she can't find you. Keep going.

C: I could just sit down with her and tell her I don't want her to ask me for things any more.

T: Yes, you could do that. What else?

C: I'm running out of ideas.

T: You could tell her you don't want to be friends with her any more.

C: I could.

Note that the therapist emphasizes quantity and variety, reinforces Christina for generating possible solutions (even impractical ones), and encourages Christina to defer judgment on the ideas for the time being. The therapist and Christina continue brainstorming until they have come up with as many possible solutions as they can. Next, they work through the decision-making stage.

T: So we have a lot of ideas here. Let's see if we can figure out which ones will be more or less effective. First, are there any on this list that just seem totally unrealistic?

C: Well, there's no way I can afford to move away so that one won't work.

T: OK, so let's just cross that one off the list. Let's talk through the pros and cons of the other ones. The first one we have here is "Say no to her when she asks for things." What would be the pros of that option?

C: It's being direct.

T: Yes, it is. So I'll write that in the "pro" column. What else?

C: It might get her to stop asking.

T: Yes, once she figures out you're saying no all the time, she might stop asking. That's another pro. How about cons?

C: Well, I guess that it might take her a long time to figure out that I'm saying no, and so she might keep asking for a while.

T: That's true. Let's write that as a con. What else?

C: It might hurt her feelings? I mean, if I just start saying no all of a sudden, she might just wonder what's up and think I'm being mean to her.

T: So that's another possible con. How would that solution make you feel?

C: I think I'd feel kind of good if she stopped taking advantage of me, and I'd feel kind of good for standing up for myself, but I'd also feel kind of bad if I thought I was hurting her feelings.

T: What do you think about your ability to start saying no to her?

C: I don't think I know how.

T: So there's a question about how realistic this is.

The therapist and Christina continue in this fashion, listing the pros and cons of each potential solution. The therapist asks questions along the way about the feasibility of the options, as well as the likely positive and negative consequences of the solutions, both for Christina and for her friend. Next, the therapist helps Christina select from among her options.

T: As we look over this list, it seems that some solutions look better to you than others. Which ones stand out as being the most realistic and having the best possible outcomes?

C: I think two of them do. I think that, first, I need to sit down with her and explain that I'm still her friend, and I really value her friendship, but that I don't want to give her money and rides anymore because it puts a strain on me and puts a strain on the friendship. So that would give her a heads-up about what I'm doing and why. And then the other is that I have to start saying no to her if she does ask me for stuff like that.

T: Yes. These seem like reasonable strategies to me. How well do you think you can pull these off right now? You've mentioned that you find it hard to have these kinds of conversations.

C: I don't feel very confident about my ability to do it.

T: So perhaps there's an intermediate step to be done, which is to get you feeling more confident in your ability to have these conversations. Perhaps it would make sense for you and me to practice it for a while, so you feel a bit stronger in that regard?

C: I think that would help.

Note that here the therapist introduces a tactic (assertion training) that will serve the larger strategy of having assertive conversations with her friend. The therapist and Christina then spend some time practicing assertive behavior, using the social skill training strategies described earlier. After several role plays, as Christina's skill and self-efficacy improve, the therapist moves to solution implementation by assigning the first conversation as a homework item. At the following session, the therapist uses solution verification.

T: So how did the conversation with your friend go?

C: It went pretty well. I sat down with her, and I just told her that I was still her friend, but that it just wasn't good for me or for the friendship for me to keep loaning her money and giving her rides.

T: Congratulations! I know that was hard for you.

C: It was. My heart was pounding and I was really nervous about it. I was worried that I'd come across like a jerk.

T: And did you?

C: I don't think so. I think she was initially kind of hurt, but I reassured her that this didn't mean that I don't like her or that I don't want to keep being friends with her.

T: Nice. So here your prediction didn't come true and it turned out better than you expected. And did she ask for anything after that?

C: No, not yet.

T: So we haven't had the opportunity to see whether part 2 of the solution, saying no, works. But overall, how well does your solution seem to have gotten you to your goal of having her not keep asking you for stuff, and you feeling resentful?

C: I think it helped a lot. She's not asking me for anything right now and I feel less mad at her.

THE ESSENTIALS

* Training in any behavioral skill involves assessing the problem, providing direct instructions, modeling, practicing (including role playing), providing feedback, and assigning real-world practice.

* Social skills can include the content of speech, paralinguistic factors, and nonverbal behaviors.

* Assertion is a subset of social skill and can be trained.

* Successful problem solving involves adopting a positive problem orientation, defining the problem and attempting to understand its cause, brainstorming multiple solutions to the problem, deciding on a solution or solutions, implementing the solution, and reviewing whether the problem has been effectively solved.

KEY TERMS AND DEFINITIONS

Assertion: A class of behaviors that includes making requests of others, refusing unreasonable requests, and communicating strong opinions and feelings.

Behavioral skill training: Teaching and practicing behavioral skills needed to engage effectively with the environment.

Problem Solving

If it seems applicable to your personal target, use the problem-solving strategies in this chapter. If it is not applicable, identify a potential problem-solving exercise for a client or other person you know.

Step 1. Write down the problem, using objective language. Be as clear as possible. Describe why this is a problem, and what you want to see happen.

My problem is _____.

This is a problem because _____.

My goal for this problem is _____.

Step 2. Write as many possible solutions to the problem as you can think of in column 1. Defer judgment on whether or not they would work or be possible; just be as creative as possible.

Potential Solution	Pros	Cons

Step 3. For each potential solution, write down the likely pros (what would be good about it) and cons (what would be bad about it). Write the pros and cons in columns 2 and 3. Consider whether the solution would work, whether you could actually do it, and what the likely effects would be on you and on others.

Step 4. Write down which solution(s) you want to try first.

I will try: _____.

Step 5. After trying your solution(s), evaluate the outcome.

Overall, how satisfied are you with the results? _____.

From *Doing CBT* by David F. Tolin. Copyright © 2016 The Guilford Press. Permission to photocopy this worksheet is granted to purchasers of this book for personal use only (see copyright page for details). Purchasers can download enlarged versions of this worksheet (see the box at the end of the table of contents).

SECTION C

COGNITIVE-LEVEL INTERVENTIONS

In this section, we discuss the cognitive-level interventions in CBT. These interventions are called for when you want to *directly* target maladaptive cognitive processes, rather than targeting those processes *indirectly* through behavior-level or emotion-level interventions.

Figure IIC.1 shows the targets for our cognitive-level interventions. Your targets here are:

- Biases in attention and memory.
- Faulty interpretations of events.
- Maladaptive core beliefs.

To affect these targets, we can select from several interventions. There are two broad ways to get at maladaptive cognitions. The first is to *directly challenge the content of thoughts.* Strategies in this group include:

- Identifying and challenging faulty interpretations.
- Identifying and challenging maladaptive core beliefs.
- Using self-monitoring to facilitate awareness and challenging of thoughts.
- Using facilitated recall to combat selective memory.

The other way takes a very different approach of challenging the person's response to thoughts, but not the content of thoughts themselves. These strategies include:

- Using mindfulness and acceptance strategies to increase tolerance of unwanted thoughts.
- Training reallocation of attention.

And remember from our core pathological process that behavioral, cognitive, and emotional systems all influence each other. So a cognitive intervention can create behavioral and emotional change as well.

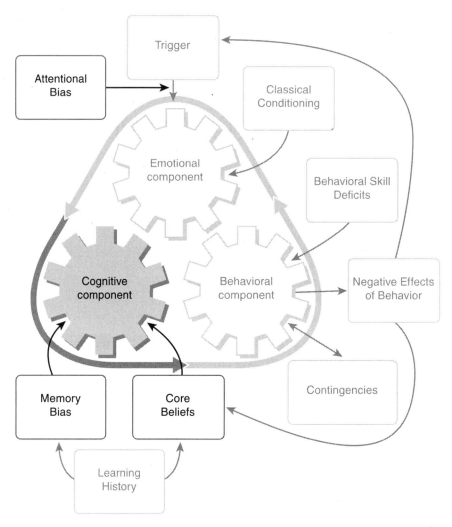

FIGURE IIC.1. The targets for cognitive-level interventions.

CHAPTER 13

What's the Client Thinking?

As you will recall from our meaty conceptualization (Chapter 5), the core pathological process comprises cognitive, emotional, and behavioral processes that mutually influence one another, for better or worse. The cognitive elements include *automatic cognitive processes* such as intrusions and information processing, *semi-automatic cognitive processes* including interpretations and core beliefs, and *effortful cognitive processes* such as thought suppression, mental compulsions, rumination, and worry. In this chapter and the next, we'll focus on interventions that directly target the semi-automatic cognitive processes: the client's interpretations that are on "autopilot" but that can, with some effort, be identified and modified.

As we discussed in Chapter 3, *cognitive distortions* are semi-automatic interpretive errors that we all make. In psychological problems, the person makes the same kind of error(s) over and over, which has a negative effect on emotions and behaviors. For example:

- Anna, our client with panic disorder, experiences dizziness and has the interpretation "I'm going to pass out." That interpretation increases her feeling of fear and her likelihood of engaging in avoidance and escape behaviors.
- Christina, our client with severe depression, experiences a minor setback and has the interpretation "I can't do anything right." That interpretation increases her feeling of sadness and decreases her likelihood of taking positive action.
- Elizabeth, our client with borderline personality disorder, experiences disappointment in a therapy session and has the interpretation "My therapist doesn't care about me at all." That interpretation increases her feelings of sadness and despair, as well as the likelihood that Elizabeth will engage in TIBs.
- Lauren, our client with schizophrenia, experiences unusual thoughts and has the interpretation "Someone is trying to control my mind." This interpretation increases her feeling of fear and the likelihood that she will avoid people or act suspiciously toward them.

- Blaise, who has a substance use disorder, has urges to use and has the interpretation "If I can't use right now, I'll never be able to feel better." This interpretation increases her sense of urgency and despair, along with the likelihood that she will use.
- Nick, whose marriage with Johanna is in distress, is experiencing some problems with child rearing and has the interpretation "This is all Johanna's fault; she is trying to make my life miserable." This interpretation increases his feelings of anger and the likelihood that his behaviors toward Johanna will be negative or hostile.
- Samuel, who suffers from insomnia, lies in bed and thinks, "If I can't fall asleep, I'll never be able to function and my day will be ruined. Maybe I'll even get fired." This interpretation increases his anxiety and decreases the likelihood of his falling asleep.
- Shari, our client with bulimia, has an episode of binge eating and thinks, "I'm so disgusting and fat." This interpretation increases her feelings of disgust, sadness, and shame and increases the likelihood that she will engage in purging behavior.

Because distorted interpretations can have a negative influence on emotions and behaviors, it could be argued that directly modifying those interpretations will have a positive influence on emotions and behaviors. So, for example:

- If Anna didn't think she was going to pass out, perhaps she would feel less fearful and would be less likely to engage in avoidance and escape behaviors.
- If Christina didn't think that she can't do anything right, perhaps she would feel less sad and would be more likely to take positive action.
- If Elizabeth didn't think of her therapist as uncaring, perhaps she would feel less sad and despairing and would be less likely to engage in TIBs.
- If Lauren didn't think that someone was trying to control her mind, perhaps she would feel less fearful and engage in less avoidance.
- If Blaise didn't think that using was the only way to feel better, perhaps she would feel less desperate and would be less likely to use substances.
- If Nick didn't blame things on Johanna and think she was trying to make his life miserable, perhaps he would feel less angry and would act more nicely toward her.
- If Samuel didn't think that the consequences of not sleeping would be disastrous, perhaps he'd feel less anxious and actually fall asleep.
- If Shari didn't think of herself as disgusting and fat, perhaps she'd feel less shame and would be less likely to purge.

Working at the cognitive level includes two somewhat overlapping procedures: *eliciting and identifying maladaptive thoughts* (which we discuss in this chapter) and *challenging and modifying maladaptive thoughts* (which we'll discuss in the next chapter).

Before we can work with the client's interpretations, we have to get them "out on the table." That is, the therapist and client must each understand what the client is thinking.

What Thoughts Are We Looking For?

Everyone has a stream of consciousness, and not all of it is clinically meaningful or helpful. I find it helpful to distinguish between *cold thoughts* and *hot thoughts* (Greenberger

& Padesky, 2016). **Cold thoughts** are descriptive and don't elicit much of an emotional response. By contrast, **hot thoughts** are emotionally evocative. They are both influenced by emotion and influence emotion. "Hmm, there goes a dog" is a cold thought. "Yikes, that dog's going to bite my face off!" is a hot thought.

As we discuss thoughts with our clients, part of our task is to weed through the cold thoughts and try to find the hot thoughts—those thoughts that are part of the core pathological process of thoughts, emotions, and behaviors.

Thoughts can be about *external events*, such as activities, other people, objects, and so on. So, for example, a depressed individual might have hot thoughts such as "No one likes me," or an anxious person might have hot thoughts such as "I'm going to get hurt."

Thoughts can also be about *emotions* or *physiological sensations*. We discussed depressive rumination in Chapter 3; a depressed individual might have the hot thought "I'm such a loser for feeling sad." That is, we have a cognitive reaction ("I'm a loser") to an emotion (sadness). Not surprisingly, the cognitive reaction loops back and fuels more feelings of sadness. In a similar fashion, a client with panic disorder might have the hot thought "That pain in my chest means I'm having a heart attack!" This is a cognitive reaction ("I'm having a heart attack") to a physiological sensation (chest pain). Most likely, the thought is erroneous—most chest pain does not signal a heart attack (M. A. Kohn, Kwan, Gupta, & Tabas, 2005)—yet the thought loops back and fuels even more feelings of anxiety (perhaps including more chest pain).

Thoughts can also be about *thoughts*, a process termed **metacognition** (Wells, 2009). That is, one can have a cognitive reaction to one's own thoughts. A really clear example of metacognition can be seen in the client with OCD who thinks "I just thought of harming my baby—that must mean I'm a murderer!" You can see in this case that there are really two thoughts going on—an *intrusion* (the image of harming a baby) and an *interpretation* of the mental image as meaning that the person is a murderer. Often, metacognitions are distorted: Most perfectly healthy people have bizarre or violent thoughts pop into their heads (Rachman & de Silva, 1978), yet that doesn't make them violent people.

Using Socratic Questioning to Elicit Interpretations

As discussed in Chapter 7, *Socratic questioning* means that we use questions, rather than statements, to help the client arrive at the conclusion. In this case, we would use a series of questions that helps the client identify his or her interpretations. Padesky (1993, p. 4) defines Socratic questioning as using questions that:

1. The client has the knowledge to answer;
2. Draw the client's attention to information that is relevant to the issue being discussed but that may be outside the client's current focus;
3. Generally move from the concrete to the more abstract, so that
4. The client can, in the end, apply the new information to either reevaluate a previous conclusion or construct a new idea.

Here, the therapist is working with Elizabeth (E), our client with borderline personality disorder and a long history of self-injurious behaviors that have resulted in multiple hospitalizations. The therapist's aim in this discussion is to help Elizabeth identify the interpretations that precede those behaviors.

T: Elizabeth, we've been talking for a while about your cutting, and it seems like we agree that it's a problem for you.

E: Definitely. I wish I could be different, I really do. But I just don't know how. It just seems like I lose it and can't control myself.

T: Yes, I can see why it would seem that way. It must be very scary to feel like you're out of control.

E: It is.

T: Maybe a good step toward helping you feel more in control would be for us to spend some time trying to understand why this is happening.

E: I don't know why it's happening. I'm just so pissed off that I can't help it.

T: Right, at this time you and I don't know why it's happening. But perhaps if we put our heads together we can come up with some ideas. Your statement about being pissed off might give us a clue here; do you think there's a relationship between being pissed off and cutting?

E: Maybe, yeah. Sometimes when I'm really mad about something I want to cut.

T: OK, maybe we're on to something here. Let's see if we can take an example from your experience and really understand it. When was the last time you cut yourself?

E: It was about a week ago. That was the one that landed me in the hospital.

T: OK, let's talk about that event and see if we can understand it a little better. Can you recall what was going on?

E: Well, I had a big argument with my boyfriend. We were really yelling at each other and stomping around the house. It was really nasty. I called him a bunch of names, and he said I was a psycho.

T: Wow, that sounds like a really crummy situation. I wonder whether him calling you a psycho was particularly hurtful?

E: It was. And then he stormed out the door and said he was going to go cool off and have a beer with his buddies and he slammed the door and left me alone in the house.

T: So let's imagine this situation. There you are in the house, by yourself, just after having this big argument. And this is when you cut yourself?

E: Eventually, yeah. First I sat there just feeling sorry for myself for a while and then I got pissed off and I just grabbed a knife from the kitchen and cut my wrist.

T: OK, let's rewind this scene just a little bit. Take me back to just after the door slammed and you were by yourself.

E. OK.

T: Right at that moment, how were you feeling?

E: I don't know. A mess, I guess.

T: What does "a mess" feel like?

E: I don't know. Just a mess.

T: Well, let's stay on this a bit. Often, we're feeling things even if we can't quite make sense of them. But if we take some time and think about it, we can often clarify what we're feeling. You mentioned earlier that you had felt pissed off; is that what you were feeling right at that moment?

E: No, I didn't feel pissed off until later. At this point I was just feeling . . . I don't know . . . just sad or something.

T: Sad.

E: Yeah, I was sad because he just walked out.

T: What was it about him walking out that made you feel sad?

E: Well, it's like he just walked out and left me all alone with no one to talk to or anything.

T: Is that the part that really bothered you? That you were alone?

E: I guess.

T: What were you thinking at that time?

E: I was just upset and sad, like I felt like crying.

T: Yes, you had the feeling of being sad, and felt like crying. That's a feeling, something that's happening in your body. I'm wondering about thoughts, like the words that go through your head. We all talk to ourselves sometimes, and I'm wondering whether you were talking to yourself then.

E: Well, I guess I was thinking that I'm all alone and it sucks to be all alone.

T: What about being all alone sucks? To ask it another way, did you say something to yourself about what it means to be all alone?

E: I don't get it.

T: Well, for example, did you say to yourself, "I'm all alone; thank goodness, now I can finally have some peace and quiet"?

E: No.

T: A lot of the time, when people are feeling really sad, they're thinking about something being hopeless—like that a bad situation is never going to improve.

E: Yeah, I thought I'm all alone and it's going to stay that way.

T: It's going to stay that way? For how long were you telling yourself it would stay that way?

E: Forever, I guess.

T: So part of what you were saying to yourself—your thought—was "I'll be alone forever"?

E: Yeah.

T: When you had that thought, how did it make you feel?

E: I don't know.

T: Well, just as an experiment, try thinking it now. Can you think to yourself, "I'll be alone forever"?

E: Yeah.

T: As you sit here and think it, how do you feel?

E: Sad.

T: So it sounds like when your boyfriend stomped out of the house and slammed the door, you had the thought "I'll be alone forever," and that's a thought that makes you feel sad.

E: (*becoming tearful*) Yeah.

T: I notice you're having some feelings right now. What just came up for you?

E: I guess I'm feeling pissed off again.

T: Like you were right before you cut yourself?

E: Yeah, kind of like that.

T: Where do you feel that, in your body?

E: Right in my chest, like it's tightening. And my face feels hot.

T: What went through your mind just then? Right before you felt pissed off?

E: I was just thinking how unfair it is. He goes out to have a beer with his buddies and I'm left home feeling like garbage.

T: So you have another thought there—"It's not fair."

E: Right.

T: Can you say more about what strikes you as unfair about it?

E: Well, if I'm feeling terrible he shouldn't be able to just walk out and see his buddies and leave me at home. He should stay and talk it out with me and be supportive of me. Instead I'm just stuck here.

T: (*Takes out a piece of paper.*) I'd like to write down a couple of the things you've mentioned, because I think they might be helpful to us. You have a couple of thoughts here. The first is the thought "I'll be alone forever." And when you have that thought, the associated feeling is sadness. And you have another thought, too, which is "It's not fair," and there are some other thoughts that go along with it, like "He should stay with me" and "I'm stuck here." And when you have those thoughts, you feel pissed off.

In this example, the therapist uses several different strategies (see Wright et al., 2006), embedded within the general framework of Socratic questioning, to elicit Elizabeth's interpretations:

• The therapist focuses on a *specific example* of the clinical problem. It's often easier to speak in generalities (e.g., "What kinds of thoughts do you usually have before you cut yourself?"), but the results are likely less reliable and less likely to evoke "hot thoughts." Instead, the therapist asks questions such as, "When was the last time you cut yourself?" "Can you recall what was going on?" The therapist also uses *imagery* by asking Elizabeth to imagine herself back in the situation and uses a *video metaphor* by asking Elizabeth to "Rewind the scene" and "Take me back to just after the door slammed and you were by yourself." This way, the therapist can pinpoint specific time frames within the larger situation.

• The therapist uses empathy and validation. Without the liberal use of empathic, validating statements, the process of eliciting maladaptive thoughts can seem critical or judgmental. Here, the therapist takes pains to strengthen the alliance with Elizabeth, using statements such as "It must be very scary to feel like you're out of control" and "Wow, that sounds like a really crummy situation."

• The therapist emphasizes *collaboration*. The principle of *collaborative empiricism* (see Chapter 1) emphasizes that the therapist and client work together to find the answers. Using statements such as "perhaps if we put our heads together we can come up with some ideas" and "maybe we're on to something here," the therapist underscores the fact that they are on the same team.

- The therapist uses *psychoeducation* to help move Elizabeth past stuck points. At times in the discussion, Elizabeth seemed not to know, or at least couldn't immediately come up with, the answer. Rather than hammering her with more questions, the therapist shifts to a more educational mode, using such statements as "Often, we're feeling things even if we can't quite make sense of them"; "We all talk to ourselves sometimes, and I'm wondering whether you were talking to yourself then"; and "A lot of the time, when people are feeling really sad, they're thinking about something being hopeless." Notice as well that the therapist helps Elizabeth distinguish between thoughts and feelings. We often use the word *feel* when we really mean *think*—for example, you might tell someone, "I *feel* like you're not listening to me right now." But that's a thought, not a feeling. Some clients need to practice distinguishing between the two.

- The therapist observes a *mood shift* in Elizabeth and makes use of the emotion to elicit more interpretations: "I notice you're having some feelings right now. What just came up for you?" Remember that emotions, behaviors, and thoughts tend to go together. So if the client exhibits a shift in emotions during the session, it is quite likely that there has also been a shift in thoughts.

Bringing the Problem into the Room

The process of eliciting "hot thoughts" is deliberately evocative. We ask pointed questions that stir up emotions and inquire about mood shifts when we observe them. We do this because the client may be uniquely able to identify maladaptive thoughts while experiencing the emotion, given what we know about mood-congruent information processing (see Chapter 3). In fact, a general principle, which we will revisit often, is that therapy works best when the client can experience some of the problem emotion in the session (Foa & Kozak, 1986).

This is not to say that we want Elizabeth's sadness and anger to overwhelm her in the session. Similarly, our aim is not for Anna to have a panic attack or for Lauren to become overtly paranoid in the session. But the client does need to be "in touch with" the emotion. CBT is not a cold and detached therapy. Rather, throughout the therapy part of our aim is to activate elements of the core pathological process, at least a bit, so that the client can identify and work on it. This is **bringing the problem into the room.** At some level, we want the client to experience some of the problem emotion during the therapy session so that we can work on it most effectively. The therapist amplifies Elizabeth's emotional experience a bit by asking her to identify not only the subjective feeling state but also the physiological sensations ("Where do you feel it?").

With any evocative therapy such as CBT, there is always a possibility that the client's cognitive, emotional, or behavioral reaction will be too strong in the session for meaningful therapy to take place. When the client is sobbing uncontrollably, pacing the room, acting in an overtly hostile manner, and so forth, it's time to shift strategies. We might use some of the *emotion regulation* interventions described in Chapters 18 and 19, for example, to help the client reduce his or her level of arousal. It doesn't mean the session has gone badly; it's just a signal to change things up. The skilled therapist watches the client carefully, pushing the emotion when appropriate and pulling back on the emotion when necessary.

Using Role Playing to Elicit Interpretations

Sometimes it's hard for the client to identify his or her thoughts using dialogue alone. As we know from our discussion on mood-congruent information processing, when one is having a calm, reasoned discussion in a quiet office, it can be difficult to retrieve memories of what you were thinking when you were more distressed (just as when you're distressed, it can be difficult to retrieve memories of what you were thinking when you were calm). In such cases, **role playing** of critical events can be helpful as a way of facilitating the thoughts' availability to consciousness. This is another way of bringing the problem into the room.

Here, the therapist is working with Scott (S), our socially anxious client. The therapist's aim in this discussion is to help Scott identify his anxious interpretations during a recent meeting with his manager at work.

T: Scott, while you were in the meeting with your boss, what kinds of thoughts were going through your head?

S: I don't know. I'm not sure I was really thinking anything. I just know I felt really anxious.

T: Yes, you were definitely anxious. And maybe it's true that you weren't thinking anything, but it could also be that you weren't paying a whole lot of attention to your thoughts at the time, or that it's just hard to recall them now, sitting here in my office.

S: That's possible. I know we've been talking about interpretations, but honestly a lot of the time I just don't really know what I was thinking. I just know how I feel.

T: That's perfectly fine. A lot of people have trouble identifying their thoughts because the feelings just dominate the picture. I wonder if we might try something a little different, though. Could we role-play a little of this meeting so we can see what comes up for you?

S: I guess. I mean, it would be kind of artificial.

T: Understood. This is just an exercise; maybe we'll learn something, maybe not. But let's find out. I'll be your boss and you be you. Can you set up the scene for me?

S: Well, first, my boss was sitting at his desk and I was on the other side of the desk.

T: OK, then let's go over to my desk here and sit like you two were. (*Sits at desk.*) Now can you set up the scene for us? What are we talking about?

S: Well, he's talking to me about a report I wrote and the fact that he found some typos on it.

T: OK. Did he have the report?

S: Yeah, it was in his hand.

T: (*Picks up a piece of paper from the desk.*) So I'll hold this and it will be the report. And what kind of tone and facial expression was he using?

S: I guess he had kind of a stern look on his face. His tone didn't sound particularly stern but his face did.

T: (*Makes a stern face.*) Like this?

S: (*Laughs.*) Yeah, that's pretty close.

T: OK, so let's try this. I want to go through this situation with you, but since I wasn't there, I might need you to coach me a little. Your job here is to pay attention to what's going on inside you.

S: OK.

T: (*in character*) Scott, I'd like to talk to you about this report you wrote. As I was reading it, I found two typos.

S: Oh, I didn't know that. Where were they?

T: There was one here, and one here. (*Points to paper.*)

S: Ah, I see them. I'm sorry for the error.

T: (*breaking character*) So right now, can you tell me what thoughts are going through your head?

S: Well, I'm thinking he's really mad.

T: At you?

S: Yeah, mad at me.

T: OK, so we have one thought here, "He's really mad at me." Let's keep going a little bit and see whether anything else comes up. (*back in character*) I'm really disappointed in this report. I think you could have done better.

S: Well, I was up really late and I was really tired. I don't usually make mistakes like that. I'm really sorry.

T: (*breaking character*) Seems like you're experiencing a little more anxiety here?

S: Yeah, I can feel myself getting red in the face and I can feel my heart beating.

T: What's going through your mind?

S: I'm thinking that he's super mad and I'm going to get fired.

T: So there's another thought. "I'm going to get fired." And you mentioned you felt your face getting red and your heart beating. Any thoughts about that?

S: I'm thinking that I'm getting really anxious and he can probably tell.

T: Hmm, so you're thinking that he can see you're anxious. And what then?

S: Well, he probably thinks that I'm just a ball of anxiety and probably incompetent so that will just make him want to fire me even more.

T: I see. So during this role play we identified several interpretations. The first one was "He's mad at me." The second is "I'm going to get fired." The third is "He can see that I'm anxious." The fourth is "He'll think I'm a ball of anxiety," and the fifth is "If he thinks I'm a ball of anxiety, he'll think I'm incompetent and will want to fire me even more." Let's write those thoughts down so we can talk about them further.

Clinical judgment is critical when using role play. If the therapeutic alliance seems fragile, or if it seems that the client needs to keep the therapist on his or her "side" during a role-play exercise, it can be helpful to bring in a third person to be the actor. I'm fortunate to have students in my clinic, and I will often bring one of them into a session (with the client's permission) to act out a role. That way, I can remain aligned with the client, pausing the scene occasionally to inquire about the client's inner experience.

Adapting the Process: *Eliciting Interpretations . . .*

. . . with high-functioning clients. Higher-functioning clients are somewhat more likely to be "psychologically minded," meaning that they can readily identify their own thoughts and feelings. Of course, there are plenty of exceptions to this, so we can't take it for granted.

. . . with low-functioning clients. Lower-functioning clients may have difficulty identifying their own thoughts and the relationship between thoughts, feelings, and behaviors. In many cases, you'll need to go over several examples with them. It might be useful to give several imaginary scenarios or examples from your own experience and quiz the client: "What was my thought in that situation?" "What was my feeling in that situation?"

. . . with children. Depending on developmental level, many kids can identify their own thoughts. But in some cases, it's difficult. I've seen therapists do great work by giving kids cartoons with empty "thought bubbles" over the character's heads and asking the child to write down what the character is thinking.

. . . in groups. Group CBT usually requires that we focus on common factors across group members. Groups can review the list of cognitive distortions, and the therapist can ask group members to provide examples of interpretations they have had that match those distortions (e.g., "Who has found themselves catastrophizing? What was your catastrophizing thought?").

. . . on the inpatient unit. Clients who are acutely ill are often highly aware of their emotions, which may facilitate identification of interpretations. Inpatient conversations are usually briefer than are those in outpatient CBT, so we often have to rely on a truncated version of the procedure to identify interpretations and beliefs. Simple questions such as "What did you make of that?" or "What did you take that to mean?" might help the client identify some cognitive processes. Most likely, a brief inpatient stay will not provide enough time to fully challenge the client's interpretations (which can be particularly entrenched for severely ill clients), although you may be able to "loosen up" the client's thinking. More on that topic in the next chapter. In many cases, inpatient interventions will emphasize behavioral over cognitive strategies. We'll get to those behavioral interventions later in this book.

Using Checklists to Identify Interpretations

At times, it's expedient to use prewritten checklists of common maladaptive interpretations. This way, the client can simply read examples of maladaptive thoughts and check which ones seem to apply. There are a number of them out there, and many can be obtained free on the Web or through your library. I list a few here, which can be found in their source articles or on online sites. These measures aren't a substitute for talking to the client about his or her thoughts—and you may recognize many of the items on these measures as feelings, rather than thoughts—but they can be a helpful way to start the conversation.

- The *Automatic Thoughts Questionnaire* (Hollon & Kendall, 1980) is a checklist of maladaptive thoughts commonly associated with depression.
- The *Anxious Self-Statements Questionnaire* (Kendall & Hollon, 1989) is a checklist of

anxious thoughts reflecting one's inability to cope and anxiety/uncertainty about the future.

- The *Children's Automatic Thoughts Scale* (Schniering & Rapee, 2002) is a measure of thoughts related to physical threat, social threat, personal failure, and hostility in children and adolescents.
- The *Post-Traumatic Cognitions Inventory* (Foa et al., 1999) is a measure of negative beliefs about oneself, the world, and self-blame following a traumatic event.
- The *Agoraphobic Cognitions Questionnaire* (Chambless, Caputo, Bright, & Gallagher, 1984) is a measure of fearful beliefs about one's bodily sensations that are common in individuals with panic and agoraphobia.
- The *Obsessional Beliefs Questionnaire* (Obsessive Compulsive Cognitions Working Group, 2005) is a measure of various maladaptive beliefs common to OCD, including threat overestimation and responsibility, perfectionism and tolerance of uncertainty, and importance of and need to control thoughts.
- The *Brief Hypomanic Attitudes and Positive Predictions Inventory* (Mansell & Jones, 2006) is a measure of beliefs that may predispose individuals to mania.
- The *Peters et al. Delusions Inventory* (Peters, Joseph, Day, & Garety, 2004) is a measure of delusional beliefs characteristic of schizophrenia and other psychotic disorders.
- The *Green et al. Paranoid Thought Scales* (Green et al., 2008) is a measure of ideas of reference and of persecution characteristic of paranoia.
- The *Eating Disorder Belief Questionnaire* (Cooper, Cohen-Tovee, Todd, Wells, & Tovee, 1997) is a measure of assumptions and beliefs associated with bulimia nervosa and anorexia nervosa.
- The *Personality Disorder Belief Questionnaire* (Arntz, Dreessen, Schouten, & Weertman, 2004) is a measure of beliefs commonly seen in individuals with avoidant, dependent, obsessive-compulsive, paranoid, histrionic, and borderline personality disorders.

Here, the therapist is working with Christina (C), our depressed client. Christina is acutely aware of her feelings of sadness, and she has been able to identify many external triggers for her sadness; however, she has had difficulty identifying her specific interpretations. The therapist administered the Automatic Thoughts Questionnaire (Hollon & Kendall, 1980) prior to the session and reviews the results with her.

T: Christina, as I mentioned before, we're in the process of trying to understand how your thinking might be contributing to your depression. Remember, sometimes people become depressed, in part, because they have fallen into a habit of thinking in a very negative or depressing way. So I asked you to complete this questionnaire as a way of helping us to see whether that's the case with you. Any reactions to filling out the questionnaire?

C: Yes, I noticed that a lot of the statements on the questionnaire seemed really true for me. I guess that means that I'm thinking in a depressing way?

T: It might, but let's take a closer look. Lots of people have depressing thoughts from time to time. The nice thing about a questionnaire like this is that it's been given to a lot of people who are depressed, as well as a lot of people who aren't depressed. So we can get a sense of whether you have more of these kinds of thoughts than the average person does. If so, that might be an important clue for us.

C: OK.

T: To get a score on this questionnaire, we add up all of the ratings. When we do that, we see a score of 80, which is about average for a person who is depressed. By comparison, the average nondepressed person scores around a 49, much lower.

C: Right, so I'm depressed?

T: Well, we pretty much knew that part already. What this questionnaire is measuring is not whether you're depressed, but whether you are having the kinds of thoughts that might be at the root of your depression.

C: OK, I think I get it.

T: Let's take a look at some specific examples. For each of these thoughts, you identified the frequency on a 1-to-5 scale from "not at all" to "all the time," and you also identified how much you believe those thoughts, on a 1-to-5 scale from "not at all" to "totally." Let's see if we can find some good examples here—items that had a particularly strong frequency or believability rating. As you review your answers, what do you find?

C: Well, there's a thought here that says "I'm a failure." I gave that a frequency of 5 and a believability of 5.

T: OK, so that looks like a really strong thought for you. Let's discuss that one a bit. What leads you to think this way?

Metaphor

Metaphors can be helpful in getting clients to recognize the impact of thoughts on emotions. Beck et al. (1979, pp. 147–148) describe the following discussion between a therapist (T) and patient (P):

T: The way a person thinks about or interprets events affects how he feels and behaves. For example, say he was home alone one night and heard a crash in another room. If he thinks, "There's a burglar in the room," how do you think he would feel?

P: Very anxious, terrified.

T: And how might he behave?

P: He might try to hide or if he was smart he would phone the police.

T: OK, so in response to a thought that a burglar made the noise, the person would probably feel anxious and behave in such a way as to protect himself. Now, let's say he heard the same noise and thought, "The windows have been left open and the wind has caused something to fall over." How would he feel?

P: Well, he wouldn't be afraid. He might be sad if he thought something valuable was broken or he might be annoyed that one of the kids left the window open.

T: And would his behavior be different following this thought?

P: Sure, he would probably go and see what the problem was. He certainly wouldn't phone the police.

T: OK. Now, what this example shows us is that there are usually a number of ways in which you can interpret a situation. Also, the way you interpret the situation affects your feelings and behavior.

In this fashion, the therapist uses examples from the questionnaire as a starting point for a discussion of specific maladaptive thoughts.

Monitoring Thoughts

Thought monitoring is an important part of cognitive intervention. After interpretations have been identified in the session, the therapist assigns thought monitoring as homework. The client is instructed to identify his or her maladaptive interpretations as they come up in the natural environment and to record them as they occur. Thought monitoring serves several purposes:

• Thought monitoring helps *identify interpretations.* Memory for anything, particularly things as fleeting as one's own thoughts, tends to be highly fallible (not to mention mood dependent). It's quite likely, therefore, that a client would experience some difficulty, in the therapist's comfortable office, identifying thoughts that occurred several days prior under stressful circumstances. The information will be clearest, and most useful, if it is captured in "real time."

• Thought monitoring helps *clarify the relationships among events, thoughts, and emotions.* By asking the client to monitor not only the thoughts but also the events that preceded the thought, the therapist is able to understand how the client's thoughts fit into the core pathological process.

• Thought monitoring *educates the client about the CBT model.* Firsthand experience is a far better teacher than any discussion. Although we spend a fair amount of time in the early sessions (and, indeed, throughout the therapy) teaching the client a cognitive-behavioral model of his or her symptoms, it is much more useful to have the client try it out as a way of increasing his or her awareness of the concept.

• Thought monitoring induces *measurement reactivity.* As discussed in Chapter 6, the mere act of measuring something tends to affect the thing you're measuring. We are directing the client's attention, on an ongoing basis, to his or her thoughts. In so doing, we are likely to start a process by which the client starts to challenge those thoughts on his or her own, even before we begin the formal process of thought challenging.

Holding Up a Mirror

Thought monitoring is a great way to hold up a mirror to the client. We often don't pay attention to our thoughts and interpretations, not because they are "unconscious" in the psychoanalytic sense but because we're not used to that kind of introspection. When we ask clients to write down their interpretations in distressing situations, we're essentially asking them to take a good, hard look at their thoughts. Although we'll talk about challenging interpretations in the next chapter, the mere act of verbalizing, writing, and reflecting the client's thoughts can help the client start to question those thoughts.

Ways of Monitoring Thoughts

The most straightforward way for a client to monitor his or her thoughts is to use a paper *thought recording form* as shown in Figure 13.1; a blank version is provided in Appendix B. Like any form in this book, you can modify the form if it seems appropriate for a given client.

Here we ask the client to record three things: the *situation*, which can be the external or internal stimuli that precede the interpretation; the *interpretation* itself; and the *emotional or physical response* to the interpretation. We also ask the client to rate the intensity of the emotional or physical reaction on a numeric scale.

In addition to the traditional paper-and-pencil methods, some other strategies of thought monitoring may also be useful:

- Some clinicians have asked clients to use audio recording devices to record their thoughts during stressful situations (Macaskill, 1996); such devices are now available on most smartphones.
- Smartphone apps have been developed that allow clients to type in their thoughts. MoodKit and iCBT are two examples.

In this example, the therapist is working with Melissa (M), our client with PTSD. They have spent the majority of their session using Socratic questioning to reveal Melissa's thoughts. The therapist now assigns thought monitoring homework.

T: Melissa, today we've covered some really important ground. We've identified a number of interpretations that seem to be associated with your feelings of anxiety, sadness, and anger.

M: Yeah, it seems like I have a lot of negative thinking.

T: Right, and it seems like there's a direct relationship between your thoughts and your feelings.

M: Definitely. When I have negative thoughts I feel worse.

T: Exactly. So I'd like to take the next step now. Having identified some of these interpretations here in our meeting, the next step is to have you start catching them as they come up in your day-to-day life. (*Takes out a Thought Monitoring Form.*) You'll see here that I have this paper divided into three columns. The first is the situation. That means whatever is going on that is leading you to feel uncomfortable. The second is the interpretations. That means the words that go through your head; the meaning you give to the situation. And the third is the feeling or emotion. That means how you feel in your body, like sad, scared, angry, and so on. Does that make sense to you?

M: I guess so. When am I supposed to fill this out?

Situation	Interpretation(s)	Emotion(s) (0–100)
Late for work	I'll never succeed in this job	Sadness 65

FIGURE 13.1. Sample Thought Monitoring Form.

T: I'd recommend we let your feelings be the guide. I'd like you to carry this piece of paper around with you, like in your back pocket, every day. Whenever you notice yourself feeling especially sad, scared, or mad, that should be your cue to pull out the piece of paper and write down what's going on.

M: OK. So should I be trying not to have negative thoughts?

T: No, the goal here is not for you to have no negative thoughts. As we've talked about, one of the problems that happens to a lot of people with PTSD is that they start trying really hard not to let bad things come into their minds. . . .

M: . . . and then they just think about it more.

T: Right. So for now, your job is just to notice these thoughts when they come up and to write them down. Then, at our next session, bring this sheet in with you and we can talk about what you wrote down.

M: Would it be OK if I left the sheet at home and just filled it out at night, instead of carrying it all over the place with me?

T: You could do that, and it's better than not doing it at all. However, I suspect you'll find that it's less effective that way. I have a few reasons for believing that. First, we know that the longer you wait, the fuzzier your memory becomes. So by that evening, your memory for the details of exactly what you were thinking and when will probably be less clear. Second, we have this idea that overcoming negative interpretations will be an important part of how you overcome PTSD. So an initial part of that process is getting you to focus more on your thinking in the moment. Over time, it would be good if you can get to the point where if something bothers you, one of your first thoughts will be, "What am I thinking right now?" But to get you there, you'll need to start practicing doing it in real time.

M: OK, I can do that.

T: Let's practice it here, just so you can get used to it. Can we use a recent example of when you felt particularly upset?

M: Yeah, I came into the living room and my roommate was watching this movie where a woman was being mistreated and I freaked out.

T: Uh-huh. You saw something that bothered you?

M: Yeah, there was just a lot of yelling and fighting and stuff like that. It really made me nervous. And I was mad at my roommate, too.

T: OK, so we potentially have a couple of different feelings here, and maybe more than one thought as well. Let's write down what happened. Can you come up with a brief way of summarizing the situation?

M: Yeah, there was a crappy movie on and I freaked out.

T: Let's put the "freaking out" part to the side for just a second. That's your emotional reaction. But here, in this column, I'd like us just to write the facts of the situation. So how about I write "Movie on TV showing abuse"?

M: OK.

T: OK, I'll write it here. (*Writes under "Situations" column.*) Now, can you recall what kind of thoughts you had—what you made of it?

M: Well, the first thing that went through my mind was "Oh crap, there's no way I can watch this."

T: Ah. Let's write that here—(*Writes under "Interpretations" column.*)—"There's no way I can watch this." Can we take that thought a little farther? Why couldn't you watch it?

M: Well, if I watched it I'd just be a basket case. I'd get super anxious and wouldn't be able to concentrate or sleep that night, and the next day I'd probably be a mess.

T: So we can add a little more detail to that thought: (*Writes.*) "I'll get so anxious I won't be able to concentrate, sleep, or function tomorrow." Now, having thought that, what was your emotional or physical reaction?

M: I was anxious. And I felt sweaty. And it felt like my heart was pounding.

T: OK, so we can write those reactions here: (*Writes under "Emotions" column.*) "Anxious, sweaty, heart pounding." On a scale from 0 to 100, with 100 being the worst it's ever been, how strong was that feeling?

M: I'd say about a 70.

T: So it was pretty strong. (*Writes.*) I'll put the number 70 next to those feelings. And do I recall that you also said you had another feeling in that situation too, about your roommate?

M: Yeah, I was mad at her for even having the movie on in the first place.

T: OK, let's have you fill this one out. It's the same situation, so we can skip that part. What would you put down for your interpretations?

M: Well, I was really mad.

T: Yes. Would you call that a thought or a feeling?

M: I guess it's a feeling.

T: Right. So you would write it here in the "Emotions" column. What were the thoughts that went with that?

M: Well, I guess I thought "She's got no right to have that movie on."

T: Great. Let's write that in the "Interpretations" column. Just like before, can we take this thought a little farther? Why did she have no right to have it on?

M: She's my roommate. She knows me and she knows what I'm going through.

T: Which means what to you?

M: Which means she should know I can't watch that kind of thing.

T: Ah, so let's write that down as well: "She should know I can't watch this." And, just to take it a little farther, if she knows you can't watch this, and turns it on anyway, what would you take that to mean?

M: That she's an inconsiderate asshole.

T: Perfect. Let's write that one down too: "She's an inconsiderate asshole."

At the following session, the therapist reviews the monitoring form with Melissa.

T: So how did the homework go?

M: It went OK. I admit that for the first couple of days I didn't write much down. But after a while I realized that I'd better get on it so I started carrying the form around.

T: Sounds just fine. I'm glad you were able to get yourself to the point where you could do that. Can we review what you came up with?

M: (*Takes out the form.*) Sure. The first example here was at work. I was late for my shift and my boss was being a real jerk.

T: OK, and I see you have that written here in the "Situation" column. But let me ask you: The part about him being a jerk, is that the situation, or is that your thought about the situation?

M: I guess that was my thought about the situation.

In this fashion, the therapist and Melissa go through her list of interpretations. The therapist notes the thoughts that come up, as well as the emotional responses that are associated with the thoughts. The therapist also corrects those areas, as above, in which Melissa had difficulty distinguishing among situations, thoughts, and emotions.

TIB Alert!

One common form of TIB is failing to complete self-monitoring assignments such as thought monitoring. As we've discussed, it is important to address TIBs every time they show up. If you fail to discuss them, you are sending an implicit message of "It's OK not to put much effort into this treatment." At the outset of treatment, you and the client made an agreement about what is expected of each of you. It is important to show that you fully expect that agreement to be upheld.

The aim here is not to chastise the client or make him or her feel bad about not doing the homework, and this fact often has to be stated explicitly (and repeatedly, for some clients). Rather, the aim is to understand what is getting in the way so that a more effective solution can be found. In the case of a thought monitoring assignment, there can be several barriers to completing the assignment:

- *Lack of buy-in.* Does the client understand, and agree with, the rationale for the assignment? If not, the homework assignment might have been premature. Additional psychoeducation is likely needed.

- *Inaccurate understanding.* Does the client understand how to complete the assignment? One common mistake is to assign the homework quickly, in the last 2 minutes of the session, without ascertaining that the client adequately understands it. Spend more time discussing it, providing examples, and practicing the assignment with the client.

- *Core pathological process rearing its ugly head.* Often, the client's presenting problem will pose an obstacle to homework completion. For example, a client who is highly perfectionistic may have fears of making a mistake on the homework, leading to avoidance. Another client who is highly pessimistic may doubt that anything will help his or her situation, leading to reduced effort. In cases such as these, psychoeducation, reassurance, and cognitive challenging (as discussed in the next chapter) may be helpful.

- *Lack of motivation.* I list this one last for a reason. It's often the first explanation we, as therapists, generate to explain why the client didn't do the assignment: "He or she just isn't motivated enough." That's true some of the time, but often it's too simplistic an explanation. What we call "poor motivation" is, in many cases, a mixture of cognitive, emotional, and environmental barriers to taking action. Understanding those various barriers is more productive than just labeling the client "unmotivated." When motivation does seem to be an issue, the therapist should temporarily fall back to the strategies in MI (see Chapter 7), including weighing the pros and cons of doing the assignment. It is entirely possible that, during the course of MI, the client decides that the cons outweigh the pros—that the hassles of therapy are greater than the problems the therapy seeks to treat. Although there are some exceptions (e.g., involuntary or court-mandated treatment), for the most part the therapist accepts the client's decisions. After all, it is ultimately up to him or her. And it is OK to stop a treatment, with no hard feelings, if the client decides he or she isn't ready to do the work.

Resolving the TIB is an important goal. And yet from time to time we will encounter a situation in which the TIB simply won't go away—for example, we could have a client who's not going to complete the thought monitoring form, no matter what we do. In such a case, the therapist has a decision to make: We could stop the therapy, or we could try something else. The decision hinges, at least in part, on whether this TIB is a "deal-breaker"; that is, can we predict that the therapy could be successful even if this TIB is not resolved? For some TIBs, such as failing to come to sessions, the answer might well be no, and it would therefore be appropriate to stop the therapy. For others, such as failing to complete thought monitoring homework, it's less clear. As mentioned earlier in this chapter, cognitive interventions may or may not be the way to go for various clinical problems, and many clients will respond very nicely to behavioral strategies. So if I think that I have a good shot at helping the client without this particular piece of homework, I will stop banging my head against the wall and shift strategies.

THE ESSENTIALS

* The first step in cognitive restructuring is to identify the client's "hot" thoughts: those thoughts that are emotionally evocative.

* "Hot" thoughts might be about external events. They might be about the client's emotions or physiological sensations. They might even be about the client's own thoughts (a process called *metacognition*).

* Socratic questioning, role playing, and using written checklists are all good ways to identify interpretations.

* Clients should be instructed to monitor their interpretations on an ongoing basis as homework.

KEY TERMS AND DEFINITIONS

Bringing the problem into the room: Eliciting elements of the problem thought, emotion, or behavior in the therapy session.

Cold thoughts: Descriptive thoughts that do not elicit significant emotional responses.

Hot thoughts: Thoughts that are emotionally evocative and are potential targets for cognitive restructuring.

Metacognition: Thoughts about one's own thoughts.

Role playing: Enacting past or future situations with the client.

Thought monitoring: Self-monitoring maladaptive or distorted thoughts.

Finding Distortions

Find a self-report cognitive checklist online or in one of the source articles and take it yourself. Pick a checklist that seems to come closest to your personal target, even if it isn't an exact match.

What are some interpretations or beliefs that you endorsed?

_____

_____

_____

_____

_____

_____

_____

Next, check whether any of the following cognitive distortions are present in the interpretations listed above and briefly indicate *why* you think it is a distortion.

Probability overestimation _____

Catastrophizing _____

Overgeneralization _____

Personalizing _____

All-or-nothing thinking _____

"Should" statements _____

Mind reading _____

Emotional reasoning _____

Minimizing _____

From *Doing CBT* by David F. Tolin. Copyright © 2016 The Guilford Press. Permission to photocopy this worksheet is granted to purchasers of this book for personal use only (see copyright page for details). Purchasers can download enlarged versions of this worksheet (see the box at the end of the table of contents).

CHAPTER 14

Restructuring Thoughts

In the previous chapter, we discussed how to get the client's interpretations out on the table. The therapist can use a number of strategies, including Socratic questioning, role play, and checklists to help the client identify his or her maladaptive "hot thoughts" and may opt to instruct the client to self-monitor these thoughts in his or her natural environment between sessions. When an interpretation is identified, the therapist repeats it back to the client, often writing it down.

The process of getting the client to rethink and revise maladaptive interpretations is called **cognitive restructuring.** As the name implies, the essential strategy is to restructure the client's system of thoughts, appraisals, and beliefs. The tactics we use fall primarily into two categories:

Holding Up a Mirror

Sometimes, the mere act of repeating a thought back to the client is sufficient to trigger some degree of cognitive change. Repeating back the client's statement, perhaps paired with a pleasant yet ever-so-slightly perplexed facial expression, followed by a bit of a pause, can often cause the client to rethink what he or she just said.

This is where clinical art comes in, however. Facial expressions and tone of voice are highly nuanced and can be easily misinterpreted (especially among clients who are prone to maladaptive interpretations and mood-congruent information processing). One common mistake for therapists is failing to take one's own *stimulus value* into account—for example, how you look and sound to the client, and how your presentation is likely to be interpreted. It might sound a bit silly to say, but if you're going to use facial expression and tone of voice as therapeutic tools, make sure you know what your face looks like and what your voice sounds like when you do it.

1. Help the client to understand what is wrong with how she or he is currently thinking.
2. Help the client reach, accept, and rehearse a more adaptive way of thinking.

Identifying What's Wrong

Before we can intervene further, the client and therapist have to arrive at a shared understanding not only of what the interpretations are (see previous chapter) but also of what is wrong with those thoughts—how they are distorted, irrational, or maladaptive.

One way to accomplish this is to refer to the list of *cognitive distortions* in Chapter 3, Table 3.2, and also provided in Appendix B. Here, the therapist works with William (W), our client with a mix of mood disturbance, interpersonal dependency, and pain.

T: We've identified some potentially important thoughts that seem to be associated with your depressed feelings. What I'd like to do now is take a good look at those thoughts and to evaluate them. Sometimes our thoughts are completely accurate. Sometimes they're not. We all make errors in our thinking sometimes—me, you, everyone. And we tend to just accept them as facts, even if they're not accurate.

W: So you're saying that my thoughts are wrong and that's why I'm depressed?

T: Well, I don't know whether your thoughts are right or wrong, or whether they're partly right and partly wrong. What would be helpful, I think, is for us to consider the possibility that there might be some parts of your thinking that aren't completely accurate, just as there are some parts of my thinking and everyone else's thinking that aren't completely accurate.

W: OK.

T: (*Takes out the list of cognitive distortions.*) When people make errors in their thinking, we call them cognitive distortions. "Cognitive" means related to our thinking, and "distortions" means, well, that they are distorted in some way.

W: Like they're wrong.

T: Possibly, but they also could just be a bit exaggerated, or they could overlook some important facts. I have here a list of some very common cognitive distortions—errors in thinking that a lot of people make. Let's take a look at this first one, which is called probability overestimation. That means that people overpredict the likelihood that some bad outcome is going to happen, even when that outcome is fairly unlikely. As you think about some of the thoughts we've identified, can you spot any probability overestimation in there?

W: Well, the example of "Everyone at the party is going to hate me" looks a little bit like how I think. That wasn't my exact thought, but I did think that my performance review at work is going to go really badly and that I'll get criticized.

T: Yes, so you were predicting what is going to happen.

W: Yeah, I was thinking about how I thought it's going to go.

T: So how might that have been probability overestimation?

W: Well, I've never gotten a bad review before, so it was probably not going to happen, but I kind of convinced myself that it would.

T: Exactly. So that's how probability overestimation goes—we talk ourselves into believing that something is going to happen, even when it's pretty unlikely. Let's take a look at the other cognitive distortions on this list and see if any of them apply as well.

There are a couple of stylistic issues to note here:

- The therapist maintains a *dialogue* with the client, rather than a monologue. Whenever we're working with forms, charts, and so on, it's easy to slip into "lecture" format. Instead, the therapist makes a quick psychoeducational statement (e.g., "That means that people overpredict the likelihood that some bad outcome is going to happen, even when that outcome is fairly unlikely") but then encourages William to join the discussion ("As you think about some of the thoughts we've identified, can you spot any probability overestimation in there?").

- The therapist takes a *neutral perspective* on the accuracy of William's interpretations (e.g., "I don't know whether your thoughts are right or wrong, or whether they're partly right and partly wrong").• The therapist *normalizes* the presence of cognitive distortions. William is highly sensitive to perceived criticism, and you can see that he often falls back to interpreting the therapist's statements as meaning that his interpretations are "wrong" or that he is to blame for his depression. The therapist makes it clear that distorted thoughts are normal (e.g., "We all make errors in our thinking sometimes—me, you, everyone") and that the presence of a distortion does not imply a global "wrongness" of his thoughts (e.g., "Possibly, but they also could just be a bit exaggerated, or they could overlook some important facts").

There are a couple of potential follow-up points here that the therapist may opt to come back to in the therapy:

- William's misinterpretation of the therapist's meaning (e.g., "So you're saying that my thoughts are wrong and that's why I'm depressed?") is an important piece of what my psychodynamically oriented colleagues call *transference*. We don't necessarily interpret the phenomenon in the same way—that is, we do not have good reason to believe that William is projecting unconscious conflicts onto the therapist—but the phenomenon is real nevertheless. Clients have a (potentially distorted) cognitive response to their therapists, just as they have a cognitive response to everything else. The therapist might choose to come back to this issue and examine William's interpretations in response to specific therapeutic interventions, perhaps working through them as an example of his larger depressive and dependent pattern.

- William gives an example of *all-or-nothing thinking* in his globalization of the therapist's comments. When the therapist introduces the idea that William's thoughts might be distorted, he replies with the statement "Like they're wrong." This might signal the fact that William believes that if his thoughts are not completely accurate, they are completely "wrong." That distortion likely helps us understand the persistence of his depressed mood.

We can also help clients identify cognitive distortions in the context of the conversation without using worksheets or forms. Here, the therapist is working with Blaise (B), our client with substance dependence.

B: I used last week. I feel terrible about it.

T: What leads you to feel terrible about using?

B: I was doing so well and was really proud of myself for staying clean, and now I just blew it.

T: So you are saying to yourself that your using last week means that you blew it.

B: Yes, like I just undid all of my progress.

T: And you feel bad about that.

B: I feel like such a failure.

T: I understand. Can we talk about "blowing it?" How do you define that?

B: Well, it means I screwed up.

T: OK, I guess what I'm wondering is how much would you have to use in order to determine that you blew it?

B: I only used once this week.

T: And that's enough to label it "blowing it."

B: Right.

T: And on the flip side of that, how clean would you have to stay in order to determine that you didn't blow it?

B: Well, if I used, I blew it, so not blowing would mean I didn't use.

T: At all.

B: Right.

T: So you have this way of looking at things here, which is "If I'm not 100% successful in my recovery, I blew it." I hear people say things like that a lot. In fact, it comes up so often that we have a name for it. We call it all-or-nothing thinking. Can you imagine what that label means?

B: Like it has to be all one way or all the other way?

T: Kind of, yes. When people have all-or-nothing thinking, they tend to create strict cutoffs, like it's either this or it's that, it's either perfect or it's terrible, I'm either clean or I've blown it.

B: I think that's what I'm doing. But isn't my goal to stay clean?

T: Absolutely. That's why we're here, after all. But let's think through the implications of the all-or-nothing thinking. When you tell yourself that anything short of perfect sobriety means you've blown it, where might that thinking lead you?

B: I guess it would lead me to have a really high standard for myself.

T: A high standard that you could reliably meet?

B: I think it would be hard. I might slip.

T: And if you slipped, and you decided "I've blown it," where would that take you?

B: I guess I'd get discouraged and hopeless.

T: I suspect you're right. And would those feelings of being discouraged and hopeless help you meet your goals, or get in the way?

B: They'd probably get in the way.

A couple of points to note from this discussion with Blaise:

- The therapist opted to target Blaise's all-or-nothing thinking in this example. Blaise also revealed another cognitive distortion in her comments. When she said "I feel like a failure," the therapist might have picked up on the *overgeneralization* and addressed that distortion in a similar fashion.

- The therapist made a point to not only identify the cognitive distortion but also to help Blaise understand *why* that distortion is harmful. The therapist drew a link between thinking, emotion, and behavior by using Socratic questioning to help Blaise recognize that her all-or-nothing thinking is likely to exacerbate her negative mood and predispose her to further substance use.

Helping the Client Reach, Accept, and Rehearse a More Adaptive Way of Thinking

Having identified the presence of cognitive distortions, the next step is to help the client to identify an alternative way of thinking. Sometimes, people erroneously believe that the aim of cognitive restructuring is to get clients to "think positive." However, this is not

Bringing the Problem into the Room

Generally speaking, cognitive restructuring (and many other CBT interventions) is most effective when the client is experiencing a bit of the problem right there in the therapy session. This doesn't mean that the client needs to feel awful; however, the problem needs to be active in the person's mind. In Blaise's example above, she leads with "I feel terrible about it." The problem—in this case Blaise's upset feeling—is in the room.

There are a few reasons why it's helpful to "activate" the problem in session. First, the "hot" thoughts we're looking for are likely to come to mind much more easily, giving us more to work with. Second, as discussed in Chapter 3, memory can be mood congruent: Material learned in a particular emotional state may be recalled more accurately when the person is in a similar emotional state. So if we want the client to be able to retrieve our cognitive intervention from memory when he or she is anxious, sad, or angry, then it makes sense for us to teach the material when the client is anxious, sad, or angry—at least somewhat. Third, when "hot" thoughts are elicited in the session and negative emotions or physiological sensations accompany them, the therapist has a unique opportunity to demonstrate the power of cognitive restructuring right there in the session. By challenging and revising a maladaptive thought, the therapist can then inquire about whether the client's negative feelings have gotten better or worse. In most cases the client finds that he or she feels a bit better, which is a valuable learning experience.

It's often not difficult to bring the problem into the room. Sometimes, simply asking the client to recall a recent, upsetting example of the problem is enough to activate the associated thoughts and emotions. If needed, we could augment the discussion with imagery—for example, "Can you imagine yourself back in that situation? What kind of thoughts and feelings are coming up for you?"

likely to be helpful. The aim is not to replace unrealistically negative thoughts with unrealistically positive thoughts. For example, if we tried to get the client to believe that everything is fine and that nothing bad can happen, we would likely fail. Bad things do happen, and uncomfortable situations do exist. Our aim is to help clients think about these things *realistically*, rather than *positively*. Thinking realistically about a bad situation is likely to lead to some normal feelings of discomfort but is unlikely to lead to serious disturbance of mood or behavior.

Examining the Evidence

One way to help identify more adaptive thoughts is by **examining the evidence** for and against the maladaptive thought. The therapist and client review the evidence that would support the distorted interpretation and then review evidence that does not support the interpretation.

This can be done on a piece of paper with a line drawn down the middle, as shown in Figure 14.1 and in Appendix B. After discussing the evidence for and against the interpretation, the therapist and client come up with a new interpretation that is more realistic and more adaptive.

A potential sticking point in this exercise is that the client will come up with more evidence for the interpretation than against it. This is hardly surprising; based on what we know about mood-congruent memory (see Chapter 3), we can predict that information that is consistent with the client's current mood state will be easier to retrieve. Part of the therapist's job is to help the client identify evidence against the thought.

Another potential sticking point is treating the evidence examination like a "vote count," in which the side with the most points wins. We are certainly interested in the quantity of evidence on either side, but we are equally interested in the *quality* of that evidence. We often find that "evidence" for an interpretation isn't particularly strong evidence for the thought at all. The therapist can help the client to critically evaluate the evidence in order to determine whether it should be believed.

Interpretation: *My boss called me in to his office because I'm in trouble.*

Evidence *for* interpretation	Evidence *against* interpretation
He has a stern look on his face.	I haven't done anything that would get me in trouble.
	I got a good performance review last month.
	Sometimes he just has a stern expression but no one gets in trouble.
New, balanced interpretation	
I really have no reason to expect that I'm in trouble. He could be calling me to his office for any number of reasons, and being in trouble doesn't seem like the most likely one.	

FIGURE 14.1. Sample worksheet for examining the evidence for interpretations.

Adapting the Process: *Cognitive Restructuring . . .*

. . . with high-functioning clients. Higher-functioning, more psychologically minded clients will usually take well to cognitive restructuring. They are usually already able to identify what they are thinking and feeling and can discuss their thoughts analytically.

. . . with low-functioning clients. Lower-functioning clients, such as those with intellectual challenges, will have varying ability to identify and challenge maladaptive thoughts (Sturmey, 2004). Slowed thinking, poor attention and memory, limited vocabulary, and problems with abstract thinking may all hamper cognitive restructuring efforts. It may be that the behavioral elements of CBT, which we'll review later in this book, will be more important than will the cognitive elements for such clients. This isn't to say it's not possible, however. Most clients with intellectual challenges can identify and link thoughts, emotions, and behaviors, although their ability to think hypothetically about thoughts and beliefs is limited (Dagnan, Chadwick, & Proudlove, 2000). Most likely, the cognitive restructuring process will need to progress slowly and at a basic level, such as described below for children (although we want to take care not to inappropriately use child-like language with adults).

Other lower-functioning clients, however, can respond well to cognitive restructuring. This includes clients with psychotic disorders (S. Lewis et al., 2002; Morrison et al., 2014; Sensky et al., 2000). Delusional beliefs, considered by many to be impervious to psychotherapy, can be modified (O'Connor et al., 2007). Kingdon and Turkington (1991) use a normalizing rationale, in which psychotic experiences such as delusions and hallucinations are discussed on a continuum with normal experiences, helping the client to feel less alienated and stigmatized. Remaining nonjudgmental and empathic, the therapist uses gentle logical probes such as "If your voices came from the radiator, why can't anyone else hear them?" (Kingdon & Turkington, 2006, p. 49). The client is encouraged to develop his or her own alternative interpretations, rather than forcing the therapist's interpretations into the client. Penn et al. (2005) incorporate cognitive restructuring in their CBT program for schizophrenia and bipolar disorder by showing video vignettes of people who "jump to conclusions" in interpersonal situations. The process of jumping to conclusions is normalized (i.e., we all do it), but the potentially adverse events of reaching an inaccurate conclusion are noted. Clients are encouraged to replace "making a guess" (considering alternatives) with jumping to conclusions to and rate their confidence in various guesses. "Checking it out" (empirical data gathering) is proposed as a strategy for identifying which guess is most accurate.

. . . with children. Although older adolescents can often respond to cognitive restructuring in much the same way that adults do, younger children may require modifications based on developmental stage (Grave & Blissett, 2004). For example, they may have difficulty in recognizing that there are other perspectives besides their own (Wadsworth, 1996) and in incorporating information that conflicts with their beliefs (Bierman, 1988). Children may do better when maladaptive thoughts are framed as "commands" the brain gives the body (Ronen, 1992) or when maladaptive thoughts are externalized as characters, such as a "bad thought monster" (Leahy, 1998). A great example of a developmental modification of cognitive restructuring can be seen in Kendall and Hedtke's (2006) "Coping Cat" program for anxious youth ages 7–13. To help kids identify and work on their anxious interpretations, they use the mnemonic "FEAR" (Feeling frightened? Expecting bad things to happen? Attitudes and actions that can help, Results and rewards). As they discuss "expecting bad things to happen," therapists ask about and watch for maladaptive interpretations and encourage kids to label them using terms such as "my worry voice" or "my hopeless voice" (Beidas, Benjamin, Puleo, Edmunds, & Kendall, 2010, p. 10).

Long lists of cognitive distortions are probably too much for younger kids to take in. Rapee, Spence, Cobham, and Wignall (2000) narrow the list down to probability overestimation and catastrophizing, the two distortions most commonly seen in the anxious children for which their program is designed. They emphasize acting like a "detective" by examining the evidence for and against an anxious interpretation, often using artificial scenarios (e.g., seeing a big dog in the street, mom coming home late, being asked to give a talk in class, meeting other kids) for demonstration.

Cognitive restructuring with children should have a distinctly fun and playful element, with concepts presented at a developmentally appropriate level and using examples with which the child is readily familiar (Stallard, 2002). As just one example from my own work, I have, at times, found myself asking younger kids questions such as "What do you think Tom Brady [the quarterback for the New England Patriots] would say about this?" or "How would Spider-Man think about it?" This is a way of introducing the strategy of considering alternatives in a child-friendly manner.

In most cases, treatment of children will include behavioral interventions, perhaps receiving more emphasis than cognitive ones (Spence, 1994; Stallard, 2002).

. . . in groups. Cognitive distortions can be discussed in a group setting, such as in the "jumping to conclusions" discussions described above in Penn et al.'s (2005) CBT for schizophrenia. In their group CBT for social phobia, Heimberg and Becker (2002) begin by having the therapist tell a story about a distressing event from his or her own life and list his or her maladaptive thoughts. The clients then generate challenging questions to ask the therapist, such as considering alternatives or examining evidence. The therapist then gives a sample anxiety-eliciting situation, such as being asked to come to a boss's office, and asks the group to identify potential interpretations and to have a group discussion about how to challenge and replace maladaptive interpretations.

. . . on the inpatient unit. Cognitive restructuring with inpatients poses a particular challenge, given the (usually) brief length of stay, the severe and acute nature of symptoms, concerns related to the hospitalization itself, and removal from the usual triggers in the person's natural environment. Ludgate, Wright, Bowers, and Camp (1993) suggest several modifications to usual treatment:

1. *Focus on symptom relief:* longer-term goals should be deferred to outpatient therapy.
2. *Adjust length and frequency of sessions:* try meeting with the client daily for 30 minutes or less.
3. *Involve ancillary therapists:* everyone who interacts with the client (e.g., nurses, occupational therapists, social workers) has the opportunity to reiterate and reinforce what the client is working on.
4. *Integrate therapeutic efforts:* the CBT therapist develops the case formulation and works with the pharmacotherapist, family therapist, consulting internist, group therapist, and other clinicians to make sure that all are working in the same direction.
5. *Assign homework in the milieu:* unit staff members should be enlisted to help the client perform homework assignments on the unit.
6. *Use the hospital setting to identify "hot" cognitions:* identify stressors that occur on the unit and guide the client through the steps of cognitive restructuring around those stressors.
7. *Take advantage of distance from environmental stressors:* the client's temporary removal from the natural environment may give a modicum of "breathing room" that allows the client to analyze and work on how he or she has been responding to those stressors.

Here, the therapist is working again with William (W), who had identified a belief that his performance review at work would go badly.

T: I'd like to take a good look at this prediction you have, that your performance review is going to go really badly and you'll be criticized. What evidence can you think of that might support that belief?

W: Well, I've been late to work a few times this month so that's not good.

T: I see. How late are we talking about?

W: Maybe 5 to 10 minutes, not terrible but someone could have noticed.

T: OK, so let's write that down here. (*Draws a line down the center of a sheet of paper and writes.*) "I've been late." What other evidence can you think of?

W: Um, I've been pretty depressed.

T: Yes. And that's evidence for the belief?

W: I suppose someone could have noticed that I was depressed?

T: Let's think about that one a bit. Do you have reason to believe that your depression was noticed?

W: It's hard to say; I'm not sure.

T: OK, so that one's a little unclear. At any rate, has the depression impacted your job performance?

W: I don't think so; not really. I mean, I still get my job done.

T: So what do you think about the likelihood that this would be something you'd get criticized for?

W: I guess it's kind of low?

T: Maybe. Let's write it here but let's also put a big question mark next to it because we're just not sure whether that tells us much about how the performance evaluation is going to go. (*Writes.*): "I've been depressed"? Any other evidence?

W: No, I think that's about it.

T: OK, let's look at the other side of it. Can you think of any evidence that might not support this belief—that is, any evidence that would suggest that the performance review will go fine?

W: Well, as I mentioned, I haven't gotten a bad review before.

T: That seems like an important piece of evidence. So let's write it here. (*Writes.*) "I've never had a bad review before." What else can you think of?

W: (*long pause*) I can't really think of anything else.

T: You mentioned a minute ago that you get the job done; can you say a bit more about that?

W: Well, I always get my reports finished on time.

T: So you get the job done on time. What else?

W: I think I usually do a decent job with them.

T: Decent, meaning what exactly?

W: Well, I think they're accurate, and I write pretty well. I don't make many mistakes or anything like that.

T: Anyone ever notice that?

W: Yeah, every now and then my manager will give me a thumbs-up and say "nice job."

T: Hmm, so we have a couple of pieces of evidence that we could add. (*Writes.*) The first is "My work is on time and pretty good quality."

W: Yeah.

T: And the other that you just mentioned is (*writing*): "My manager has complimented my work."

W: That's true.

T: So we have some evidence here on both sides of the thought. As you look at the evidence for the thought, and the evidence against the thought, what's your view of this?

W: I guess the thought isn't really true.

T: Yeah, the evidence doesn't really seem to support it, does it?

W: No, not really when I look at it like this.

T: So what would be a more helpful way to think about your performance evaluation?

W: It's going to go just fine?

T: Well, let's think about that one for a minute. Do you know that it's going to go just fine?

W: No, I don't know that. I think it probably will.

T: But that's different from knowing that it will.

W: Yeah.

T: So what's the truth?

W: The truth is, I guess, that it will probably go fine, but I can't know for sure.

T: That would seem to be a little more realistic. Is it OK that you can't know for sure?

W: I'd like to know for sure.

T: Absolutely. But can you manage anyway, even if you can't know?

W: Yeah, I guess I can manage not knowing.

T: So perhaps for a more balanced thought we could write it this way. (*Writes.*) "My review will probably go fine. I can't know for sure, but I can manage not knowing."

How to do cognitive restructuring poorly	How to do cognitive restructuring like a champ
Debate the client. Get into arguments with the client about the validity of his or her interpretations. Point out how ridiculous the interpretations are.	*Collaborate with the client.* During cognitive restructuring, we take a rather neutral stance on the client's interpretation. It could be right, it could be wrong, or it could be somewhere in between. Be curious about the client's interpretations and ask him or her to look at the available evidence.
Encourage positive thinking. Try to get the client to say positive statements to him- or herself, regardless of whether those statements are accurate or not.	*Encourage realistic thinking.* Not all realistic thoughts are positive. However, taking a realistic view of a situation—even an objectively bad situation—tends not to result in severe psychological symptoms.

Don't worry about homework. There's no need for clients to keep track of their thoughts. After all, you can ask about the thoughts in session.	*Encourage ongoing thought monitoring.* Cognitive restructuring takes significant effort on the client's part, and discussing the accuracy of interpretations once per week in a therapist's office isn't likely to make enough of a dent. To be successful, the client needs to monitor and work with his or her thoughts on an ongoing basis.

Considering Alternatives

Another way of disputing maladaptive thoughts and introducing more adaptive ones is to encourage the client to **consider alternatives.** Like examining evidence, considering alternatives is not specific to any particular kind of cognitive distortion, so it too is broadly applicable.

The basic idea in considering alternatives is to invite the client to step outside of his or her frame of reference and consider other ways of thinking.

Here, the therapist continues to work with Blaise (B) about her substance use lapse.

T: We've identified a couple of important thoughts here. The first is thinking "I've blown it" after you used. And the other is thinking "I'm a failure" because of it. I'd like us to think about these beliefs a little more. Are they true?

B: Well, they feel true to me.

T: Yes, they feel true to you. But my question is a little different: In reality, are they true? Is that really how it is?

B: Kind of. I mean, I did blow it, and that's a failure, isn't it?

T: I wonder, is there another way to look at it?

B: I dunno, I guess there could be.

T: What might that other way be? I'm not necessarily asking you to believe that other way, either, but I'm just wondering what you could come up with?

B: Well, I guess another way of looking at it would be that slip-ups happen and that doesn't necessarily mean I've blown it.

T: That would be another way, yes. But right now that's not how you're thinking about it.

B: Not really, no. I mean, I guess it could be true.

T: Well, let's imagine that someone else was there and saw what happened. Who's someone whose opinion you really trust?

B: My mom. She's pretty smart.

T: OK, let's imagine that your mom saw this go down.

B: She'd be really disappointed.

T: Perhaps. If I talked to your mom after that and asked, "Did Blaise blow it? Is she a failure?" What do you think she would say?

B: I don't think she'd say I was a failure.

T: She wouldn't? What would she be more likely to say?

B: She'd probably say that I made a mistake.

Metaphor

Sometimes the process of cognitive restructuring (and other interventions) can be easier when we get the client in the habit of identifying his or her thoughts as an external entity of some kind. Just saying something like "That's my addiction talking" or "That's an OCD thought" can help the client feel a bit detached from the thought and feel a greater sense of control over it. Otto (2000, p. 169) has used a metaphor of a "depression gargoyle":

> I would like you to picture a gargoyle on your shoulder. Because gargoyles are made of stone, this gargoyle of depression weighs you down, makes it harder to do things and harder to feel motivated. In addition, this gargoyle is whispering in your ear. The gargoyle wants you to blame yourself for the weight that you feel, rather than turning your attention toward getting rid of it. . . . And remember, because you are depressed, many of the messages whispered by the gargoyle will feel true. The trick is to make sure you do not buy into the gargoyle's message . . . when you hear this voice, I want you to label it as the voice of the "depression gargoyle."

In a similar vein, March and Mulle (1998, pp. 64–65) describe the use of an externalizing metaphor in their work with children who have OCD:

> It is kind of like the brain gets the hiccups, which you experience as OCD. In your case, OCD gives you a *big* fear message concerning normal everyday experiences. For example, when you go into public restrooms, your brain might tell you to be *extra, extra* careful and wash your hands many times. . . . While we are working together, I will be like your coach and teach you how to boss back OCD. . . . The first thing we'll do is give OCD a nasty nickname. . . . Do you have any name in mind?

T: But not that you were a failure.

B: No. She'd probably say something more like "it's a setback, but she just has to keep working at it."

T: So perhaps that's our alternative way of thinking about it—it's a setback and something you have to keep working on, but it doesn't make you a failure.

Interventions for Specific Cognitive Distortions

Addressing Probability Overestimation and Minimizing by Doing the Math

When people engage in probability overestimation, they are mistaking a low-probability event for a high-probability event. In minimizing, the person is doing the opposite: mistaking a high-probability event for a low-probability event.

The aim of cognitive restructuring for probability overestimation is not to convince the overestimating client that this event *won't* happen—in many cases, there is some possibility that it will—nor to convince the minimizing client that this event *will* happen—in many cases, there is some possibility that it won't. Rather, we're trying to help the client take a more realistic view of the actual probability.

Doing the math means that if the client's thinking is distorted by bad estimates of probability, we want to help the client make better estimates of probability. One straightforward way to do this is to provide a basic math lesson. Here, the therapist is working with Suzanne (S), our client with GAD and benzodiazepine dependence. Suzanne is fearful to fly on an airplane and usually relies on heavy benzodiazepine use to get through air travel. They are discussing Suzanne's upcoming flight to visit her daughter.

S: I just can't shake this worry that the plane's going to crash.

T: So your thought about flying is, "the plane is going to crash," and you're anxious in response to that thought. So let's take a look at this thought. How accurate does it seem to you?

S: Well, if I'm getting on a plane, it seems really accurate. And the plane makes all of those noises, too, and that really makes me even more afraid that it's going to crash.

T: Yes, the noises on a plane can be scary if you don't know what they mean. But let's start with looking at the basic level of risk here. What do you think is the actual probability that a plane will crash? If a 0% chance means that the plane is absolutely not going to crash, and a 100% chance means that the plane is absolutely going to crash, when you get on a plane, what do you think is your probability?

S: I'm not sure; maybe 20%?

T: So when you get on a plane there's a 20% chance that it will crash?

S: Yeah, maybe.

T: Let's think about that a little more. A 20% chance of a plane crashing would mean that on average, one out of every five planes crashes. Does that seem accurate?

S: Well, no, I guess that's not right.

T: Seems high. So we could know the real probability by finding out how many planes crash, and divide that by how many planes are in service, right?

S: Right.

T: (*Looking up the web page on a smartphone.*) The National Transportation Safety Board posts its statistics over the past 10 years on the Internet. Over the past 10 years, there were 42 commercial plane crashes. It also shows that over that same time frame, there were 191,355,969 commercial flights. So if we divide 42 by 191,355,969, we get two hundred-thousandths of 1% percent, or about one out of every 4.5 million flights.

S: Wow, that's a lot smaller than I thought.

T: Certainly less than 1 out of every 5, right?

S: But even if the chance is one in 4 million, it still seems scary.

T: Well, let's try to put that into perspective. How do you get to the airport?

S: I drive.

T: What do you think is more likely to kill you, the drive to the airport, or the flight?

S: I guess the drive.

T: Are you afraid of the drive?

S: No.

T: So your fear is misaligned a bit there. When you get on the plane, how do you manage your anxiety?

S: I take a Xanax and sometimes I'll have a glass of wine, too.

T: What do you think is more likely to kill you, the Xanax and wine, or the flight?

S: The Xanax and wine.

T: Right. Now, I'm not trying to instill new fears in you, but I want us to see the basic point. There are risks all around us, some of which are much more likely than others. Part of healthy living means adjusting your fear reaction to the actual risk rather than the made-up risk.

In many cases, you can follow a similar therapeutic course without doing formal math problems. Rather, you can point to the client's own experiences.

Decatastrophizing

Catastrophizing occurs when the client engages in one (or both) of these two kinds of errors:

1. Believing that the consequences of an event would be completely devastating, when in all likelihood they would probably be less serious.
2. Believing that he or she would be completely unable to cope with an event, when in all likelihood he or she would be able to cope with it.

The aim of decatastrophizing, therefore, is to reduce the perceived negative impact of an anticipated event and/or to increase the client's sense of coping self-efficacy should the event occur.

The **downward arrow** (e.g., Greenberger & Padesky, 2016) is one way to decatastrophize a dreaded event (there are other applications of the downward arrow as well, which we discuss later on). The basic idea of the downward arrow is that the therapist uses a series of "if–then" questions that lead the client toward a conclusion of reduced event impact and/or adequate coping capacity.

Here, the therapist is working with Anna (A), our client with panic disorder and agoraphobic avoidance.

T: So we've identified the thought that "If I feel sick to my stomach, I'll throw up." For the moment, let's just assume that does indeed happen—you throw up. What would bother you about that?

A: Well, I don't want to throw up.

T: No, I wouldn't imagine you would. I wouldn't either. But what do you find particularly bad about throwing up?

A: If I were in a public place it would be embarrassing.

T: I can imagine. So let's just go with that for a minute. If you do throw up in a public place, what would be the result of that?

A: I don't know; I've never thought about it. I just know it would be awful.

T: It's interesting that you know it would be awful, yet you haven't thought about it. That could be part of the problem—you've assumed it would be awful, but do we really know that to be a fact?

A: Well, I guess I don't know that for sure.

T: Well, let's think it through a little bit more. Imagine this with me: Here you are, in a public place, and you just threw up in front of a bunch of people. What would happen?

A: I'd feel humiliated.

T: For how long would you feel humiliated? Would you feel that way for the rest of your life?

A: No, I guess not. I'd probably feel humiliated for the rest of the day, though.

T: Right, you'd feel bad but not forever. Would your feelings of being humiliated be so bad that you wouldn't be able to cope with them?

A: I feel like I wouldn't.

T: Let's keep thinking it through. How would you react, really?

A: I guess I'd just go home and clean up and then eventually get on with things?

T: That seems pretty likely. I'm not trying to say that you wouldn't feel bad about it, but when we really think about it, it sounds like you'd handle it and not feel bad forever.

A: Yeah, I'd deal with it.

T: What about the people who saw you throw up? How do you imagine they would respond? For example, would they point and laugh at you?

A: Some might.

T: That's true, some might. Would that be how most people responded?

A: Maybe not. Maybe some people would ignore it.

T: Maybe. Is it possible that anyone might express concern for you?

A: Yeah, maybe someone would help.

T: So my question to you is, if you threw up in a public place, would it be the end of the world? Or would it just be an unpleasant experience?

A: It would just be unpleasant.

Note that the therapist could also have addressed the *probability overestimation* in Anna's thinking by asking her to recall how many times she has felt sick to her stomach and, of those times, how often she has and has not thrown up.

Decatastrophizing can be used for lots of feared negative outcomes. Obviously some feared outcomes, such as being killed, are inherently pretty catastrophic, and decatastrophizing probably won't help much (although Albert Ellis is said to have quipped, "If you die, you die"). When the feared outcome is *truly* catastrophic, I'm likely to target probability overestimation (e.g., "Yes, that would be terrible, but it's highly unlikely"). In most other cases, however, the feared outcome is bad but not catastrophic, lending itself to a decatastrophizing approach. Failing a test, making a mistake at work, and breaking up with a partner are all examples of feared outcomes that can be decatastrophized.

Challenging Overgeneralizing by Finding the Exceptions

When people overgeneralize, they make sweeping conclusions about something based on fairly limited evidence. We can challenge overgeneralizing by **finding the exceptions** to those sweeping conclusions.

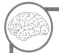

Engaging the Frontal Lobes

Emotional distress comes from the limbic regions of the brain, particularly the *amygdala*. When we engage in cognitive restructuring (sometimes called *reappraisal*), areas from our frontal lobes (which are responsible for thinking and more complex processing of information) engage and temper the more emotional parts of the brain (e.g., Kalisch, 2009; Ochsner, Silvers, & Buhle, 2012; Ray & Zald, 2012). In particular, several areas of the prefrontal cortex (PFC) become more active during reappraisal; as they do so, the amygdala becomes less active (Diekhof, Geier, Falkai, & Gruber, 2011). So when we ask clients to think about things in a different way, we're teaching them a new means of controlling their out-of-control emotions, which is an important part of emotion regulation (J. J. Gross & Thompson, 2007). Bear in mind, the primary goal of cognitive restructuring is not necessarily to eliminate cognitive distortions, nor is it necessarily to get the client to believe things that are more healthy. The act of identifying problems in the thought process, considering alternatives, examining evidence, and doing other kinds of "thinking about thinking" seems to shift clients out of a more automatic and extreme mode of cognitive responding into a more thoughtful, controlled, and flexible mode. Research suggests that this shift may be an important factor in recovering from psychological problems—perhaps even more so than simply getting clients to "think logically" (Barber & DeRubeis, 1989; Teasdale et al., 2001).

Here, the therapist is working with Nick (N), who is feeling highly pessimistic about his marriage.

T: We have this thought that comes up for you a lot: "My marriage is broken." Can you tell me how you came to that conclusion?

N: Well, we argue a lot. And we just get on each other's nerves over every little thing.

T: I see. So there's arguing, and you get on each other's nerves, and you take that to mean that the marriage is broken.

N: Yeah. I mean, happy couples don't act this way.

T: Happy couples don't argue with each other or get on each other's nerves?

N: Well, I guess they do. But not as much as we do.

T: Do we know that for sure? I mean, do you know how often happy couples argue?

N: No, I guess I don't know that.

T: Let's look at the other side of it. What's good about the marriage?

N: What's good about it? Nothing, I think.

T: For example, has anything good ever happened between the two of you?

N: Ever? Well, sure.

T: Like what?

N: We used to like to go hiking together. But we haven't done that in a long time.

T: But there's at least some common interest there? Anything else?

N: Well, lately I haven't been up for doing much, but we do like watching movies on TV together. And sometimes we talk about the movie afterward.

T: That sounds like it might be nice.

N: Yeah, I suppose it is.

T: Are your interactions always arguments?

N: No, sometimes we treat each other decently.

T: What would be an example of that?

N: Well, when I get home she asks me how my day was, and I ask her how hers was.

T: OK, that sounds promising. What else?

N: I guess sometimes I'll offer to help her with things like cooking dinner, and she seems to appreciate that. And sometimes she'll listen to me when I'm feeling depressed.

T: So I think I'm hearing that there are some things about the marriage that you definitely don't like—the arguments and getting on each other's nerves. And I'm also hearing that there are some times when you two have shared interests and are pretty nice to each other. I wonder whether it would be more accurate to say that the marriage is completely broken, or whether it would be more accurate to say that there are some things you want to work on in the marriage?

N: It's more like we have things I want to work on.

Note, in this case, that the therapist does not dismiss the real problems in the marriage. Those problems can be worked on in a productive manner, but first it was necessary to help Nick assume a more constructive mind-set about the marriage.

Challenging Personalizing by Identifying External Factors

Personalizing can take two forms:

1. Believing that one is to blame for events that are not entirely under one's control. Depressed individuals frequently attribute negative outcomes to their own short-comings, overlooking other important contributions (Seligman, Abramson, Semmel, & von Baeyer, 1979).
2. Believing that external events are related to oneself. A clear example of this form of personalizing is seen in the delusions of reference among clients with psychotic disorders, such as believing that things on television represent special messages. However, less extreme variations of this distortion can be seen in many forms of psychopathology, such as misinterpreting another person's facial expression or tone of voice to mean something personal.

We can challenge personalizing by **identifying external factors** that might provide alternative explanations.

Here, the therapist is working with Lauren (L), our client with schizophrenia. Lauren has persecutory delusions that she is being monitored by a government agency.

L: I saw that white van on my street again yesterday.

T: And that got you thinking that you were being monitored?

L: Yeah. They're there all the time. I think they're sitting in that van listening to me, like in the movies.

T: I would imagine that's frightening.

L: It's terrifying.

T: How sure are you that the van was there to monitor you?

L: I'm positive. That van is always there on my street.

T: OK, I'm open to the possibility that the van was there to monitor you. But can we think of any other reasons that the van could have been there?

L: I can't think of any.

T: Well, let's brainstorm a bit. What are some reasons that a van might be parked on a street?

L: Um . . . it might belong to someone who lives there?

T: Yes, that's possible. What are some other reasons?

L: I guess it could be like workers working on someone's house?

T: Could be. Anything else?

L: Maybe it could just be someone visiting a lot like someone's boyfriend or something?

T: Maybe. So one possibility is that the van was there because someone wanted to monitor you. Some other possibilities are that the van is there because it belongs to someone who lives there, or someone who is working on someone's house, or someone who is visiting. How sure are you that the van was there to monitor you?

L: I guess I'm not so sure.

Time for a quick reality check. It's unlikely that the cognitive restructuring will completely resolve Lauren's delusional belief. However, it is quite possible to "loosen up" her delusions so that she can be more open to alternatives and willing to try other therapeutic strategies.

Challenging All-or-Nothing Thinking Using Scaling

All-or-nothing thinking refers to viewing events, people, or oneself in terms of dichotomous categories. For example, things are either perfect or they are terrible, as seen in individuals with perfectionism (Shafran, Cooper, & Fairburn, 2002), or people are either all good or all bad, as seen in the idealization and devaluation in individuals with borderline personality disorder (Napolitano & McKay, 2007).

There are three potential problems with all-or-nothing thinking:

1. The "good" category usually is so rigid or so unattainable that people or things inevitably end up in the "bad" category.
2. The determination that anything is completely "good" or "bad" can lead to an *attentional bias* (see Chapter 3) such that the person disproportionately attends to stimulus characteristics that are consistent with the label while selectively ignoring stimulus characteristic that are inconsistent with the label. These extremes in labeling therefore become self-perpetuating.
3. Extreme cognitive appraisals tend to contribute to extreme emotional and behavioral responses.

The extreme categorization of all-or-nothing thinking can be challenged using **scaling,** in which the therapist helps the client to see shades of gray rather than just black and white.

Here, the therapist is working again with Blaise (B), who had thought that she had "blown it" and was a "failure" because of her substance use relapse.

T: Let's talk more about this idea of failure. We've talked about this idea that you are either successful in your sobriety or you are a failure.

B: Right.

T: I wonder whether it has to be either/or? Is there something in between?

B: What do you mean, something in between success and failure? Isn't that just failure?

T: Well, let's think about it. Let's imagine we have a scale of some kind—let's call it the Fail-O-Meter. And the Fail-O-Meter gives us a number ranging from 0 to 100, with 100 being a total and complete failure—the worst failure the world has ever seen. And 0 means the complete opposite of failure, a total success. What would your number be?

B: (*Pauses.*) I guess it would be like a 70?

T: Not 100? Why not?

B: Well, I have been sober for a while. I went almost 3 weeks without using before I slipped up.

T: Right, so that's worth noticing. Why else?

B: I guess there's the fact that after I slipped up I called you and I didn't use again.

T: True, it could have been worse. So I wonder, how accurate is it to label you a "failure"?

B: I guess it's not that accurate.

T: What would be a more accurate way to describe you?

B: Working on it?

T: That sure sounds a lot better. Does it feel better to think that way?

B: Yeah, it does.

Challenging "Should" Statements by Questioning the Rule

The psychoanalyst Karen Horney (1950) wrote of the "tyranny of the shoulds" as part of a central conflict in neurosis, in which individuals can never live up to certain standards. Similarly, David Shapiro (1989) has suggested that many neurotic individuals act according to what they think they *should* want and feel, rather than what they *actually* want and feel.

The concept of irrational rule setting has been continued in models of CBT. Many clients have specific, if unspoken, beliefs about how they should feel, think, and behave; how others should act; and how the world should be. And, of course, those "shoulds" are rarely met.

Albert Ellis (2001) frequently told his clients to stop "musterbating": believing that things *must* be a certain way. He might also have come up with the term "you're shoulding all over yourself," although I associate that one a bit more with the *Saturday Night Live* character Stuart Smalley. (If you're not an SNL fan or are too young to remember it, Stuart Smalley was a wannabe therapist who kept repeating the mantra "I'm good enough, I'm smart enough, and doggone it, people like me!").

I challenge "should" statements by **questioning the rule.** For example, I might ask questions such as:

> "Is it really true that your coworkers *should* respect you? Is that a rule? Or would it be more accurate to say that is your *strong preference?*"
>
> "You're saying that you *shouldn't* feel upset about that, but obviously you do. Have you broken a rule of some kind? Where is it written that you're not allowed to feel upset?"
>
> "Where is it written that your wife *should* be more affectionate toward you?"

The aim of questioning the rule is to encourage the client to reframe "shoulds" into "preferences." We want to help the client arrive at more adaptive beliefs such as:

> "I would like it a lot better if my coworkers respected me, but I can survive if they don't."
>
> "I'd rather not feel upset, but I do feel upset, and I can live with it."
>
> "I would prefer my wife to be more affectionate toward me, but I can cope if she isn't."

When the "should" is changed to a preference or desire, rather than a rule, the belief carries less emotional baggage—it is less likely to evoke strong negative emotions, helps the client to recognize that the world will not end if his or her preferences are not met, and positions the client to take a more pragmatic, problem-solving approach to the problem. So now the client can entertain practical questions such as:

> "Because I would like it a lot better if my coworkers respected me, how could I change their attitudes or behavior?"
>
> "Because I'd rather not feel upset, what can I do to help myself feel better?"
>
> "Because I would prefer my wife to be more affectionate toward me, how can I improve the intimacy and affection in our relationship?"

Here's an example of rule questioning from a conversation with our client Elizabeth (E), who has borderline personality disorder and a lot of problems with interpersonal relationships.

> E: I got so pissed at my boyfriend yesterday. I was feeling really upset and he didn't even try to help me or make me feel better. I just felt all alone. I'm still pissed.
>
> T: I see. So what was it about your boyfriend's actions that really bothered you?
>
> E: Well, it's like he wasn't even interested in the fact that I was suffering. You know, like if I'm having a hard time, feeling really down, that's not the time for him to be all cheerful, like nothing's going on.
>
> T: Ah. So we have a thought here that he should have done something to help you. What should he have done?
>
> E: I don't know, just something.

T: So maybe another part of this thought is that he should know what to do. Sounds like you don't know, but he should have known?

E: I guess . . . well, hearing you say it like that makes it sound a little weird.

T: Weird how?

E: I guess weird that I would expect him to know what to do when I myself don't know.

T: Yeah, you're seeing something kind of illogical about that. Tell me, did you ask him for help?

E: Well, no. I mean, why do I need to ask for help? He's my boyfriend.

T: And he should have known.

E: Yeah.

T: So look at all of the "shoulds" you have lined up here. He should have known that I needed help. He should have known what to do. And he should have done it. Do I have that right? Is that how your thinking goes?

E: I guess so, yeah.

T: So when you use a word like *should,* it makes me think that there's a rule here. So your boyfriend broke some rules.

E: Yeah.

T: And so, naturally, you got angry at him. It's really annoying when people break rules, isn't it?

E: Definitely.

T: So is that really a rule? I mean, is there a law written down somewhere about how boyfriends are supposed to behave?

E: Well, no, it's not a law. But everyone knows how boyfriends should act.

T: They do? Everyone knows that boyfriends are supposed to be able to read you and know when you need help? I don't think I was aware of that rule. Is this something he could get arrested for?

E: No, he wouldn't get arrested.

T: Oh. Well then, was it more like a spiritual kind of rule, like one of the Ten Commandments? I don't recall that one; was there a "thou shalt read thy girlfriend at all times and know what she needs?"

E: (*Laughs.*) No.

T: So is that really a rule? Or a preference?

E: I guess a preference. A strong one.

T: Yes, a strong one, but it's a preference, not a rule. You want things to be a certain way, and you want it very much. But when things don't go the way you want, that doesn't mean someone has violated a rule. So could you instead say "I would have preferred that he could read me and know what I needed?"

E: I would have preferred that he could read me and know what I needed.

T: When you say it that way, what happens to your anger? Does it go up or down?

E: Down.

Note that it's perfectly acceptable to infuse your cognitive restructuring with a little humor. That's part of the artistic science. You have to know your client and what kinds of things will resonate with him or her and what won't. In this case, the therapist had a solid relationship with Elizabeth and knew she could tolerate some gentle teasing.

Challenging Mind Reading and Emotional Reasoning
Using Socratic Questioning

Mind reading and emotional reasoning share the common characteristic of inferring the truth about a situation based on one's own feelings, intuition, or hunches. Of course, feelings, intuition, and hunches are all important and worthy of our attention. But clients run into trouble when they automatically accept these as factual, rather than as hypotheses. In addition to the other strategies in this chapter, such as examining the evidence, *Socratic questioning* can be used to help decrease the client's belief in his or her feelings as facts and help him or her to consider those feelings as one of several possible hypotheses.

Here, the therapist is working again with Elizabeth (E) concerning her reactions to her boyfriend stomping out of the house after an argument.

T: Let's talk more about what you thought right when he left the house. What did you take that to mean?

E: I just figured, he's done.

T: He's done; what does that mean?

E: He's done with me. He's finally fed up and he doesn't love me anymore and he's not coming back.

T: OK, so you thought that he was fed up and didn't love you anymore. How did you arrive at that conclusion?

E: Well, I just knew it in my gut.

T: So your gut was telling you that he was fed up and didn't love you. Did anything else tell you that?

E: Well, he was really angry and he was yelling and the way he stomped out of the house, I knew he had finally decided it was over.

T: So he was looking very angry, and your gut was telling you he'd made up his mind. Is your gut always right about these things?

E: A lot of the time it is, yeah.

T: All the time?

E: Well, not all the time.

T: Mine, neither. Sometimes I think I know what someone else is thinking and feeling, but I really don't. Has that ever happened to you?

E: Oh sure, plenty of times.

T: So how certain can we be about what he was thinking?

E: I guess I'm not completely certain.

T: No. You have a hunch about what he was thinking. And that hunch could be accurate, or it could be inaccurate. What else might he have been thinking?

E: He might have been mad but not necessarily that the relationship was over.

T: Possibly. What about not loving you?

E: He might not have stopped loving me. He could have just been mad.

What If It's Not a Distortion?

What if the evidence actually supports the interpretation? For example, what if, after looking at all of the available evidence, William and the therapist both agreed that he was probably going to get a bad review? In such a case, we have at least identified the most likely outcome, which is a good thing, and we can now shift our emphasis to figuring out how to help William cope with it.

The same point can be made for any of the cognitive "distortions" we're talking about here. What if we find out that Anna really is at high risk of a heart attack? Or we find that Nick and Johanna's marriage really is unfixable? Or we find that Elizabeth's boyfriend really is fed up and planning to leave? Well, if any of those things are really true, we'd want to know it. So going through the cognitive restructuring exercises is still helpful. But once we have determined that an interpretation is not distorted, we are then faced with the challenge of helping the person effectively deal with the reality of the situation.

Remember, it's only paranoia if they're not actually out to get you.

Using Thought Change Records

The therapy session is used to practice strategies for challenging maladaptive thoughts. However, as is the case with many other aspects of therapy, durable change often does not occur until the person applies these strategies repeatedly in daily life. In order to accomplish this, the therapist might opt to use a **Thought Change Record,** as shown in Figure 14.2 and in Appendix B. This form is an extension of the Thought Monitoring Form introduced in Chapter 13.

Thought Change Records accomplish several aims:

- They help the client practice identifying and challenging maladaptive thoughts in the natural environment. Doing it in the therapy session is great, but doing it outside of the therapy session can be immensely more productive for producing long-lasting change.
- They help keep the client attentive to his or her interpretations throughout the day, making it more likely that these thoughts will be detected and challenged.
- They help illustrate for the client the link between cognitive change and emotional change.

Here, the therapist introduces the Thought Change Record to Suzanne (S).

T: We've talked a lot in today's visit about cognitive distortions and how they can influence how you feel. For example, when we were talking about your upcoming trip, we identified the fact that you were overestimating the probability that the plane would crash. I'd like to have you continue thinking about this issue by doing some homework. If you look at this form, you'll see that it has a place for you to write down the situation, your interpretations, and how you felt, just as you did before. But now there are some other parts. In this column, I'd like you to reread the interpretations you wrote down and check whether you can spot any cognitive distortions. Let's try that together. Let's imagine you're thinking about your upcoming flight. Where would you write that part?

S: Here, in the "triggering event" column.

Triggering event	Interpretation	Emotion(s)	Intensity of emotion(s) (0–100)	Cognitive distortions (check all that apply)	New interpretation	Emotion(s)	Intensity of emotion(s) (0–100)
Late for work	I'll never succeed in this job. I'm such a screw-up. I'll probably get fired.	Sadness Anxiety	65 50	☑ Probability overestimation ☑ Catastrophizing ☑ Overgeneralization ☐ Personalizing ☐ All-or-nothing thinking ☐ "Should" statements ☐ Mind reading ☐ Emotional reasoning ☐ Minimizing	This is an isolated incident. There's no reason to believe it will keep happening. Being late doesn't make me a screw-up. I actually do a lot of things well. I have no reason to believe I'll be fired.	Sadness Anxiety	30 20

FIGURE 14.2. Sample Thought Change Record.

347

T: Right. So write it there: "thinking about the flight." (*Suzanne does so.*) Now, the fearful interpretation that comes to mind is what?

S: That the plane's going to crash.

T: Yes. And you would write that where?

S: In the "interpretations" column. (*Does so.*)

T: Very good, and now can you write the emotion you feel when you think that way, and the intensity of that emotion?

S: OK, I'm writing "fear" and a severity of 80.

T: Perfect. Now let's look at the next column. From our discussion, what cognitive distortion could you identify?

S: I guess that would be probability overestimation?

T: Yes. So check that one. (*Suzanne does so.*) Now, thinking back to our conversation, what's the alternative, more realistic interpretation?

S: That the plane's probably not going to crash.

T: Right. Can we guarantee that the plane is not going to crash?

S: No. There are no guarantees in the world.

T: But it's really unlikely. So let's have you write that down.

S: OK. "The plane's really unlikely to crash." Maybe I should say more? Like "the chances are less than one in a million"?

T: Sounds good. Now, having written that, read that new interpretation a couple of times to yourself, and write how you are feeling.

S: Still some fear, I think, but it's less. Like maybe 50.

T: OK, so you would write "fear" and "50" in the next columns. (*Suzanne does so.*) Perfect. Now, what I'd like you to do this week is to keep a copy of this form on you at all times—in your purse, in your pocket, wherever it's convenient. The time to write on this form is any time you notice yourself feeling anxious. Just like we did here, I want you to stop what you're doing, if you can, and write down what you're thinking and how you're feeling, and then see if you can detect any cognitive distortions. If you do, write a possible alternative interpretation and see what effect, if any, that has on how you feel.

Using Behavioral Experiments to Challenge Thoughts

One of the most potent ways to modify maladaptive interpretations is through the use of **behavioral experiments.** In keeping with the empirical philosophy of CBT, we want to convey to clients that their interpretations are simply hypotheses (rather than facts) and that the best way to determine what is true is to go find out through some kind of observation.

Behavioral experiments are particularly useful when the client's maladaptive thoughts contain a prediction about what will happen (e.g., probability overestimation, minimizing, or catastrophizing). The idea is to engage in a different kind of behavior with the aim of determining whether the prediction comes true.

Here, the therapist is working with Scott (S), our socially anxious client.

T: You've been thinking about going to the party, but you've been fearful of that. Can you tell me what you're afraid of specifically?

S: Well, I just think that if I go there people will see how nervous I am.

T: And then?

S: I'd make a bad impression. No one would want to talk to me.

T: I see. What do you think they would notice?

S: I guess they'd notice that I was stuttering when I talked—I always do that when I'm nervous. And they might see that I was sweating. They'd know I was a wreck.

T: OK, you have a couple of predictions here. Specifically, you are predicting that if you go to the party, people will see that you are stuttering and sweating. And you then go on to predict that if they see that, they won't want to talk to you. I wonder how we could find out whether your predictions are accurate.

S: Well, I guess I could go to the party?

T: You could. What would you want to look for there, as a way of checking your predictions?

S: I could look to see whether anyone is talking to me?

T: Yes, that would probably be informative. But what about the stuttering and sweating you're worried about?

S: I'm not sure . . . I could see if I'm stuttering and sweating?

T: You could do that, although I suspect that paying a lot more attention to yourself and how you think you are coming across might end up just making you more anxious.

S: That's true.

T: What if you took a bold step and stuttered on purpose?

S: You mean do it deliberately?

T: Right. What if, at some point in the conversation, you made a point of stuttering?

S: That would be scary.

T: Yes, I imagine it would be. But let's think through what might happen. I guess one possibility is that the person you're talking to decides to stop, wraps up the conversation quickly, and walks away. That would be consistent with your prediction. But what else could happen?

S: I guess they might not even notice? Or maybe they'd notice but not make a big deal about it.

T: Yes, that could happen, too. And if that happened, what would that tell us about your prediction?

S: That it was wrong. That I was just getting anxious for nothing.

T: So at least we'd know, one way or the other. What if you did the same thing for sweating? Like perhaps you went into the bathroom and dabbed a little water on your forehead, just enough to look a little sweaty?

S: Yeah, and then I could talk to someone and see if they notice.

Astute readers may note that this behavioral experiment looks a lot like exposure therapy (see Chapter 11). And they'd be right. There is a point at which behavioral and cognitive interventions converge.

We can think of lots of ways that behavioral experiments could help our clients. For example:

- Anna, our client with panic disorder, experiences dizziness and has the interpretation "I'm going to pass out." So how could we create a behavioral experiment to test that prediction? We could have her deliberately get dizzy in the therapist's office or elsewhere and see whether or not she passes out.
- Blaise, who has a substance use disorder, has urges to use and has the interpretation "If I can't use right now, I'll never be able to feel better." How could we test that? In the therapist's office, we could stimulate urges to use—perhaps by having her think of her substance of choice, or by exposing her to stimuli that trigger cravings—and then have her see whether she starts to feel better over time or with the use of emotion regulation strategies (e.g., Chapters 18 and 19).
- Bethany, our client with OCD, thinks "I'm going to lose control and kill someone." As a result, she avoids being around knives or sharp objects. How could we test that? The therapist could hand her a knife and see whether she is able to maintain

TIB Alert!

Most clients respond quite well to cognitive restructuring. Of course, every client is different, and some clients have adverse reactions to having their thoughts and beliefs questioned in this way. One client, for example, reported feeling like Socratic questioning was an effort to "trap" her. Other clients seem to want to prove to the therapist that they are right and adopt an adversarial stance.

As we discuss below, cognitive restructuring may or may not be critical, and certainly for some clients it's not needed. However, a client's adverse reaction to this or any other intervention might be construed as a clinically relevant behavior (see Chapter 9): an example of the client's problem enacted in the session. That's not necessarily a bad thing, if it's informative about the problem and gives you an in-session target. It's just an example of bringing the problem into the room. Perhaps, for example, the client who thinks that Socratic questioning is a "trap" is suspicious of others in general or has a general tendency to view things as a threat to personal autonomy. The client's in-session reaction would yield a fruitful topic of discussion and an opportunity to evaluate, challenge, and work through a long-standing maladaptive pattern of interpersonal behavior.

Also, it's important to remember that cognitive restructuring is not intended to be an argument, or even a debate. It's intended to be a collaborative process between two (or more) people who are trying to figure things out together. So if it starts feeling like you and the client are arguing with each other, put the brakes on. Step back, reiterate the aims of what you're trying to do, and deal with any potential alliance ruptures that may have occurred (see Chapter 7).

Finally, remember that, in most cases, you have time on your side. You might not get a big "a-ha" moment in a single session. It's nice when that happens, but much of the time cognitive restructuring is a slow process of chipping away at a belief, loosening up the client's mental "grip" on the belief, over the course of several sessions.

control of herself. (Remember, we know that Bethany has OCD and is not a violent person. We need to show that to her).

Using Coping Cards

We all remember mood-congruent memory from Chapter 3. People selectively recall things that are congruent with their current mood state. One problem with mood-congruent memory is this: You might be able to come up with balanced, rational, adaptive thoughts during a comfortable therapy session; however, there's no guarantee that the client will actually remember these in daily life under stressful circumstances.

To facilitate the transfer of material from the therapy session to the natural environment, it can be helpful to use **coping cards,** in which the client writes down the adaptive thought on a piece of paper to carry with her or him (e.g., in a wallet or purse) or to put in places where the symptoms are likely to occur (e.g., in the car or on the refrigerator door). Coping cards could also contain information about desired behaviors, which would be consistent with the idea of *stimulus control* we discussed in Chapter 8. Once an adaptive thought has been identified, I sometimes ask the client to write that thought on a small card in session and to carry it with her or him, with instructions to take it out and read it during stressful daily experiences.

THE ESSENTIALS

* The aim of cognitive restructuring is to help the client think more realistically (which is not necessarily the same thing as thinking positively).
* Helping clients identify their cognitive distortions is a helpful first step.
* Therapists can challenge distorted interpretations by:
  * Examining the evidence for and against an interpretation.
  * Asking the client to consider alternatives to the interpretation.
  * Doing the math to reach realistic probability estimates.
  * Using the downward arrow technique in cases of catastrophizing.
  * Finding exceptions to overgeneralized interpretations.
  * Identifying external factors in cases of personalizing.
  * Using scaling to counteract all-or-nothing thinking.
  * Questioning the rules behind "should" statements.
* Behavioral experiments are a powerful way to challenge distorted interpretations.
* Coping cards and Thought Change Records are useful homework exercises for challenging distorted interpretations and rehearsing new, more realistic interpretations.

KEY TERMS AND DEFINITIONS

Behavioral experiment: Testing the validity of a thought by making specific predictions and then engaging in a behavior that would allow a determination of whether or not the prediction came true.

Cognitive restructuring: The process of identifying, challenging, and revising maladaptive thoughts.

Considering alternatives: Inviting the client to identify other, potentially more adaptive, thoughts and interpretations.

Coping card: A portable, written document, to be used outside of the therapy setting, that reminds the client of specific adaptive thoughts and/or desired behaviors.

Doing the math: Challenging probability overestimation by considering actual probabilities.

Downward arrow: A Socratic method using a series of "if–then" questions to challenge catastrophizing.

Examining the evidence: Identifying facts that might confirm or disconfirm a thought or belief.

Finding the exceptions: Challenging overgeneralization by helping the client identify exceptions to the global thought or belief.

Identifying external factors: Challenging personalizing by helping the client identify external (nonpersonal) factors responsible for a given situation or outcome.

Questioning the rule: Challenging "should" statements by raising questions about the validity of internal "rules."

Scaling: Challenging all-or-nothing thinking by using a numeric scale or other method of considering a continuum rather than extreme categories.

Thought Change Record: A self-monitoring form used to identify interpretations, document the relationship between interpretations and emotions, challenge cognitive distortions, and identify more realistic interpretations.

Restructuring Thoughts

For a period of 24 hours, monitor and challenge any maladaptive interpretations that contribute to the personal target.

Triggering event	Interpretation	Emotion(s)	Intensity of emotion(s) (0–100)	Cognitive distortions (check all that apply)	New interpretation	Emotion(s)	Intensity of emotion(s) (0–100)
				☐ Probability overestimation ☐ Catastrophizing ☐ Overgeneralization ☐ Personalizing ☐ All-or-nothing thinking ☐ "Should" statements ☐ Mind reading ☐ Emotional reasoning ☐ Minimizing			
				☐ Probability overestimation ☐ Catastrophizing ☐ Overgeneralization ☐ Personalizing ☐ All-or-nothing thinking ☐ "Should" statements ☐ Mind reading ☐ Emotional reasoning ☐ Minimizing			

From *Doing CBT* by David F. Tolin. Copyright © 2016 The Guilford Press. Permission to photocopy this worksheet is granted to purchasers of this book for personal use only (see copyright page for details). Purchasers can download enlarged versions of this worksheet (see the box at the end of the table of contents).

CHAPTER 15

Leave Them Thoughts Alone

The Art of *Not* Challenging Thoughts

If you recall, way back in Chapter 1, I talked about how CBT, because of its emphasis on the scientific method, is constantly evolving. We're constantly learning about how thoughts, feelings, and behaviors interact, and from that knowledge we're developing new ways to help clients. Over the past two decades, a lot of researchers and clinicians have been trying a new approach to maladaptive thoughts.

The science of emotion regulation puts strategies into two broad categories: *antecedent-focused* (i.e., primarily affecting things that happen before the emotional response) or *response-focused* (i.e., primarily affecting things that happen after the emotional response has begun; J. J. Gross, 1998; Werner & Gross, 2010). The cognitive restructuring strategies described in Chapter 14 are largely antecedent-focused. They are based on the idea that maladaptive interpretations come before (and perhaps cause) the emotion and that, therefore, if you challenge the interpretation, you can head off the onset of the negative emotion.

Several innovative clinicians have taken a more response-focused approach to dealing with negative thoughts. The idea here is not so much that they want to change the thoughts themselves; rather, they want to change the person's cognitive, emotional, and behavioral *responses* to those thoughts. So in these newer variations of CBT, traditional antecedent-focused cognitive restructuring is deemphasized. Indeed, a central premise of one newer form of CBT, *acceptance and commitment therapy* (Hayes et al., 2012), is that individuals' efforts to get control of thoughts and emotions are part of the problem. Such control efforts are called **experiential avoidance:** attempts to avoid or escape from aversive internal experiences.

Other recent variants of CBT take a less hard line on the subject—they don't necessarily argue that efforts to control thoughts are inherently part of the problem—but they do point out that clients can sometimes get too hung up on the internal struggle against their own thoughts and suggest alternatives to cognitive restructuring. *Dialectical behavior therapy* (Linehan, 1993) and *mindfulness-based cognitive therapy* (Segal, Williams, & Teasdale, 2002) are both based, in part, on the notion that clients may want to change their internal experiences but can often become trapped in a self-perpetuating cycle of negative thoughts and feelings when they try to do so. *Metacognitive therapy* (Wells, 2009) posits that emotional distress is maintained by maladaptive effortful cognitive processes such as worry, rumination, and fixated attention. The basic idea is that the problem has less to do with the content of maladaptive thoughts than with how the person responds and relates to those thoughts. So generalized anxiety is conceptualized as "worry about worry," depression is conceptualized as "sadness about sadness," panic is conceptualized as "fear of fear," and so on.

Note that these conceptualizations differ substantially from that of the traditional cognitive elements of CBT. The traditional cognitive conceptualization posits that pathology results when the *content* of thoughts is distorted or irrational and causes emotional distress. These alternative variations, however, suggest that the *content* of the thoughts is not the problem, but rather the person's *mental, emotional,* and *behavioral reactions* to their thoughts.

We can certainly see examples in our clients of how one's relationship to one's thoughts can cause more harm than the thoughts themselves:

- Melissa, who suffers from PTSD, attempts to suppress her intrusive traumatic memories. This attempt at *thought suppression* backfires, making the memories occur more frequently and preventing Melissa from being more comfortable with the memories.
- Christina, our depressed client, has the negative thought "my life sucks." She then gets mad at herself, thinking, "What's wrong with me? Why am I so depressed all the time? Why can't I snap out of this?" This *rumination* deepens her feelings of depression.
- Anna, who has panic disorder, worries that she's going to have a heart attack. She accepts this thought as a fact and avoids feared situations to prevent it from happening. This *avoidance* prevents her from learning that the situations are safe and therefore causes her maladaptive beliefs to persist.
- Bethany, who has OCD, engages in constant mental compulsions such as self-reassurance, counting, and praying in order to cope with obsessive thoughts. Although these compulsions provide momentary relief, they have become "crutches" that she relies on, instead of recognizing that her obsessions are illogical.

From this different conceptualization come different interventions, aimed not at altering the *content* of thoughts but rather at altering the person's *reactions* to those thoughts. Dialectical behavior therapy (Linehan, 1993), developed with borderline personality disorder in mind, does not eschew cognitive restructuring but adds a component of *mindfulness training*. Mindfulness-based cognitive therapy (Segal et al., 2002), as its name implies, also emphasizes mindfulness training. **Mindfulness,** drawn in part from Eastern meditation practices, is defined as attending to one's experiences (including thoughts, feelings, and behaviors) in the present moment without making any judgments as to their meaning or value (Baer, 2003; Brantley, 2003; Kabat-Zinn, 1994; Linehan, Armstrong, Suarez, Allmon, & Heard, 1993). In mindfulness training (Linehan, 2015; Segal et al., 2002), clients use meditation strategies to practice:

- Observing current experiences (sensations, emotions, thoughts, and behaviors) without necessarily trying to terminate them when unpleasant.
- Describing events, emotions, thoughts, and behaviors in words.
- Refraining from judging (e.g., labeling as "good" or "bad") events, emotions, thoughts, and behaviors.
- Focusing the mind on, and participating completely in, the current moment's activity (sometimes called "being present" or "being in the moment").

Metacognitive therapy (Wells, 2009) also incorporates mindfulness training, which Wells refers to as "detached mindfulness" (p. 71). This variant of mindfulness does not use the formal practice sessions seen in dialectical behavior therapy or mindfulness-based cognitive therapy. Clients receiving this form of mindfulness training practice:

- Being aware of their thoughts as they occur.
- Recognizing that their thoughts are mental processes, rather than facts.
- Switching attention among thoughts, emotions, and external events.
- Refraining from efforts to understand the meaning of thoughts or to avoid or escape from erroneous threats.
- Taking an observer perspective toward one's thoughts.

Acceptance and commitment therapy (Hayes et al., 2012) takes a stronger position against cognitive restructuring (i.e., attempting to alter the content of thoughts). In this model, the core intervention is **acceptance,** defined as "allowing, tolerating, embracing, experiencing, or making contact with a source of stimulation, particularly private experiences, that previously provoked escape, avoidance, or aggression" (Hayes & Pankey, 2003, p. 4). In acceptance, the client moves away from viewing thoughts and feelings as reality or things that need to be changed and toward embracing them simply as internal events (Hayes et al., 2012; Roemer & Orsillo, 2003). Acceptance has a long tradition in humanistic psychotherapies such as Gestalt therapy (e.g., Perls, 1973). Acceptance has also been emphasized in certain substance abuse treatments, such as in the concept of "urge surfing" (e.g., Marlatt & Gordon, 1985). In acceptance training, clients practice:

- Detecting and challenging experiential avoidance responses such as thought suppression, cognitive challenging, rumination, or behavioral avoidance.
- Exposing oneself to previously avoided thoughts and emotions, noticing specific bodily sensations or mental activity but not attempting to control them.
- Using more adaptive responses to thoughts and emotions, emphasizing a willingness to experience these thoughts and emotions.
- Using **cognitive defusion** (Luoma & Hayes, 2003), defined as detaching from the literal meaning of thoughts and focusing instead on the thoughts as a product of ongoing mental processes, using strategies such as repeating thoughts over and over, noticing and describing the thoughts, and being willing to coexist with the thoughts without acting on them.

So from the previous chapter and this chapter, it's clear that we have two basic, seemingly discrepant conceptualizations about the role that thoughts play in the maintenance of psychological problems and about how best to address maladaptive thoughts. The first, which is the more traditional CBT approach, posits that the content of thoughts is distorted and that these distortions lead to emotional suffering and maladaptive behaviors.

A core intervention, therefore, is to challenge the accuracy of these thoughts and generate alternative, more balanced thoughts.

The second conceptualization reflects the role of mindfulness and acceptance. As you can see, although these two interventions are different in some respects, they share a common idea that psychological problems stem less from the content of the thoughts than from one's emotional, cognitive, and behavioral responses to those thoughts. A core intervention across these interventions, therefore, is to help the client to be aware of the thoughts and to refrain from direct attempts to change them. A potential mechanism of acceptance is *cognitive defusion*, in which the thought is stripped of its literal semantic meaning and is viewed as merely a thought (some authors have used the term *decentering* to describe a similar process).

In short, the distinction could be summed up as "change the thoughts" versus "change how you *respond to* the thoughts" (Hofmann & Asmundson, 2008).

A concrete example of the difference between these two conceptualizations can be seen in Table 15.1.

TABLE 15.1. A Comparison of Traditional Cognitive and Acceptance Perspectives on Maladaptive Thoughts

	Traditional cognitive perspective	Acceptance perspective
The thought is . . .	• "I'm such a failure."	• "I'm such a failure."
The problem here is . . .	• The thought is inaccurate or exaggerated. • The inaccurate thought leads to emotional distress.	• The person treats the thought as a fact rather than as just a thought. • The person pays excessive attention to the thought and tries to change it, feel better about it, avoid it, or act on it.
And so the solution is . . .	• Demonstrate that the thought is a source of emotional distress. • Help the client to understand that the thought is inaccurate or exaggerated. • Help the client to identify and practice a new, more adaptive and realistic thought.	• Help the client to focus awareness on the thought in the present moment. • Teach the client to experience the thought without judging it, analyzing it, feeling better about it, or trying to control it. • Help the client to recognize that this is just a thought. • Redirect the client's efforts away from attempts to control or change thoughts and toward value- or goal-oriented activity.
And this should work because . . .	• Cognitive reappraisal helps the client view things more realistically. • Realistic beliefs are less emotionally distressing. • Thinking realistically allows for better problem-focused coping strategies.	• Cognitive defusion helps the client recognize that thoughts are not "real" in a literal sense. • When thoughts are perceived as less "real," the client is better able to respond appropriately to situations. • Stopping maladaptive control efforts will likely reduce emotional distress.

Critical elements of the acceptance conceptualization are:

- Unpleasant or unwanted thoughts are an unavoidable part of life and need not be a source of significant emotional distress.
- Distress does not necessarily come from the *content* of unwanted thoughts—that is, whether a thought is accurate or inaccurate is not the central concern—but rather from how one *responds to* their unwanted thoughts.
- Distressed people are characterized by excessive "buy-in" of their interpretations. Rather than viewing them as thoughts, they view them as facts to be acted on.
- In many cases, the person treats the thoughts themselves as if they were the problem, rather than just mental reactions to a problem. So instead of dealing with actual problems in life, they spend a lot of time and energy trying to suppress or "fix" unpleasant or unwanted thoughts. These efforts end up doing more harm than good and distract the person from actually dealing effectively with real problems or pursuing their own goals and values.
- Emotional distress can come from either paying too little attention to one's thoughts (in which case we may act on them automatically) or from "buying into" those thoughts and interpreting them as rules or facts.

And from the acceptance conceptualization come the following acceptance interventions:

- Clients should be taught, through words or through metaphors and exercises, that their efforts to control their thoughts are a major part of the problem.
- Clients should learn to pay attention to their thoughts and to identify them as thoughts (rather than as facts, rules, etc.).
- Clients should accept their thoughts without judging them, labeling them as "good" or "bad," or attempting to gain control over them.

 Things That Might Bug You about This

It's easy to misunderstand what we mean by *mindfulness* and *acceptance*. Sometimes, when we think of mindfulness or other meditative strategies, we think that the aim is to achieve a state of physiological relaxation, or to have an "empty mind." Clients will often think at first that this is what they're supposed to strive for. In reality, we're not looking to empty the mind of thoughts or to clear the body of tension. Rather, we're trying to undermine the client's maladaptive secondary reactions *to* those thoughts and feelings by having him or her practice noticing them without judging, evaluating, or changing them.

Sometimes we interpret the word *acceptance* to mean a form of passivity, just allowing bad things to keep happening. Acceptance does adopt a passive stance, but only toward thoughts and feelings. The idea here is that you're unlikely to win in a struggle against your own internal experiences, so you're better off not even getting into that fight. But there's nothing passive about how we address behavior. Here, we are very active, vigorously encouraging the client to take meaningful action to make life better. In short, work on fixing your life, rather than fixing your thoughts and feelings.

- Clients should learn to direct their attention toward the present moment, rather than the past or the future.
- Clients should redirect their efforts away from trying to gain control over their thoughts and toward engaging in behaviors that are consistent with meaningful goals and personal values.

Less Thinking, More Doing: Value-Based Action

As mentioned above, many people with psychological problems place a premium on feeling better (or sometimes thinking better). That is, people with anxiety disorders want to feel less anxious; people with depression want to feel happier; people with OCD or PTSD want intrusions out of their heads; and so on. That's certainly understandable; but is that the best priority? Hayes et al. (1999, p. 217) ask clients, "imagine that you can write anything you want on your tombstone that says what you stood for in your life. What would you want to have there, if it could be absolutely anything?" Perhaps not surprisingly, few clients will answer "He never had any bad thoughts" or "She was prepared for threat" or "He didn't feel sad." Rather, asking this kind of question forces clients to think about what's really important to them: being a good parent or partner, having a good network of friends, adhering to spiritual beliefs, helping other people, being good at their jobs, and so on.

But having identified those values, we see just how far many of our clients have strayed from the pursuit of those values. They spend much of their time up in their own heads, trying to think and feel better, while life passes them by. As just a few examples:

- Anna is so consumed with trying not to panic that she has stopped attending her classes, despite the fact that graduating from college was one of her life's ambitions.
- Melissa, who has PTSD, has avoided others even though she would like to have more friends. She stays away from what feels threatening because that feels safer.
- Johanna and Nick have become so consumed with being "right," blaming each other for their problems, and trying to feel better about their marriage that they have stopped attending to their own family behaviors—Johanna being the best wife she can, and Nick being the best husband he can, and both of them being the best parents they can be to James.

So what would acceptance look like for our clients? That is, what would happen if these clients accepted their thoughts, rather than fought them, and redirected their efforts toward **value-based action**?

- Suzanne, our client with generalized anxiety, might be willing to have her scary thoughts without trying to worry them away or chase them off with benzodiazepines.
- Melissa might accept her intrusive memories of abuse. That doesn't mean she'd like them, but she would recognize that they are just images in her head, nothing more. She would make a point of actively building friendships with people, even when she feels uneasy.
- Christina, our depressed client, would notice when her depressive internal voice started talking and would treat that voice with a bit of sympathy rather than

rumination and trying to "snap out of it." She would also reengage in church, which had previously been a source of inspiration and fulfillment for her, but which she has lately been neglecting.

- Johanna and Nick would accept the fact that they have negative thoughts about each other and about the marriage. They would acknowledge that the thoughts are there, without necessarily taking those thoughts as evidence of trouble—they are just thoughts. They would instead focus more of their attention on being the best partners and parents they can be.
- Bethany, our client with OCD, would recognize that her obsessive thoughts about hurting someone were just "brain farts" and that, although they were part of her, they weren't something she needed to do anything about (such as compulsions and avoidance).
- Lauren, our client with schizophrenia, would notice when her voices showed up, say a mental "hi, voices" to them, and get on with her activities of daily living.
- Samuel, our client with insomnia, would catch himself in the act of worrying about how he was not sleeping and gently remind himself that this was just part of his thought process. He would then focus on doing the activities that he knows are likely to help with sleep and stopping activities that interfere with sleep.

The Science behind It

What's more effective: cognitive restructuring or acceptance? In laboratory research:

- Cognitive reappraisal was more effective than was acceptance in moderating acute feelings of anxiety during a public-speaking task (Hofmann, Heering, Sawyer, & Asnaani, 2009).

- Reappraisal and acceptance were both superior to suppression instructions in reducing eye-blink startle reflex (a measure of physiological anxiety) but did not differ from each other (Asnaani, Sawyer, Aderka, & Hofmann, 2013).

- Reappraisal and acceptance instructions led to comparable reductions in emotional distress after viewing emotionally evocative film clips in healthy control participants (Wolgast, Lundh, & Viborg, 2011); a similar study using clients with schizophrenia found that reappraisal yielded greater reductions in emotional distress, although any differences were temporary (Perry, Henry, Nangle, & Grisham, 2012).

- Among adolescents, reappraisal of a recent stressful event led to greater decreases in negative affect than did acceptance (Rood, Roelofs, Bogels, & Arntz, 2012).

- Among women with body shape dissatisfaction, repeating a negative thought over and over "until the meaning of the word disappears and all that is left is just a sound" and reappraisal produced equivalent improvements in body shape dissatisfaction (Deacon, Fawzy, Lickel, & Wolitzky-Taylor, 2011).

- Among clients with anorexia nervosa and body dysmorphic disorder, both acceptance and cognitive reappraisal led to similar decreases in the frequency of body-related negative thoughts and similar increases in acceptance of those thoughts (Hartmann, Thomas, Greenberg, Rosenfield, & Wilhelm, 2015).

So, in tightly controlled laboratory studies, interventions based on the model of acceptance/defusion seem to produce results that are more or less equivalent to interventions based on the model of cognitive restructuring/reappraisal. What about the use of these strategies in actual clinical contexts?

- A young but substantial literature suggests that acceptance-based interventions can be helpful for a range of problems, such as borderline personality disorder (Kliem, Kroger, & Kosfelder, 2010), mood disorders (Harley, Sprich, Safren, Jacobo, & Fava, 2008; Teasdale et al., 2000; van Aalderen et al., 2012; J. M. G. Williams et al., 2008), anxiety disorders (Arch et al., 2012; Craske et al., 2014; Hoge et al., 2013; Neacsiu, Eberle, Kramer, Wiesmann, & Linehan, 2014; Roemer, Orsillo, & Salters-Pedneault, 2008; van der Heiden, Muris, & van der Molen, 2012; Wells et al., 2010), eating disorders (C. F. Telch, Agras, & Linehan, 2001), substance use disorders (Linehan et al., 1999; Stotts et al., 2012), psychosis (Bach & Hayes, 2002; Chadwick, Hughes, Russell, Russell, & Dagnan, 2009; Gaudiano & Herbert, 2006), and chronic pain (Garland et al., 2014; Morone, Greco, & Weiner, 2008; Thorsell et al., 2011).

- When we compare acceptance-based interventions to other forms of CBT, no significant differences in outcome are observed across studies, either at posttreatment or at follow-up (Öst, 2014). Evaluation of differences between variations of CBT is difficult, however, as many interventions contain multiple interventions.

- Some evidence suggests that even though traditional CBT (incorporating cognitive restructuring) and acceptance-based strategies yield comparable outcomes, they may work for somewhat different reasons: Although clients receiving both treatments demonstrate decreases in negative thoughts, among clients receiving acceptance-based treatments, treatment response is associated with increased acceptance and decreased experiential avoidance (Forman, Herbert, Moitra, Yeomans, & Geller, 2007; Niles et al., 2014).

As you can see from the "Science behind It" sidebar, we have a bit of a conundrum here. The client comes in with a negative, distorted thought. Do we help him or her to challenge that thought, examine the evidence, and develop a new, more balanced thought? Or do we encourage him or her to notice the thought, recognize that it's just a thought, and refrain from trying to change it?

We have little science to guide us on this issue, so my answer is somewhere between "it depends" and "I don't know." Those are probably not the answers you were looking for, but at the time of this writing, that's an open and hotly debated question in CBT research. We have two viable approaches to negative cognitions here, and they both seem to be helpful. I'll tell you what I do clinically, but I reserve the right to be wrong about this.

Recall from Chapter 3 our discussion of automatic cognitive processes, semi-automatic cognitive processes, and effortful cognitive processes.

- *Automatic cognitive processes* include attention (e.g., one's attention is drawn toward something negative), memory (mood-congruent events are remembered), and intrusions (ideas, pictures, memories, or impulses that "pop" into the person's head involuntarily). I tend to use acceptance here. So, for example, when Bethany, our teenage client with OCD, experiences an intrusive thought that she's going to murder someone, I'm unlikely to spend much time in verbal discussion of the validity of that thought (though I might do some of that up front). I am much more likely to take the position that this is just a thought, that Bethany doesn't have to behave in an avoidant manner because of it, and that she should practice doing what's important to her despite the presence of the obsession. Similarly, when Melissa, our client with complex PTSD, has an intrusive memory of her childhood abuse, that situation seems to call less for cognitive restructuring than for acceptance. I might discuss with Melissa how these memories are inevitable for someone who has been through trauma but that at the end of the day they are just unpleasant memories (rather than present-time threats). They can't hurt her.

• *Semi-automatic cognitive processes* include interpretations and core beliefs. Here's where the available evidence is most gray and where there is room for the greatest amount of debate. I use cognitive restructuring and acceptance, with varying emphases, for different clients. Sometimes, the cognitive distortion is abundantly clear and provides a good target for intervention. When Christina tells me that her situation is hopeless, and she's going to lose her job and her family and end up destitute, I'm likely to evaluate the evidence and take on the catastrophizing. In other cases, the distortion is less clear, or the client is a bit less receptive to the kind of back-and-forth discussion that cognitive restructuring entails. Here I might encourage the client to recognize that "these are just thoughts." There are other clients who seem so "up in his or her head" that they have become compulsive about appraising and reappraising their own thoughts. Lots of clients spend an awful lot of time and mental energy trying to evaluate the accuracy and validity of their own thoughts, often fruitlessly. I take that as a sign that cognitive reappraisal might not fit well with this client's psychology and might steer him or her toward acceptance.

• *Effortful cognitive processes* such as rumination, worry, and thought suppression are an easier target for intervention. Here, we want the client to stop (or at least decrease) the process so that he or she doesn't add more fuel to the fire. I might talk to Melissa, for example, about the paradoxical effects of trying to suppress her traumatic memories. I might coach Suzanne, our client with GAD, to refrain from rehearsing potential disasters (worrying) and instead focus on productive problem solving (see Chapter 12). I might steer Christina and William away from depressive rumination, in which they exert excessive time and effort wondering why they feel the way they do and berating themselves for not feeling better, and toward activities that are more in line with their overall goals and values.

Engaging the Frontal Lobes

Do cognitive restructuring and acceptance work in a similar fashion, biologically speaking? There are some differences in brain activity when people reappraise versus accept unpleasant stimuli, emotions, or thoughts (Grecucci, Pappaianni, Siugzdaite, Theunick, & Job, 2015; Hölzel et al., 2011). However, acceptance and mindfulness still seem to activate the prefrontal cortex (Farb et al., 2010; Farb et al., 2007), which, in turn, helps modify signals from limbic regions such as the amygdala. So in acceptance, even though we're not telling the client to try to think differently, he or she inevitably is. The mere act of looking at a thought, discussing it, and even "playing" with it likely engages the frontal lobes in its own way, creating a different perspective and allowing for greater emotional control.

In the previous chapter, we saw a cognitive restructuring approach with William, our client with a mix of depression, dependent personality characteristics, and pain who had identified a belief that his performance review at work would go badly. Let's try a different approach for the same problem. Over the next several vignettes, the therapist uses acceptance to address William's thoughts.

Giving Up the Struggle

The first challenge is getting William (W) to notice his maladaptive efforts to control his thoughts, to recognize that they are not working, and to give up the fight against them.

T: When you've had these kind of thoughts in the past, how have you dealt with them?

W: Sometimes I just tell myself to get over it. You know, like "Quit your whining."

T: Being stern with yourself. How has that worked overall?

W: That doesn't work well at all.

T: No, I'm not surprised. Perhaps that even makes you feel worse?

W: It probably does, in the long run.

T: So you've tried being stern with yourself, and that hasn't actually relieved you of these depressing thoughts and sad feelings. Why do you suppose that is?

W: Maybe I'm not trying hard enough? Or maybe just not consistently enough?

T: Well, that's one possibility. But on the other hand it seems that more of the same would be kind of unlikely to produce better results. Let me suggest an alternative to you. Could it be that being stern with yourself about your thoughts is actually part of the problem?

W: I'm not sure what you mean.

T: Well, I'm wondering whether in the long run these things actually make you feel worse. So, for example, if I just told you, "Whatever you do, don't have any negative thoughts," could you do it?

W: Probably not.

T: No, I couldn't, either. In fact, that might even make things worse. Try an exercise with me. For the next 30 seconds or so, don't think about elephants. Not even a little bit. I'll time us. (*after 30 seconds*) What was your experience?

W: Well, I started going over my grocery list to try to distract myself.

T: OK, so you tried distracting yourself. And where was the elephant while you were distracting yourself?

W: It would just kind of pop up every so often.

T: Hmm. I wonder why that is?

W: I guess because I knew I wasn't supposed to be thinking about elephants, so just knowing that made me think about elephants.

T: Right. That's what happens to most of us. When we try not to think about something, the very act of not thinking about it . . .

W: Makes you think about it.

Show Me, Don't Tell Me

Note that in this discussion, the therapist uses an exercise to teach William about the paradoxical effects of thought suppression. This topic could have been handled purely by discussion, but by having William actually see for himself, the lesson is much more salient and more likely to "stick" in his mind. The therapist can then refer back to this in future sessions, for example, "Remember the elephants?"

Other creative exercises can be employed to illustrate the futility of effortful cognitive processes that reflect maladaptive control efforts. For example, Kuehlwein (2000, p. 185) writes about how he addressed the problem of rumination with a depressed client:

> I asked her to stand up and stretch out her hands face up. I then placed a large book in her hands and asked her to imagine that carrying this weight represented the experience of being depressed. I next placed several other large books on top of these, saying things like, "God, I'm such a weakling for being depressed!" and "What the hell's the matter with me? Why can't I just snap out of it?" I asked her how she felt then. She reported that the burden was now heavier and smiled. I further asked, "How easy would it be to function now? How easy to work on your depression?" She remarked on how difficult it would be and we both observed that the original depression (the first book) was now obscured by the self-blame.

T: Right. But perhaps you weren't trying hard enough? I mean, what if we really raised the stakes here, and I told you that I had your chair wired to shock you every time you thought about an elephant?

W: I guess I'd probably just think about them more. I'd get shocked.

T: And so what if I told you, for example, not to think any depressing thoughts?

W: I'd think about them more?

T: And that would make you feel better or worse?

W: Worse.

T: So we have a problem here. You try and try not to think these negative thoughts, but it seems like the harder you try, the more you think about them. It seems that the more you struggle with these thoughts, the more trapped you become—like being in quicksand.

W: It does feel that way. Like I can't get out.

T: You can't. At least not this way.

Metaphor

Here, the therapist uses a metaphor of quicksand to help illustrate the futility of William's internal struggle against his negative thoughts. This metaphor nicely conveys the idea that the more William struggles, the more mired in the problem he will become.

Hayes et al. (2012) provide several clever metaphors that convey the same idea—that struggling with thoughts can be counterproductive. One is the image of Chinese handcuffs, the woven tube that catches your index fingers when you insert them into the tube. The harder you try to pull your fingers out of the tube, the tighter it gets. The only way to get your fingers out is to push them into the tube, which causes it to expand. Thus, sometimes we must "push into" our thoughts rather than try to "pull out" of them. Another metaphor used for a similar purpose is to have the client imagine that he or she is driving a bus and that his or her negative thoughts are represented by nasty, scary-looking passengers who are barking orders and otherwise being obnoxious. To deal directly with these passengers requires stopping the bus, which defeats the whole purpose of the trip—in other words, to struggle against your negative thoughts requires stopping other, more important activities, which defeats the whole purpose of life. The bus driver's best option is to continue driving and learn not to take the passengers too seriously. And the client's best option is to get on with the activities of life and not take his or her negative thoughts too seriously. They are just thoughts, after all.

Watching Your Thoughts

Having pointed out the futility of William's internal struggle, the therapist now has to help William find another way to respond to his thoughts. The aim here is to get William to notice and observe his thoughts, without necessarily buying into them or responding to them.

> T: So how about we try an alternative? Let's try something for a few minutes. It might seem a little weird, but I'll do it with you, so we'll be weird together. Let's close our eyes and just pay attention to our thoughts. We're not going to try to think anything, or not think anything. We'll just see what comes up.
>
> W: (*closing eyes*) OK.
>
> T: Here's how I'd like to do it. When a thought comes to mind, I'd like you to envision it floating by you, like you're watching clouds in the sky. You might notice some unpleasant thoughts come up; let them float by. You might notice some pleasant thoughts as well; let them float by, too. You might even notice some thoughts about what we're doing, like "This is dumb," or "I'm not doing this right." Let those float by, too. Ready? OK, start. (*Lets a few minutes pass.*) OK, when you feel ready, you can open your eyes. What did you experience?
>
> W: Well, for the most part I think I was able to just let random thoughts float by.
>
> T: For the most part? Were there some times that were more difficult?
>
> W: Yeah, there was a time in there when I thought maybe I wasn't doing what I was supposed to do. I wasn't sure I understood the instructions.
>
> T: I see. And did those thoughts float by, too?
>
> W: No, not really. It kind of took me out of the exercise and I tried to figure out what I was supposed to be doing.
>
> T: That's a good example of what can happen. You had a thought that you weren't doing it right; that you were screwing it up somehow. And you bought it.
>
> W: I bought it?
>
> T: You took it literally and instead of being just a thought that you could let float by, it became something that you had to deal with somehow. You had to work it out.
>
> W: Yeah, I felt like I needed to make sure I was doing it right.

T: Can you appreciate that this idea of "I'm not doing it right" was just a thought, too?

W: I guess so.

T: So what would happen if you said, "OK, I just had that thought that I'm not doing it right; I can let that thought float by along with the others"?

W: That would be tough.

T: At first, yes. You're used to reacting to your thoughts. It's hard to just let them be there.

W: I know, but with something like this, knowing that I'm screwing it up, shouldn't I do something about it?

T: Look how quickly you went from "I had the thought that I am screwing up" to "I know that I'm screwing up." See what you just did there? You started treating that thought as if it were a fact, and not just a thought in your head. But what's the real fact here? Were you screwing up?

W: I don't know.

T: There are two different things here. One is screwing up, actually doing a task wrong. And the other is thinking about screwing up. Those aren't the same. Which one is more important?

W: Actually screwing up.

T: When a thought about screwing up comes to mind, do you need to do something about that?

W: Well, I'd rather not have thoughts about screwing up.

T: Can you control your thoughts?

W: No.

T: What can you control?

W: Whether or not I actually screw up.

T: Yes. You can control what you do, but not what you think. And when we get hung up on fixing our thoughts, we just have more negative thoughts and feel worse.

W: So how do I not get hung up on fixing my thoughts?

T: What about learning to live with them?

W: Live with them? Like just be depressed forever?

 Metaphor

In this example, the therapist introduced William to the idea of noticing his thoughts without responding to them by describing them as if they were clouds in the sky. Lots of other metaphors for a similar process have been suggested, including the image of standing in a train station and watching trains go by (Wells, 2009), standing by a stream and watching leaves drift by, or watching soldiers marching in a parade, perhaps holding signs that represent the client's stream of consciousness (Hayes et al., 2012).

T: No, I'm not saying that. What I am saying is that it is possible to have negative thoughts but not to be depressed about them. And the way to stop being depressed about your thoughts is?

W: To stop trying to fix them.

Making Friends with Your Brain

If we are prepared to conclude that struggling against one's thoughts is counterproductive, what's the alternative? One answer might be *acceptance*: a willingness to experience all thoughts, even the really, really unpleasant ones.

Now, I should be clear about what I do and don't mean here. I don't mean that our clients need to give up working on their problems. Rather, these unpleasant thoughts are just products of our own brains—they are part of us. And since they're part of us, perhaps we should learn to get along with them. We could even make friends with them. This is a response-focused emotion regulation strategy, in which we work on eliminating maladaptive *responses* to our negative thoughts, rather than the thoughts themselves.

Let's come back to the example of the therapist working with William.

T: So we know that struggling against your thoughts is a good way to get stuck and a good way to keep feeling crummy. What if, as an alternative, you were willing to have those thoughts? To just let them be there?

W: So I should just be stuck in these thoughts and feel like crap?

T: No, not at all. What I mean is that it seems from your experience that these thoughts are going to keep showing up, whether you want them to or not. All the unwillingness you can muster doesn't seem to be able to keep them away. The stuckness, and the feeling like crap, those are by-products of your unwillingness to have the thoughts.

W: I don't think I get it.

T: Well, think of it this way. The more unwilling you are to experience these unpleasant thoughts, the more you struggle against them by ruminating, avoiding, being

Metaphor

Hayes et al. (2012) use a great metaphor to illustrate the idea of acceptance. They ask the client to imagine that he or she is hosting a party and has invited the whole neighborhood. Joe the Bum, who lives behind the dumpster, has also shown up, and his presence isn't welcome. Here the client has several options. He or she could kick Joe out and then stand guard by the front door to make sure he doesn't come back in. Or he or she could follow Joe around the party, making sure he doesn't misbehave. But in either case, the client is missing out on the party that's going on. Hayes et al. ask, "Are the bums welcome? Can you choose to welcome them in, even though you don't like the fact that they came? If not, what's the party going to be like?" In this metaphor, the party is the client's life, and Joe the Bum is an unwanted thought. Since exerting energy to keep the "bad" thoughts out means missing out on important things in life, they encourage an attitude of willingness and welcoming.

stern with yourself, and so on—and the worse you feel. So if you were more willing to have the thoughts—not like you really have much choice in the matter, anyway—then you wouldn't need to fight so hard, and you wouldn't keep falling into that depression trap. Maybe the unpleasant thoughts could just become like background noise—a noise that perhaps gets fainter and fainter over time, but only if you don't try so hard to make it go away.

W: OK, I guess that makes sense.

T: There's a very old Buddhist quote that goes, "Pain is inevitable. Suffering is optional." If we think about that in terms of your thoughts and feelings, we might say that the initial pain—the negative thoughts that intrude into your mind—is inevitable. But the suffering—the feeling stuck and feeling like crap—is something that you definitely don't have to experience. Imagine what life would be like if you had a negative thought but didn't feel bad about it and didn't feel stuck because of it.

W: It's hard to imagine.

T: Yes, I can appreciate that. Let's try something. I want to write a really depressing thought on this piece of paper here. From our previous discussion, you identified "I'm going to fail miserably" as a really unpleasant thought. So I'll write that on here. (*Does so.*) Now, we don't like this thought, and it's really ugly. But can you also see that it's just some words?

W: Yeah.

T: So what would happen if you folded up this paper and put it in your pocket and carried it around with you the rest of the day?

W: I think it would be depressing.

T: I suppose you could depress yourself over it if you chose to. You could struggle against it. You could try to convince yourself it's not true. You could try to forget it's there. You could kick yourself for thinking it in the first place. You could curse me for giving it to you. All of those responses would be pretty depressing. And, of course, none of them would actually make the thought go away. So then you would be a guy who has this thought *and* is depressed. But what if you tried the willingness alternative? What if you just said to yourself, "OK, I have this. No big deal. Let me get on with my day now." Then you would be a guy who has this thought and is *not* depressed.

W: I can try that.

 Show Me, Don't Tell Me

The therapist used an exercise of having William carry a piece of paper with a negative thought written on it to illustrate the concept of willingness to experience thoughts. As with other exercises, this will likely stick in William's memory better than a dry discussion. Hayes et al. (2012) have come up with several exercises that illustrate a similar point, including writing several negative thoughts on cards and tossing them onto the client, instructing the client to either swat them away (experiential avoidance) or let them fall where they may (willingness).

THE ESSENTIALS

✱ An alternative way of dealing with negative thoughts is to focus not on the content of those thoughts but rather on the person's mental, emotional, and behavioral reactions to the thoughts.

✱ The basic principles of acceptance are:
- Negative thoughts are normal and unavoidable.
- Distress comes less from negative thoughts than from how the person responds to the thoughts.
- Efforts to gain control over negative thoughts may do more harm than good.

✱ The key elements of acceptance interventions are:
- Teaching the client to decrease efforts to control, label, judge, fix, or avoid negative thoughts.
- Teaching the client to pay attention to his or her thoughts and to label them as just thoughts.
- Having the client pay attention to the present moment.
- Redirecting the client's energy away from thought control and toward value-based action.

KEY TERMS AND DEFINITIONS

Acceptance: Willingness to experience and tolerate aversive internal experiences (e.g., thoughts, emotions, or physiological sensations).

Cognitive defusion: Appreciating and understanding thoughts as a product of the mind, rather than as facts.

Experiential avoidance: Efforts to avoid or escape from aversive internal experiences (i.e., thoughts, emotions, or physiological sensations).

Mindfulness: Attending to one's thoughts and feelings in the present moment without making any judgments as to their meaning or value.

Value-based action: Behaviors consistent with, and in pursuit of, one's personal values and long-term goals.

Cognitive Acceptance

Step 1: Identify a negative or maladaptive thought related to your personal target.

Step 2: For a period of 5 minutes (set a timer so you don't have to keep checking), close your eyes and imagine seeing all of your thoughts float past your field of vision, as if you were watching clouds in the sky. Do not judge or evaluate your thoughts; just notice them. If a maladaptive thought related to your personal target shows up, notice that, too, but let it float by with the other thoughts.

What was your experience in Step 2? Specifically: How hard or easy was it? When did it become hard? Did thoughts related to your personal target show up? What was your response to the thoughts? Did your response change over time?

Step 3: For a period of 24 hours, notice any thoughts related to the personal target, but do not judge or evaluate them. Do not attempt to determine whether they are good or bad, accurate or inaccurate, distorted or not. Do not attempt to change them. Do not attempt to avoid them.

What was your experience in Step 3? Specifically: How hard or easy was it? When did it become hard? Did thoughts related to your personal target show up? What was your response to the thoughts? Did your response change over time?

From *Doing CBT* by David F. Tolin. Copyright © 2016 The Guilford Press. Permission to photocopy this worksheet is granted to purchasers of this book for personal use only (see copyright page for details). Purchasers can download enlarged versions of this worksheet (see the box at the end of the table of contents).

CHAPTER 16

Going Deeper with Core Beliefs

Finding Core Beliefs

As was the case with interpretations (see Chapter 14), the first step in working with core beliefs is to get them "out on the table" so that the therapist and client can discuss them openly and frankly. Because core beliefs are below the threshold of ordinary awareness (meaning that the person is not used to thinking about them explicitly), we often have to use some strategies to get to them.

Connecting the Dots: Finding Core Beliefs Using Pattern Detection

Often, as you learn about the client's interpretations, a pattern begins to emerge. Like the dots in a connect-the-dots puzzle, the individual interpretations all seem to be part of a larger whole. The trick is for you and the client to use **pattern detection** to discover what they have in common. That common theme may be a maladaptive core belief.

Here, the therapist is working with Suzanne (S), our client with GAD and benzodiazepine abuse. They have been discussing Suzanne's interpretations over the past few sessions, and the therapist wants to move toward addressing Suzanne's core beliefs using pattern detection, combined with our old standby of Socratic questioning.

> T: I'd like to take a moment and review some of the thought monitoring forms you've filled out over the last couple of weeks. You've come up with several good examples of negative interpretations: "My husband probably had a car accident"; "We'll lose our retirement money because of the stock market"; "If I'm late for the meeting, everything will fall apart"; and "Because I can't keep up with the chores, the house will be a wreck, and we'll never be comfortable." These are the thoughts that went through your head during different stressful situations.
>
> S: Right. I just get anxious about all of these things.
>
> T: I wonder whether you see a pattern here?

S: They're all really anxious and worried?

T: Well, that's true. I guess what I'm wondering is whether there's a way that we could sum all of these thoughts up—a belief, or a way of seeing the world, that would be consistent with all of them.

S: I guess they all share the general idea that something bad is going to happen.

T: Yes, I see what you mean. They all seem to indicate some kind of looming threat, don't they?

S: Yes. "Looming threat" is a good way to put it.

T: Let's talk a bit more about looming threat. How would someone who saw looming threats everywhere describe the world?

S: Um . . . I suppose someone who saw looming threats everywhere would say that the world is dangerous?

T: So the world is dangerous. What might the word *looming* imply?

S: I guess *looming* means that the threat is right around the corner and getting closer and closer.

T: So it's not just that the world is dangerous; it's that the danger is growing by the minute?

S: Yes, that sounds right.

T: And what would that person say about the future?

S: The future is not good?

T: In what way? What specifically is not good?

S: Everything's going to go badly.

T: So the world is dangerous, the danger is growing by the minute, and everything's going to go badly. I wonder whether those ideas are part of how you think.

S: Yeah, I guess I do.

T: And that set of beliefs serves as your filter for how you look at things.

S: It does, but a lot of that is probably true. I mean, things have gone badly for me.

T: That's true; they have. I wonder, though, whether that means that they always *will* go badly.

S: I think they will.

T: You could be right about that. After all, I can't predict the future. At the moment, you believe this pretty strongly. That's fine. As we go, however, I may want to come back and ask you a bit more about it.

These core beliefs—"the world is dangerous," "the danger is growing by the minute," and "everything's going to go badly"—are probably not Suzanne's only maladaptive core beliefs. From what we know about her dependent personality characteristics, we might hypothesize that she also has maladaptive core beliefs about her own competence and her need to rely on others. The therapist might opt to pursue these core beliefs as well.

Note that Suzanne clings to her core belief fairly strongly and brings up some evidence that seems to support the belief. This is not surprising. The therapist opts not to challenge it too strongly at this point, choosing instead just to notice it, validate it as part of Suzanne's experience, and agree to revisit it. Part of the art of CBT is striking a balance between challenging and validating.

Holding Up a Mirror

Pattern detection is a good way to help the client take a good look at his or her interpretations and what they might indicate about core beliefs. Remember that core beliefs are usually never verbalized or thought about directly; rather, they serve as the unspoken "program" that influences the interpretations of daily events. By reflecting the client's interpretations back to him or her in a specific manner (e.g., linking them together as variations on a possible theme), we help put the client in a better position to look at the underlying assumptions and beliefs that he or she might never have thought about previously.

"If That Were True, What Would That Mean?": Finding Core Beliefs Using the Downward Arrow

In Chapter 14 we discussed using the downward arrow strategy to "decatastrophize" interpretations. The downward arrow can also be used to uncover core beliefs. As described previously, the downward arrow is a series of "if–then" questions, each assuming (for the sake of discussion) that the client's previous statement is true. In this application, however, the aim is to ask questions directed toward *meaning*, rather than toward what would happen. So the therapist is repeatedly asking variations on the question "If that were true, what would that mean?"

Here, the therapist uses the downward arrow with Melissa (M), our client with complex PTSD and interpersonal difficulties secondary to chronic abuse when she was a child.

M: I don't know why I can't just have a normal relationship.

T: Define *normal.*

M: You know, like just date someone, and have a nice time together, and just love each other, you know?

T: That does sound nice. What's preventing you from having that?

M: It's just that whenever I start to like someone I just mess it up. Like I pick a fight or I decide that they're not right for me, or whatever.

T: And you think this is what's going to keep happening.

M: Right.

T: So you have this thought that "If I like someone, I'll mess it up somehow."

M: Yes.

T: Let's assume for the moment that that's true—let's assume that you will indeed mess it up. If that's the case, what would that tell you?

M: That I'm just no good at relationships.

T: OK, and if that's true, that you're no good at relationships, what would that mean to you?

M: That I just have something wrong with me that makes me unable to be with people.

T: And if that were the case, that there's something wrong with you like this, what would that say about you?

M: That I'm . . . I don't know . . . damaged.

Metaphor

Padesky (1994, p. 273) uses the topic of prejudice to illustrate for clients the nature of core beliefs, the effect of core beliefs, and factors that maintain core beliefs. When someone is prejudiced against a certain group of people, he or she tends to maintain those prejudicial beliefs despite contradictory evidence. Certain information that might contradict the prejudice gets ignored, distorted, or reasoned away. So it is with core beliefs. We could ask the client to think about someone he or she knows who has a particular prejudice and use that as an example for how we understand core beliefs. It becomes clear to the client, through this discussion, that the prejudice (and belief) will only be overcome when the person starts actively looking for, and incorporating, belief-incongruent information.

T: I see. So perhaps part of what's bothering you is the fact that underneath it all, you believe that you are damaged.

M: Yeah, I think so.

Finding Core Beliefs Using Checklists

As was the case with eliciting interpretations, sometimes it's helpful to use a written checklist to help clients identify their core beliefs. There are a few well-validated, commercially available questionnaires that you can use. Alternatively, I have created one, the Core Beliefs Checklist, which is provided in Appendix B. Please note that this measure has not been subjected to psychometric study and should not be considered a definitive measure of anything. Rather, think of it as a conversation starter.

Engaging the Frontal Lobes

Although there's not much data to tell us exactly what happens in the brain when someone identifies and challenges a core belief, we can make an educated guess that part of what is happening is that we are activating the "thinking" parts of the brain to deal with material that had not previously been processed in that manner. In keeping with our previous discussions, just about anything that gets the person looking at his or her thoughts, beliefs, and cognitive processes in a new way is a good thing. So the mere act of identifying a core belief, putting words to it, and having the client consider the meaning and implication of those words probably helps start them down the path toward thinking differently. So if we ask the client to dispute the core belief, that's probably helpful. If we ask him or her to test out the core belief and gather data, that's probably helpful. If we ask the client to "play with" the core belief by writing or talking about it, that's probably helpful. If we ask the client to notice and be mindful of the core belief, that's probably helpful—because all of these interventions are basically creating the same process in the brain: getting those frontal lobes engaged where they had previously been quiet.

Finding Core Beliefs by Finding Stuckness

Often, the client's core beliefs will become apparent through "stuck points" in therapy. You may find, for example:

- The client continuously says things like "I know it's true rationally; I just don't *feel* it." I tend to rephrase this back to the client as "You know what the right words are, but you don't really *believe* them." In other words, despite using various cognitive restructuring strategies (see Chapter 14), the client has a hard time letting go of a particular cognitive distortion.

- Despite an acceptance of the rationale for performing a new behavior, adequate skills to perform the behavior, and appropriate motivation for behavioral change, the client continuously reverts back to old behavioral patterns. Often, he or she can't fully articulate the reasons for doing so.

- We see stuck points in the therapeutic relationship itself. Either the relationship can't seem to get started in a positive direction, or it starts to derail over the course of treatment. The client, for example, might resist the therapist's suggestions, either directly or indirectly. That could be a sign that the therapist has misjudged the client's stage of change (see Chapter 7), and/or it could reflect the fact that certain core beliefs are being activated during the therapy. Alternatively, the client may show difficulty establishing and maintaining a collaborative, warm relationship with appropriate therapeutic boundaries— the client may seem guarded, overly clingy or reassurance seeking, chronically disgruntled, dramatic, and so forth (Prasko et al., 2010). These patterns similarly may suggest that the therapy, or the therapist, is activating maladaptive core beliefs.

Bringing the Problem into the Room

Remember that some of our greatest therapeutic opportunities take place when the client's problem is right in front of us, staring us in the face. So a client getting "stuck" represents a great opportunity to learn more about the client and work on core beliefs.

This is true when the therapeutic relationship gets "stuck," as well. Our psychodynamic colleagues invite transference reactions (Gabbard, 1994), and many psychotherapists have suggested that *alliance ruptures,* which could be brief "blips" in the therapeutic relationship or more serious or chronic relational problems, provide an opportunity to link the rupture to characteristic patterns in the client's life (e.g., Safran et al., 2011; Safran & Segal, 1990). That's not to say alliance ruptures shouldn't be fixed—indeed, when a rupture is detected, the therapist needs to manage the relationship extra carefully—but it's important to see the opportunity that lies beneath the problem. We wouldn't use the same kinds of transference interpretations that would be used in a psychodynamic therapy; however, we would ask the client to describe his or her cognitive and emotional reactions to the therapist, the therapy, or a specific therapeutic procedure and query whether those reactions are part of a larger, long-standing pattern (see Chapter 7 for additional discussion). So, for example, a client who behaves suspiciously toward the therapist might hold the core belief that "people can't be trusted." With that hypothesis in mind, the therapist might ask the client to describe his or her thoughts about the therapy and the therapist and start a discussion about whether the client has similar reactions to other people in his or her life.

Restructuring Core Beliefs

Do You Go There?

There are different schools of thought about the importance of addressing core beliefs in CBT. Some suggest that CBT should be all about core beliefs (Young et al., 2003), whereas others make little mention of core beliefs at all or suggest that core beliefs should be addressed only after symptom reduction has been achieved.

There are certainly some cases in which it does not make much sense to attempt to restructure core beliefs.

• In an inpatient setting, for example, you usually have a limited amount of time to work with the client, and that time would likely be better spent pursuing other goals, such as immediate symptom relief, functional improvement, and preparing to transfer treatment gains to the natural environment (Ludgate et al., 1993).

• At times, the aims of the therapy are highly focal. As an extreme example, if I'm treating someone with an uncomplicated phobia, there is little reason to go into the person's core beliefs—the therapy works extremely well and has quite durable results without doing so (Öst, 1989). One could make an argument that there are many other examples of treatment for fairly focal (even if serious) problems in which the treatment goes fine without having to dig into the person's underlying core belief system.

• Sometimes, the amount of behavioral work to be done diminishes the relative importance of addressing core beliefs. In some cases, for example, what's really important right now is boosting the client's behavioral skill repertoire (see Chapter 12), improving patterns of maladaptive behavior through direct prescriptions such as activity scheduling or exposure (see Chapters 10 and 11), or rearranging contingencies to promote more adaptive behavior (see Chapter 9). That doesn't mean that the client should *never* address his or her core beliefs; rather, when time is limited, core beliefs may be a bit lower on the hierarchy of needs.

• I am less likely to go the core beliefs route with children and adolescents than I am with adults. This isn't to say kids don't have core beliefs. But their core beliefs tend to be less well formed and entrenched than those of adults, making other strategies more appealing.

In other cases, however, it makes a lot of sense to go after core beliefs. Maladaptive personality traits, which are commonly conceptualized in terms of core beliefs and schemas, seem particularly well addressed by this strategy (A. T. Beck & Freeman, 1990; Young, 1999). Even for those disorders previously referred to as "Axis I" (i.e., not personality) disorders, an argument has been made that addressing core beliefs or schemas can improve results and reduce risk of relapse (Young et al., 2003), though empirical evidence for that assertion is slim (e.g., N. S. Jacobson et al., 1996).

When Do You Target Core Beliefs?

Young's model of *schema therapy* (Young, 1999; Young et al., 2003) starts assessing and challenging core beliefs right away. Beck's model of *cognitive therapy* (A. T. Beck, Emery, & Greenberg, 1985; A. T. Beck & Freeman, 1990; A. T. Beck et al., 1979), on the other hand, holds off on challenging core beliefs until after the client has learned to identify and challenge interpretations and has begun experiencing some symptom improvement, usually in mid- to later stages of therapy.

When I do address core beliefs, I tend to do it closer to Beck's style. I work on interpretations and behavioral patterns first. As time allows, and as the material presents itself in the therapy, I start to work in the idea of core beliefs, identifying and challenging them along the way.

. . . And I always have exceptions to the rule. Sometimes the core belief really does seem to be part and parcel of the presenting problem, and it's just sitting there right in front of me. So in a case like that, I'll often go for it, regardless of what other work we have or have not already done. There's no strict schedule that needs to be followed here, as long as we are broadly following a reasonable hierarchy of treatment goals (see Chapter 7), usually along the lines of: (1) threats to safety of self or others, (2) therapy-interfering behaviors, (3) problems that have an immediate negative impact on functioning or quality of life, and (4) problems that are likely to worsen and cause a negative impact on functioning or quality of life.

The Process of Modifying Core Beliefs

The strategy for modifying core beliefs parallels that of modifying interpretations. Broadly speaking, we want to help the client to identify the core beliefs and to understand how they might be maladaptive, then employ various strategies to undermine the strength of belief and introduce new ways of thinking. The difference between challenging interpretations and challenging core beliefs is largely one of scope, given the broader influence of the core beliefs.

It should also be noted that changing core beliefs is often a longer and more labor-intensive process (for the client and the therapist) than is changing interpretations. As noted in our meaty conceptualization (see Chapter 5), core beliefs are highly entrenched. The client often believes these things at a basic or "gut" level and has likely never even considered the fact that they exist, let alone that they might be inaccurate or unhelpful. Significant cognitive biases have likely developed that serve to "confirm" the core belief.

Identifying What's Wrong

As was the case with interpretations, we are most likely to be successful when the core belief is articulated verbally and discussed freely between the client and the therapist. One way to help the client understand the maladaptive nature of the core belief is to identify and articulate its pros and cons.

Here, the therapist works with William (W), our client with a mix of depression, pain, and dependent personality characteristics. Having worked on his interpretations and maladaptive behavior patterns for a while in therapy, William is starting to feel considerably better, and the therapist wishes to direct the discussion toward his long-standing core beliefs. In this case, William has completed the Core Beliefs Checklist in Appendix B (although a similar discussion might occur had the therapist used the pattern detection, downward arrow, or finding "stuckness" strategies).

T: As I look over this checklist, I see a bunch of statements that seemed to ring true to you.

W: Yeah, I realized as I was going through it just how many negative thoughts I have.

T: If we look at the items for which you circled "I totally believe this," do any jump out at you as being especially important?

W: I think "I am helpless" seems important.

T: Tell me why that one seems particularly important.

W: I guess it just seemed like that one captures a lot of the other ones.

T: Like it's bigger, somehow.

W: Maybe.

T: OK, for now let's just treat it as a guess. So we can guess that you have this belief that "I am helpless." It seems to me that this belief really has a lot to do with how you think a lot of the time. We have a name for this: We call it a core belief. We use the word *core* here to mean that you have become very strongly attached to this belief, or it has become very attached to you, and so you're kind of always walking around with it. Does that seem to describe it for you?

W: Well, I'm not sure if it's really a belief. It's not like I just repeat that to myself.

T: No, you don't. You're not actively thinking it. What I'm thinking is that even when you're not literally saying the words "I am helpless" to yourself, you're carrying it around with you. It's just become part of how you regard yourself, and how you engage with the world. Does that make sense?

W: Maybe, I'm not sure.

T: Well, let's look at it this way. Would you say that you often feel like a person who believes he is helpless?

W: I guess I feel down a lot.

T: OK. Do you often act like a person who believes he is helpless?

W: Yeah, I definitely act like that at least some of the time.

T: So you feel and act like a person who believes he is helpless. Would it be reasonable for us to guess that somewhere deep down, even though you might not say it, this is what you believe?

W: Yeah, I guess so.

T: It's sounding that way to me, too. In some ways, that belief forms a basic filter that you view everything through. With that core belief, it's no wonder that you have some of the interpretations that you do. Perhaps we can see an example of that happening. When we were talking a while back about your marriage, you were having the thought that "my marriage is broken." How could that core belief of "I'm helpless" have played a role in your thoughts about your marriage?

W: I'm not sure.

T: Well, let's think about it a bit. Imagine someone who is always walking around with the core belief "I'm helpless." And then that person goes home and things aren't going very well with his husband. How would he be likely to respond, mentally?

W: He'd feel helpless?

T: Yes, probably so. How might that be reflected in what he thinks about?

W: I guess he'd focus on all of the things that are wrong.

T: And that are out of his control?

W: Maybe.

T: So what would he not be thinking about?

W: The things that he actually can control.

T: Right. So we can take a guess here that when you walk around with this core belief of "I'm helpless," that changes how you respond to things. You are likely to focus in on negative things that are outside of your control and are likely not to pay attention to things that you can control.

W: I get it.

T: Now, I'm not asking you to believe otherwise just now. But for a moment, can we talk about the advantages and disadvantages of viewing yourself as helpless? (*Draws a line down the center of a piece of paper.*) On this side of the paper, let's list the advantages. What can you think of?

W: Advantages? I can't really think of any.

T: Oh, surely there must be some advantages; otherwise, why believe it?

W: Well, I guess in some ways it lets me off the hook.

T: That's good. (*Writes.*) By perceiving yourself to be helpless, there's less responsibility on you. Anything else?

W: I think that's it.

T: OK, let's think of the disadvantages. What comes to mind?

W: (*long pause*) I guess it keeps me stuck.

T: Keeps you stuck. Can you elaborate on that?

W: Well, it means that I'm going to keep having negative interpretations and I'll keep feeling depressed.

T: (*Writes.*) It sets you up to be depressed.

W: Yeah. And I guess that if I'm not thinking of the things that are under my control, then I won't really do much to make things better.

T: (*Writes.*) So you get kind of paralyzed out of helplessness, and don't take action.

W: Right.

T: Anything else?

W: That's all I can think of.

T: On balance, then, do you get a sense that this core belief of being helpless is doing more good than harm, or doing more harm than good?

W: I think it's doing more harm than good.

Challenging Core Beliefs

Through therapy (and often over the course of many sessions), we want to undermine the core belief—to begin to lessen the degree to which the client clings to it and to raise doubts about its accuracy and necessity. We want, over time, to help the client arrive at and practice adopting a new, more realistic core belief.

Challenging Core Beliefs by Examining the Evidence

As was the case with interpretations, we can challenge core beliefs by *examining the evidence* for and against the belief. This can be done on a piece of paper with a line drawn down the middle, as shown in Figure 16.1; a blank version is provided in Appendix B. After discussing the evidence for and against the core belief, the therapist and client come

Core belief: _I'm basically incompetent_

Evidence _for_ core belief	Evidence _against_ core belief
I screw up a lot of things.	I do a lot of things right.
My wife often has to fix my errors.	I often come up with an answer when no one else does.
I didn't do well in school.	My poor school performance was partly because I had attention problems that no one recognized.

New, balanced core belief
Like everyone, I have strengths and weaknesses. I do some things well and some things not so well. But I'm basically a competent person.

FIGURE 16.1. Sample worksheet for examining the evidence for core beliefs.

up with a new, more adaptive core belief (with the understanding that the new belief will likely seem foreign and hard to accept at first).

We potentially run into the same sticking points in examining evidence for core beliefs that we do in examining evidence for interpretations. For example, the client may (quite understandably) come up with more evidence for the core belief than against it, in which case part of the therapist's job is to help the client identify evidence against the belief. We can also have a sticking point in which the "evidence" for a core belief isn't particularly strong evidence for the belief at all. The therapist can help the client to critically evaluate the evidence in order to determine whether it should be believed.

Here, the therapist is working again with Melissa (M), our client with complex PTSD. During the downward arrow discussion, Melissa identified the core belief "I am damaged."

T: So we have this core belief of "I am damaged," and it seems that you think this belief might not be so good for you.

M: No, it's not. I hate having to feel this way all the time.

T: Understood. It's hard for me to imagine someone with that belief really feeling very happy. So is that belief true?

M: It feels true.

T: Meaning you pretty much believe it.

M: Yeah.

T: When we were talking about interpretations, we took a look at the evidence for and against. Remember that?

M: Yeah, it was helpful to look at things from another perspective that way.

T: Well, let's try the same thing here. Let's look at the evidence for and against the idea that you are damaged. (_Draws a line down the center of a piece of paper._) What evidence can you think of that supports that belief?

M: Well, I was abused.

T: You were, yes. And that's evidence for you being damaged?

M: It feels like it.

T: (*Writes.*) OK, let's add it here although I might want to come back and talk about that one some more. But for now, it feels like evidence to you, so we'll add it. What else?

M: My relationships are a mess. You know, I push people away and I make stupid choices.

T: (*Writes.*) OK, I'll add that one here. What else can you think of?

M: Well, I just feel like crap all the time. I'm depressed, I get angry, it's like I'm never in control of my feelings.

T: (*Writes.*) So that one can go here as well, that you feel like crap and not in control of your feelings. Anything else?

M: I can't think of anything else.

T: So let's look at the flip side now. Any evidence that would not support this belief? That is, any evidence that might suggest that you're not so damaged?

M: (*long pause*) I'm having a hard time thinking of anything. When I look at my life, all I see is a train wreck.

T: It's true you've had a lot of bad experiences, and you have felt very bad for a long time. I guess what I'm wondering is whether you can see anything undamaged about yourself? Any good or healthy qualities, for example?

M: Um . . . sometimes I'm a nice person. But a lot of the time I'm not; I get into arguments and I mess up whatever relationships I have.

T: Yes, we captured some of that information over on this side of the page, but I think I heard you say that sometimes you're a nice person? How so?

M: Well, sometimes I do nice things for people. Like I helped out my neighbor when she was recovering from her surgery. I gave her rides and brought her meals and stuff.

T: Hmm, that's worth noting. (*Writes.*) So sometimes you really are nice to other people.

M: I guess.

T: Seems like you're having a hard time buying this right now.

M: Maybe a little. Bringing some meals over to a neighbor doesn't really make me feel like I'm not damaged.

T: I understand, and I'm not at all surprised. After thinking a certain way for a long time, and having that belief be so important in your life, we're not going to change it with a few words. That's OK. You can keep this belief for as long as it suits you. Right now we're just coming up with ideas.

M: OK.

T: What other evidence would not support the belief that you are damaged?

M: I guess there are some things I do all right.

T: Such as?

M: I take care of my kids.

T: That you do. They're fed, clothed, go to school. What else; do you provide a safe environment for them?

M: Yes. I keep them safe.

T: What about love?

M: They get a lot of love from me.

T: You sound like a pretty good mom.

M: I guess I am.

T: (*Writes.*) So maybe "I'm a good mom" can be some evidence against the belief. What else do you do all right?

M: I have a job.

T: Yes, you have a job. What does that tell you?

M: I guess it tells me that someone would hire me.

T: Well, it does tell us that. Anything else it tells us?

M: That I can do it?

T: Seems so. You didn't just get the job; you kept it, despite feeling like crap.

M: I did, yeah.

T: (*Writes.*) So having a job could be some evidence against the belief as well. As we look over this evidence for and against, what are you thinking about the belief "I'm damaged?"

M: I guess maybe it's not 100% true.

Challenging Core Beliefs by Considering Alternatives

Considering alternatives to the core belief is another helpful strategy. In essence, just as we did with interpretations, we're trying to encourage the client to step outside of his or her frame of reference and consider other ways of thinking. We probably won't get the client to believe these alternatives, at least not right away. But the first step is just to get them out there for consideration.

Here, the therapist is working with Suzanne (S), our client with generalized anxiety disorder and benzodiazepine abuse. Previously, Suzanne had identified core beliefs of "The world is dangerous," "The danger is growing by the minute," and "Everything's going to go badly."

T: Let's talk about this idea that the world is dangerous. Is that accurate?

S: Well, there are a lot of dangerous things out there in the world.

T: That's true; there are. Would someone else look at the world, with those dangers, and reach the same conclusion, that the world is a dangerous place?

S: They might.

T: They might. Would that be a guarantee?

S: Maybe not a guarantee, no.

T: So they might reach a different conclusion. What different conclusion might they reach?

S: I don't know. Maybe that it's not so dangerous?

T: I guess that's possible. If I took a survey of people and asked them to tell me their thoughts about the world, in terms of safety and danger, what kind of results do you think I'd get?

S: I guess you'd have some people say that the world is a dangerous place, but maybe some other people would say that there are some dangerous things in the world but that doesn't make the world dangerous overall.

T: Yes, they might say that. If you weren't anxious—I know this might be a little difficult for you to imagine—but if you weren't anxious, do you think you would still believe that the world is dangerous?

S: I guess I wouldn't. Or at least not so much.

T: What would you believe?

S: I'd believe that the world is pretty safe, even though there are dangers.

T: Safe enough?

S: Safe enough, yes.

Here, the therapist continues the conversation with Melissa (M), who had examined the evidence for the core belief "I am damaged."

T: If we think now that the belief "I am damaged" is not 100% true, is there another belief that might be more truthful? I'm not asking you to believe it just now; I just want to see if we can identify one. What could you believe about yourself other than "damaged"?

M: Um . . . I've been through a lot but . . . (*Pauses.*)

T: . . . but . . .

M: I survived and kept some things together?

T: "I'm a survivor"?

M: Maybe.

T: "I'm basically competent"?

M: Maybe. I just don't know if I believe those things.

T: No, I wouldn't expect you to. Not yet, anyway. But let's write them down so we remember them.

Challenging Core Beliefs Using Scaling

Core beliefs tend to be fairly extreme in their wording. Because they are so deeply ingrained and unexamined, they tend to have an all-or-nothing quality to them. *Scaling* can be used to help the client adopt a more nuanced view of things.

Let's go back to William (W). Here, the therapist uses scaling to challenge the all-or-nothing quality of his belief that he is helpless.

T: So we have this core belief of "I'm helpless," and it seems that this belief is really at the heart of a lot of your reactions to things.

W: Right.

T: I wonder whether we could determine how helpless you believe yourself to be. What's the most helpless thing you can think of? You know, completely and totally helpless.

W: Hmm . . . maybe a turtle on its back.

T: Oh, that's a good one. That's very helpless. Now how about the opposite of that—the least helpless thing you can imagine? Something completely in control and all powerful.

W: Um . . . maybe someone who has complete control over everything, like an emperor or something.

T: OK, very good. So let's think about there being a spectrum of helplessness and control, ranging from a turtle on its back, on one extreme, to an emperor on the other extreme.

W: OK.

T: And all of us are somewhere on that spectrum. Where are you on that spectrum?

W: Hmm. Well, I'm not as helpless as a turtle on his back. Maybe somewhere in the middle? Like maybe halfway between the middle and the turtle.

T: So about a quarter of the way up from a turtle on his back.

W: That sounds about right.

T: It's interesting that you didn't put yourself closer to the turtle. Why not?

W: Well, it's not like I'm completely helpless. I feel that way a lot, but I know that I'm capable of doing some things for myself.

TIB Alert!

Therapy-interfering behaviors (TIBs) are common when you work with core beliefs. By definition, core beliefs are resistant to change. All of us, therapists and clients alike, act in ways, or put ourselves into situations, that seem to confirm what we "know" to be true. We pay particular attention to information that seems to prove us right, ignoring information that might contradict our core beliefs. When faced with information that seems to go against what we believe, we have a whole armamentarium of cognitive distortions that will twist and filter that information until it seems to fit, or at least until it doesn't seem contradictory.

We need to recognize that changing core beliefs takes time and effort and not a small amount of mental discomfort from the client. Changing long-standing ways of viewing oneself and the world is hard and unsettling. Whereas interpretations might collapse like a house of cards when we challenge them, changing a core belief is a little bit like chipping away at a brick wall. It's doable, but it takes time and consistent effort. You're probably not going to change a deeply held belief in a single session.

Sometimes, when faced with TIBs, it's tempting to shrug our shoulders and conclude that the client "wants" to keep believing what he or she believes. I've heard jaded therapists conclude that a client "just wants to be miserable." Nonsense. No one wants to be miserable. Linehan (1993), who has spent a lot of time treating clients with the often-maligned diagnosis of borderline personality disorder and who are often accused of "wanting" to be miserable, has stated that "all people are, at any given point in time, doing the best they can" (p. 106). It's a pretty powerful statement, when you think about it. It means that the client doesn't want to be suffering but that various influences (both internal and external to the person) have placed limits around what he or she can accomplish. Our aim, then, is not simply to admonish the client to "try harder," nor is it to imply that he or she doesn't really want to feel better. Rather, our aim is to identify, understand, and eventually overcome those influences that are maintaining the TIB.

Notice that the therapist uses a little trick of speech here. The therapist asked William why he was unlike the turtle, not why he was unlike the emperor. He did something similar using scaling for interpretations in Chapter 14, when he asked the client why she did not rate herself as *more* of a failure. This strategy is borrowed from motivational interviewing (W. R. Miller & Rollnick, 2013). By asking William to distance himself verbally from the "unhealthy" (turtle) side of the scale, he is structuring the discussion in a manner that is conducive to having William talk about his areas of competence.

Challenging Core Beliefs by Keeping Core Belief Diaries

Self-monitoring in the form of **core belief diaries** can be useful for addressing core beliefs. Here, the aim is to help the client observe him- or herself or the world over time, looking for evidence that does and does not support the maladaptive belief.

These diary forms can be created "on the fly" by the therapist, in collaboration with the client. As just one example, here the therapist is working with Lauren (L), our client with schizophrenia. Through a series of strategies, the therapist and Lauren arrived at the core belief "Others will hurt me, manipulate me, or take advantage of me."

T: So we have this core belief that people will hurt you, manipulate you, or take advantage of you. And that belief, whether true or not, seems to have a strong influence on you.

L: Yes, it seems like whatever I do, that's my assumption.

T: Of course, you spend most of your time at home by yourself.

L: Well yes, that's because I don't want to get hurt.

T: Understood. No one wants to get hurt, so I can't blame you, having this belief, for wanting to stay home. But there's a potential down side to staying home, as well. You don't really get a chance to see whether your belief is accurate or not.

L: I guess that's true.

T: I wonder whether we could come up with some homework that would allow you to evaluate this belief?

L: You mean, see whether people hurt me and so on?

T: Yeah, something like that. Let me show you what I have in mind. (*Takes out a piece of paper and writes [see Figure 16.2].*) I'd like you to try going places and doing things where you might encounter other people.

L: That would be scary.

T: Yes, it probably will be, at least at first. But I'd like you to do your best with this. Remember, what's scaring you is a belief that seems very true to you, but then again you haven't had much opportunity to actually check it out. If it goes badly, you can always stop and we can try something else. Would you be willing to try this, just as an experiment?

L: OK, I guess I could try it.

T: I think it makes sense to do this in places that most people would consider more or less safe. So, for example, I don't think I'd advise you to go to a really dangerous part of town. But maybe some place like a grocery store or a shopping mall—things that the average person doesn't feel threatened by.

Date	Activity	With whom did I interact?	How did they act towards me?	Did they hurt, manipulate, or take advantage of me?
				Yes No
				Yes No
				Yes No

FIGURE 16.2. Sample "on the fly" core belief diary.

L: OK.

T: Each time you go out, I'd like you to write down the date and what you were doing here. Then I'd like you to write down who you encountered. Maybe you know that person's name, or maybe you just write "a guy with a hat." What's really important is that you write down how that person acted toward you—that is, did they smile, frown, talk to you, and so on.

L: OK, I think I get it.

T: And then in this last part, I'd like you to circle whether, in your opinion, that person or those people hurt you, manipulated you, or took advantage of you. This part's really critical, because it gives us direct evidence for or against the belief. So I'd like you to come up with your best "yes" or "no" on this one.

In the next session, the therapist follows up on Lauren's homework.

T: Let's talk about the homework from last week. How did it go?

L: It was interesting. I did what you suggested and I went out to some places. Like I went to the grocery store and then I walked around the mall.

T: Congratulations! I know you were scared of that idea so it's great that you had the courage to give this a try. And so what did you record when you went out?

L: Well, no one tried to hurt me or manipulate me or take advantage of me.

T: That's certainly good. How did they act?

L: Really pretty friendly. The sales clerk smiled and said "have a nice day."

T: I see. What about other people, like people you just passed by at the mall or in the store?

L: Mostly they just ignored me. They didn't seem to be paying attention to me.

T: OK, so you went out and found some evidence here that at least some people are friendly, and at least some people are just wrapped up in their own business and aren't paying attention to you.

L: Yes.

T: How does that affect your core belief?

L: I guess it seems a little less true. But I still think there are people out there who would hurt me.

T: Well, there are. People aren't 100% nice, and so it doesn't make sense to be 100% trusting. But perhaps people also aren't 100% malicious, and so it doesn't make sense to be 100% mistrustful.

L: Maybe.

Now, this conversation, like any other conversation, could have gone in several different directions. Lauren could, by virtue of her biased perceptions, have misinterpreted a clerk's smile and "have a nice day" as a veiled threat and therefore taken it as evidence in favor of her core belief. She could have been hypervigilant for threat (attentional bias) and directed her attention toward the most hostile-looking people in the mall, rather than more benign attentional targets. She could even have encountered someone who was indeed malicious. All of these things are possible, yet none of them are a good reason not to do this kind of exercise. A skilled therapist tries to arrange the exercise in a way that maximizes the client's chances of success (e.g., advising Lauren to go to a reasonably safe shopping mall or grocery store, rather than to a dangerous part of town). When biases of attention or interpretation seem to be present, we make therapy out of them. So, for example, if Lauren misinterpreted the cashier's behaviors as being threatening, the therapist can use the cognitive restructuring strategies described in Chapter 14 to help Lauren evaluate and challenge her interpretations about the cashier; alternatively, the therapist could use acceptance strategies (see Chapter 15) to help her notice and detach from those interpretations.

Challenging Core Beliefs by Acting the Opposite

At times, after a core belief has been identified, it can be helpful to encourage the client to try **acting the opposite,** that is, behaving in a manner that seems to be the opposite of the belief. For example, a client with the core belief "I'm incompetent" might be encouraged to perform an activity which he or she has a high likelihood of doing competently. A client with the core belief "I should never show weakness" might be encouraged to deliberately show some form of weakness to other people. A client with the core belief "Things need to be perfect" might be encouraged to deliberately do things imperfectly.

Acting the Opposite

Notice that acting the opposite is a behavioral intervention for a cognitive target. CBT has a lot of those—remember that behaviors, thoughts, and emotions all influence each other. Here, having identified a maladaptive core belief, we ask the client to behave *as if* the belief were not true. We're not directly challenging the belief; rather, we're encouraging him or her to "test drive" a new attitude and to notice his or her reactions. So, for example, we might ask Melissa to go somewhere or do something and act *as if* she were not damaged, or we might ask Suzanne to act *as if* the world were not so dangerous.

Sometimes, the client will balk at the idea of doing a complete 180-degree turn on the core belief, even when it's framed as an experiment. That's OK – baby steps. In such cases, we might compromise by having the client act in a manner that represents a less extreme version of the core belief, such as deliberately introducing tiny, hard-to-notice imperfections.

And, of course, the therapist always needs to use common sense. We select exercises that have a high probability of success (even though such success can never be guaranteed). So we don't ask the perfectionistic client to make a bunch of huge mistakes that could get him or her fired, and we don't ask the timid client to go for a walk at night through murder alley.

This strategy overlaps considerably with the topics of direct behavioral prescriptions (see Chapter 10) and exposure (see Chapter 11), and we'll talk more about them there. Remember, you can achieve cognitive change with behavioral strategies.

Challenging Core Beliefs by Talking to Them

In their schema therapy, Young et al. (2003) take an interesting approach, derived from the **empty chair technique** in Gestalt therapy (Perls, 1973). They ask the client to talk to the core belief, often pretending that the belief is a separate person sitting in another chair in the room. Then they have the client take the role of the core belief and talk back. The "dialogue" can go back and forth like this, with coaching from the therapist, in order to weaken the strength of the core belief.

I like this idea for a couple of reasons. First, the idea of "talking to" the core belief serves to externalize the belief (here the effect diverges from the aims of Gestalt), enabling the client to evaluate it a bit more critically. Even adopting the role of the core belief and talking back seems to have an externalizing effect because it is framed in the context of role playing. Behaving, during an exercise, as if you believe in the core belief 100% may actually raise additional doubts in the client's head—speaking in extremes often causes opposite thoughts to come to mind more readily (Hayes et al., 2012). Second, I have often found empty-chair-style strategies to be quite emotionally evocative. Because it's different from the usual mode of thought, and because thoughts are articulated in a "raw" form, there can be a more visceral reaction—which can be helpful for the overly cerebral client.

Here, the therapist is working again with Melissa (M), our client with complex PTSD. As you may recall, Melissa had identified the core belief "I'm damaged."

> T: I'd like to see if we can have a conversation with this core belief that you're damaged. Can we try something here? I'd like to have you pretend to be this core belief and articulate your opinions—really try to be persuasive about them. And then I'd like you to be the healthier side of you, and see how you might answer what the belief has to say.

M: OK.

T: So let's start by having you be the belief. Say what you think about Melissa.

M: (*as the belief side*) Um . . . Melissa is really damaged. After everything that's happened to her, she's just a mess. She can't do anything right and she can't have a decent relationship with anybody.

T: OK, now be the healthier side of Melissa. What do you have to say about that?

M: (*as the healthy side*) I guess I'd have to say that I'm not that damaged. I mean, I do take care of my kids, so that's got to mean something. And I still have my job. A really damaged person wouldn't be able to do that.

T: Now go back to the belief side again.

M: (*as the belief side*) You take care of your kids, but only barely. Yes, you do feed them and clothe them, but that doesn't make you Mother of the Year. These kids are growing up with a train wreck for a mother, and that's going to cause problems for them later in life.

T: Now be the healthy Melissa side.

M: (*as the healthy side*) I don't need to be Mother of the Year. I love the kids and they know that. How they turn out, I just won't know for a long time, so there's no reason to get super upset about it now.

T: See if you can answer that issue, though. It's true that we won't know about how the kids turn out for a long time, but can you see if you can come up with an answer?

M: (*as the healthy side*) If I meet the kids' needs and show them enough love, I think they'll turn out fine.

T: But what about Melissa's relationships? Take the belief side and talk about that.

M: (*as the belief side*) You screw up every relationship you're in. What's that saying, "All of your failed relationships have one thing in common—you"? Well, that's true.

T: Now be the healthy Melissa side.

M: (*as the healthy side*) It's true that my relationships haven't gone well. I just . . . maybe that's not all my fault? I don't know.

T: How about there's no way that could be all your fault, and even if it was all your fault, that doesn't make you a damaged person?

M: (*as the healthy side*) It takes two people to screw up a relationship. Maybe I've picked people who weren't good for me, and yes, maybe I wasn't in a good place to be in a relationship myself. But that doesn't mean I'm a damaged person.

T: Now be the belief side again.

M: (*as the belief side*) Of course it means you're a damaged person. That's the definition of "damaged." If you can't even manage a simple relationship, what else could that mean? And what good are you, anyway?

T: Now be the healthy Melissa side.

M: (*as the healthy side*) What good I am is that I'm more than just my relationships. And if I make bad choices about who I date, that's something I need to work on. And if I get into relationships that I'm not ready for, well, that's something I need to work on, too. But that doesn't say anything about what kind of person I am globally.

Devil's Advocate

An alternative to the "empty chair" dialogue could be a dialogue between the therapist and the client, in which the therapist takes the role of the maladaptive belief and asks the client to respond. The therapist has a bit more control over the discussion this way and can even ask the client to respond to outrageous exaggerations of the belief (e.g., "Well, I can tell you that you are the most damaged person who ever walked the face of the earth! What do you say to that?" or "The world is so very dangerous that you shouldn't even go outside or talk to anyone, ever, because you're doomed!"). Now, there is of course a lot of scientific art that goes into this. You need to know your client and have a decent sense of what kind of conversation he or she can tolerate. The client who is really concrete and can't take you with a grain of salt might not take well to that kind of challenge. But if the client is willing to think a bit objectively about the core belief and has a modicum of a sense of humor, exaggerating the core belief can get him or her articulating the opposite side of the argument.

THE ESSENTIALS

✽ Not all clients require challenging of core beliefs. When core beliefs are to be challenged, I often do this later in therapy, after addressing interpretations and behavioral patterns. In some cases, however, challenging of core beliefs can begin right away.

 The process of challenging core beliefs begins with identifying them. This can be done by:

- Detecting patterns among interpretations.
- Using the downward arrow technique.
- Using written checklists.
- Identifying "stuck" points in the therapy.

✽ The therapist should help the client to understand how his or her core belief might be maladaptive.

 Therapists can challenge distorted core beliefs by:

- Examining the evidence for and against a core belief.
- Asking the client to consider alternatives to the core belief.
- Using scaling to counteract overgeneralized beliefs.
- Encouraging the client to keep a core belief diary to collect evidence.
- Encouraging the client to try acting in a manner that is the opposite of the belief.
- Having the client "talk to the belief" in the session.

Acting the opposite: Challenging core beliefs by instructing the client to experiment with acting in a manner that is incompatible with the core belief.

Core belief diaries: Self-monitoring forms, to be used outside of the therapy session, developed to capture evidence consistent and inconsistent with a core belief.

Empty chair technique: Challenging core beliefs by instructing the client to have a two-sided "dialogue" between the core belief and a more adaptive belief.

Pattern detection: Identifying core beliefs by noting common themes across interpretations over time.

Identifying and Challenging Core Beliefs

Step 1: See if you can identify a maladaptive core belief that is related to your personal target. You can use one or more of these strategies:

- You can use the Core Beliefs Checklist in Appendix B for suggestions.
- You can use *pattern detection* to see what your interpretations have in common with each other.
- You can use a *downward arrow* to elaborate on the implications and meanings of your interpretations.
- You can *find "stuckness"* by identifying a thought or feeling that seems to be particularly resistant to change and thinking about what underlying beliefs or rules might underlie the "stuckness."

My maladaptive core belief is:	And I identified it this way (be specific):

Step 2: Try one of the interventions in this chapter to address this core belief. You can use one or more of these strategies:

- You can *examine the evidence* for and against the core belief.
- You can *consider alternatives* to the core belief.
- You can use *scaling* to address the all-or-nothing nature of the belief.
- You can keep a *core belief diary* in which you look for evidence.
- You can *act the opposite* of the core belief.
- You can try *talking to the belief* and having a dialogue between the belief and your healthy self.

I used this strategy (be specific):	And my experience of it was:

From *Doing CBT* by David F. Tolin. Copyright © 2016 The Guilford Press. Permission to photocopy this worksheet is granted to purchasers of this book for personal use only (see copyright page for details). Purchasers can download enlarged versions of this worksheet (see the box at the end of the table of contents).

CHAPTER 17

Addressing Information-Processing Biases

Attentional Deployment

In Chapter 3, we talked about the concept of *attentional bias* in psychological problems. Specifically, people tend to deploy attention disproportionately toward stimuli that are congruent with their current beliefs or mood states. So, for example, people with anxiety- or fear-based problems selectively (though often involuntarily) seek out and attend to threat-related information, such as a person with panic disorder being hyperaware of his or her heartbeat, or a client with a fear of flying being overly attentive to the noises of the airplane. Some people (e.g., those with GAD) engage in *worry*, in which they focus their attention on thoughts of future, anticipated negative events. Some (e.g., those who have depression) often engage in *rumination*, in which they selectively focus on their unpleasant feelings and negative past experiences. They also tend to evaluate those events, thoughts, and feelings negatively.

So we see a client who appears to have an attentional bias toward stimuli that get the core pathological process going. For example, Nick, our client who is in a distressed marriage with Johanna, pays close attention to signs that his marriage is failing (e.g., lack of affection) and that he is helpless but pays little attention to positive facets of his marriage and factors he can control.

One possible strategy would be to use *distraction*—keeping the mind busy. One could imagine, for example, asking Anna, our client with panic and agoraphobia, to do math problems in her head while walking through a crowded supermarket. Distraction such as this can be tricky business. A little bit of distraction may work fairly well as a short-term strategy to help people get through tough situations (Campbell-Sills & Barlow, 2007). However, the problem is that many clients start to rely excessively on distraction as a coping strategy. When used chronically, distraction probably does more harm than good—it prevents the person from getting used to the situation, challenging his or her maladaptive thoughts about the situation, or taking meaningful, problem-solving action (Hunt, 1998). So I tend to discourage the "La-la-la-I'm-not-paying-attention" style of distraction for most clients, particularly those with anxiety and mood disorders, although I might retain it for some clients with particularly severe emotional dysregulation, such as borderline personality disorder.

There are other potential ways to get at attentional deployment that don't involve unhealthy distraction. One group of strategies is called **attentional control training** (see C. T. Taylor & Amir, 2010, for a review). In the most well-studied of these strategies (Wells, 2009), clients are taught, in the therapist's office, to develop better control over their attentional processes. The idea is that by strengthening attentional control, the person will be less likely to have his or her attention hijacked by emotion. Steps in attentional control training include:

- *Selective attention.* The client practices focusing on one sound in the office, picking it out from competing sounds.
- *Rapid attention switching.* The client practices shifting attention between individual sounds with progressively increasing speed (e.g., every 10 seconds, then every 5 seconds).
- *Divided attention.* The client practices paying attention to multiple sounds simultaneously.

Here, the therapist is working with William (W) in an effort to target his chronic pain, using a process adapted from that described by Wells (2009).

T: We've talked about how your attention can feed into your pain. Specifically, when you start to notice some pain in your body, you end up focusing much of your attention on how you feel.

W: Right. And then I get so focused on the pain that I don't really pay attention to anything else, and the pain just gets worse and worse.

T: Exactly. And right now, your attention is pretty much out of your control. That is, you don't just decide, "I'm going to focus all of my attention on my pain."

W: No, it's automatic. It just happens.

T: So what I'd like to try is to see if we can give you a bit more control over your attention. That way, you, not your pain, can decide what you pay attention to. The aim here is not for you to distract yourself away from unpleasant feelings, though. If you have unpleasant feelings, for now I'd like you to just let them be there.

W: OK.

T: Let's try an attention exercise. You see that dot on the wall? (*Points to a spot on the wall across the room.*) I'd like you to just focus your eyes on that dot. As we go through the exercise, I'll ask you to pay attention to different sounds while you just look at the dot.

W: OK.

[Selective attention:]

T: To start, I'd like you to focus on the sound of my voice. Pay close attention to it. No other sound matters right now, so if you hear other sounds, just ignore them and listen to my voice. Just focus on this one sound. This is the one thing I want you to pay attention to right now. Now I want you to listen to the sound I'm making as I tap on the desk (*tapping fingers on the desk*). I want you to focus all of your attention on the tapping sound. No other sound matters right now. If you hear any other sounds, just ignore them and pay attention to the sound of the tapping. Keep listening to this sound. Now focus on the sound of the ticking clock over on the shelf. Pay very close attention to that sound. No other sound matters right now. Keep listening to that sound. If you hear other sounds, ignore them and return your attention to the sound of the clock. Put all of your attention on that sound. (*Continues for four more sounds, including some sounds outside of the office, each time directing William to focus all of his attention on the individual sounds.*)

[Rapid attention switching:]

T: Next, I'm going to ask you to shift your attention quickly among different sounds. First, focus on the sound of my fingers tapping on the desk. No other sound matters. Now switch your attention to the ticking of the clock on the shelf. Pay close attention to it. No other sound matters. (*Continues, switching among the seven different sounds previously identified.*)

[Divided attention:]

T: Now I want you to work on expanding your attention. I want you to pay attention to all of the sounds, in all of the locations, that we've been paying attention to during this exercise. Try to hear them all at the same time. See how many different sounds you can hear at the same time.

A variation on this theme would be to have William practice focusing his attention outward, toward the task at hand. So, for example, the therapist and William could engage in activities that elicit mild to moderate pain, while William practiced paying attention to the content of the discussion, the look and sound of the therapist, and so forth, which would presumably redirect attentional resources away from his self-focus (Bögels, 2006).

The Science behind It

Some researchers have worked on a high-tech strategy for attentional deployment as an emotion regulation strategy. **Attention modification programs (AMP)** are computer-based exercises that systematically train attention away from threatening stimuli. I won't go into all of the details here, although you can find more information in the articles cited here below.

The jury's still out on whether these programs really work and how well they work. AMP appears to reduce anxiety, at least in the short term, in college students with social anxiety (Amir, Weber, Beard, Bomyea, & Taylor, 2008; Klumpp & Amir, 2010), obsessive–compulsive anxiety (Najmi & Amir, 2010), and general anxiety (Eldar & Bar-Haim, 2010). More recent studies suggest that computerized attention modification decreases anxiety among clinic clients with GAD (Amir, Beard, Burns, & Bomyea, 2009) and social anxiety disorder (Amir, Beard, Taylor, et al., 2009; Schmidt, Richey, Buckner, & Timpano, 2009). In two of these studies, the anxiety-reducing effects were still seen at 4-month follow-up (Amir, Beard, Taylor, et al., 2009; Schmidt et al., 2009). On the other hand, across studies, the effect on anxiety and mood symptoms appears to be fairly small and unstable (Hallion & Ruscio, 2011).

Modifying attention is something that, for most clients, will require quite a bit of practice. In William's case, the therapist audio-recorded the attention modification exercise for William and encouraged him to practice it daily at home. Other therapists might adopt meditation strategies that accomplish similar aims by having clients practice focusing and shifting attention.

Facilitated Recall

Part of our aim in cognitive restructuring is to help the client draw on his or her past experiences in order to correct faulty interpretations. However, memory bias can often make that process difficult. Remember the phenomenon of mood-congruent memory from Chapter 3. People tend to disproportionately recall information that is consistent with their current mood states or with their preexisting beliefs. So, for example, when anticipating a dreaded outcome, clients may selectively recall past experiences of that outcome, while failing to recall the times that the outcome did not happen. Part of overcoming that problem is **facilitated recall,** in which we help the client recall mood- or belief-incongruent information to arrive at a more accurate probability. Asking the client to recall how many times the anticipated outcome has occurred, and then asking him or her to recall how many times the anticipated negative outcome has *not* occurred, helps balance the client's understanding of the actual likelihood.

Here, the therapist is working with Blaise (B), who seems to be minimizing the likelihood of an aversive outcome from substance use.

B: I think I can handle going out for drinks with my friends. It's not going to make me start using again.

T: So your thought here is that "If I go out for drinks, nothing bad is going to happen." Let's look at that idea carefully. I'm not telling you what to do or what not to do; I just want to make sure we're looking at this as objectively as we can.

B: OK.

T: Who are the friends you're thinking about going out with?

B: Kate and Brigette, old friends of mine.

T: These are the friends that you've used with in the past.

B: Yeah, but that doesn't mean it'll happen again.

T: No, not necessarily. Let's think it through a bit. How many times would you estimate that you've gone out for drinks with Kate and Brigette?

B: Jeez, I dunno . . . a hundred times, maybe, over the years.

T: OK. About how many times have those get-togethers for drinks ended up with you using, and about how many times have you walked away without using?

B: Um . . . most of the time we would end up using. We'd go to Kate's house when we left the bar.

T: You say "most of the time." What proportion are we talking about? Like a percentage?

B: I'd say maybe 80 or 90% of the time we would go use after hitting the bar.

T: 80 to 90%. Leaving 10 to 20% of times that you didn't use?

B: Yeah, that sounds about right.

T: OK. Now, I'm not a gambler, but let's say I was. And so I'm gonna bet on whether or not Blaise is gonna use tonight. And I look at her history and I see that over time, these get-togethers have an 80 to 90% likelihood of leading to her using. What bet should I make, if I'm a smart gambler?

B: I guess you'd go with the odds.

T: Which are what?

B: That I'm gonna use.

T: Yeah. Now the question I have for you is: What bet are you gonna make? Thinking about what you're betting—your sobriety—would you want to put that on a four-to-one bet?

B: No, I guess not.

✴ THE ESSENTIALS ✴

✴ Information-processing biases are often addressed indirectly using other strategies, but they can be direct targets of intervention.

✴ Attentional control training is used to help clients practice selective attention, rapid attention switching, and divided attention.

✴ Facilitated recall is used to counteract memory bias. Clients are asked to recall experiences that are inconsistent with current beliefs and interpretations, with cues from the therapist.

✴ KEY TERMS AND DEFINITIONS ✴

Attention modification programs: Computerized programs that systematically train clients to allocate attention away from negative stimuli.

Attentional control training: CBT interventions that are designed to facilitate the person's control over his or her attention.

Facilitated recall: Helping the client to recall information that is inconsistent with a current mood state or belief.

Addressing Information-Processing Biases

See if you can identify and address one or more information-processing biases that are related to your personal target.

Do you have an *attentional bias* (i.e., you disproportionately allocate attention to things that are consistent with your emotions and beliefs)? If so, describe what you pay excessive attention to and what you tend not to pay attention to.

_____

_____

Do you have a *memory bias* (i.e., you disproportionately recall things that are consistent with your emotions and beliefs)? If so, describe what you tend to recall, and what you tend not to recall (if you can).

_____

_____

Attentional retraining exercise:

- For 5 minutes, close your eyes and focus on one sound in the room, picking it out from competing sounds.
- For 5 minutes, practice shifting attention between individual sounds with progressively increasing speed (e.g., every 10 seconds, then every 5 seconds).
- For 5 minutes, practice paying attention to multiple sounds simultaneously.

Facilitated recall exercise: Try to recall five events that are *inconsistent* with your emotions and beliefs.

_____

_____

_____

_____

_____

_____

What did you notice or experience during these exercises?

_____

_____

_____

_____

_____

From *Doing CBT* by David F. Tolin. Copyright © 2016 The Guilford Press. Permission to photocopy this worksheet is granted to purchasers of this book for personal use only (see copyright page for details). Purchasers can download enlarged versions of this worksheet (see the box at the end of the table of contents).

EMOTION-LEVEL INTERVENTIONS

In this section, we'll discuss the emotion-level interventions in CBT. These interventions are used when you want to target maladaptive emotional processes *directly*, rather than targeting those processes *indirectly* through behavior-level or cognitive-level interventions.

Figure IID.1 shows the targets for our emotion-level interventions. Your target here is the emotion itself. However, you'll note that I've also highlighted the cognitive and behavioral aspects of the core pathological process. The reason is that, as we'll see later, affecting an emotion sometimes involves addressing how the person thinks and acts in response to his or her emotion.

Just as was the case with the cognitive-level interventions (Part IIB), there are two broad ways to affect these targets. The first of these is *emotion modulation*, in which we try to change the person's emotional experience. Usually, emotion modulation strategies are designed to decrease the client's level of physiological arousal. They include:

- Relaxation training.
- Breathing retraining.

The other way of addressing maladaptive emotion is to teach *distress tolerance*. That is, we are aiming to affect how the person responds to his or her emotions, rather than trying to change the emotions themselves. These strategies include:

- Acceptance.
- Directing the client to behave in a manner that is incompatible with the emotion.
- Prescribing value-based action.

And remember from our core pathological process that behavioral, cognitive, and emotional systems all influence each other. So an emotion-level intervention can create behavioral and cognitive change as well.

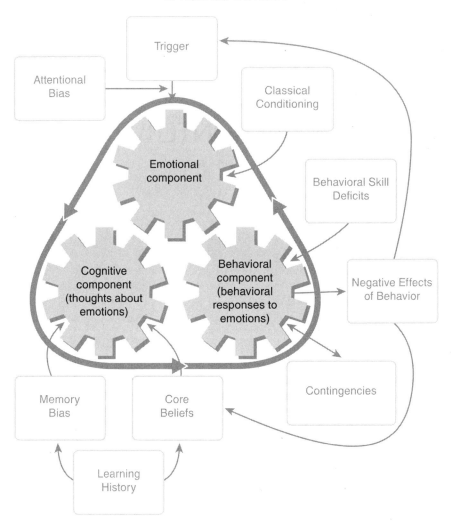

FIGURE IID.1. The targets for emotion-level interventions.

CHAPTER 18

Modulating Emotion

Often we find it helpful to intervene at the level of maladaptive emotions. As described in Chapter 4, "emotions" as we define them include both subjective feeling states (e.g., scared, sad, angry) and internal physiological sensations (e.g., increased heart rate, muscle tension, tiredness). Emotions are considered maladaptive when they (1) do not remit with a change of circumstances, (2) are markedly out of proportion to the situation, or (3) impair performance.

Turning again to the broad model of *emotion regulation* (J. J. Gross, 1998), when we are trying to intervene directly at the emotional level, we are often trying to down-regulate a negative emotion. For example, when we are treating our depressed client Christina, our aim might be to help her feel *less sad*.

Simultaneously or alternatively, we might be trying to up-regulate a positive emotion. For example, with Christina, we might be interested in helping her to feel *more happy*. Although that might seem like simply the flip side of "less sad," it's not. We know from research that positive and negative affect (emotions) can operate separately and that the absence of one does not necessarily imply the presence of the other (L. A. Clark & Watson, 1991).

There may even be times when we are trying to down-regulate a positive emotion. Some clients with bipolar, addictive, or impulse control disorders could experience maladaptive levels of positive emotions, such as excitement, thrill, or anticipation. Sometimes we want to help clients keep those emotions in check so that they are less likely to lead to maladaptive behaviors.

Gross and Thompson (2007) propose a multistage model of emotion regulation, much of which has been (or will be) covered in other chapters in this book. Their stages, and associated interventions, include:

- Situation selection and situation modification (see Chapter 8).
- Attentional deployment.
- Cognitive change (see Chapter 14).
- Response modulation.

So some of the emotion regulation strategies involve *indirect* modification of emotions by selecting or changing situations (the event level of change), by modifying thoughts and beliefs (the cognitive level of change), or by changing behaviors (the behavioral level of change). In this chapter, we talk about strategies for directly targeting and modulating emotional response.

Emotional Response Modulation as an Emotion Regulation Strategy

In many cases, the behavioral strategy for response modification involves *acting the opposite*, that is, in a manner that is somehow inconsistent with the emotion (Ellard, Fairholme, Boisseau, Farchione, & Barlow, 2010; Linehan, 1993). As discussed previously in this book, people can deal with fear by acting not fearful, they can deal with sadness by acting not sad, and so forth.

Sometimes, however, we want to make a direct modification of the emotional response itself. This has been particularly emphasized in treatments of hyperarousal-based disorders such as anxiety and anger. Two ways that we might do this are *relaxation training* and *breathing retraining*.

Relaxation Training

Relaxation training (Bernstein & Borkovec, 1973) is one of the oldest CBT interventions, initially developed when Edmund Jacobson (1929) found that anxious clients could feel less anxious by achieving a deep state of muscle relaxation. His approach, called **progressive relaxation,** involved systematically contracting, then relaxing, skeletal muscles of the body. The original progressive relaxation was a very long treatment, often requiring 50 or more training sessions. It has subsequently been shortened and has been used as a stand-alone treatment for conditions such as generalized anxiety/tension (Borkovec & Costello, 1993; Borkovec, Grayson, & Cooper, 1978); arousal-based somatic concerns such as insomnia, chronic pain, irritable bowel, and headache (Carlson & Hoyle, 1993); and excessive anger (Deffenbacher, Lynch, Oetting, & Kemper, 1996; Deffenbacher & Stark, 1992). It has also been combined with other treatments, such as the combination of relaxation and exposure in systematic desensitization (Wolpe, 1961; see Chapter 11) and is found as a component of many multi-intervention programs such as anxiety management training (Suinn & Richardson, 1971), stress inoculation training (Meichenbaum, 1977), anger management therapy (Deffenbacher, 2011; Kassinove & Tafrate, 2002), and numerous behavioral medicine applications (Edinger, Wohlgemuth, Radtke, Marsh, & Quillian, 2001; Glombiewski et al., 2010; Olatunji, Tolin, & Lohr, 2004).

Progressive relaxation usually goes something like this:

- Have the client sit in a comfortable chair with a relaxed posture (e.g., arms and legs not crossed, leaning back).
- Have the client close his or her eyes if he or she is willing and if doing so does not cause increased anxiety.
- Minimize distractions in the room (e.g., sounds).
- Select one muscle or muscle group at a time. Have the client tense the muscle for about 5 seconds (not necessarily as hard as possible; moderate tension seems to work fine) and then relax it for 10 seconds or more. Tensing the muscle first yields

demonstrably greater relaxation results than does simply encouraging the client to relax the muscle (Borkovec et al., 1978).
- Follow the tension–relaxation cycle for each muscle group in the body.
- Encourage slow, controlled breathing during the process.
- Often, some kind of imagery is used (e.g., visualizing tension leaving the body).

Here is an example of a progressive relaxation script:

"We're going to do an exercise that teaches you how to relax your body and your mind. The way we'll do this is to tighten a muscle group, and then relax it, going muscle by muscle over your entire body. I'll ask you to tighten a specific muscle group for about 5 seconds, and then I'll ask you to relax that muscle group. If tensing the muscle hurts, you can skip that part, or try tensing it a little less.

"To start, let's have you sit as comfortably as you can in the chair. Have both feet on the floor, and allow your hands to rest in your lap or on the arms of the chair. Lean back comfortably against the back rest.

"If you feel comfortable doing so, close your eyes. Just take a moment and be aware of your body. As we go through this exercise, you'll be paying attention to your body. If your mind wanders or you get distracted, that's OK; just bring your attention back to your body.

"Pay attention to your breathing. Notice the air going into your lungs, and notice the air coming out. In and out. Make your breaths nice and slow and relaxed. Every time you exhale, you can imagine a little bit of tension leaving your body. Keep breathing as we go through the exercise.

"Let's start with your facial muscles. Raise your eyebrows as high as you can so that your forehead wrinkles up. Hold them there. Notice that feeling of tension in your forehead. Now, all at once, relax. Let the eyebrows go back to their natural position. Feel the tension melting away from your forehead. That's good. Let the tension go. Notice how different that feels; how much better it feels. Keep breathing nice and slow and relaxed. (*Wait 5–10 seconds before progressing to the next muscle group.*)

"Now let's tighten the muscles of your mouth. Smile as widely as you can, really stretching your mouth. Clench your jaw while you're doing it. Notice all of that tension; feel the tension in every muscle. Now, all at once, relax. Relax your lips, your cheeks, your jaw. Feel all of the tension melting away. Notice how different it feels to have those muscles relax. Keep breathing nice and slow and relaxed.

"Now tighten the muscles around your eyes by squeezing your eyes shut. Squeeze them as tightly as you can. Notice how tense those muscles feel. Now, relax. Relax your eyes, your eyelids, the muscles around your eyes. Let go of the tension. Notice the difference between tense and relaxed. Notice how much better relaxed feels. Keep your breathing going. In and out. Nice and slow and relaxed.

"Let's move down now to your shoulders. Lift your shoulders up, like you're trying to touch your ears with your shoulders. Like you're shrugging. Notice the tension in those shoulder muscles. Notice what that tension feels like. And now . . . relax. Let the shoulders drop back down. Feel the tension melting away. Notice how different it feels to let those muscles relax. As you breathe in and out, you can imagine that tension coming out through your breath.

"And now let's go to your upper back. Tense those upper back muscles by pulling your shoulders back, trying to make your shoulder blades touch each other. Really feel the tension in those muscles. Hold it. And now . . . relax. Let it go. Notice the muscles relaxing; notice how much better it feels. Keep breathing nice and slow and relaxed.

"And keep going down to the lower back. You can tense those muscles by arching your back. Hold it there. Notice the tension in your lower back. And . . . relax. Let all of that tension go, coming out through your breath, as you breathe nice and slow. Notice the relaxed feeling.

"Let's move to your chest muscles. Tighten those muscles by pulling your shoulders forward. You can bring your upper arms together in front of you to pull those muscles tight. Hold it. Notice that tension. And now . . . relax. Relax the chest. Your arms flop back to where they were. Notice the feeling of relaxation. Breathing nice and slow and relaxed.

"Move down to your stomach muscles. Make your stomach tight, like you're trying to show off your six-pack. Tighten them up and hold it. Notice how that feels. And . . . relax. Let the stomach muscles relax. It becomes easier to breathe this way, nice and slow and relaxed.

"Let's do your hands next. Make fists with both your hands. Hold them tight, really tight. Hold it and notice the tension in all of those hand muscles. And . . . relax. Let the hands relax, your fingers get floppy and relaxed. Imagine the tension melting out of your hands and your fingers. Breathing nice and slow.

"Tighten your bicep muscles now, like you're flexing. Tight and flexed. Notice the tension here. And now . . . relax. The arms get loose, and you can feel the tension melting away. Let it go. Breathe the tension out.

"Tighten your buttock muscles now. This should lift you up out of your chair a little bit. Make those muscles really tense. Notice the tension. And . . . relax. Let your body sink into the chair. Nice and relaxed. Notice how different that feels. Breathing is nice and slow and relaxed.

"Now you can tighten your thighs by pushing your knees together, like you're trying to hold a penny between your knees. Hold it tight. And now . . . relax. Relax those thighs. Let the tension melt away. Notice the difference. Breathing in . . . and out.

"We'll flex your calf muscles by pointing your toes forward. Really feel the tension in your calves. Hold it. And . . . relax. Let all of the tension go. Notice how different the relaxation feels. Your breathing is nice and relaxed.

"Tense your feet by curling your toes, like you're making fists with your feet. Hold that. You can feel the tension in all of those foot muscles. And . . . relax. Let the toes go back to normal. Feel the tension melting away from your feet and toes. Keep breathing nice and slow and relaxed.

"When you want to, you can open your eyes, but you can keep feeling relaxed in your body."

The exact set of muscle groups, and the exact sequence, isn't a magic formula. It probably doesn't matter much, as long as you follow the basic principles described above.

Progressive relaxation training in the therapy session is usually followed by a homework assignment. I generally instruct the client to do the relaxation exercise at least twice per day. In order to accomplish this, I often find it helpful to record the session (or I can have a premade recording of myself doing the exercise). Recording the instructions on the client's smartphone, using a freely downloadable voice recording app, is one straightforward way to do it that ensures portability. At first, I'm not looking to have the client use this strategy in difficult or stressful situations. Rather, I encourage the client just to pick a time of day when he or she knows it can be done without being interrupted.

Sometimes clients want to do this in bed before going to sleep. That's fine (especially if insomnia is a concern), although in most cases I don't count that toward the homework. Falling asleep right after the exercise defeats the purpose of helping them to feel more relaxed during their daily activities.

Notice in the script above that the therapist makes liberal use of the word *relax*. That's deliberate. The therapist is making sure to say "relax" right at the moment when the client abruptly lets go of the tension. Over time, the idea is that the client will associate the word with the feeling and will therefore be better able to achieve a relaxed state by thinking the word *relax*. That's called **cue-controlled relaxation,** and it's based on the principles of classical conditioning we discussed in Chapter 4. The word *relax* is the conditioned stimulus, and muscle relaxation is the conditioned response. Over time, we can instruct the client to use the word *relax* during in-home practice and during stressful situations (Bernstein & Borkovec, 1973).

Whenever we're using an exercise-based intervention such as relaxation, we have to pay careful attention to **generalization** of the treatment. That is, it's all well and good for the client to be able to relax in our office, or in a quiet room at home. But as you might imagine, that skill by itself probably won't be terribly helpful in the client's day-to-day life. We can never expect that just because a client learns something (be it behavioral, cognitive, or emotional learning), he or she will reliably apply it in daily activities (Stokes & Baer, 1977). So once the client can do the relaxation exercise in a controlled setting fairly well, it's time to bring that skill out into his or her world. So we can encourage the client to do abbreviated versions of progressive relaxation in different stressful situations. A student in a classroom, for example, can practice relaxing the muscles of his or her face, shoulders, and hands while breathing slowly (Poppen, 1998). Reminders to relax (see the discussion of *stimulus control* in Chapter 8), such as strategically located stickers or signs or beeps on a watch alarm, can help prompt the use of these exercises.

Breathing Retraining

Who would think that someone would need to learn how to breathe? Doesn't it just come naturally? Well, it turns out that for some clients, maladaptive breathing patterns may play a role in the maintenance of their symptoms, and correcting those breathing patterns may help interrupt the core pathological process.

A really clear example of a maladaptive breathing pattern is **hyperventilation,** in which the person breathes more rapidly or more deeply than needed. Another is *irregular breathing,* in which the person engages in breath holding, sighing, or other variations that prevent regular oxygen flow. Hyperventilation and irregular breathing seem to be common among people with panic disorder (Abelson, Weg, Nesse, & Curtis, 2001; Caldirola, Bellodi, Caumo, Migliarese, & Perna, 2004; J. M. Martinez et al., 2001; Wilhelm, Trabert, & Roth, 2001), and among people with panic disorder, breathing abnormalities appear to precede the occurrence of panic attacks (Meuret et al., 2011; Papp et al., 1997; Rosenfield et al., 2010). Breathing abnormalities have also been noted in individuals experiencing anger, with deeper and more rapid breaths (S. Bloch, Lemeignan, & Aguilera, 1991).

The problem with hyperventilation and irregular breathing is that they can trigger a cascade of bodily sensations such as increased heart rate, lightheadedness, dizziness, and muscle tension (Gilbert, 1999). Paradoxically, hyperventilation and irregular breathing can even induce feelings of suffocation (Klein, 1993), resulting in even more hyperventilation (Dempsey, Forster, Gledhill, & doPico, 1975). So it's not hard to imagine how bad breathing patterns can set someone up to experience anxiety and panic. Similarly, given the increase in muscle tension associated with hyperventilation, one can easily imagine how an angry individual can "ramp up" his or her anger level, much in the same way that any angry behavior can increase angry emotions (as discussed in Chapter 2).

Many researchers have therefore examined whether **breathing retraining** can reduce physiological and emotional arousal. Variations of breathing retraining have been used in the treatment of panic disorder (Craske & Barlow, 2001), GAD (Borkovec & Ruscio, 2001), PTSD (Foa & Rothbaum, 1998), anger management (Deffenbacher, Filetti, Lynch, Dahlen, & Oetting, 2002), behavioral medicine applications (Fried, 1993), and overall stress reduction in clients ranging from the "worried well" to those with severe mental illness (Key, Craske, & Reno, 2003). It's been applied across the lifespan, including with younger children (Bothe, Grignon, & Olness, 2014). Interestingly, in one study of clients with panic disorder, normalization of respiratory function preceded and predicted changes in panic-related cognitive distortions (Meuret, Rosenfield, Hofmann, Suvak, & Roth, 2009), lending further support for the idea that the three elements of the core pathological process (thoughts, behaviors, and emotions) all influence one another.

Breathing retraining commonly targets two different aspects of dysfunctional respiration:

1. *Rate.* First and foremost, hyperventilation is characterized by rapid breathing. One aim of breathing retraining, therefore, is to slow the rate of breathing. Usually we aim for a rate of one breath cycle (in and out) every 5–10 seconds (Bonn, Readhead, & Timmons, 1984; Salkovskis, Jones, & Clark, 1986), although some clients may need to approach this target in a gradual fashion.

2. *Depth.* Sometimes people mistakenly think that the way to breathe properly is to take in huge "cleansing breaths." Not a great idea, unless you're conducting a hyperventilation exposure (which we sometimes do, as discussed in Chapter 11). Rather, we want the client to breathe less from the chest and more from the diaphragm. Diaphragmatic breaths tend to involve greater airflow but are also slower than breathing from the chest and therefore can reduce arousal sensations (Ley, 1985). Using the nose, rather than the mouth, for inhalation can help reduce the amount of oxygen being taken in (nostrils are smaller than the mouth). When individuals are engaging in chest breathing, their shoulders will often rise, or their chests will expand. Conversely, when individuals are engaging in diaphragmatic breathing, their shoulders and chests will be relatively still, and their abdomens will expand. Some clients have a hard time figuring out how to breathe from the diaphragm. Sometimes it's easier if one lies down on the floor, face down, with his or her hands folded under his or her head. I get right down there with them, by the way. Once they figure out how to do it, they can return to practicing in a chair.

Here's an example of a breathing retraining script:

"We're going to focus on your breathing now. To start, let's have you sit as comfortably as you can in the chair. Have both feet on the floor, and allow your hands to rest in your lap or on the arms of the chair. Lean back comfortably against the back rest. If you feel comfortable doing so, close your eyes.

"Concentrate on taking breaths from your stomach. Put one hand on your stomach, and the other hand on your chest. Your chest should be fairly still while you breathe in and out. When you breathe in, your stomach should expand, like a balloon inflating. When you breathe out, your stomach should contract, like the balloon is deflating.

"Breathe slowly and smoothly. No sudden breaths in or out. No holding your breath. Just a nice, easy, in and out of a continuous stream of air down to your stomach, and then back out.

"Breathe in through your nose, and out through your mouth. In through the nose, out through the mouth. Still breathing from your stomach.

"I'd like you to count to yourself so that you can pace your breathing. I'll start by counting for you. I'll count to 4 while you breathe in through the nose, and I'll count to 6 while you breathe out through the mouth. Breathe in through the nose . . . 1 . . . 2 . . . 3 . . . 4 . . . and out through the mouth . . . 1 . . . 2 . . . 3 . . . 4 . . . 5 . . . 6. In through the nose . . . 1 . . . 2 . . . 3 . . . 4 . . . and out through the mouth . . . 1 . . . 2 . . . 3 . . . 4 . . . 5 . . . 6. In through the nose . . . 1 . . . 2 . . . 3 . . . 4 . . . and out through the mouth . . . 1 . . . 2 . . . 3 . . . 4 . . . 5 . . . 6.

"Now you count in your head. In through the nose [pause for 4 seconds], and out through the mouth [pause for 6 seconds]. In through the nose [pause for 4 seconds, and out through the mouth [pause for 6 seconds]. Keep going just like that."

Like relaxation training, we want to make sure clients are practicing breathing retraining outside of the therapist's office. This can be done by simply having clients set aside time each day to focus on slow, diaphragmatic breathing. It is often helpful to provide an audio recording to help the client time his or her breath cycles. Some have used more high-tech strategies, such as a portable biofeedback device that monitors respiration rate and exhaled CO_2 levels (Meuret, Wilhelm, Ritz, & Roth, 2008).

Adapting the Process: *Relaxation . . .*

. . . with children. For children, relaxation exercises should be kept simple and short, perhaps no longer than 5 minutes. The therapist might opt to demonstrate each step to the child in order to show how it's done. Kids may respond well to incorporating relaxing imagery such as lying on a beach or floating in space—whatever the child would find relaxing. After a relaxation exercise, kids might be asked to color a human figure, using red to show the body parts that were very tense, yellow to show the body parts that were a bit relaxed, and blue to show the body parts that were very relaxed (Rapee et al., 2000).

. . . with medical patients. Relaxation exercises can be helpful in cases of chronic pain, although there are some clients for whom the exercises seem to exacerbate the pain (Bakal, Demjen, & Kaganov, 1981). In such cases, breathing exercises, rather than progressive muscle relaxation, might be selected. For clients with chronic pain, it is often helpful to discuss the mutually escalating relationship among muscle tension, anxiety, and pain. The concept of relaxation through pain can be discussed using examples such as childbirth classes, in which mothers-to-be are taught that tensing up during pain only exacerbates the pain, whereas deliberately relaxing muscle groups can lessen the sensation of pain (Turk, Meichenbaum, & Genest, 1983). For some patients, electromyographic (EMG) biofeedback has been a promising way to induce a state of physiological relaxation, although it is not clear whether the additional "gizmos" of biofeedback produce a stronger effect than do traditional relaxation strategies (Flor & Turk, 2011).

The Science behind It

How well do these "calming down" interventions work? There's no question that relaxation and breathing retraining are helpful interventions. They're broadly applicable, easy to understand, have a demonstrable impact on arousal levels, and have been used in all kinds of CBT packages. Across studies, relaxation training is associated with moderate to high effects for clients with anxiety disorders (Manzoni, Pagnini, Castelnuovo, & Molinari, 2008) and moderate effects for clients with physical concerns such as headache, hypertension, and the side effects of chemotherapy (Carlson & Hoyle, 1993). In the treatment of GAD, it yields results that are roughly comparable to those of cognitive strategies (Siev & Chambless, 2007). Plus it's relatively easy to do, and clients generally like it. So, broadly speaking, I give relaxation and breathing retraining a thumbs-up for arousal-based problems.

. . . And, of course, there are always exceptions. One possible example is in clients with panic disorder. Relaxation does have a demonstrable benefit for clients with panic disorder (Öst & Westling, 1995), as does breathing retraining (Meuret et al., 2008). However, across studies, clients with panic disorder seem to do less well with relaxation than they do with strategies such as *cognitive restructuring* and *exposure* (Siev & Chambless, 2007). One dismantling study of CBT for panic disorder (Schmidt et al., 2000) may be particularly informative. All clients received cognitive restructuring and exposure. Some of the clients also received instruction in breathing retraining. In general, the addition of breathing retraining did not improve treatment outcomes, and some data suggested that breathing retraining may have been associated with *poorer* outcomes.

Now, that one is a puzzler, because we already know (as described above) that breathing retraining and relaxation have a documented track record of efficacy in the treatment of panic. So why, when you combine it with other CBT interventions, might breathing retraining *detract* from the treatment? One possibility is that clients may have used the breathing exercise as a *safety behavior*, in which they tried to avoid feeling anxious by clinging to an exercise. Doing so might have undermined the therapy's ability to teach the clients more valuable lessons, such as that anxiety will not last forever, that panic attacks are not dangerous, and so on. Furthermore, as safety behaviors tend to do, the breathing exercise could have become a "crutch" that decreased clients' rehearsal of more adaptive coping strategies.

Why I Don't Use Relaxation and Breathing Training with Everyone

As discussed in the "Science behind It" sidebar, relaxation and breathing training have robust effects on problems of hyperarousal, and that's why I use them. But at the same time, there's some reason for pause. First, it's not entirely clear how well "calming down" interventions interact with other elements of CBT. They have at least a moderate effect on their own, but for at least some people (e.g., those with panic disorder), they may actually run counter to some of the lessons we're trying to teach the client. For example, it's hard to tell the client that his or her physical sensations are not dangerous and that he or she doesn't have to react to them while simultaneously having the client practice a strategy designed to get control over his or her physical sensations (Schmidt et al., 2000). And then, of course, when the relaxation fails (as is likely when a panic attack is coming on), we may have even added fuel to the fire because now the client thinks, "Even my relaxation exercise didn't work! I'm doomed!" Generally speaking, when I'm treating someone with anxiety, I find it most helpful to limit the use of *safety behaviors* (see Chapter 11).

I also think that sometimes we run into the problem of what economists call *opportunity cost*. Basically, the client has a limited amount of time and money to invest in treatment. That means we are obligated to select our interventions carefully, emphasizing interventions that will produce the strongest results in the shortest amount of time. As discussed above, there are some cases in which relaxation and breathing retraining do really well, and by all means you should use them. Some of our clients would probably do well with relaxation or breathing exercises. For example:

- Suzanne and Blaise are both struggling with some degree of substance misuse, albeit at different levels and with different substances. But in both cases, they seem to use substances as a form of self-medication, in which they attempt to control physiological arousal by taking drugs to calm down. Offering relaxation and breathing exercises might provide an alternative that could reduce the perceived need to use substances.

- Melissa and Elizabeth both have significant emotional dysregulation, and their emotions often feel out of control. For them, it might be useful to teach them a strategy such as relaxation or paced breathing as a way of helping them feel a bit more in control of themselves.

- Johanna and Nick, our distressed couple, frequently feel emotionally "flooded" (Gottman, 1999) when they start to argue. They become highly aroused, which causes their interpretations of each other to become distorted and their problem-solving capability to break down and fuels increased hostile behavior. It might be helpful for us to build in a "time-out" in which they can separate briefly and relax before restarting the conversation.

- Samuel, our insomniac client, might do well to try some relaxation and controlled breathing prior to attempting to go to sleep. Usually, when he gets into bed he's fairly wound up, which is not conducive to sleeping, so relaxing before bed might help get him on the right track.

However, in other cases, strategies such as *cognitive restructuring* (see Chapter 14) and *exposure* (see Chapter 11) give you more bang for your buck (Siev & Chambless, 2007). In such cases, your limited time and resources are better spent elsewhere. When my case conceptualization doesn't suggest a strong role of physiological arousal in the person's problem (as, for example, could be the case for many clients with depression), I would probably skip relaxation and spend my time on more promising interventions such as *activity scheduling* (see Chapter 10) and perhaps cognitive restructuring (see Chapter 14). Even when arousal is an issue, some conditions, such as specific anxiety disorders or OCD, respond really well to exposure with response prevention (see Chapter 11), so much so that I'm hesitant to give up any "exposure time" to do a relaxation exercise.

THE ESSENTIALS

- ✱ *Emotion regulation* refers to strategies aimed at decreasing negative emotion or increasing positive emotion.
- ✱ Many emotion regulation strategies are indirect, with the direct targets being other aspects of the system such as interpretations, behaviors, and attentional deployment. However, emotions can be the direct target of interventions as well.

✴ Progressive relaxation is a commonly used emotion modulation strategy that involves systematically tensing and relaxing the muscles of the body.

✴ Breathing retraining, which can address both the rate and depth of breaths, can help counteract the tendency to hyperventilate.

✴ With any emotional modulation strategy, it is important not to create maladaptive safety behaviors.

KEY TERMS AND DEFINITIONS

Breathing retraining: Teaching and practicing slow, controlled breathing from the diaphragm.

Cue-controlled relaxation: The pairing of muscle relaxation with a specific word or phrase, which is subsequently used to elicit relaxation.

Generalization: The degree to which learning that occurs during therapy sessions can transfer to real-world situations.

Hyperventilation: Breathing more rapidly or deeply than needed.

Progressive relaxation: A systematic approach to muscle relaxation that involves contracting and then relaxing the skeletal muscles.

Relaxation and Breathing Retraining

For at least 10 minutes, use the progressive relaxation exercise described in this chapter. Because you'll be keeping your eyes closed, you might wish to play recorded instructions, such as those at *http://media.dartmouth.edu/~healthed/p_muscle_relax.mp3.*

- Sit in a comfortable chair with a relaxed posture.
- Close your eyes.
- Minimize distractions in the room (e.g., sounds).
- Tense (at least 5 seconds) and relax (at least 10 seconds) the following muscle groups:
  - Forehead
  - Mouth
  - Eyes
  - Shoulders
  - Upper back
  - Lower back
  - Chest
  - Stomach
  - Hands
  - Biceps
  - Buttocks
  - Thighs
  - Calves
  - Feet
- Practice breathing slowly (4 seconds in, 6 seconds out) from your diaphragm (a hand on your stomach should feel expansion as you inhale and contraction as you exhale).

What was your experience with this exercise? Specifically: How hard or easy was it? When did it become hard? Did your emotions or physical sensations change over time?

From *Doing CBT* by David F. Tolin. Copyright © 2016 The Guilford Press. Permission to photocopy this worksheet is granted to purchasers of this book for personal use only (see copyright page for details). Purchasers can download enlarged versions of this worksheet (see the box at the end of the table of contents).

CHAPTER 19

Distress Tolerance

Is Calming Down Overrated?

In the previous chapter, we discussed the fact that relaxation training can be helpful for certain problems. However, we're still not sure exactly *why* it works. There doesn't seem to be a clear, direct link between muscle tension and subjective anxiety, nor is there a clear, direct link between the reduction of muscle tension and the reduction of anxiety (Conrad & Roth, 2007). Therefore, some have suggested that relaxation's mechanism of action might not be calming the person down. Rather, they suggest that relaxation improves the client's sense of self-efficacy to manage anxiety. Or it might work by *defusion*, the concept introduced in Chapter 15, through which clients learn to recognize their thoughts and feelings as internal events, rather than threats that need to be acted upon (Hayes-Skelton, Usmani, Lee, Roemer, & Orsillo, 2012).

In Chapter 15, I talked about the acceptance alternative to cognitive restructuring. As you may recall, the basic idea of acceptance is that, for many people, the problem isn't

Try This

Remember the white bear example of thought suppression in Chapter 3? We saw that when you try to suppress a thought, it tends to occur even more over time. The same phenomenon happens with emotions. Try an exercise: Think of something that's really bothering you. Imagine it vividly. Now, for 1 minute, try to force yourself to feel better about it. Make it critical that you feel better right now. Tell yourself that if you don't feel better *right now*, you're a mess.

What happened? If your response was at all like mine, you probably found that you couldn't simply force yourself to feel better. In fact, you might have found that trying in that way actually made you feel worse. That's because the very act of trying not to feel a certain way leads you to compare how you feel with how you think you "should" feel, which makes you feel worse (M. Williams, Teasdale, Segal, & Kabat-Zinn, 2007).

their thoughts and feelings; rather, it's how they *respond* to their thoughts and feelings. In particular, some people get so wrapped up in attempts to avoid or escape from aversive internal experiences (*experiential avoidance*) that they make the problem worse (e.g., Hayes et al., 2012).

We can certainly imagine a lot of ways in which our clients' efforts to avoid or control emotions or physical sensations could compound the problem, such as:

• Anna, who has panic disorder, thinks, "I'd better relax, or else!" and then when she doesn't relax, thinks, "Oh, no, something might be really wrong with me because I can't relax!" Or she thinks, "I'd better control my breathing!" and then proceeds to hyperventilate herself into a panic attack.

• When Elizabeth, our client with borderline personality, feels angry, she thinks, "I'd better get this anger out of my system!" and then proceeds to pace around or drink alcohol, strategies that not only don't work but that may even increase her feelings of anger.

• Melissa, who has PTSD, avoids objectively harmless situations because they bring up feelings of fear. That avoidance allows the fear to persist.

• Nick, who is angry at his wife, Johanna, thinks, "It's not appropriate to feel angry toward my spouse—I should only feel love!" and then tries to suppress any angry feelings, waiting for the love to emerge (which, naturally, doesn't happen).

• Christina, our depressed client, thinks, "I'm too sad to go out today," and spends the rest of the day at home, lying in bed and waiting to feel better. And, as we might predict, she gets increasingly depressed.

• When William experiences feelings of physical pain, he *catastrophizes* (see Chapter 3), thinking, "This is going to get worse and worse until I can't stand it anymore!" He also thinks, "I'd better take it easy today; I don't want my pain to get worse." So he spends much of his time inactive, which causes him to be increasingly deconditioned and more susceptible to noticing pain.

Distress Tolerance as a Potential Target

In addition to understanding the amount of distress a client is experiencing, it's also important for us to understand the client's level of **distress tolerance.** Distress tolerance is defined in two ways: (1) the person's *perceived* capacity to withstand negative emotional or physical states and (2) the *behavioral act* of withstanding negative emotional or physical states (Leyro, Zvolensky, & Bernstein, 2010). People exhibit good distress tolerance when they can resist the desire to escape (negative reinforcement) from aversive internal states. Poor distress tolerance, conversely, consists of several overlapping constructs, including the following.

• Some people have **intolerance of uncertainty,** meaning that they have a negative emotional, cognitive, or behavioral reaction to situations or events that are uncertain (Dugas, Freeston, & Ladouceur, 1997). Our client Suzanne, who has GAD, is highly intolerant of uncertainty. When she doesn't know what's going to happen or doesn't have all of the information in front of her, she gets highly anxious and is motivated to engage in certainty-seeking behaviors such as calling her husband, checking the locks on the doors and windows, and so forth.

- Some show **physical discomfort intolerance,** defined as difficulty withstanding uncomfortable physical sensations (Schmidt, Richey, Cromer, & Buckner, 2007). Our client William, who is diagnosed with fibromyalgia, has physical discomfort intolerance. When he experiences feelings of pain, he engages in catastrophizing, finds the pain intolerable, and is highly motivated to escape or avoid situations or activities that trigger pain. A related construct is **anxiety sensitivity,** in which people react fearfully to anxiety-related bodily sensations due to beliefs that these symptoms have harmful physical, psychological, or social consequences (Reiss, Peterson, Gursky, & McNally, 1986). Anna, our client with panic disorder, has a high level of anxiety sensitivity. When she starts noticing her heart rate increasing, or she starts to feel dizzy, she fears that she's going to have a heart attack, is going to go crazy, or is going to embarrass herself.

- Some have poor **emotional distress tolerance,** meaning that they have difficulty tolerating negative emotions, view negative emotions as unacceptable, and pay excessive attention to negative emotions (Simons & Gaher, 2005). Our client Elizabeth, who has borderline personality, perceives her negative emotions, such as anger and sadness, to be unacceptable and intolerable. She believes that she shouldn't feel this way, and when she does, she focuses all of her attention on how rotten she feels. At times, she engages in risky or self-damaging behaviors to try to rid herself of, or distract herself from, her negative feelings.

- Some have poor **frustration tolerance,** which makes them believe that aversive situations are intolerable (Kassinove, 1986). Blaise, our substance-abusing client, believes that she is incapable of withstanding her urges to use. She also tends not to persist at tasks that are difficult and seems to insist that life should be easy and comfortable. She is unlikely to do things unless there is a promise of immediate reward.

All of these constructs have a common theme. Some people can have unpleasant feelings and still get on with their lives. Other people have unpleasant feelings and become paralyzed by them. They react to their feelings with maladaptive thoughts and behaviors, which makes things even worse (see Figure 19.1).

One could argue, therefore, that we can best help our clients by increasing their distress tolerance, rather than simply focusing on reducing their distress. What would that look like? For the clients we discussed above, it might be that:

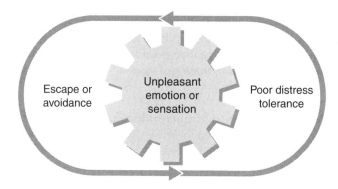

FIGURE 19.1. A conceptual model of maladaptive secondary reactions to unpleasant emotions.

- Suzanne shows greater tolerance of uncertainty. When she doesn't know what's going to happen or doesn't have all of the information in front of her, she accepts the fact that she doesn't have all of the answers and does not feel compelled to engage in certainty-seeking behaviors.
- William shows improved physical discomfort tolerance. When he experiences feelings of pain, he accepts the fact that he is not feeling good, yet he does not engage in excessive avoidance behavior.
- Anna shows decreased anxiety sensitivity. When she starts noticing her heart rate increasing, or she starts to feel dizzy, she recognizes that these are just unpleasant feelings and does not catastrophize or try to escape from the situation.
- Elizabeth has better emotional distress tolerance. When she feels angry or sad, she recognizes that these feelings are acceptable and remembers that she is able to tolerate these feelings. She notices her feelings but does not dwell excessively on them.
- Blaise's frustration tolerance improves. When she experiences an urge to use, she is aware of the fact that she does not need to act on that urge. She keeps going with things that are hard, recognizing that her efforts will probably pay off eventually.

Acceptance of Emotions

Acceptance is one way to build up a client's distress tolerance. Critical elements of the acceptance conceptualization of unpleasant emotions or physical sensations are:

- Unpleasant feelings are an unavoidable part of life, and one need not be significantly distressed about them.
- Distress does not necessarily come from the unpleasant feeling but rather from how one *responds to* that unpleasant feeling.
- Specifically, distressed people are characterized by excessive and maladaptive cognitive and behavioral efforts to suppress or "fix" unpleasant feelings; these efforts end up doing more harm than good and distract the person from actually dealing effectively with real problems or pursuing his or her own goals and values.
- Emotional distress can come from either paying too little attention to one's feelings (in which case we may act on them automatically) or from taking them too seriously and believing that they must be acted upon.

And from the acceptance conceptualization come the following acceptance interventions:

- Clients should be taught, through words or through metaphors and exercises, that their efforts to control their feelings are a major part of the problem.
- Clients should learn to pay attention to their feelings and to identify them as feelings.
- Clients should accept their feelings without judging them, labeling them as "good" or "bad," or attempting to gain control over them.
- Clients should learn to direct their attention toward the present moment, rather than the past or the future.
- Clients should redirect their efforts away from trying to gain control over their feelings and toward engaging in behaviors that are consistent with meaningful goals and personal values.

The Science behind It

There's good reason to believe that acceptance is a viable way to manage unpleasant emotions and physiological sensations. Several studies demonstrate that when people accept their current emotional states, they feel better than they do when they are instructed to suppress their emotions (Asnaani et al., 2013; Hofmann et al., 2009) or when they are given no specific instructions about what to do with their emotions (Wolgast et al., 2011). Similar findings have been reported when the physical sensation is largely outside of the person's direct control, such as chronic pain (Viane et al., 2003). In one study, teaching healthy volunteers to accept feelings of pain (electric shocks) helped them tolerate the pain better than did teaching them to challenge pain-related thoughts and feelings (Gutierrez, Luciano, Rodriguez, & Fink, 2004).

A concrete example of the difference between these two conceptualizations can be seen in Table 19.1.

As we saw with interpretations in Chapter 15, the therapist has a bit of a dilemma here. Some people say that when arousal-based emotions and physical sensations are present, you should use relaxation strategies to decrease them. And other people say that arousal-based emotions and bodily sensations, and indeed all unpleasant emotions and bodily sensations, are best handled with acceptance strategies. So your client comes in

The Science behind It

What's more effective: relaxation or acceptance for maladaptive emotions? Research tells us:

- Among students in a stress-reduction program, participants receiving *mindfulness-based stress reduction* (Kabat-Zinn, 1982) and those receiving progressive relaxation and breathing retraining showed roughly equal decreases in emotional distress, although the mindfulness group showed greater decreases in distractive and ruminative thoughts (Jain et al., 2007).

- Clients with OCD receiving *acceptance and commitment therapy* (Hayes et al., 1999) showed significantly greater symptom improvement than did those receiving progressive relaxation (Twohig et al., 2010).

- Clients with GAD receiving acceptance and commitment therapy showed similar outcomes to those receiving progressive relaxation (Hayes-Skelton, Roemer, & Orsillo, 2013).

- Among clients with chronic pain, those receiving self-help acceptance and commitment therapy reported greater increases in activity engagement and willingness to experience pain than did those receiving self-help progressive relaxation, although no significant differences between the groups were seen in life satisfaction, pain intensity, level of function, depression, or anxiety (Thorsell et al., 2011). In another study, clients with pain who used an acceptance-based intervention demonstrated greater overall functioning than did patients who received instructions for controlling pain (Vowles et al., 2007).

TABLE 19.1. A Comparison of Traditional Relaxation and Acceptance Perspectives on Unpleasant Emotions

	Traditional relaxation perspective	Acceptance perspective
The unpleasant emotion is . . .	• Anxiety	• Anxiety
The problem here is . . .	• The emotion is out of proportion to the situation. • The unpleasant emotion leads to maladaptive behavior.	• The emotion is normal. • The person treats the emotion as if it were a problem, rather than as just a feeling. • The person pays excessive attention to the emotion and tries to change it, feel better, avoid it, or act on it.
And so the solution is . . .	• Demonstrate that the emotion is a source of maladaptive behaviors. • Help the client to understand that the emotion is out of proportion. • Help the client to learn and practice strategies for reducing the unpleasant emotion.	• Help the client to focus awareness on the emotion in the present moment. • Teach the client to experience the emotion without judging it, analyzing it, feeling better, or trying to control it. • Help the client to recognize that this is just a feeling. • Redirect the client's efforts away from attempts to control or change emotions and toward value- or goal-oriented activity.
And this should work because . . .	• Relaxation reduces physiological arousal. • Decreased physiological arousal reduces maladaptive thoughts and behaviors. • Decreased physiological arousal allows for better problem-focused coping strategies.	• Defusion helps the client recognize that emotions are only internal events, rather than threats. • When emotions are perceived as nothing more than internal events, the client is better able to respond appropriately to situations. • Stopping maladaptive control efforts will likely reduce emotional distress.

with a bunch of arousal-based emotions and sensations, such as anxiety, anger, tension, or pain. Do you help him or her to relax and decrease physiological arousal? Or do you encourage him or her to notice the emotion or sensation, accept it, and refrain from trying to change it?

As is clear in the "Science behind It" sidebar, at this stage of the research I think it's a scientific toss-up. We can probably say with some confidence that relaxation won't be very helpful for clients with OCD, but beyond that, the research results generally suggest that the results of relaxation versus acceptance are more similar than they are different. So again, I'll tell you what I do clinically.

• Sometimes I run both treatment rationales by the client. I explain that both relaxation and acceptance strategies have been demonstrated to be helpful and provide a brief description of what's involved. I try to determine which strategy seems more compatible with the client's preferences and expectations. The more "buy-in" I have from the client at the outset, the easier my job will be.

• I also base my selection, in part, on what else I am likely to be using. For example, the rationale for acceptance of unpleasant emotions doesn't fit well with the rationale for cognitive restructuring of interpretations (it's tough to explain to a client why he or she should change his or her thoughts, but not his or her emotions). So if I'm planning to use cognitive restructuring for thoughts, I might opt for relaxation for emotions. Conversely, if I'm planning to use acceptance for thoughts, it's a fairly easy transition to use acceptance for emotions as well.

• For those clients who seem particularly prone to scramble for safety behaviors (see Chapter 11), I'm less likely to give them relaxation and breathing exercises that will serve as "crutches." Highly compulsive clients, for example, may be so preoccupied with the need to "fix" their emotions that they might benefit from an alternative approach (acceptance) that teaches them to accept, rather than try to fix, how they feel. Similarly, clients with urges (e.g., those with impulse control disorders or substance use disorders) might be good candidates for a strategy, such as acceptance, that helps them "ride the wave" of their urges rather than trying to control them.

• Some clients appear to be avoidant of emotions in general. The concepts of "affect phobia" in psychodynamic therapy (McCullough et al., 2003) and "emotion phobia" in dialectical behavior therapy (Linehan, 1993) parallel that of experiential avoidance in many ways. When clients seem generally reluctant to experience emotions, acceptance can be a useful way to build emotional tolerance.

• The intensity of the experienced emotion might also serve as a guide. When the arousal is so intense that the person's functioning is significantly limited, relaxation exercises may provide a good shorter-term solution to allow him or her to function better. On the other hand, when the arousal is less intense, it might be preferable to teach some

Metaphor

Noting the role of the brain's limbic system (e.g., the amygdala, often described as the brain's "fear center"), Otto (2000, p. 171) provides a metaphor of the "Limbic Kid" in the treatment of a client with PTSD who has excessive fear reactions to objectively safe situations:

> When your limbic system perceives these cues, your limbic system will start to shout "Danger, danger!" In its reaction the limbic system will be somewhat like a child who is frightened and can't tell whether a cue simply looks frightening or is truly dangerous. During our treatment of PTSD, you are going to be in the position of parenting this Limbic Kid. . . . It is important that you don't try to overcontrol the Limbic Kid. Overcontrol may just lead the Kid to become even more frightened (similar to how a real kid might react if you were to try to control her or him too much when she or he was scared). Instead, your job is to understand the symptomatic shouting, and gently soothe yourself and the Kid by explaining what is happening.

degree of emotion tolerance. So your selection of relaxation versus acceptance need not be either–or (no black-and-white thinking here). It may be that you teach your client to relax in certain situations but to accept emotions in others.

There are lots of ways that the acceptance approach to emotions can be employed. As described previously, *dialectical behavior therapy* (Linehan, 1993) and *mindfulness-based cognitive therapy* (Segal et al., 2002) use formal meditation exercises, whereas *metacognitive therapy* (Wells, 2009) and *acceptance and commitment therapy* (Hayes et al., 1999) are less likely to use formal exercises than to incorporate mindfulness and acceptance principles into other conversations and activities. We don't have a scientific basis to tell us which approach is better. I tend to incorporate acceptance into other things, as illustrated by the case example below. However, if you'd like to learn more about doing formal mindfulness meditation, there are a number of good published resources out there (*http://marc.ucla.edu/body.cfm?id=22* is a good free website for this).

Here, the therapist is working with Suzanne (S), our client with GAD. The therapist uses a metaphor to explain how difficult it can be to get one's physical arousal under control.

T: Suzanne, I know that when you feel anxious, you tend to try very hard to get that emotion under control. You try to distract yourself away from it, or you try to think happy thoughts, or you just tell yourself to get over it.

S: That's right. I just get so upset that I can't stand it. I don't want to lose control of myself.

T: I certainly understand not wanting to lose control. Nobody likes feeling out of control. But I wonder whether trying to just erase your anxiety is really helping here. It seems like it kind of invalidates the fact that you're anxious, like it tells you that it's not OK to feel that way.

S: It's not OK. It's not good to get anxious. I should have better control over my feelings.

T: I'm not sure I see it the same way you do. To me, it seems perfectly fine to feel anxious, and feeling a certain way doesn't mean that you're out of control. What's really important is how you react to that feeling, what you do about it. Let's break the process down a little bit. When something makes you anxious, what is the first thing that you notice?

S: I guess I notice that my heart starts going faster. And I feel kind of tense in my shoulders.

T: OK, so something troubling happens and then you have this automatic physical reaction where your heart speeds up and you feel tense in your shoulders. What do you do to cope with that?

S: I try taking a deep breath and thinking about something else.

T: I see. And how effective has that strategy been for you?

S: Not very effective, I guess, because I keep getting more and more worked up.

T: So even though you try to get your physical sensations under control, they just get worse. I wonder whether that's the best strategy for you, then?

S: No, I guess not, but then how am I supposed to get my anxiety under control?

T: Maybe you don't. Well, let me clarify that a little. Maybe you don't get it under control by trying to control it. Let's imagine, just for a second, that I hook you up to a heart rate monitor and then do something to make you anxious. What would happen?

S: You'd see my heart rate go through the roof.

T: Yes, that's a good bet. Now how about if I told you, right then, that you had to get your heart rate to go back to normal? Could you do it?

S: No. I've tried.

T: Well, what if I tell you that it's very, very important that you get your heart rate under control right now? Like the fate of the world depends on you making your anxiety go away and making your heart slow down? Then could you do it?

S: I'd try.

T: Yes, you'd try. And what would be the result of that trying? If you tried really, really hard to control your heart rate—and you tried taking deep breaths, thinking about something else, all that—what would happen?

S: I guess I'd just get more anxious and worked up.

T: Right. So the harder you try to control anxiety . . .

S: The worse it gets?

T: Exactly. And I wonder whether that's just what happens to you when something makes you anxious. You start trying to control your feeling of anxiety and it just gets worse. So what if we try something completely different? What if we try an exercise in not controlling your anxiety at all?

S: I'd worry that I would just get so anxious that I couldn't stand it. Or maybe I'd just lose my mind.

T: That's your prediction. And it may or may not be true. Only one way to know for sure. Would you be willing to try an exercise with me, so that we can see whether not controlling anxiety really leads it to become unbearable and you losing your mind?

S: I guess I could try something.

T: OK. If your anxiety does become truly unbearable, let me know. This isn't meant to be awful, although it's quite likely that you will experience anxiety. I'd like you to take a few minutes and tell me about something that worried you recently, something you'd rather not think about because it makes you anxious. Would you be willing to do that for a few minutes?

S: OK.

T: And your job is going to be not to try to control your anxiety. Your anxiety is what it is. All of your feelings are what they are. If your heart rate increases, what I want you to do is to notice that your heart rate is increasing. Just notice it, and tell me what you notice. But don't try to change it. And if your muscles get tense, just notice your muscles getting tense. But don't relax them. Don't try to make them feel any better than they do. We'll just notice them and talk about them.

S: Um . . . I think I'm already noticing my heart speeding up.

T: OK, that's fine. Let's just notice your heart speeding up. It can go as fast as it wants to. Let your heart do its thing, and tell me the story.

S: I guess I'm thinking about how my daughter keeps overspending. She doesn't save any of her money, and I worry that she's going to end up destitute.

T: Right now, what are you noticing in your body?

S: My heart's definitely racing.

T: OK, let it race for now. What else do you notice?

S: My heart's going a mile a minute. And my shoulders feel really tense. Like I want to run away. My face is hot.

T: You feel anxious.

S: Yes.

T: Can you just feel that anxiety and that tension right now, without doing anything?

S: I'm feeling like I want to get rid of it.

T: Yes, that's understandable. Let's try staying with it for the moment. Is it unbearable?

S: No. It feels pretty bad, but it's not unbearable.

T: You can stand it.

S: Yeah.

T: That doesn't mean you like it, but you can stand it. I want you to see that you can sit with this feeling of anxiety, that racing heart, that tension, that hot sensation in your face. Just notice those feelings, notice what they feel like. Allow them to be there. Make some room for them.

S: OK. I'm noticing them. It actually feels like they're coming down a little bit.

T: Are you doing something to make them come down?

S: No.

T: So that's important for us to notice. When you try to fix your anxiety or get away from it, it feels worse. And when you just notice it without fixing it . . .

S: It starts to get a little better.

Note that in this exercise, Suzanne's distress level started to come down. That's nice, but not critical. A client might not experience much of a decrease in distress or could even

Metaphor

I often use exercise metaphors to explain the concept of distress tolerance. When we exercise—for example, when we go running—it often doesn't feel good. It tires us out, makes us sweaty, and makes our muscles sore. So if we went running with the idea that we should feel great immediately afterward, we're missing the point. And we wouldn't judge the success or failure of a run by whether or not it made us feel good. We judge the success of running over time, by whether we are able to endure more and more of it. That's how we know we're stronger: Where we used to be able to run only half a mile, we can now run a 5K. So it is with distress tolerance. When we do exercises in therapy or as homework, we don't do them to feel better. We do it to build up our "tolerance muscles" so that emotions are less and less likely to derail us over time.

Show Me, Don't Tell Me

In mindfulness-based stress reduction (M Williams et al., 2007) and dialectical behavioral therapy (Linehan, 1993), the concept of mindfulness is often introduced with a simple sensory activity such as eating a raisin. As clients look at, feel, smell, chew, and swallow the raisin, they are encouraged to notice what they are experiencing carefully, perhaps as if they had never seen or tasted a raisin before, without trying to influence or judge what is happening. Some clients find it difficult at first to simply notice their perceptions without labeling them or otherwise judging them. This lesson then is used to illustrate how the client can respond to emotions—dispassionately, from an observing perspective.

experience an increase in distress when shifting away from controlling and toward noticing feelings. It's not surprising that addressing one's feelings in a new way and giving up old habits can in itself be a source of distress. In acceptance, we deemphasize the importance of making distress decrease in the short term, instead emphasizing the importance of building up distress tolerance in the long term.

Emotion Regulation as a Potential Target

Both emotional modulation and emotion tolerance strategies are emphasized in the relatively new area of **emotion regulation training.** Emotion regulation is a fuzzy concept that is not well defined (L. Bloch, Moran, & Kring, 2010); and various authors have suggested their own definitions (Berking et al., 2008; Gratz & Roemer, 2004; J. J. Gross & Thompson, 2007; Mennin, 2006). Across definitions, some common features of emotion regulation include:

- The ability to recognize and accurately identify one's emotions.
- The ability to recognize external or internal triggers for emotions.
- The ability to alter one's environmental context in order to change emotional response.
- The ability to use strategies to modulate and/or accept negative emotions.
- The ability to act in a manner that is incompatible with negative emotions.

Note that emotion regulation does not necessarily imply emotional *control* or emotion *elimination* (Gratz & Roemer, 2004). Rather, successful emotion regulation strategies generally modify the intensity or duration of the negative emotion, rather than changing the kind of emotion that is experienced (R. A. Thompson, 1994). In other words, successful emotion regulation means (for example) going from very sad to less sad, or from persistently sad to briefly sad, rather than going from sad to happy.

Many clients have difficulty identifying and describing their emotions, a phenomenon which has been termed **alexithymia** (Sifneos, 1973, 1996), which literally translates to "no words for feelings." Alexithymic individuals not only have difficulty recognizing their own emotional states, but also often have difficulty interpreting the emotional states of others (Cook, Brewer, Shah, & Bird, 2013; Grynberg et al., 2012). Though the term was originally coined within a psychoanalytic model and characterized as a personality dimension (G.

J. Taylor & Bagby, 2013), from a CBT perspective we can think of alexithymia as a skill deficit. As you might imagine, it's hard to regulate an emotion if you don't know what that emotion is (or, in some cases, whether you're even *having* an emotion).

As discussed in Chapter 3, clients frequently rely on maladaptive effortful cognitive processes to modify emotional experiences. Depressed individuals, for example, tend to use *rumination* strategies, in which they try to feel better by analyzing (and reanalyzing) what's bothering them and what's wrong with them. Anxious people may use *worry* strategies, in which they try to stave off anxiety by mentally rehearsing everything that could possibly go wrong (whether those events are likely or not). Clients with a range of problems may use *suppression* strategies, in which they attempt to shut themselves off from negative emotions and "snap out of it." None of these strategies are particularly effective; indeed, there's ample research showing that they all tend to make negative moods worse (Johnson-Laird, Mancini, & Gangemi, 2006; Llera & Newman, 2010; Nolen-Hoeksema & Morrow, 1993).

Behaviorally, clients usually engage in mood-congruent behavior, rather than behavior that might alter their emotional experiences. Depressed individuals withdraw and become inactive. People who are fearful avoid. People who are angry vent. People in pain move gingerly or avoid activities that they think will hurt. And, as we know, these behaviors don't really improve things. Although the person may feel a bit of short-term relief, these behaviors aren't cathartic, and they aren't an adaptive way of working through an

 The Science behind It

Though alexithymia was originally described as a contributor to somatoform disorders (perhaps due to older psychoanalytic conceptualizations of hysteria), the problem doesn't seem to be specific to any particular psychiatric disorder (G. J. Taylor, 1984). Rather, it appears to be a dimensional characteristic that can be seen in a broad range of clients, including those with somatoform disorders (De Gucht & Heiser, 2003; Gulpek, Kelemence Kaplan, Kesebir, & Bora, 2014), depression (Leweke, Leichsenring, Kruse, & Hermes, 2012), anxiety disorders (de Berardis et al., 2008; Izci et al., 2014), OCD (de Berardis et al., 2005), PTSD (Frewen, Dozois, Neufeld, & Lanius, 2008), personality disorders (de Panfilis, Ossola, Tonna, Catania, & Marchesi, 2015), substance use disorders (Shishido, Gaher, & Simons, 2013; Thorberg, Young, Sullivan, & Lyvers, 2009), schizophrenia (O'Driscoll, Laing, & Mason, 2014), and marital distress (Frye-Cox & Hesse, 2013). Across diagnostic groups, the prevalence of high alexithymia is approximately one in five clients (Leweke et al., 2012).

Alexithymic individuals show faulty decision making; for example, people with high levels of alexithymia make poorer decisions in a simulated gambling task (Aite et al., 2014; Kano, Ito, & Fukudo, 2011) and report greater impulsivity when experiencing negative emotions (Shishido et al., 2013). It seems likely that healthy decision making requires accurate perception of emotional feedback (Bechara & Damasio, 2007); without the ability to decipher such feedback, decision making becomes impulsive.

There's also reason to believe that alexithymia moderates the relationship between traumatic experiences (e.g., those occurring in childhood) and adult psychiatric symptoms (Mazzeo & Espelage, 2002; Ogrodniczuk, Joyce, & Abbass, 2014)—that is, among people experiencing aversive or traumatic life events, those who are able to identify their feelings and put them into words end up much healthier than do those who lack this ability.

emotion. Rather, as we've discussed, in the long run they tend to worsen negative emotions and physical sensations.

Likely as a result of the aforementioned problems (alexithymia and maladaptive cognitive and behavioral emotion regulation strategies), many clients will present with **emotion dysregulation** (Westen, 1994; sometimes called *affect dysregulation*). That means that when they experience negative emotions, the emotions feel particularly strong and take a long time to return to baseline levels. These clients will often feel as though their emotions are spiraling out of control or changing rapidly. Their emotional expressions tend to be intense and unmodified, their cognitive function is diminished. Emotion dysregulation has been commonly associated with borderline personality disorder (Conklin, Bradley, & Westen, 2006), although the phenomenon is not limited to clients with that diagnosis (Mennin, Heimberg, Turk, & Fresco, 2005).

Gratz and Roemer (2004), who developed their theory largely on the self-reports of clients, define emotion regulation somewhat differently from Gross and Thompson (2007), whose model emerged from basic science on emotion. The Gratz and Roemer (2004) model conceptualizes emotion regulation problems as consisting of:

- *Nonacceptance of emotional responses:* a tendency to have negative secondary emotional responses to one's negative emotions or nonaccepting reactions to one's distress.
- *Difficulties engaging in goal-directed behavior:* difficulties concentrating and accomplishing tasks when experiencing negative emotions.
- *Impulse control difficulties:* difficulties remaining in control of one's behavior when experiencing negative emotions.
- *Lack of emotional awareness:* inattention to, and lack of awareness of, emotional responses.
- *Limited access to emotion regulation strategies:* the belief that there is little that can be done to regulate emotions effectively, once an individual is upset.
- *Lack of emotional clarity:* not knowing (and being clear about) the emotions one is experiencing.

 ### The Science behind It

An emotion regulation training program for clients with borderline personality disorder and self-injurious behaviors found that training, when added to existing therapy, resulted in decreased self-injury and other impulsive behaviors, as well as decreased symptoms of borderline personality disorder and depression and improved quality of life, with gains maintained or even strengthened at a 9-month follow-up (Gratz et al., 2013). Among depressed inpatients, those receiving emotion regulation training with CBT showed greater reductions in depression and improved well-being, compared with clients receiving standard CBT alone (Berking et al., 2013). Clients with alcohol dependence who reported drinking in negative affect conditions showed decreased alcohol consumption and a greater number of abstinence days when receiving CBT plus emotion regulation training, compared with clients receiving CBT plus healthy lifestyle psychoeducation (Stasiewicz et al., 2013). When clients with PTSD received emotion regulation training prior to other CBT, they showed decreased PTSD symptoms and were less likely to drop out of treatment (Bryant et al., 2013; Cloitre et al., 2010).

Teaching Clients to Regulate Emotions

Just as there is no clear consensus as to what constitutes emotion regulation, there are varying definitions of emotion regulation training. Existing models (Berking et al., 2013; Bryant et al., 2013; Gratz & Gunderson, 2006; Greenberg, 2004; Kemeny et al., 2012; Levitt & Cloitre, 2006; Linehan, 2015; Mennin, 2006; Schuppert et al., 2012; Stasiewicz et al., 2013) often draw heavily from mindfulness and acceptance interventions, yet allow for the selection of emotion-modulation strategies such as relaxation, breathing retraining, and cognitive restructuring. Some common themes emerge from these various emotion regulation approaches:

- *Clients should be taught to identify their emotions.* This directly targets alexithymia, whether severe or mild. To do this, clients are often asked to pay close attention to bodily sensations as a signal of emotions. Having the client close his or her eyes in session and "scan" his or her body for sensations is one way to accomplish this. Clients might also be encouraged to identify thoughts as emotional "clues." That is, when an individual's thoughts revolve around themes of hopelessness and self-deprecation, the emotion of sadness might be present; similarly, when an individual's thoughts focus on potential threats, fear might be the dominant emotion (see Chapter 3). Having identified somatic or cognitive clues about emotions, clients then practice labeling those emotions verbally.

One twist on emotion labeling is distinguishing between "primary emotions" and "secondary emotions" (Greenberg & Safran, 1987). Primary emotions, which Hayes et al. (1999) label *clean discomfort,* refer to natural, biologically driven, and often adaptive emotional reactions. Emotion theorists describe the primary emotions as anger, disgust, fear, happiness, sadness, and surprise (Ekman, 1992a). Feeling sad in reaction to loss or feeling fearful in reaction to a threat are examples of primary emotions. Secondary emotions, which Hayes et al. (1999) label *dirty discomfort,* are more complex emotional reactions to the primary emotions (i.e., they are "meta-emotions," or emotions about emotions). So, for example, when one feels angry in reaction to feeling hurt, or feels afraid or guilty about feeling angry, those are examples of secondary emotions. It has been suggested that adaptive emotion regulation requires identifying, discussing, and validating the primary emotion (Greenberg, 2004).

- *Clients should be educated about the adaptive and maladaptive aspects of emotions.* Emotions serve an inherently adaptive purpose, providing motivation, allowing for the activation of innate and automatic responses, and communicating with others (e.g., Keltner & Gross, 1999; Levenson, 1999). On the other hand, unregulated emotions may lead

Metaphor

Mennin and Fresco (2013) use a nice metaphor of asking clients to imagine a pristine snowball (representing the primary emotion) rolling down a hill. As it rolls, it picks up dirt and twigs (secondary emotions), eventually becoming a hard, icy mess. The idea to get across to the client is that primary emotions are natural, often quite valid, and relatively easy to deal with, compared with secondary emotions (*meta-emotions* or *dirty discomfort*).

Bringing the Problem into the Room

Mennin (2006) brings the problem into the room by encouraging clients to experience uncomfortable emotions in session, using emotionally evocative strategies such as the downward arrow (see Chapter 14) or empty chair technique (see Chapter 16), and then by practicing selecting and applying acceptance or modification strategies.

to poor decision making, self-perpetuating cycles, and other complications (see Chapter 4). Clients practice identifying the adaptive and maladaptive aspects of their emotional experiences.

- *Clients should be taught acceptance strategies for negative emotions.* As described previously in this chapter, clients should practice observing their emotions as if from a distance, without judging them as good or bad and without attempting to influence or otherwise control them.

- *Clients should be taught emotion modulation strategies such as relaxation and cognitive reappraisal.* As described in Chapters 14 and 18, these strategies aim to temper the emotional experience.

- *Clients should be taught to select flexibly from modification and acceptance strategies.* One selection criterion might be to employ acceptance strategies toward primary emotions (*clean discomfort*) and to use modification strategies toward secondary emotions (*meta-emotions* or *dirty discomfort*), although this is not a hard-and-fast rule. The client's own experience with these strategies (e.g., what has helped in the past) may also be a useful guide.

- *Clients should practice behaving in a manner that is incompatible with secondary* (dirty discomfort) *emotions.* In many cases, this intervention involves promoting actions that are consistent with the person's greater goals and values, as discussed in the section on acceptance of emotions in this chapter. In other cases, this may mean encouraging actions that validate the primary emotions—for example, if a client feels justifiably angry about being slighted by someone, the client might learn and practice assertive communication skills; if a client feels anxious about a potentially solvable problem in living, he or she might learn and practice problem-solving skills (see Chapter 12).

Adapting the Process: *Acceptance . . .*

. . . with high-functioning clients. One of the challenges with acceptance for higher-functioning clients is keeping them from overanalyzing the process. This was my problem when I tried doing acceptance. Maybe it's my science background, but I'm used to a logical, analytic, linear way of addressing problems. So when a negative thought would come into my head, it was hard for me to resist the temptation to analyze it, challenge it, and somehow "fix" it. The problem with that approach is that it's hard to be analytic and experiential at the same time. That is, it's difficult to feel something and analyze it simultaneously. I needed to

be reminded (a lot) that this was not an equation to be solved; it was something to be experienced and worked through.

   . . . with low-functioning clients. Linehan's (1993) dialectical behavior therapy for clients with borderline personality disorder, many of whom are chronically suicidal or self-injurious, employs the concept of *radical acceptance*, which she describes as "acceptance of what is" (p. 99). Clients practice experiencing emotions without judging them or trying to control them. With clients suffering from severe, chronic, and complex disorders such as schizophrenia, although some of the metaphors may need to be simplified depending on the client's cognitive function (e.g., capacity for abstract thinking), the experiential exercises in acceptance can be helpful. In one novel application, clients with schizophrenia were taught an acceptance response to auditory hallucinations ("voices"). They practiced simply noticing the voices without acting on them, accepting voices even though they were unpleasant, and accomplishing valued goals in the context of ongoing voices (Bach & Hayes, 2002; Gaudiano & Herbert, 2006; Shawyer et al., 2012). Interestingly (and consistent with the general model of acceptance), although clients did not report a decrease in the hallucinations themselves, they reported believing them less and had a much lower rate of rehospitalization than did clients not receiving the intervention (Bach & Hayes, 2002). Lower-functioning clients may require shorter mindfulness exercises, combined with significant emphasis on managing daily "hassles" with problem-solving training (see Chapter 12), in order to keep them engaged in the treatment (Deckersbach et al., 2012).

   . . . with children. Emotional acceptance with children often requires creative use of metaphors and stories. For example, Saltzman and Goldin (2008) encourage children to give names to their various emotions and to describe where they are felt in the body. They also describe whether the feelings have colors or sounds and to ask the feelings what they want.

   . . . in groups. The experiential exercises used in many acceptance interventions lend themselves to a group setting. Some interventions, such as mindfulness-based cognitive therapy, were originally designed to be provided in groups; others, such as dialectical behavior therapy, use a mix of individual and group treatments. After the group leader introduces an exercise, group members can discuss their shared and unique reactions to the exercise. During discussion of metaphors, group members may have their own unique interpretations and real-life examples that can serve as fuel for a group discussion.

   . . . with medical patients. Acceptance is a promising intervention for chronic pain. Clients discuss their values, and the topic of value-oriented behavior (despite the presence of pain) is raised. The overall aim is to enhance "willingness to have discomfort in the service of meaningful living" (Vowles, Wetherell, & Sorrell, 2009, p. 57). As part of this, *exposure* (see Chapter 11) is used to gradually increase the client's behavioral repertoire to include activities that cause some pain but increase the client's overall quality of life (Wicksell, Dahl, Magnusson, & Olsson, 2005). Mindfulness practice is thought to help clients detach from the pain: Clients are taught to notice and observe their pain, as well as any accompanying thoughts or emotions, thus potentially "uncoupling" the pain from its attendant alarm reaction (Kabat-Zinn, 1982).

▰▰▰▰▰▰ THE ESSENTIALS ▰▰▰▰▰▰

✳ An alternative way of dealing with unpleasant emotions is to try to increase the client's distress tolerance, rather than trying to lessen the emotions themselves.

✳ The basic principles of acceptance for emotions are:
  • Unpleasant emotions are normal and unavoidable.
  • Distress comes less from unpleasant emotions than from how the person responds to the emotions.
  • Efforts to gain control over unpleasant emotions may do more harm than good.

✳ The key elements of acceptance interventions are:
  • Teaching the client to decrease efforts to control, label, judge, fix, or avoid unpleasant emotions.
  • Teaching the client to pay attention to his or her feelings and to label them as just feelings.
  • Having the client pay attention to the present moment.
  • Redirecting the client's energy away from emotional control and toward value-based action.

✳ Emotion regulation training involves the following steps:
  • Helping the client accurately identify pleasant and unpleasant emotions.
  • Educating the client about adaptive and maladaptive aspects of emotions.
  • Teaching acceptance strategies for thoughts and emotions.
  • Teaching modulation strategies such as relaxation and cognitive restructuring.
  • Teaching and practicing the flexible selection of acceptance versus modulation strategies.
  • Encouraging the client to behave in a manner that is incompatible with secondary emotions (though the behavior may be consistent with primary emotions).

▰▰▰▰▰ KEY TERMS AND DEFINITIONS ▰▰▰▰▰

Alexithymia: Difficulty identifying and describing emotional states.

Anxiety sensitivity: Fear of anxiety-related bodily sensations due to a belief that these sensations will have negative physical, psychological, or social consequences.

Distress tolerance: The perceived and/or behavioral capacity to withstand negative emotional or physical states.

Emotion dysregulation: A deficit in the ability to modulate emotion, resulting in a sense that emotions are spiraling out of control, in rapidly changing emotions, in intense and unmodified expression of emotion, and in impaired cognitive function.

Emotion regulation training: A collection of interventions aimed at improving clients' ability to modify or otherwise cope with negative emotions and the behavioral expression thereof in distressing situations.

Emotional distress tolerance: The ability to withstand negative emotions.

Frustration tolerance: A belief that aversive situations are intolerable.

Intolerance of uncertainty: Reacting negatively to uncertain situations or events.

Physical discomfort intolerance: Difficulty withstanding uncomfortable physical sensations.

Acceptance of Emotions and Physical Sensations

Step 1: Try to create a feeling or a physical sensation related to your personal target. To do this, you might try thinking about a situation related to the target, or doing something that makes you feel uncomfortable.

Step 2: For a period of 10 minutes, close your eyes and notice your feelings and physical sensations. Do not judge or evaluate your feelings; just notice them. Describe them to yourself in your mind but don't try to explain or understand them. Just notice.

What was your experience in Step 2? Specifically: How hard or easy was it? When did it become hard? What was your response to your feelings? Did your response change over time?

Step 3: For a period of 24 hours, notice any emotions or sensations related to the personal target, but do not judge or evaluate them. Do not attempt to determine whether they are good or bad. Do not attempt to change them. Do not attempt to avoid them.

What was your experience in Step 3? Specifically: How hard or easy was it? When did it become hard? What was your response to your feelings? Did you notice any attempts to control or "fix" the emotion? Did you notice any attempts to avoid the emotion? Did your response change over time?

From *Doing CBT* by David F. Tolin. Copyright © 2016 The Guilford Press. Permission to photocopy this worksheet is granted to purchasers of this book for personal use only (see copyright page for details). Purchasers can download enlarged versions of this worksheet (see the box at the end of the table of contents).

PART III

Putting It All Together

In this section, we review the complete CBT for three of our clients: William, who is dependent on others and experiences chronic pain; Anna, who experiences unexpected panic attacks and is becoming increasingly avoidant; and Elizabeth, who has been diagnosed with borderline personality disorder and has been in the hospital repeatedly for suicidality and self-injury.

By reading the transcripts, you'll get a sense of how the therapist interacts with the clients. The therapist fosters a sense of collaborative empiricism, enjoining the clients to act as "coinvestigators" as they try to develop an understanding of what's happening. At times, the therapist employs strategies from MI in order to boost clients' readiness to work on the problem. You'll also see that the therapist keeps the empathy, genuineness, and unconditional positive regard coming, from start to finish.

As you read these case examples, pay attention to how the therapist conceptualizes the cases. Diagnoses matter, and do come into play; however, knowing the client's diagnosis is less important than having an understanding of why the client continues to suffer, day in and day out. You'll see that the meaty conceptualization is always a work in progress and that the therapist is constantly referring back to and modifying the conceptualization with the client. The therapist focuses in on the critical questions we discussed way back in Chapter 1:

- Under what circumstances does this problem occur?
- What are the *behavioral* elements of the problem?
    - How do external and internal *contingencies* (e.g., reward and punishment) influence his or her behavioral responses?
    - Does the person lack specific *behavioral skills* needed to adapt successfully to the environment?
    - What are the negative effects of the person's behaviors?
- What are the *cognitive* elements of the problem?
    - To what extent does this person have *interpretations* that are unhelpful?
    - To what extent do this person's *core beliefs* shape his or her thinking in difficult situations?

- To what extent do *information processing biases* distort how information is attended to and remembered?
- To what extent does this person engage in *maladaptive mental coping strategies?*
  - What are the *emotional* elements of the problem?
    - What are the subjective feeling states experienced?
    - What physiological sensations are associated with those emotions?
    - To what extent have emotional responses been *classically conditioned* through paired associations?
  - How has the person's *learning history* shaped his or her thoughts, emotions, and behaviors?

Finally, note that there are several decision-making points in the treatments. After developing a meaty conceptualization, the therapist must select specific targets and use specific interventions designed to address those targets. Behavior-level interventions were used in each case; CBT is unlikely to gain much traction without them. Varying cognitive- and emotion-level interventions were used, depending on how well the clients were responding to the behavior-level interventions. At times, these interventions attempted to modify thoughts and emotions; at other times, however, the therapist encouraged the client to practice accepting unwanted thoughts and emotions and refocus on more pertinent, value-based goals.

CHAPTER 20

Putting It All Together

William's CBT

In this chapter, we review the treatment of our client William. Figure 20.1 shows when various interventions were introduced into the therapy. As you can see, William was treated for a total of 20 outpatient sessions, with most delivered once per week. Dark gray shading shows that a strategy was heavily emphasized during that session; light gray shading shows that a strategy was present, but not heavily emphasized.

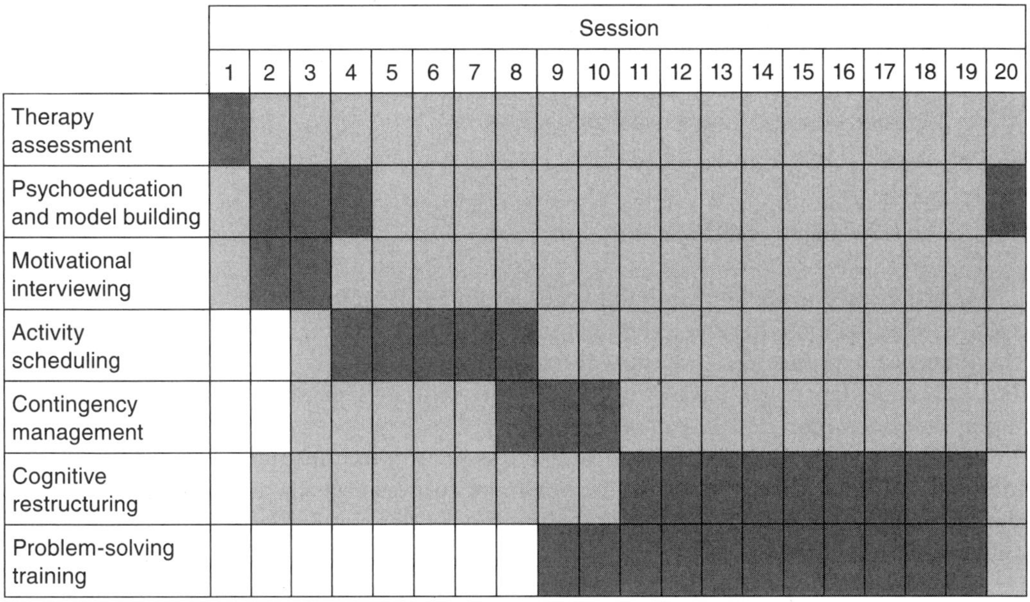

FIGURE 20.1. Session-by-session description of William's CBT.

Therapy Assessment

The therapist opens the initial session by providing structure and getting a general sense of William's presenting concerns.

T: Welcome, William. It's nice to meet you.

W: Nice to meet you too.

T: What I have in mind for today is to get a bit of a sense of what's been bothering you and ask you a lot of questions. I'd also like to see if we can start to think of a plan for how we might be able to make things better and to start to develop an overall strategy. Does that agenda sound OK to you?

W: Yes, whatever you think is best.

T: OK. So what's been going on?

W: Well, I'm just bummed out all the time, and I have a lot of pain.

T: Bummed out and in pain.

W: Yeah.

T: Tell me about the bummed out part. What do you experience?

W: I guess I just feel really pessimistic and that everything is going wrong, and I can't seem to get along with my husband, and I don't really want to do anything anymore.

T: And you'd like to work on that.

W: I guess, yeah. My husband thought it would be a good idea.

T: OK. And tell me a bit about the pain. What's going on there?

W: Well, I have fibromyalgia, and so a lot of the time I can't do stuff because of the pain. It just hurts too much to move sometimes. And my husband just doesn't seem to understand that. It's like he doesn't get how much pain I have, and he expects that I can still do everything.

T: I see. So there's a lot of pain, and it sounds like that's been a source of some conflict between you and your husband.

W: Yeah.

T: OK. I'd like to go through some specific questions that will help me understand these problems a little better.

The therapist made some mental notes about William's in-session behaviors. Specifically, William seemed quite deferential and didn't bring up much detail unless prompted. The therapist hypothesized that these might be unhealthy CRBs. The therapist also noted that although depressed mood and pain were William's presenting complaints, there might have been more to these problems.

The therapist conducted a diagnostic assessment, which included a thorough history and review of symptoms. William did not meet full criteria for any DSM-5 psychiatric disorder, although he did endorse some symptoms of dependent personality disorder and somatic symptom disorder with predominant pain.

To help gather information, the therapist used structured diagnostic interviews, as well as two freely available questionnaires, the Short-Form McGill Pain Questionnaire–2 (SF-MPQ-2; Dworkin et al., 2009) and the Depression Anxiety Stress Scales (DASS;

Lovibond & Lovibond, 1995). William's score on the SF-MPQ-2 was 4, in the middle of the possible range of 0–10. His DASS Depression subscale was 26, which is in the severe range (the average score for people without depression is 6, and the best cutoff between populations with and without depression is 14). The therapist also reviewed the presence of risk factors and determined that William was at not high risk of suicide, although he did express high levels of hopelessness.

Here, the therapist provides a bit of psychoeducation and asks William about his goals and expectations.

T: William, we've gone over a lot of information today about your pain and your mood, and how these things have been affecting you. It looks like your level of pain is moderate, compared to other people who have pain-related problems, and I certainly get the fact that it seems to get in your way a lot. It also seems that you're experiencing quite a bit of depression. On this questionnaire you completed, as just one example, you answered the questions in a way that is usually seen in people who are severely depressed, and very different from what we see from people who are not depressed. But of course, these are just questionnaires. Let me ask you: Do the results of these questionnaires seem accurate to you? Would "moderately in pain" and "severely depressed" be an accurate way to describe you right now?

W: Yeah, I think so. The pain is pretty bad. I guess I hadn't really thought about how severe the depression is; I've noticed that I was feeling bummed out, but I didn't know if it was really bad.

T: Let's talk a little bit about what you'd like to see happen as a result of coming to see me. How would you like things to be?

W: Well, I'd like to be less depressed.

T: OK. Anything related to your pain?

W: Well, I wish you could do something about my pain.

T: OK, so that's one thing. What else?

W: I guess I wish you could just make my husband understand that when I'm in pain, he should just leave me alone and not keep insisting that I do things.

T: OK. Now, let's talk about what's realistic to expect. I probably can't do much to make your pain go away. But you and I might be able to figure out ways that the pain can be less of a problem for you, make it not get in your way so much. Would that be a reasonable thing for us to shoot for?

W: I don't know what can be done about that. I mean, when I hurt, I hurt.

T: Understood. And I can appreciate that right now it might be hard to imagine what we could do. You and I will have to do some thinking around that. But for the moment, can we at least have it on our list of things we'd like to have happen?

W: Yeah, I guess I'll just have to trust your judgment.

T: No need to trust my judgment. We'll see for ourselves. And we also know that you'd like to feel less depressed. Let's see if we can put a finer point on that. If we were able to get you feeling less depressed, and if we were able to have pain be less a problem for you, how would we know that we had succeeded?

W: I guess I'd just feel better.

T: You would, yes. Staying with that idea for a moment, if I came to see you when you were no longer depressed, and pain was no longer controlling you, what would I see that was different? How would you be different?

W: Um . . . I guess I'd be doing more stuff, like getting together with my friends.

T: Ah. What else?

W: I wouldn't be sitting on the couch all day. And maybe my husband and I would be getting along better.

T: OK, so we have the overall goal of having you feel less depressed and having pain control you less, and part of that goal, really, is that you'd be spending less time on the couch, and doing more things with friends, and getting along better with your husband. Do I have that right?

W: Yeah.

T: I wonder whether these specific activities—getting off the couch, doing more, and so on—might be something we could try in order to see how that affects your pain and your mood.

W: We could try, but I mean, when I'm having pain, it's hard to do things.

T: Sounds like you're not completely convinced.

W: Well, I'm just not sure how it's going to go.

T: That's understandable. If we think about your goals of making pain have less control of you, feeling less depressed, doing more stuff, getting off the couch, getting along better with your husband, and so on, how successful do you think we're likely to be?

W: I don't know. I just don't know if anything's going to work.

T: So, kind of pessimistic and doubtful.

W: Yeah, I guess.

T: Of course, we can never predict perfectly how successful treatment is going to be. But the kind of treatment I have in mind, which is called cognitive-behavioral therapy, or CBT for short, has a very good track record. Here's what we know: Most people who receive CBT end up feeling significantly better. That doesn't necessarily mean that they are depression-free for life, or that they never have problems with pain again. But it does mean that on average, people who receive CBT feel a lot better and find that life goes better for them as well.

W: OK, well, that's good to know, but I still don't know if it's going to help me.

T: No, can't know that for sure. But if you are willing to try, we can see for ourselves. Let me describe a bit about what's involved with CBT. As the name suggests, the treatment is cognitive, meaning it involves looking at how you think, and behavioral, meaning it involves looking at what you do. Now, I understand that the main reason you're here talking to me is because of how you feel, and we definitely want that to get better. But we often find that the best way to feel different is to think differently and act differently. Does that make sense to you?

W: I guess so.

Note that the therapist uses a variation of the "miracle question" (de Shazer, 1988) to help William articulate his initially vague goal in more concrete terms. In keeping with the spirit of empiricism, the therapist presents a summary of the research data in understandable terms and frames suggestions as testable hypotheses (e.g., "If you're willing to try, we can see for ourselves").

The therapist continues to note William's CRBs. First, he continuously defers to the therapist, phrasing his goals as things that he wants the therapist to "fix." The therapist immediately begins countering this CRB by using "we" statements, indicating that this is a collaborative effort, not something the therapist will do to William. This also implies a fair amount of responsibility on William's part. Second, William repeatedly refers back to his pain, using it as a reason for not doing things. The therapist sidesteps this by pointing out that even if they cannot make the pain go away, they might be able to improve his functioning despite the presence of pain.

The therapist has secured an initial buy-in from William, but it's also not clear whether he is fully on board with the idea just yet, and it seems that his expectations for improvement are rather low. The therapist will continue to monitor William's agreement with the treatment rationale and plan. Here, the therapist obtains a bit more information about William's motivation to change, using strategies derived from motivational interviewing (W. R. Miller & Rollnick, 2002):

T: You have these goals of feeling less depressed and having the pain control you less. What is the downside to working on this? What do you stand to lose, for example?

W: Um . . . I guess it would be a lot of work.

T: Yes, that's important for us to note. It would take work. What else?

W: It would also take time. And money for these meetings.

T: Yes, that's true, too. So working on this pain and depression would require an investment of effort, time, and money. I can see how those would be important things to consider. Anything else?

W: Nothing that I can think of.

T: As you think about a life less depressed, with you, rather than the pain, in the driver's seat, is there a downside to living that kind of life?

W: I'm not sure what you mean.

T: Well, as one example, would people's reactions to you, their expectations of you, and so on, be different in some way?

W: I guess people would probably expect more of me.

T: Yes, they might. And is that a pro or a con of working on the problem?

W: I guess a con.

T: OK, so let's note that too. How about the flip side? That is, can you tell me why working on the pain and depression is important to you?

W: Well, I guess I'd just like to feel better.

T: Yes, you'd like to feel better than you currently do. Besides being more pleasant for you, what else would be good about overcoming these problems?

W: I think my marriage would be better.

T: Ah, OK. So that's important. What else would be good about it?

W: I guess I'd have more friends and just a more satisfying life.

T: That's important, too. Anything else?

W: I think that's about it.

T: So there are some pros and some cons here. On one hand, working on the pain and depression would involve an investment of effort, time, and money. And on the other hand, you'd like to feel better, and you'd like your marriage to go better, and you'd like to have more friends and have a more satisfying life. On balance, what do you think makes the most sense for you right now?

W: I think I should probably work on it.

T: If we imagine a scale from 0 to 10, with 0 being "I'm not ready to work on my pain and depression at all," and 10 being "I'm totally ready to work on my pain and depression," where would you rate yourself right now?

W: I think I'm about a 6 or 7.

T: That's interesting. Why not lower than that? I mean, why not a 2 or a 4?

W: Well, because I really don't like feeling this way, and I really do want my marriage to be better, and I just want to feel better about myself and have something to look forward to, instead of every day just feeling like the same old depressing routine.

T: And that's what's really important to you.

W: Yeah.

From this discussion, the therapist surmised that William was waffling between the contemplation and action stages of change (Prochaska & DiClemente, 1982). The therapist therefore elicited from William the pros and cons of changing. The therapist also used a Readiness Ruler (Biener & Abrams, 1991), asking William to rate his motivation on a scale from 0 to 10. The therapist's follow-up question ("Why isn't it lower?") framed the discussion so that William would have to reply by further articulating his reasons for wanting to make a change. Note that had the therapist asked the follow-up question differently ("Why isn't it higher?"), William would have had to reply by further articulating his reasons for not wanting to change. Because the therapist's goal was to nudge William from the contemplation stage of change to the action stage of change, it was helpful to set up a discussion in a manner that encouraged William to make as much "change talk" as possible. Note as well that the therapist follows the MI principles of autonomy, collaboration, and evocation—the therapist does not tell William what to do, and instead uses questioning to evoke from William his reasons for wanting to change. The therapist uses open-ended questions, affirmations, reflective listening, and summarizing as a way of minimizing resistance and encouraging collaboration.

Note from Figure 20.1 that the therapy assessment never completely ends. The therapist continuously monitored William's level of motivation, expectancies for improvement, and agreement with the treatment rationale and plan, adjusting the treatment as needed. The therapist and William also agreed to monitor William's pain and depression on a weekly basis by having William complete the SF-MPQ-2 and DASS in the waiting room prior to every session.

Initial Treatment Planning

William did not fit neatly into any diagnostic category. The therapist therefore looked at *anchor diagnoses*—that is, diagnoses or problems that seemed closest to what William was describing. The therapist determined that although William did not meet criteria for dependent personality or somatic symptom disorder with predominant pain, his problems seemed to be in the general ballpark of those diagnoses. Therefore, the therapist started looking into treatments that could be helpful for those problems. At *www.psychologicaltreatments.org*, the therapist was able to determine that multicomponent CBT was effective for chronic pain from fibromyalgia. Examination of online materials gave the therapist some initial hypotheses about what might be effective for William.

That site did not provide information about dependent personality disorder, the other anchor diagnosis. Next, the therapist searched the primary source literature at *www.pubmed.com*. No luck there, either—the search did not reveal a body of research on CBT or any other psychotherapy for dependent personality. The therapist had to get more creative. Broadening the search to personality disorders and CBT, the therapist found a review article that was freely available online. Examination of that article revealed that, although there was little research on the treatment of dependent personality disorder, there had been several positive studies of CBT for other "Cluster C" (to use DSM-IV-TR categorization) personality disorders (i.e., avoidant and obsessive–compulsive personality disorders). It seemed, from that review, that there was a significant amount of overlap in the treatments for these disorders. It seemed reasonable to hypothesize, therefore, that some of the CBT interventions used for anxious personality disorders in general might be helpful for William. The therapist also consulted existing manuals for treating personality disorders—not necessarily as a "script" for therapy, but rather to generate ideas about what kinds of interventions and therapeutic styles might be effective.

Based on reviewing the available literature, the therapist hypothesized that the following treatment elements *might* be effective:

- Developing a positive, collaborative working relationship.
- Activity scheduling.
- Contingency management both inside and outside of the session.
- Training in effective problem solving.
- Cognitive restructuring of interpretations and core beliefs.
- Relaxation or other modulation strategy for pain.

Of course, at this stage, these were just hypotheses. The therapist was open to the possibility that these ideas could be wrong and that, as things progressed, the plan would need to be altered.

Psychoeducation and Model Building

The therapist engaged William in a model-building discussion of his pain and depression. This served two primary aims. First, by demystifying these problems, it was hoped that William's level of self-efficacy would increase. Second, identification of the factors maintaining William's pain and depression was hoped to make productive therapeutic targets more apparent.

T: I'd like to see if we can get a better understanding of how your pain and depression are related, and why these things are happening. Do you have a sense of it?

W: Well, my pain is depressing.

T: Yes, I can imagine. Let's see if we can flesh out our understanding a bit more. Can you think of a recent time that you got a really strong sad or depressed feeling, or you experienced a flare-up of your pain?

W: Yeah, I was having a lot of pain and depression this morning when I was getting ready to leave for work.

T: OK, can you walk me through that scene? What was going on?

W: Well, my husband was being kind of cranky and he was just hurrying to get us both out the door for work. And I wasn't feeling very good physically; I was having some pain, and I was just hoping that he'd slow down a little. But he just seemed to get more and more impatient. And I was hoping he would at least come over and kiss me goodbye and he didn't. He just kind of mumbled "see you after work" and left.

T: I see. So it seems like that's when you got the strong feelings of depression?

W: Yeah.

T: And what did you notice going on with your pain then?

W: It seemed like it got worse.

T: (*Taking out a piece of paper, shown in Figure 20.2.*) Let me see if I can draw a diagram of how this went. I'll write this here, as a possible trigger: "Having pain and feeling

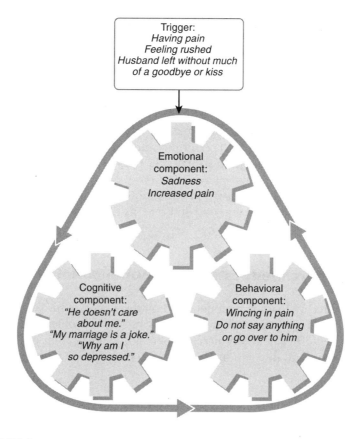

FIGURE 20.2. Initial conceptualization of William's episode of pain and depression.

rushed; husband left without much of a good-bye or a kiss." What did you notice then?

W: Well, I was just really depressed.

T: You felt depressed. What did that feel like, exactly?

W: Just, I don't know, sad. Like he doesn't even care about me.

T: We have two different things here. One is a feeling, an emotion. That's sad. That's something you feel in your gut. And then the other thing is a thought, words that you say to yourself in your mind. You thought, or said, to yourself, "He doesn't care about me." So I'll write that over here. Do you see the difference between a feeling and a thought?

W: I think so.

T: Sometimes it's tricky, but you can think about it this way. Feelings come from our guts and we feel them in our bodies. Thoughts come from our minds and they are words, or sometimes pictures—that's us interpreting the situation, trying to figure out what it means.

W: OK, I think I get it. So then another thought was that my marriage was a joke.

T: Right, that's a thought, too, so I'll write it here with the other thought. What did you do during this scene?

W: What do you mean? I guess I didn't really do anything.

T: You didn't, for example, go after your husband and ask to kiss him, or give him a good-bye?

W: No, I just stood there in the kitchen.

T: So maybe standing there and not taking action was part of this, too?

W: Maybe.

T: That's an action, so I'll write that over here. So here you are, standing there in the kitchen, and are you doing something to try to get this sorted out or to make it better?

W: I was just trying to figure out where things went wrong.

T: Can you elaborate?

W: I guess I just stood there for a while trying to understand why he didn't love me anymore, and how I might have let him down, and why I was just so depressed all the time.

T: Ah. We have a word for that kind of thinking. We call it *rumination*. It's reflecting over and over again about how you feel and what's gone wrong. So that's part of your thinking, too. Looking back at your actions, was there any other communication you did?

W: I didn't, no. But he did say "I hope you feel better" right before he left.

T: How would he know you weren't feeling better?

W: I think I was wincing from the pain. He could see I hurt.

T: And then he said something about it. Did that help at all?

W: Well, I guess I knew he wasn't completely ignoring me; like he might have cared a tiny bit.

T: OK, so wincing was another action. I'll write it here. Now, can you see how all of these things—your feelings, your thoughts, and your actions—are all interconnected, like gears in a machine?

W: Yeah. I guess that means they all influence each other?

T: Exactly. As one of these things is happening, it tends to make the other things happen, as well. So let's think this one through based on that model. If you think "He doesn't care about me" and "My marriage is a joke," what's likely to happen to your feelings and actions?

W: Um . . . I guess I would feel more depressed and sad, and I would just stand there.

T: Right. And maybe more pain, too?

W: Maybe.

T: And if you felt really sad, and were having a lot of pain, what would happen to your thoughts and actions?

W: I would think more pessimistically?

T: Yeah. Maybe just freeze in place, wincing?

W: I guess.

T: And if you just stand there and wince, what can we expect for your thoughts and feelings?

W: Worse.

T: Exactly. Now, let's think about it in the other direction. Let's say, for example, that you made a change here, in your actions. You didn't just stand there and wince. Instead, let's say you went after him and kissed him and gave him a nice good-bye. What would be the impact on your thoughts and feelings?

W: Um . . . I actually probably would have felt better, as long as he kissed me back.

T: Right. And if you didn't think that he doesn't love you? What then?

W: I guess I would feel less sad and I'd do something different besides stand there?

T: Right. That's CBT. We want to try to reverse this cycle that you're in.

Tracking William's Progress

From the initial session, the therapist kept track of William's SF-MPQ-2 total score and his DASS Depression score. This often served as the initial focus of the session:

T: Let's take a quick look at your score. Looks like it's coming down a bit from last week. Does that seem accurate to you?

W: I think so. I did notice myself feeling a little better this week.

T: What specifically have you noticed is better?

After the first visit, William's depression score decreased (see Figure 20.3), which is not uncommon once someone starts therapy—just the relief of talking to a professional can cause some reduction in symptoms, even if temporarily. By the third session, however, his depression had returned to close to its baseline level. His pain level had increased somewhat as well.

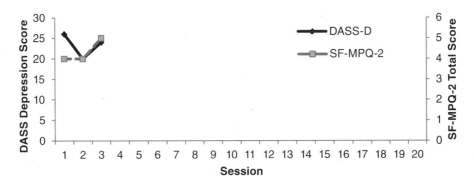

FIGURE 20.3. William's pain and depression graph at Session 3.

Activity Scheduling

In the second and third sessions, it was becoming evident that William's behavioral passivity and inactivity were playing a major role in the maintenance of both his pain and his depression. As various external triggers came up, William's response appeared to follow a fairly consistent pattern.

Figure 20.4 shows a model that the therapist and William drew collaboratively in Session 3 after William reported becoming distressed about an unpaid bill. You can see that his behavior was similar to that described in the example with his husband: William responds to stressors by being inactive, not taking the initiative to solve problems, and complaining of increased pain. Here, the therapist works with William to flesh out the model a bit more.

T: It seems that there's a pattern here, in which you kind of freeze up and ruminate instead of taking positive action.

W: Yeah, that's pretty much what I do.

T: So how well is that strategy working?

W: In what sense?

T: Well, I guess I'm wondering whether it seems that this way of responding has helped you be happier, or has it gotten in the way of your happiness?

W: I think it's gotten in the way.

T: I suspect so. But is there something you get out of it? I mean, is there a purpose or payoff of some kind to doing this?

W: Not that I know of.

T: Well, think about it this way. If you did take it on yourself to fix this problem of the unpaid bill, what would that feel like right then and there?

W: I guess it would be kind of uncomfortable because that's not what I usually do.

T: OK, so doing something new and different is uncomfortable, and you can avoid that discomfort by freezing up.

W: I guess. But it's not like I'm freezing up just because I want to avoid doing things.

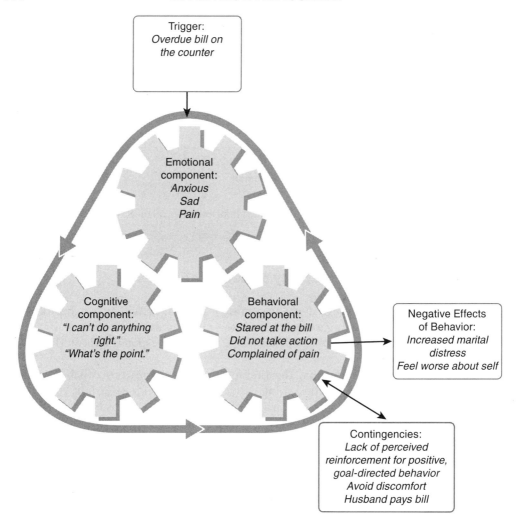

FIGURE 20.4. Expanded model for William showing the function of behavior.

T: No, I wouldn't imagine so. Depression has a lot of moving parts, as you can see in the diagram. You freeze up because you feel anxious and sad, and because you think you can't do anything right and what's the point anyway, and because you can avoid discomfort by freezing. And there are probably more factors involved as well that we haven't discussed yet. This is just one part of the puzzle. Let me ask another question: In the past, what's happened when you have taken appropriate action? Like, for example, when you've paid a bill yourself?

W: Sometimes I've screwed it up, like not paying the right amount, and so we get another overdue notice.

T: I see. And how does your husband respond when you've taken the initiative?

W: Well, he used to yell when I'd mess it up, saying things like "How could you get it wrong?" And lately he just kind of takes over because he's just better at it and it's easier for him to just do it.

T: OK. And when you've taken the initiative, how have you responded in your own mind? Did you say, "Attaboy, good job"?

W: No. When I do it I wonder what I might have screwed up this time, and when it turns out I messed up, I just kick myself and think what an idiot I am.

T: I see. So when you've taken the initiative, you don't reward yourself. Your husband doesn't reward you. The bill collectors don't reward you. I don't blame you for not doing it any more. I'm not sure I'd do it, either, if that was my experience. So we have another problem, which I'll write down here: You haven't really experienced much payoff from taking the initiative and fixing problems as they come up, and in fact some of the time you end up with a slap on the wrist, either from someone else or from yourself.

W: Yeah.

T: And it seems that when you tell your husband about your pain, he might step in and just do it for you, to help you out.

W: Yeah.

T: So these are very short-term payoffs for freezing up and talking about your pain, which is that you can avoid being uncomfortable and maybe get your husband to step in and take over. But how about in the long term? What's the effect?

W: Well, I can feel it in my marriage, because my husband just gets more and more stressed out, like he can't handle everything himself and he wishes that I were doing better.

T: Yes. I'll write that down here as a consequence. And how about your sad and anxious feelings? Does freezing and ruminating make those feelings better, or worse?

W: Worse.

T: And your belief that you can't do anything right? Does freezing and ruminating make that belief stronger or weaker?

W: Stronger.

To further explore the hypothesis that William's inactivity was part of the problem, at the end of Session 3 the therapist asked William to self-monitor his activities using the Activity Monitoring Form in Appendix B. William was to record, for one entire week, his activities on an hourly basis. They reviewed his forms in Session 4.

T: I'm curious to know how the activity recording went.

W: Well . . . I think I'm not doing much.

T: Yeah, from these forms it looks like you spent quite a bit of time in front of the TV.

W: I didn't really realize how much until I had to write it down. But I just had so much pain this week, it was hard to do much.

T: I notice as well that on these mastery and pleasure ratings, your numbers are really low. Not much above a 3 here. Would it be fair to say that there's not much going on in your life right now that gives you a sense of pleasure, or a sense of accomplishment?

W: I'd say that's fair. Life is just kind of . . . blah.

T: What do you suppose the impact of that blah life is on you?

W: I don't feel good about it.

T: No, I wouldn't imagine so. I wonder how this impacts your mood?

W: I get depressed and then I just don't really feel like doing much.

T: Yes, I get that. So your pain and depressed mood impact your activities. I'm wondering about the reverse: How do your activities impact your pain and your mood? For example, do you find that this lifestyle helps you feel happier or more comfortable?

W: Well, I think that I'd have a lot of pain if I got up and did more stuff.

T: You might, in the short term. How about the long term? Does it seem that this is resulting in a long-term improvement in how you feel?

W: No, it's not. I think it's making it worse.

T: I suspect you're right. This is what happens to a lot of people who are struggling with pain and depression. They feel rotten, so they do less, but then life gets less rewarding and their bodies get out of practice, so they feel even worse.

W: Like a vicious circle.

T: Exactly. So if sitting in front of the TV is making you feel worse, then what might a solution be?

W: Do something else?

T: Yes. The question is, what should that something be? If we need to boost the amount of mastery and pleasure you get out of life, what kind of activities would we be talking about?

W: I don't know. Right now it's hard to imagine anything being fun or anything that wouldn't hurt.

To help stimulate William's thinking about possible mastery and pleasure activities, the therapist showed William the Mastery and Pleasure Checklist from Appendix B. William found it hard to imagine any of the activities on the list being particularly enjoyable but was able to identify some activities that he had enjoyed when he was less depressed: fishing, photography, and walking. The therapist and William negotiated a schedule in which he would do one of these activities per day for at least 30 minutes. William had some concerns about how walking might affect his pain:

W: I just don't know how much walking I can do. Sometimes my body just hurts and I don't feel like I can continue.

T: I understand. We're going to have to have some trial and error here to figure out what works for you. Here's what I have in mind. I'd like you to push just a bit outside of your normal comfort zone. By "just a bit," I mean that this isn't meant to be an excruciating endurance exercise. We're not here to torture you. But at the same time, it's important that you push beyond what you'd normally be comfortable doing. So if you're doing it right, you'll experience some pain, but it won't be more than you can stand. What could you do if you were walking and you started experiencing pain?

W: Stop?

T: Yes, you could stop and take a break. And then what? Do you go home or keep going?

W: I guess I should keep going.

T: Right, you would keep going at a pace that's comfortable for you. Remember, we want to get you out there, outside of your comfort zone, but if you need to slow down or take breaks, that's fine.

William also raised a concern about the fishing activity, which the therapist addressed using informal cognitive restructuring:

W: But when I used to go fishing, it was always with my buddies. I just don't keep in touch with them anymore.

T: I understand. And if we made it dependent on having your buddies with you, I suspect it would be hard to actually make this happen. So what's stopping you from doing it by yourself?

W: I don't know; it's just usually something you do with a friend. I mean, I'm just going to sit there on the dock fishing by myself?

T: Why not? What would be wrong with that?

W: It would be weird, wouldn't it? I mean, everyone's out fishing with their friends on a nice day, and I'm just by myself? I'd look like I don't have any friends.

T: Ah. You think that people will be paying attention to you.

W: Yeah.

T: And noticing that you're by yourself.

W: Right.

T: And making evaluations of you based on that.

W: I guess so.

T: Do you think that's true? Do you think people will really be paying attention to you and evaluating you in that way?

W: I don't know. Maybe not.

T: Maybe, maybe not. When you're fishing, is that what you're doing? Looking around and trying to figure out who has friends and who doesn't?

W: No, I'm just paying attention to fishing.

T: So what do you think the other people will be doing when you go fishing?

W: Probably paying attention to fishing.

T: Seems pretty likely. But just for the sake of discussion, let's assume someone does pay attention to you and does notice that you're by yourself and does decide that you don't have any friends. What of it?

W: Well, I wouldn't like someone judging me that way.

T: No, I wouldn't, either. But would that affect you in some way?

W: I guess not. I wouldn't know what someone was thinking anyway, so how could it affect me?

T: Well, let's take it a step further and imagine that this guy is really going to confront you about this, so he starts pointing, and yelling "Hey, loser with no friends!"

W: I'd hate that.

T: Would that be the end of the world?

W: It would be really unpleasant.

T: Yes. How unpleasant? So bad you couldn't stand it?

W: I would feel that way.

T: Would it be that way?

W: I guess not. He'd just be a jerk.

At the next session, the therapist checked in on William's homework.

T: So tell me about the activities.

W: You know, it wasn't that bad.

T: No?

W: Yeah, I mean, it's not like it was completely fun, but I guess I felt kind of good about getting off the couch and doing something.

T: How was the walk?

W: I did have some pain. But I took a break and slowed down, and it was OK.

T: I'm particularly curious about the fishing by yourself, because I know you had some concerns about that. How did that go?

W: It was actually kind of nice. Peaceful. I really missed doing that.

T: No one called you a loser with no friends?

W: (*Smiles.*) No. Nothing like that.

T: You know, I think that's the first time I've seen you smile. It's a good look on you.

Over the next several sessions, the therapist and William continued to schedule mastery and pleasure activities, plugging more and more activities into his day. As shown in Figure 20.5, his depression scores showed a progressive decrease. They were still high, so William was clearly not out of the woods yet, but both William and the therapist were encouraged by his progress. William's pain scores showed an initial decrease, followed by an increase as he increased his activity level. The therapist had warned William that some temporary increase in pain was likely, and William was not particularly discouraged by this.

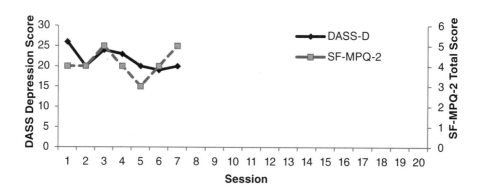

FIGURE 20.5. William's pain and depression graph at Session 8.

Contingency Management

Although William was doing well with mastery and pleasure activities, the therapist had noted two other patterns in William's behavior. First, William tended to be passive and to rely on his husband for many tasks and decisions. Relatedly, William increased his facial grimacing and pain-related complaints when he felt that a task was too difficult and wanted help.

The therapist hypothesized that these behaviors were contributing to the maintenance of the problem. Specifically, it was thought that William's overreliance on his husband and his overuse of pain behaviors fostered a low sense of self-efficacy, deprived him of a sense of mastery, and contributed to maladaptive core beliefs about himself. The therapist also suspected that because William's husband couldn't read his mind and know what he needed all of the time, William often came away from interactions with his husband disappointed and strengthening his sense of hopelessness and pessimism about his marriage. The therapist therefore decided to address this pattern directly, first using contingency management strategies.

The first step was for the therapist and William to identify the desired and undesired target behaviors in a manner that was objective, clear, and complete. Here, the therapist starts that discussion, using observations from the therapy sessions and William's previous descriptions of his marital interactions:

T: There's something I've noticed as we've been talking about your marriage. It seems like perhaps there's a pattern here between you and your husband, but I'd like to get your take on it. It seems like a lot of the time, when you're discouraged about the relationship, you're waiting for him to do something and he ends up not doing it, or not doing exactly what you had hoped he would do. Like, for example, when you were hoping he would kiss you good-bye and he didn't, or when you were waiting for him to bring up the subject of how your kids are doing in school, and he didn't. Is that something you've noticed?

W: I don't know. I guess I hadn't really thought much about it.

T: Well, let's think about it now. Overall, who seems to take the lead in the relationship? That is, who tends to make the decisions, make sure things get done, and so on?

W: That would definitely be my husband. He's the boss of the house.

T: I see. And this is something you're satisfied with?

W: Well, yeah, I guess so, most of the time. I mean, he's really good at handling things, and I know that I just mess a lot of things up when I do them.

T: OK, so the overall thinking in the relationship is your husband is the more competent one, and so he handles things.

W: Yeah, kind of.

T: And you're the less competent one.

W: I guess.

T: I wonder what the impact of that is on you. I mean, to have this system in place in which you see yourself as the less competent one. Does that seem like it's pointing you toward happiness or toward unhappiness?

W: I guess it's pointing me toward unhappiness.

T: So perhaps you're not completely satisfied with the way things are.

W: No. I mean, I like being able to count on him and I like knowing that he can do things. But I don't really like thinking of myself as incompetent. And I know I don't like how I feel at home.

T: So let's think about this issue a bit more. You get into this pattern with him in which you're kind of "one down." When you're in "one-down" mode, how does that get reflected in your actions?

W: Um . . . I guess I wait for him to do stuff.

T: Like take the initiative.

W: Yeah.

T: And when you wince with pain or tell him how much pain you're having, is that part of what leads him to take the initiative?

W: Yeah, I guess so.

T: So when you wince with pain or tell him about your pain, you're also telling him something else, right? What is that?

W: I need you to do it?

T: I need you to do it because . . .

W: . . . because I can't.

T: Yeah. Now, can I share an observation with you? I've noticed in our meetings that a lot of the time it seems like you're waiting for me to bring things up, rather than bringing them up yourself. Have you noticed that?

W: I guess so, yeah.

T: Is that part of the same pattern? That is, are you finding yourself in that "one-down" mode here with me sometimes?

W: Maybe. But I mean, you're the professional, right? You know how this is supposed to go.

T: That's true in a way. I have done this a lot, and I do have a pretty good understanding of depression, and I have a good understanding of how to help people with depression. At the same time, though, that doesn't mean that I will know what's on your mind at any given time, or what's important to you, or exactly how you're feeling and what you're thinking. You're the expert on those things.

W: I guess you're right.

T: So let's make a note of this pattern: "Waiting for someone else to initiate." Let's flip it around for a moment. How about when you're not in "one-down" mode? That is, are there times when you're feeling competent?

W: I guess when I'm fishing or doing my photography, I feel pretty competent. And I feel pretty competent when I'm doing my work in my office.

T: OK, so there are times that you feel competent. These are mostly solitary activities?

W: Yeah.

T: What about with other people? Are there times when you're in "competent" mode?

W: Not really. I think it's kind of a pattern.

T: Let's use our imaginations for a moment. Can you imagine yourself feeling competent at home? I'm not actually asking you to feel that way; I just wonder if you can imagine it.

W: I can imagine it, I guess.

T: So stay with this for a bit. As you imagine yourself feeling competent at home, what kinds of things do you imagine doing?

W: I guess I would just do stuff. You know, without waiting for him to do them. I'd just handle it.

T: Let's flesh that out a little bit. What kind of stuff would you be doing?

W: Um . . . like chores and things?

T: OK, so chores are one thing, but why would you be doing those things?

W: Well, there would be a lot less arguing, because my husband really wants that stuff to get done.

T: I agree that the chores are an issue, but I wonder if this is exactly on the mark. It seems that part of what you'd be doing is making your husband happier and doing what he wants you to do. Would that really combat this "one-down" pattern you're in?

W: I guess not.

T: To be clear, I'm not saying don't do chores, and I'm not saying don't make your husband happy. But I wonder whether it's helpful for us to make that our specific priority. If you were really feeling competent at home, and not at all feeling "one down," what would you do?

W: I guess I would just do what I thought needed to be done.

T: For example?

W: Well, like actually making decisions about things, like some of the budgeting decisions, what to buy and how much to save, and that sort of thing.

T: That's something your husband does now.

W: Yeah. And I guess if I were really feeling competent, I wouldn't rely on him so much for that stuff.

T: OK. What about here, in our meetings? If you were really feeling competent and not "one down" in our meetings, what would you be doing?

W: Um . . . I guess bringing up things that were important to me?

T: Yes, that could be one thing. Let's think of some more.

The therapist and William continued in this fashion for much of the remainder of the session, identifying specific unwanted behaviors (i.e., those that fed into William's belief that he was incompetent) and desired behaviors (i.e., those that would foster a sense of competence). At the conclusion of the session, the therapist asked William to self-monitor "competent" behaviors, as well as their antecedents and consequences. William came to the next session with no such behaviors recorded, indicating that the desired behaviors weren't occurring naturally. That meant that some degree of *shaping* would be needed: They would need to start slowly, having William do small versions of the desired behaviors and reinforcing successive approximations until William was able to engage in fully "competent" behaviors.

The therapist faced a decision point here. One option at this stage would have been to bring William's husband into the session, get his perspective on things, and enlist his aid in the contingency management process. However, because the overall target was to help

William rely less on his husband and more on himself, the therapist opted to encourage William to use *self-control* strategies for the time being, keeping the option of joint sessions as a backup possibility.

In Session 9, William created a *contingency contract* with the therapist's help. William agreed that if he made a decision without consulting his husband or another person, he would buy himself a specialty coffee drink. In subsequent sessions, additional items would be added to the contract, but for now, the therapist started small.

The therapist also emphasized reinforcing clinically relevant behavior in session. Having discussed the presence of unhealthy CRBs (e.g., waiting for the therapist to bring up topics, deferring unnecessarily to the therapist's expertise) and envisioned possible healthy CRBs (e.g., bringing up topics and stating opinions), the therapist paid close attention to William's in-session behavior, calling his attention to unhealthy CRBs and reinforcing healthy CRBs.

For reinforcement, the therapist used behaviors that approximated a good environmental response to the healthy CRB. Specifically, when William brought up a topic for discussion, the therapist made sure to listen carefully and acknowledge it, even if the therapist didn't find it to be spot-on. Getting William's rate of healthy CRBs up was more important that making sure the discussion was always focused and on track. When William stated an opinion, even one that the therapist disagreed with, the therapist made a point of listening carefully and acknowledging the validity of the opinion.

For unhealthy CRBs in session, the therapist avoided anything that would be perceived as punitive. Rather, the therapist called attention to the behavior, discussed its effects on the therapy session, and suggested William use one of his healthy CRBs (*differential reinforcement of other behavior* [DRO]). Here's an example from the beginning of Session 9.

> T: Let's set the agenda for our meeting today. I'd like to take a look at your pain and depression scores and review your homework to start. What else do you have on your agenda?
>
> W: Um, nothing else, really.
>
> T: I wonder whether this is an example of you waiting for me to bring things up, like we talked about last week.
>
> W: I dunno. Maybe.
>
> T: It's hard for me to know what's going on with you when that happens. Perhaps this would be a good time for you to reflect on what's on your mind, and bring it up. (*Waits.*)
>
> W: (*long pause*) I guess I had a nasty encounter with my boss that's been bugging me.
>
> T: OK. That sounds important, and I'm glad you brought it up. Let's plan to spend some of our session talking about that.

Relaxation Training

The therapist hypothesized that some training in progressive muscle relaxation would help William cope more effectively with his pain. In Session 9, the therapist introduced the idea this way:

T: As we've been discussing how you respond to your pain, I think I hear a pattern in which you feel some pain, and then you tighten up your body in reaction to that pain. Do I have that right?

W: Yeah, sometimes it almost feels like I could double over.

T: And even if you don't double over, you've mentioned that you'll do other things like clench your jaw and your fists and shrug your shoulders up high. What do you suppose the long-term impact is of tensing up like that?

W: My muscles feel sore.

T: So potentially more pain. It's common for people to want to tighten up when they feel pain, but that's not very helpful. Are you familiar with childbirth classes, like Lamaze?

W: Yeah. That's where they do the natural childbirth thing so the women don't feel so much pain.

T: And how do they instruct the women to respond to pain?

W: To breathe?

T: Yes, to regulate their breathing. And what about tightening up?

W: Um . . . I think they tell them not to do that.

T: Right. So the same thing applies here. It seems that your pain management might be more effective if, instead of tightening up when you feel pain, that you practice a relaxation response—to relax your muscles and regulate your breathing. I have an exercise that I'd like to try with you, to see if you can learn to relax your body a bit more, and then we can see whether that helps with your pain. Can we try that together?

William was enthusiastic about trying relaxation. The therapist followed the progressive muscle relaxation and breathing retraining program described in Chapter 18. In William's case, the therapist took care not to let William overtense the muscles that were particularly painful, so as not to exacerbate the problem. William's homework for the next 2 weeks was to practice the relaxation exercises twice per day, even when he wasn't experiencing acute pain. In subsequent sessions, the use of relaxation as a direct response to pain was introduced.

Problem-Solving Training

As William was trying to make more decisions around the house, he encountered some pushback from his husband. He wasn't used to William's taking the initiative and had a tendency to take over, assuming that William was just going through the motions and didn't really intend to do much. This was frustrating to William.

Again, the therapist had a decision to make. This problem could have been addressed in a couple's session, but given William's maladaptive pattern of dependent behavior, the therapist opted to try to resolve the issue individually with William first (keeping the option of a couple's session as a backup plan).

William seemed frozen. He couldn't think of what to do and had a tendency to revert to feeling hopeless about the situation. The therapist recognized this as a *negative problem orientation*. The therapist opted, beginning in Session 9, to employ *problem-solving training* for William. The first step was to bring the problem-solving deficit up for discussion and to promote a *positive problem orientation*. The therapist began by diagramming the situation (see Figure 20.6).

T: As you're describing this problem to me, it seems that it was hard for you to know what to do.

W: Well, what could I do? He just took over.

T: Right. And you felt sort of paralyzed.

W: Yeah.

T: I think it's actually pretty common for people to have this kind of problem. Whenever we make a behavioral change, especially when they involve how we interact with another person, the other person might not fully understand and appreciate what we're doing.

W: He definitely doesn't.

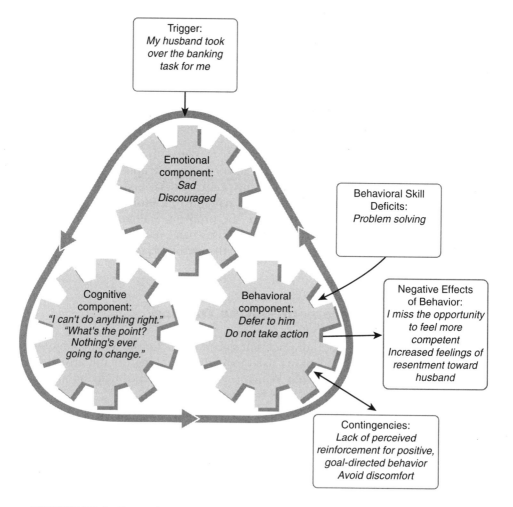

FIGURE 20.6. Expanded model for William showing the presence of skill deficits.

T: And so they expect us to go back to our old way of doing things. Maybe they even exert some pressure on us to go back.

W: That's exactly what he's doing.

T: I suspect that this is a solvable problem, but we can see whether I'm right about that. One thing I'll mention is that problem solving can be hard for any of us when we're stressed out. Have you noticed that in yourself?

W: Yeah, when I'm stressed out I just feel like I have no clue what I'm supposed to do.

T: I won't claim to know what you're supposed to do; maybe there's no "supposed to" here. Perhaps the more critical issue is just that it's hard for you to think it through and make a decision that will be satisfactory to you. So all of us find it harder to solve problems when we're under stress. We can also see that when someone is depressed, that makes problem solving even harder. Does that seem true for you?

W: I think so.

T: It wouldn't surprise me if that's the case. So here you are, stressed and depressed, and you're trying to make a change, and your husband pushes back and says "Oh, just let me do it." Not surprising that you'd feel stuck right then. So let's add that to our model of this incident, right here. Problem solving is a skill, and each of us has a varying ability to use that skill in any given situation. Seems like in this particular moment, you were having a hard time using your problem-solving ability. That's not to say that you're not good at solving other kinds of problems, or that in a better frame of mind you couldn't solve this problem, too. Let me suggest a basic framework for responding to these kinds of challenging situations. The acronym is SSTA, which stands for *stop, slow down, think,* and *act.* Let's talk about how each of these ingredients might help you respond more effectively.

The therapist and William reviewed the SSTA steps described in Chapter 12. Using the Problem-Solving Worksheet in Appendix B, the therapist first worked with William on defining the problem objectively and concisely.

W: Well, I think the basic problem is that my husband just assumes that I can't do anything and so he won't let me try.

T: OK, that's a start. Let's see if we can be more specific about what we mean by that. What exactly is the thing your husband is doing that bugs you? That is, rather than trying to infer what he thinks, can you say exactly what he does?

W: He takes over rather than just letting me try.

T: Right. And how about your contribution to this? What can you say about your actions in this situation?

W: I just let him.

T: Yes. It's easier just to let him do it. So perhaps we can define the problem as "My husband takes over tasks for me, and I don't say anything about it." What gets in your way?

W: Well, it's just easier not to rock the boat, you know what I mean? Why get into an argument over it?

T: So to rephrase that slightly, part of what gets in the way is thinking that if you did say something, that would start an argument.

W: Yeah.

T: And that would be bad because . . .

W: Because I just want to have a happy relationship, you know? And I might not even really know what I'm talking about; I mean, I'm not some banking genius or anything. I can barely even balance a checkbook.

T: So there are some really negative beliefs here. Let's try something. I want to say those beliefs to you, and I'd like to see if you can respond to them. So William, I say, you shouldn't say anything because it's just going to rock the boat and then your relationship will be unhappy and you'll probably screw up anyway.

W: Um . . . I don't know how to respond to that.

T: I'll go one further. You should let him handle everything, because he's competent, and you're not.

W: Well, no, I wouldn't go that far.

T: Tell me why not.

W: Well, I'm not entirely incompetent. I mean, I don't really know how to do the finances very well, but then again that's partly because I haven't done it in a long time.

T: Well, you shouldn't rock the boat. You should never have an argument with your husband; it will just lead to misery.

W: I don't think that's true. Every couple argues sometimes. And maybe it's even good for a relationship sometimes because people need to be able to say what's on their mind.

T: No, one should never, ever, disagree with one's husband.

W: That's definitely not true. If I never disagreed, then it would be like I never had an opinion.

T: Ah. Good point. So addressing this problem might be a good idea after all. What's your goal for this problem?

W: I guess I'd like to speak up?

T: Well, that's one strategy, and it could be the right one, but for now, I want to focus on the goal itself. After all is said and done, how do you want things to be in the house, related to this issue of his taking on tasks and you letting him?

W: Um . . . I guess I'd like to just be able to make some reasonable decisions in the house without having someone else come and just do everything for me. I want to feel more like I'm contributing and being an adult, not being treated like a child.

The therapist and William then used the Problem-Solving Worksheet to brainstorm several potential alternatives, as described in Chapter 12. After eliminating the obviously ineffective alternatives, they then weighed the pros and cons of each one. William selected the strategy of speaking with his husband about his efforts to take on more responsibility for household decision making and to ask for his cooperation.

The problem-solving strategy became an ongoing aspect of sessions through the remainder of William's therapy. The therapist would inquire about William's homework from the previous week, which was to implement one or more chosen solutions, and to evaluate whether the solution seemed to have been effective and satisfactory. As new problems were identified, they would define the problem, brainstorm alternatives, weigh the pros and cons, select a desired solution, and apply it as homework for the following week.

Cognitive Restructuring

Over the next few sessions, although William's pain was decreasing somewhat as he got used to his activities, his depression appeared to plateau (see Figure 20.7). Although he seemed to be solving daily problems more effectively and continued to engage in daily mastery and pleasure activities, he continued to feel depressed and to express ideas of pessimism and self-doubt. The therapist therefore decided to address William's negative thinking more directly.

You may note from the previous sessions that the therapist had been eliciting and identifying William's negative thoughts, using *Socratic questioning*, from the start of therapy, challenging them along the way. The therapist called particular attention to William's *hot thoughts*, those thoughts that had a noticeable impact on his emotions and behavior. Sometimes, William's hot thoughts would be about external events, such as his husband or his work. Sometimes they would be about his emotions, such as when he would describe himself as a "loser" for being "sad all the time." Here's an example from Session 3:

> T: It sounds like you got really upset when your husband left without saying good-bye or giving you a good-bye kiss. What did you take that to mean?
>
> W: Well, it just made me mad. I just wish he had.
>
> T: Yes, I understand that's how you felt. I want to ask about something slightly different, which are your thoughts in that situation. These are the words we say to ourselves in our heads. Often, they are our interpretations of what's going on. When he left the house, what did you say to yourself about that in your head?
>
> W: I guess I just thought about what a mess the relationship is. It's not supposed to be this way.
>
> T: So two thoughts came to mind: "My relationship is a mess" and "It's not supposed to be this way." Anything else?

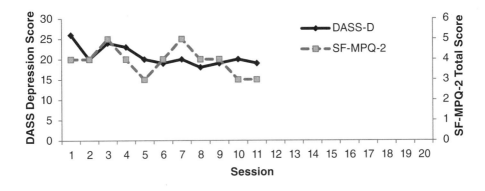

FIGURE 20.7. William's pain and depression graph at Session 11.

W: Um . . . maybe that he didn't feel the same way about me that I feel about him.

T: In what way?

W: Well, I don't know . . . he's just really important to me and I really care about him.

T: You love him.

W: Yeah.

T: And if he feels differently about you than you feel about him, how do you think he feels?

W: He doesn't love me, I guess.

T: So that's part of the thinking, too? "He doesn't love me?"

W: Yeah.

As homework, the therapist asked William to perform *thought monitoring* throughout the week, noting instances of interpretations that were associated with increases in depressed mood using the Thought Monitoring Form in Appendix B.

The therapist used *cognitive restructuring* to challenge William's maladaptive thoughts. Using the list of *cognitive distortions* in Appendix B, they went through his interpretations and identified the presence of distortions for each one (see Chapter 14). They then used the strategy of *examining the evidence* for and against each thought. William's homework in subsequent sessions included monitoring and challenging his thoughts in real time, using the *Thought Change Record* in Appendix B. Here's an example of a discussion based on examining the evidence from Session 11:

T: You have this thought that your husband thinks you can't do anything. We've talked about mind reading, and I wonder whether that's what's going on here.

W: Yeah, maybe it is. But I think maybe that's really how he thinks.

T: It might be. But can we know that for sure? Do we know what he's thinking?

W: No, I guess not.

T: Let's take a look at the evidence and see if that helps us. What evidence might suggest that he thinks you can't do anything?

W: Well, he does everything.

T: Everything?

W: Most things. He handles most of the finances, and the decisions around the house, stuff like that.

T: OK. What else can you think of?

W: Um . . . well, he just acts like I can't do anything.

T: Mind reading again. What does he actually do?

W: I don't know. I guess I assume that he does the stuff in the house because he thinks I can't.

T: OK, that's an assumption, but is it a fact?

W: It feels like a fact.

T: Is it a fact?

W: I guess not.

T: Any other evidence? Facts, that is?

W: Well, we're not really close to each other right now.

T: And that seems like evidence that he thinks you can't do anything.

W: Maybe.

T: Any other possible explanation here?

W: Um . . . maybe we're not close because of other stuff.

T: Like?

W: Like we're both stressed out and maybe I haven't really been acting close either.

T: Perhaps. How about the other side? Any evidence to suggest that he doesn't think that you can't do anything?

W: Well, sometimes he does ask me to do things.

T: I see. And presumably he wouldn't do that if he thought you couldn't. What else?

W: Well, he knows I do a pretty good job at work, and he knows I got promoted last year, and he seemed pretty proud of that.

T: Yes, that seems like he recognizes that you can do some things.

The more the therapist spoke with William, the more the therapist suspected that even though he had not said it directly, he had a *core belief* of being incompetent. Such a core belief might help explain William's persistent pattern of negative self-directed interpretations, as well as his dependent pattern of behavior, which might reflect both a surrender to the belief and an avoidance of activating it. Rather than assuming, however, the therapist opted to check it out using *pattern detection* and *downward arrow* (see Chapter 16).

T: Can I point something out to you? I've noticed what seems to be a theme in the things you're saying. You've made several references to the likelihood that you're going to screw something up. Have you noticed that?

W: Yeah, I guess I think that a lot.

T: You've also told me a couple of times about how someone is better than you at something, like how your husband is better at the finances, or how your coworker is better at certain aspects of the job than you are.

W: Well, sometimes they are.

T: Perhaps, but the fact that these things come to mind so readily for you makes me wonder whether they are all part of the same general theme, a global way that you think about yourself. Do you have a sense of what that theme might be?

W: Um . . . just that a lot of people are better at stuff than I am.

T: Let's assume for the moment that this is true. A lot of people are better at a lot of things than you are. What bugs you about that?

W: I guess because I wish I could do the things that they can do.

T: But you can't.

W: No.

T: So if you can't do the things you wish you could do, what does that mean? What's bad about that?

W: (*becoming tearful*) I just thought I could do more. I should do more. I should be able to do more.

T: And if you can't do what you should be able to do, what do you take that to mean about you?

W: That I'm . . . I don't know . . . just a screw-up. I can't do anything.

T: Incompetent.

W: (*tearful*) Yeah.

As the discussion progressed, the therapist and William modified his model to include the core belief of incompetence (see Figure 20.8). That discussion led to several important insights, which were also added to the model:

- William's core belief that he was incompetent helped explain his tendency to doubt his ability to perform tasks correctly.
- William's avoidant behavior, and the negative effects of his avoidance, strengthened his belief that he was incompetent.
- As William looked back on his recent and distant past, he had a tendency to selectively recall examples of failure. Successes did not come readily to mind, even though he had been successful in several aspects of life.
- William's learning history may have helped shape his core belief. He was not particularly good in school (although it was not entirely clear whether this was due to lack of ability or due to failing to apply himself). He had three older siblings, and as the "baby" of the house, he was not given much responsibility; his siblings often treated him as if he were incompetent.

Over the next several sessions, the therapist used several strategies for challenging William's core belief (see Chapter 16), including:

- Discussing the advantages and disadvantages of believing himself to be incompetent.
- Examining evidence for and against the belief that he is incompetent.
- Using scaling to help modulate William's all-or-nothing perceptions of competence and incompetence.

In Session 13, the therapist developed an "on the fly" *core belief diary* for William's homework. The aim was to help William look for and retain information that would support or not support his belief that he was incompetent. For each task William attempted, he was to note how competently he performed (see Figure 20.9).

The therapist followed up on William's monitoring.

T: I'm interested to hear about your competence and incompetence diary. What kinds of things did you notice?

W: It's funny; I think that when I really looked at things objectively, there were some times that I was more competent than I thought I would be.

T: Yeah, a lot of the time when we don't pay attention to these things, we end up just having a global and general recollection of things not going well. What are some examples of where you seemed competent?

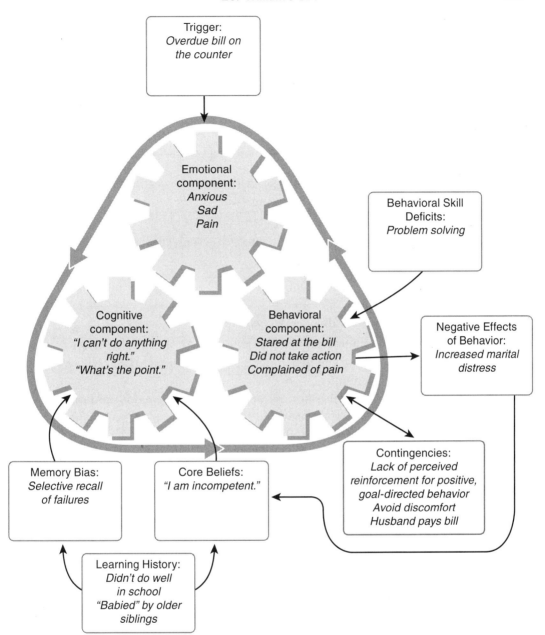

FIGURE 20.8. Expanded model for William showing the presence of core beliefs.

Date	Activity attempted	How competently did I act?
		0 ·· 100 Completely Completely incompetent competent
		0 ·· 100 Completely Completely incompetent competent
		0 ·· 100 Completely Completely incompetent competent

FIGURE 20.9. "On-the-fly" core belief diary for William.

W: Well, at work I was assigned a new project, and I had to gather information about it.

T: I see. And how competent did you rate yourself as?

W: I gave myself a 70. I thought I did pretty good.

T: OK, very good. I see there's an item ranked really low, though. Looks like a 10? Can you tell me about that one?

W: Yeah, I was trying to fix the lawn mower and I just screwed it up. I didn't know what I was doing, and oil leaked out all over the garage.

T: I see. I've had that happen, too, and it's no fun. Your rating of 10, though, seems to suggest that you perceived yourself as being incompetent?

W: Well, yeah, a more competent person would have done the job right instead of making a mess.

T: I guess it depends on how you define competence. Was there reason to believe that you should have known what to do, and that you should have done the job right, without making a mistake?

W: I don't follow.

T: Well, is this a job you have a lot of experience with?

W: No, not really. I'm not much of a repair guy.

T: So you take on a new and challenging task that you don't have much experience with. And you make a mess. And that reads to you as incompetence.

W: I guess I wasn't considering alternatives like we were talking about a couple of sessions ago.

T: Well, can we consider them now? Is there another explanation for what happened, besides you being an incompetent person?

W: I was just new at it. People make mistakes when they do something new. But isn't that the same thing as incompetence?

T: I don't think so. I think that incompetence reflects our opinion about the person and his overall capability, not whether he's well practiced at something. But let's see how that fits with your thinking. When you rated yourself as incompetent, were you making a judgment about yourself? Or just about this exact task and your skill level at it?

W: I guess about myself.

After a few sessions of core belief discussions, William's depression began to decrease again (see Figure 20.10), falling below the cutoff between populations with and without depression. Therefore, William's depression had showed *clinically significant change* (see Chapter 6). Similarly, his pain ratings decreased markedly.

At Session 17, the therapist introduced the possibility of termination. Given William's pattern of dependent behavior, the therapist hypothesized that William might have some negative thoughts and feelings about terminating treatment. At that time, William did not identify any negative reaction, stating that he was feeling better and that perhaps it was time to consider terminating, although he wanted to think about it some more. The therapist made a mental note to inquire about it at the next session.

At the next session, William's depression score had increased, furthering the therapist's hunch that William was having a negative emotional reaction to the idea of terminating therapy. This would not be terribly surprising, given William's core belief that he was incompetent. Though he was actively working on this belief and feeling more competent, a core belief can easily be reactivated under new circumstances. The therapist took the opportunity to use this as a means to challenge William's beliefs further.

T: Seems like your pain is down, but it also looks like you're experiencing some more depression today. What's up?

W: I don't know; I guess after our conversation last week about stopping therapy I started feeling really worried and hopeless.

T: Worried and hopeless. What kind of thoughts were you having?

W: It's just that I've come a long way with these sessions with you, and I just think how can I keep the progress going without you?

T: I see. You know, this is very normal. People often get distressed when they think about ending therapy. After all, your work here has been very important to you, and you and I have spent a lot of time talking and getting to know each other, so I can understand why the thought might bother you.

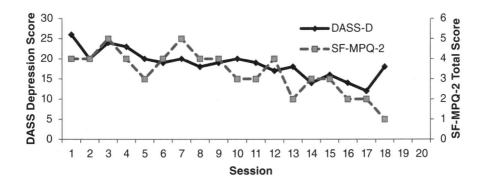

FIGURE 20.10. William's pain and depression graph at Session 18.

W: Yeah. I mean, I really like the progress I've made and I just don't want it to slip away.

T: Let's think this issue through a bit more. We know all too well that you have this core belief about being incompetent, and that other people are much better than you, and you need them to help you. I wonder, is that part of what you're experiencing now?

W: Maybe. Yeah, I think so.

T: So maybe, just to fill it in a bit, you have a belief that you're only feeling better because you keep coming to see me. And therefore, if you don't see me, you won't feel better any more.

W: Yeah, I guess that's it.

T: Can you challenge that belief, using the strategies we've been discussing?

W: Um. . . . Well, I could examine the evidence for and against the belief. The evidence for is that I felt rotten before seeing you and now I feel better. And the evidence against . . . I just don't know what that would be.

T: Well, here's one way to think about it. When you first came to see me, you didn't really know how to feel better, right?

W: Right.

T: And now you do.

W: Yeah, I guess I do.

T: So that is something you are competent to do.

W: That's true.

T: So who is now responsible for your feeling better? Me or you?

W: I am.

T: Right. You feel better now because of your own efforts, not because of me. I taught you the stuff, but now you're the one who's actually doing it.

W: Yeah, you're right. I'm doing it.

T: Let's try an experiment. I know we've been seeing each other on a weekly basis, but how about if, instead of meeting next week, we meet in 2 weeks, and see how it goes? So if it's me keeping you better, we would predict that everything will fall apart and your depression score will shoot up. And if it's you keeping you better, we would predict that you'll stay the course.

W: Yeah, OK, we can try that.

T: And if you stay the course at the next visit, let's stretch it out even further and meet in 4 weeks. That will really be a good test of how well you can manage on your own.

W: OK, that sounds reasonable.

Relapse Prevention

At the following session 2 weeks later, and at the next session 4 weeks after that, William's depression levels resumed their previous decreasing course (see Figure 20.11). The therapist used the last session for **relapse prevention.** Relapse prevention is not a unique intervention; rather, it is the application of CBT strategies (particularly cognitive restructuring

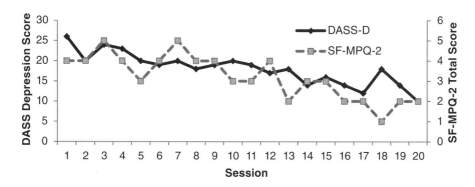

FIGURE 20.11. William's pain and depression graph at Session 20.

and problem solving) to ongoing maintenance of treatment gains. Specifically, the therapist emphasized:

• *Decatastrophizing "lapses."* The therapist reminded William that mood and pain can fluctuate from time to time and cautioned that the presence of a "lapse" (a return of pain or depressed feelings) does not necessarily imply that William is back to square one or that his hard-won gains had "worn off." Some of this discussion may take place early in therapy, so that the client can anticipate (and not catastrophize) some ups and downs during treatment. It's brought up here as something for William to think about going forward.

• *Using lapses as a cue for restarting CBT skills.* The therapist reviewed with William several possible stressful scenarios that might cause him distress in the future and suggested how he might reintroduce some of the strategies he had learned in CBT, such as activity scheduling, problem solving, and cognitive restructuring.

• *Making plans for additional treatment.* The therapist reminded William that the door was never closed completely. People with a history of pain and depression have a higher than average likelihood of experiencing such problems again, and William's core beliefs likely constituted an ongoing vulnerability factor. The therapist discussed these facts openly and realistically with William and let him know that if he experienced similar problems in the future and was unable to resolve them through his own efforts, he would be welcome to schedule a follow-up appointment.

KEY TERM AND DEFINITION

Relapse prevention: Strategies aimed at reducing the likelihood of relapse after termination of therapy.

CHAPTER 21

Putting It All Together

Anna's CBT

In this chapter, we review the treatment of Anna, our client with panic disorder. Figure 21.1 shows when various interventions were introduced into the therapy. Anna was treated with 12 outpatient sessions, delivered once per week. Dark gray shading shows that a strategy was heavily emphasized during that session; light gray shading shows that a strategy was present, but not heavily emphasized.

Therapy Assessment

The therapist opens the initial session by providing structure and getting a general sense of Anna's presenting concerns.

T: Anna, I'd like to start today by getting an understanding of what's been happening, and see if we can start to figure out why it's happening. I'd also like to start working on a plan for how you and I might make things better. How does that sound to you?

A: That sounds good. I've been having these terrible anxiety attacks and they're just the worst, so I'm really hoping to get rid of them.

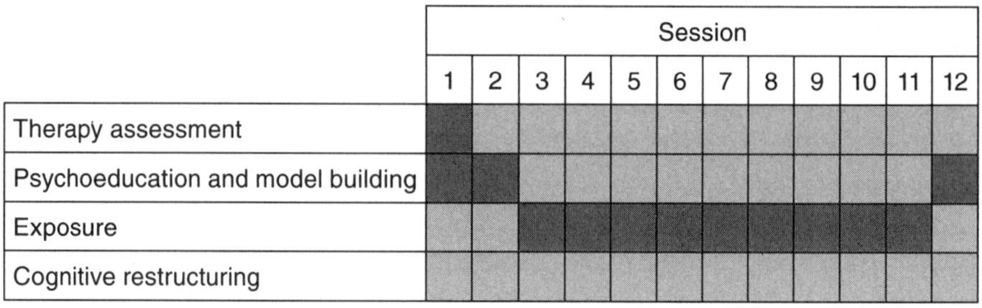

	Session											
	1	2	3	4	5	6	7	8	9	10	11	12
Therapy assessment												
Psychoeducation and model building												
Exposure												
Cognitive restructuring												

FIGURE 21.1. Session-by-session description of Anna's CBT.

T: OK. Tell me a little bit about these attacks. What do you experience when they happen?

A: Well, it's like my heart is going a million miles an hour, and I just feel dizzy, like I'm going to pass out.

T: I see. So you notice that your heart is racing, and you feel dizzy. It also sounds like you have some thoughts that you might pass out. Anything else happen during these attacks?

A: Um . . . I feel really hot. And I have like a pain in my chest, like someone's crushing me. And it feels like I can't breathe.

T: Wow, they sound scary. When you have that pain in your chest, do you ever wonder what that's about?

A: I guess sometimes I think maybe I'm going to have a heart attack or something.

T: OK. I'd like to go through some specific questions that will help me understand this problem a little better.

Note here that the therapist has already begun assessing the presence of maladaptive interpretations. Anna has described two so far: a thought that she will pass out, and a thought that she will have a heart attack. The therapist hypothesized that these thoughts were fueling Anna's feelings of fear.

The therapist conducted a diagnostic assessment, which included a thorough history and review of symptoms. The therapist also inquired about possible medical contributions to the problem. Anna had recently had a physical examination and was found to be in good physical health. She had also had several electrocardiograms (EKGs), as she visited the emergency room frequently; all had been negative. Anna met DSM-5 criteria for both panic disorder and agoraphobia.

To help gather more detailed information, the therapist used structured diagnostic interviews, as well as the self-report version of the Panic Disorder Severity Scale (PDSS; Houck, Spiegel, Shear, & Rucci, 2002). Anna's score on the PDSS was 18, which is in the severe range (remission is defined as a score of 5 or less).

In the first treatment session, the therapist clarified Anna's goals for treatment and provided psychoeducation about her condition.

T: I think I'm getting a pretty good sense of what's happening. I understand that these panic attacks are really bothersome to you, and that most of the time you're not even sure what's causing them. And I also understand that you've had to limit your life quite a bit in order to compensate for the attacks—for example, not driving by yourself, not going to church, and so on. As we think about starting treatment for this, what would you like to be the result of our treatment? How do you want things to be when we're done?

A: I'd like to just not be anxious anymore.

T: I see. I wonder, though, whether that's realistic. After all, everyone feels anxious from time to time.

A: Yeah, I know. I guess really I just don't want to have these attacks anymore.

T: OK, that seems very reasonable. So you'd like to not have panic attacks, even if that means you might still experience feelings of anxiety at times.

A: Yes.

T: And what about your life activities? What would you like to see happen there?

A: Well, I don't want to feel limited by my anxiety anymore.

T: If you weren't limited anymore, what would life look like? What would be different?

A: I guess I'd be able to go to all of my classes and be able to drive myself places without freaking out.

T: OK, these seem like very good goals. So we'll know we have succeeded when you don't have these panic attacks, and you can go to class, drive yourself, and do other things independently without having more attacks. Sound about right?

A: Definitely.

Note that the therapist redirected Anna's initial goal of "not feeling anxious" to a set of concrete behavioral goals that were more realistic. At this time, Anna seems very motivated for treatment, appearing to be in the action stage of change (Prochaska & DiClemente, 1982). The therapist remembered, though, that readiness for change can fluctuate, so Anna's motivation can never be taken for granted. As part of ongoing assessment, the therapist would periodically check on Anna's readiness, as well as administering the PDSS in the waiting room prior to every session.

Initial Treatment Planning

The therapist began by looking for evidence-based treatments for panic disorder. At *www. psychologicaltreatments.org,* the therapist saw that CBT had strong research support for that condition. On the website, the therapist found descriptions of panic-focused CBT.

The therapist also consulted a published CBT manual for treating panic and agoraphobia. As we've seen elsewhere, the manual was not necessarily intended to be followed session by session; rather, the manual gave the therapist important information about the specific interventions that were most likely to help and that therefore should be included in the treatment.

Based on reviewing the available literature, the therapist hypothesized that the following treatment elements *might* be effective:

- Developing a positive, collaborative working relationship.
- Exposure to feared body sensations and avoided activities.
- Reduction of safety behaviors.
- Cognitive restructuring of misinterpretations of body sensations.
- Relaxation or other modulation strategy for pain.

It was not clear, however, whether all of these interventions would be necessary for Anna; many studies suggested that simpler treatments were just as effective as more complex treatments for panic disorder. So the therapist opted to start with the core interventions that seemed most promising: exposure to feared body sensations and exposure to avoided activities. Modulation-based strategies (cognitive restructuring and relaxation) were kept in the "back pocket" to be introduced only if the initial intervention was not optimal.

Psychoeducation and Model Building

The therapist hypothesized that a major contributor to the maintenance of Anna's panic attacks was their unpredictability and perceived uncontrollability. Anna's panic attacks seemed to come out of nowhere, and she could not understand why they were happening. The therapist used psychoeducation and model building to take the mystery out of the process and help Anna understand why these attacks were happening.

T: Let's take a recent panic attack as an example, and see if we can understand why it happened. Can you recall a recent panic attack?

A: Absolutely. I had one just last night. I was just sitting there watching TV and all of a sudden I was panicking.

T: So it just seemed to come from out of nowhere.

A: Yeah, just one minute I was sitting there on the couch, and the next minute I was in the middle of a horrible anxiety attack.

T: Nothing was going on at the time that was particularly bothersome to you?

A: No, it was really just a regular, normal evening up to that point.

T: And the TV show you were watching? It wasn't something scary?

A: No, it was just a sitcom.

T: OK, so let's go through this scene bit by bit. You're on the couch, just watching TV. What was the very first thing you noticed that suggested something might be wrong?

A: The first thing I noticed was that my heart was speeding up.

T: I see. When you noticed your heart speeding up, what did you interpret that to mean?

A: I guess I just thought "Uh-oh, here it comes again."

T: What's the "it" that you're referring to?

A: One of my attacks.

T: Gotcha. Anything else?

A: No, not really at that moment.

T: OK, and what did you notice then?

A: Well, then I was starting to feel dizzy and kind of lightheaded, like I was going to pass out.

T: So now you're having more physical sensations, and did I also hear you say that you told yourself, "I'm going to pass out"?

A: Yeah. And then it was like my heart was really racing and it just felt like a heart attack. So I picked up the phone and called my boyfriend to come over in case I needed to go to the emergency room.

T: I see. Did you do anything else to try to cope with the situation?

A: I tried to breathe deeply, like making sure I had enough oxygen so I wouldn't pass out.

T: (*Taking out a piece of paper, shown in Figure 21.2*) Let me see if I can draw a diagram of how this went. Up here, the very first thing you noticed was increased heart

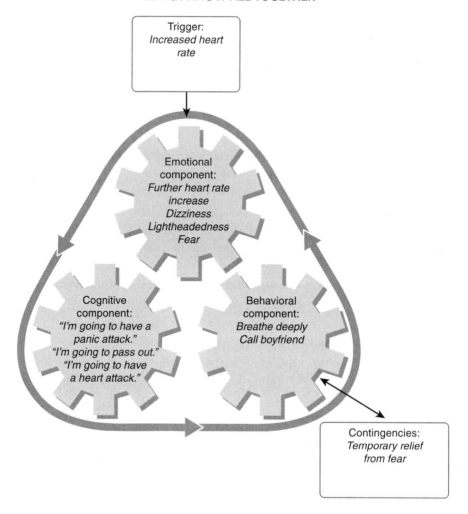

FIGURE 21.2. Initial model developed during Anna's therapy assessment.

rate. And then you had a thought about that—"I'm going to have a panic attack." And you felt more fearful then, and you were noticing your heart going even faster, and you felt dizzy and lightheaded, and then you started thinking things like "I'm going to pass out" and "I'm going to have a heart attack." And you felt even more fearful. Sound right so far?

A: Yeah, that's it.

T: And so then to cope, you started taking some deep breaths. But one thing we know about people who have panic attacks is that they often hyperventilate—they breathe too hard, which can make them feel dizzy and lightheaded. So we might guess that taking deep breaths in this instance only made you feel worse.

A: It definitely didn't make me feel much better.

T: Right. And so you end up calling your boyfriend so that he can take you to the emergency room if needed. And did calling your boyfriend make you feel less scared?

A: A little. At least I knew help was on the way.

T: We call that a "safety behavior." Meaning it's a behavior that helps you feel safer and less scared. The downside of safety behaviors, though, is that you come to rely on them.

A: That's true.

Tracking Anna's Progress

From the initial session, the therapist kept track of Anna's PDSS score. Changes in her scores, for better or for worse, often became the starting point of the session and allowed for discussion of what was going well and what was going not so well.

Anna's panic score didn't change much by the second session (see Figure 21.3). In Session 2, the therapist continued the psychoeducation and model building, using examples of panic attacks that had occurred the previous week.

T: As we've been discussing the panic attack that happened at the mall over the weekend, I'm wondering whether we can use this experience to learn more about how this problem works. Let me draw out what I'm thinking about [see Figure 21.4]. We've talked about how your feelings, thoughts, and actions all interact and play off of each other. So I'll draw those things here, just like we did last week. And I'll also note here that when you left the mall, that resulted in your fear decreasing.

A: That's right.

T: Take me back to when you were in the mall, but before your panic attack started. Can you recall what you were paying attention to?

A: What do you mean?

T: Well, some people pay a lot of attention to their bodies, looking for signs of something wrong. Does that describe you in this instance?

A: Oh, definitely. I'm always on the lookout for signs that it's going to happen again.

T: I see. So that's something we can write here. We call it an *attentional bias*. Even though you're walking through the mall, a part of you is scanning your body, looking for signs of danger.

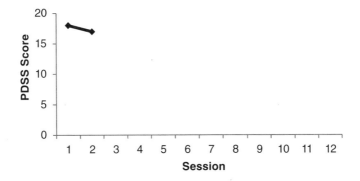

FIGURE 21.3. Anna's panic graph at Session 2.

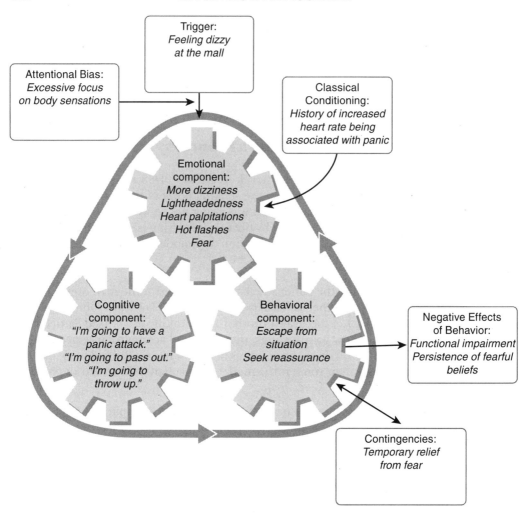

FIGURE 21.4. Expanded model for Anna.

A: Absolutely. That's what I do.

T: What do you suppose the impact of that attentional bias is?

A: I don't know.

T: Well, let me give you an example of what I'm getting at. Can you hear the clock on the wall ticking right now? (*Pauses, hearing the clock.*)

A: Yeah.

T: Had you heard it before?

A: Not really, no.

T: So why are you hearing it now? Did the clock get louder?

A: No, you just pointed it out.

T: Yes, and so now you're paying attention to it. Listen to it for a bit. (*Pauses.*)

A: Yeah, I definitely hear it now.

T: And so now here I am, talking to you, and we're doing this exercise together. But are you still hearing the clock?

A: Yeah, it's in the background.

T: And so therefore some of your brain is listening to me, and some of your brain is listening to the clock. What I'm getting at is that things can seem more or less prominent, depending on how much attention we pay to them. Something can go completely unnoticed at one moment, but then, if we shift our attention toward it, it starts to seem very noticeable, even bothersome. Still hearing it?

A: Yeah, it's like it's competing with you.

T: Right. That clock's been there the whole time. It was there last week, too. But it didn't become an issue for you until you started paying attention to it. Now take this example and tell me how it might relate to your attention to your body sensations in the mall.

A: Um . . . the more I paid attention to them, the more I noticed them, and the worse they seemed to get?

T: Exactly. Let's look at another aspect of the incident: your leaving the mall. We've discussed the upside of it, which is that you feel less scared. But is there a downside?

A: Well, I didn't get my shopping done.

T: That's right. By leaving the mall, you missed out on doing something that you wanted to do.

A: That happens all the time. I want to go to the mall, or to the movies, or to class, but a lot of the time I can't.

T: So the fear doesn't just bother you, it impairs you by way of avoidance.

A: Yeah.

T: There's another aspect to this as well. You had these thoughts that you were going to pass out or throw up. Did those things actually happen?

A: No. They felt like they were, though.

T: Why do you suppose they didn't happen? Why didn't you pass out or throw up?

A: I don't know.

T: If you had stayed in the mall, would your expectation of passing out and throwing up have increased or decreased?

A: I guess they would have increased.

T: So if staying in the mall would increase your belief that you were going to pass out or throw up, then leaving the mall would decrease it?

A: Yeah, that makes sense.

T: And so if I could speak to the anxious part of your brain right now and ask, "Why didn't Anna pass out or throw up?" what would the anxious brain's reply be?

A: Because she left the mall.

T: Right. So your brain comes away with the understanding that the reason things turned out OK was because you left the mall, not because those things probably weren't going to happen in the first place.

Exposure

Starting in Session 2, the therapist introduced the idea of *exposure*. Specifically, because Anna's problem was conceptualized as largely being a fear of her own body sensations, the therapist used *interoceptive exposure* as a main aspect of treatment.

T: We have this idea that part of what is going on is that you are having a fearful reaction to sensations in your body. For example, when you notice your heart rate increasing, that scares you because you worry it could be a heart attack, or when you notice yourself feeling dizzy, that scares you because you worry it could mean that you're going to pass out or throw up.

A: Right.

T: So let's go with that theory for a moment: You have a fear of certain body sensations like racing heart and dizziness. How does one overcome a fear of something?

A: Um. . . . I don't know . . . I guess just tell yourself it's not that bad?

T: You could do that, and that might be an important piece of the puzzle. But is there more to it than that? For example, have you ever overcome a fear of something else, like when you were a kid?

A: I used to be afraid of swimming when I was a kid.

T: But not anymore?

A: No, not anymore.

T: How did you overcome that fear?

A: I don't know. . . . I guess I just got in the water and it turned out OK.

T: I see. So you got in the water, and that's how you got over the fear of the water. How did you get in the water? Like, did you jump in?

A: No, I think I got in the shallow end and just practiced going a little deeper, and put my face in the water. My dad helped me with it.

T: That's a great example. Let me ask: Could you have overcome your fear without going in the water?

A: No, you have to go in.

T: Yes, that's right. So you overcame a fear of water by going in the water. And you can overcome a fear of dizziness by . . .

A: By being dizzy?

T: Right. And you can overcome a fear of racing heart by . . .

A: Having my heart race. But that already happens to me when I'm anxious, and it just makes me feel worse.

T: That's right, it does. You mentioned that your dad helped you overcome your fear of the water by helping you go gradually, controlling the process. What if he had just thrown you in the water without warning you? Would that have helped?

A: No, it would have freaked me out and made it worse.

T: Right. So when you have a panic attack, that's the same thing. You're not controlling it, and you can't even predict it well. I'm talking about something more like going in the shallow end, on your own terms, taking it step by step until you feel more comfortable. We call this *exposure*. Let me show you a little example of what

I'm talking about. I'm just going to roll my head around in a circle, like this. (*Does so.*) Can you do that with me?

A: I guess so. (*Does so.*)

T: OK, so here we are rolling our heads. What kind of physical sensation does that give you?

A: I feel a little dizzy.

T: Yes, me, too. Any feelings of fear, or thoughts that you're going to pass out or throw up?

A: Maybe a little.

T: And can you see that those things are not actually happening?

A: Yes.

T: Can you recall a time in your life when this was actually fun?

A: Yeah, I used to like going on rides at the amusement park when I was a kid.

T: Same kind of sensation, but you didn't label it as a threat back then.

In the next few sessions, the therapist worked on more focused *interoceptive exposure* exercises with Anna (see Chapter 11). Here, they work on confronting her fear of increased heart rate.

T: I'd like to try an exercise to see if we can help you feel more comfortable about the experience of racing heart. Let's start by standing up. (*They do so.*) Now, let's jog in place together. (*They do so.*) Keep those knees up; we really want to get our hearts racing. (*They run in place for 1 minute.*) OK, let's pause. What are you noticing?

A: My heart's definitely racing. And I feel a little out of breath.

T: Me, too. What's your fear level right now, from 0 to 100?

A: About a 70.

T: Ah. Is your brain telling you something scary about this?

A: Yeah, it's telling me that I might panic or have a heart attack.

T: I see. And are you panicking or having a heart attack?

A: No.

T: So your brain is telling you something that might not be true.

A: Right.

T: Let's keep running and I'll check in again with you in another minute or so.

Over the next few sessions, Anna's panic score decreased considerably (see Figure 21.5), although it remained in the clinically elevated range, so the therapist knew there was more work to do. The therapist next added *in vivo exposure* to the intervention.

T: You're doing a great job of learning to be less fearful of your body, Anna. And it seems like this is paying off for you.

A: Yeah, I definitely don't have nearly as many panic attacks and I feel less anxious in general.

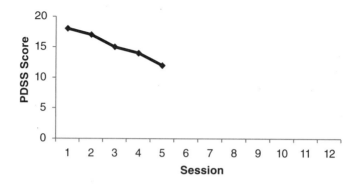

FIGURE 21.5. Anna's panic graph at Session 5.

T: That's really great. I want to add a piece to our work together. You've been avoiding a lot of activities because you worry about having panic attacks. And as we've discussed, that avoidance probably contributes to keeping you stuck. So is it time for us to do something about that avoidance?

A: (*Sighs.*) Yeah, I guess it is. I'm scared, though.

T: That's understandable. You've been avoiding for so long, how could you not feel scared? But remember, the aim is to build up gradually, with you in control of the process. Like getting over your fear of swimming.

A: OK.

T: I'd like to start by just brainstorming some activities and situations that make you feel scared and that you would tend to avoid if you could. What can you think of?

A: Well, going to the mall is definitely one of them.

T: OK, so let's imagine that you go to the mall—right smack into the middle of the mall, on a busy, crowded day. What would your fear level be?

A: About an 80.

T: Pretty high. What else?

In this fashion, the therapist and Anna developed an *exposure hierarchy* of feared and avoided activities. They included going to the mall, going to class and sitting in the middle of the room, going to the movies and sitting far from the exit, driving on a highway, and driving unaccompanied. They then ordered the situations according to the anticipated fear level.

T: I see that driving on a highway with a passenger is the lowest item, but with a fear level of 40, it's still fairly significant. Shall we start there?

A: OK, I guess so.

T: So let's do something a little different. How about we take a drive together?

A: OK, sounds weird, but we can do it.

The therapist then accompanied Anna to her car and sat in the passenger seat as Anna drove. The therapist directed her toward the interstate highway nearby.

T: As we're approaching the highway, what's your level?

A: About a 40. I feel kind of nervous.

T: Yes. Still OK to move forward?

A: Yeah, I can move forward.

T: Great. Let's get on the highway then.

A: OK. (*Merges onto highway.*)

T: What's your level now?

A: About 60. It's higher than I thought it would be.

T: OK, it went up. Too much for you to manage?

A: No, it's bad but I can manage it.

T: Is your brain telling you something scary?

A: I guess I'm wondering what would happen if I had a panic attack right now; like would I crash the car?

T: So that's a question. Often, it's the answer to the question that is the scariest, not the question itself. Is your anxious brain suggesting an answer to that question?

A: Yeah, it's telling me that it's going to happen.

T: Ah. So your brain is saying, "I *am* going to have a panic attack right now, and I *am* going to crash the car"?

A: Yeah.

T: So let's drive a bit and see if those things actually happen. (*Waits a few minutes.*) Are you having a panic attack?

A: No.

T: Are you crashing the car?

A: No.

T: So again your brain was trying to fool you into thinking something bad was going to happen.

A: Right. It's not really happening.

T: So we don't really need to listen to those thoughts much, right?

A: No, we don't. It's just my anxiety.

T: Can I share an observation? Your knuckles are white, like you're gripping the steering wheel really tightly.

A: (*Laughs nervously.*) Yeah, I guess they are.

T: What's that for?

A: I guess to feel more in control of the car.

T: I see. Does gripping the steering wheel like that really increase your control of the car?

A: No, not really.

T: So that's one of those safety behaviors we talked about. What would happen if you just relaxed your grip?

A: Nothing, I guess. (*Relaxes grip.*)

T: Car's still not crashing?

A: No, still not crashing.

The therapist used some "on-the-fly" *cognitive restructuring* during this exercise. Importantly, Anna didn't stop the exposure exercise, do some cognitive restructuring, and then go back to exposure. Such an approach might have simply fostered yet another avoidance strategy. Rather, the therapist addressed Anna's fearful thoughts and asked her to examine the evidence *during* the exposure.

You'll also note that the therapist encouraged Anna to reduce her use of *safety behaviors* during exposure. In subsequent sessions, they had more extensive discussion about her safety behaviors, and it turned out that she had a lot of them. In addition to gripping the wheel tightly while driving, she also asked her boyfriend or other people to accompany her places, tended to sit near exits and aisles in public places, carried a bottle of benzodiazepine medications wherever she went, and was never without her cell phone. The therapist therefore instructed Anna to drop these behaviors when conducting exposure exercises so that their presence would not teach a lesson of *conditional safety*.

What if Anna had actually crashed the car? First, let's remember the discussion from Chapter 11 about safety. Nothing in life is 100% safe; rather, we are looking for *safe enough*. As Anna did not have a history of crashing cars, the risk was thought to be fairly low. Furthermore, although Anna's fear was that panicking would cause a car accident, there is little reason to believe that this would have happened. People do not routinely crash because of anxiety and panic. Finally, despite all that, let's say that for whatever reason, Anna actually *did* crash the car. The therapist and Anna would have reviewed what happened, and why. If it was revealed that Anna had a *behavioral skill deficit* in her ability to drive, then the therapist might have recommended a remedial driving course. If it was just pure bad luck, then they would have had a cognitively oriented discussion about probability and risk. Overall, the benefits of this exposure exercise greatly outweigh any risks.

Over the next several sessions, Anna did both interoceptive and *in vivo* exposure exercises in session and as homework. In session, the therapist and Anna practiced becoming dizzy (by spinning in a chair), increasing her heart rate (by running in place and up and down stairs), feeling lightheaded (by deliberately hyperventilating), feeling hot (by wearing winter coats with the heat cranked up), and feeling chest pressure (by lying on the floor with heavy books stacked on her chest). She was instructed to practice interoceptive exposure every day for at least 30 minutes. For *in vivo* exposure, Anna had a new homework assignment each week, which included going to the mall, going to class and sitting in the middle of the room, going to the movies and sitting far from the exit, driving on a highway, and driving unaccompanied. In each instance, Anna was instructed not to use safety behaviors. For example, she was encouraged to leave her medications and cell phone at home when she went to the mall or to class.

As shown in Figure 21.6, by Session 8 Anna's panic scores were coming down nicely, and this was reflected in her feelings of decreased fear, improved well-being, and decreased avoidance behavior. To help Anna improve further, the therapist asked Anna to start doing combinations of interoceptive and *in vivo* exposure. For example, when driving, Anna was to deliberately overbreathe in order to achieve a feeling of lightheadedness. At the mall, she was to have a double latte in order to cause increased heart rate.

Anna's panic scores decreased more sharply at this point, as shown in Figure 21.7, passing the cutoff point for remission. Qualitatively, by this time, Anna reported that she was not feeling substantially impaired by her fears and was doing activities such as driving

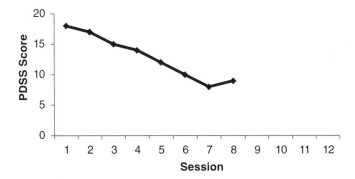

FIGURE 21.6. Anna's panic graph at Session 8.

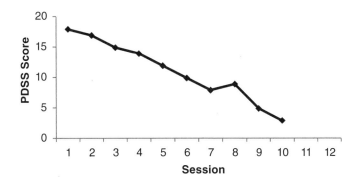

FIGURE 21.7. Anna's panic graph at Session 10.

on the highway and going to class with relative ease. She was no longer experiencing panic attacks, although she did report occasional, fluctuating feelings of anxiety. The therapist raised the question of termination.

T: Let's review where things are for you. Your panic scores look nice and low. In fact, these are in the range that we would usually associate with someone who doesn't have panic disorder. How well does that seem to reflect what's happening?

A: I think pretty well. I mean, I really feel a lot better. I have some anxiety, but it feels a lot more manageable now.

T: And no more panic attacks.

A: And no more panic attacks.

T: Let's go back to the goals we set in our very first session. You mentioned that you wanted to stop having panic attacks and that you wanted to do things like go to church and drive by yourself without feeling excessively anxious. How well does it seem that we've met those goals?

A: I think we've pretty much met them. I mean, I'm not panicking, and I'm going to church now, and I'm driving by myself. I think I still get kind of anxious when I have to drive on the highway by myself, though. That one's still kind of tough for me.

T: So let's discuss how we would like to proceed. I wonder whether we might be getting close to the point of deciding that we've done what we set out to do and that it's time for us to stop having our meetings. But at the same time, you still have some lingering fear of driving on the highway by yourself, so perhaps what would make sense for us to do would be to plan on a couple more meetings and really focus on nailing that fear into the ground by having you do lots of highway driving exposures, like every day taking a nice long drive on the highway without any safety behaviors. Then after a couple of sessions we can see where things stand, and if you're doing well, we might opt to stop at that time. Of course, if you're not doing well for some reason, we can rethink our plan. How does that sound to you?

A: That sounds good.

By Session 12, after doing much more intensive exposure to highway driving, Anna's panic scores had come down even further (see Figure 21.8), and she and the therapist both agreed that she was ready to terminate therapy (with the understanding that should her symptoms return, she would be welcome to recontact the therapist).

Relapse Prevention

Session 12 was primarily dedicated to *relapse prevention*. As discussed in the previous chapter, the therapist emphasized decatastrophizing "lapses," using lapses as a cue for restarting CBT skills, and making plans for additional treatment if needed.

Roads Not Taken

I conclude the discussion of Anna's treatment by highlighting some of the things that the therapist didn't do but could have. Selecting CBT interventions is always a judgment call, but ideally it's a judgment call based on the best available science, as well as an empirical approach to the individual client.

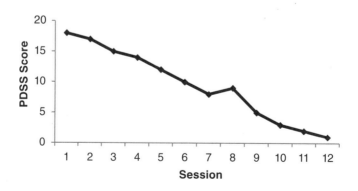

FIGURE 21.8. Anna's panic graph at Session 12.

Relaxation/Breathing Retraining

As discussed in Chapter 18, there is scientific evidence that relaxation and breathing retraining can be beneficial for clients with panic disorder (Meuret et al., 2008; Öst & Westling, 1995). However, in general it appears that exposure-based interventions are more effective (Siev & Chambless, 2007) and that combining relaxation interventions with exposure interventions may actually diminish the efficacy of the exposure by fostering yet another safety behavior (Schmidt et al., 2000). As described previously, the therapist kept relaxation in a "back pocket," but Anna's response to exposure-based therapy was going well enough that addition of new interventions seemed unnecessary (and potentially counterproductive—more is not always better).

More Formal Cognitive Restructuring

Cognitive distortions, particularly those relating to "fear of fear," are prominent in clients with panic disorder, and altered "fear of fear" beliefs are likely a key mechanism by which panic clients recover (Smits, Powers, Cho, & Telch, 2004). The critical question, however, is whether formal cognitive restructuring is the best way to do that. Research suggests that for most clients, adding cognitive restructuring does not add to the effects of exposure therapy for panic (Öst, Thulin, & Ramnero, 2004). Cognitive interventions for panic have proven helpful (Arntz, 2002; D. M. Clark et al., 1999), although these interventions still included some degree of exposure as a "behavioral experiment." Formal cognitive restructuring was therefore considered a reasonable backup plan should exposure alone have failed. Instead, the therapist opted to use "on the fly" cognitive restructuring rather than the full package of thought monitoring, identifying distortions, and so on.

Addressing Core Beliefs

It may well be that additional conversations with Anna would have identified the presence of maladaptive core beliefs, perhaps related to a sense of vulnerability, safety of the world, or her need to rely on others. This was one of those cases, however, in which it didn't seem necessary to go there. Anna's problem, as assessed using the PDSS and clinical interviews, seemed to be responding just fine to the more straightforward exposure therapy. Had Anna's progress stalled, the therapist might have considered evaluating and addressing core beliefs.

Including Anna's Boyfriend in Treatment

Couple therapy can often be a useful format for the treatment of agoraphobia (Barlow, O'Brien, & Last, 1984; Daiuto et al., 1998). In particular, many have found it helpful to employ the assistance of the client's partner in encouraging independent action and reducing accommodation behaviors. In most cases, however, panic and agoraphobia can be treated quite effectively at the individual level. Furthermore, the inclusion of the (usually male) partner in the treatment of the (usually female) agoraphobic client is based on gender roles that are now rather outdated, and its relevance to current, more independent roles of women is less clear. Had the couple's dynamic appeared to be particularly dysfunctional, or had Anna been unable to make sufficient progress on her own, the therapist might have considered addressing the agoraphobia within the context of behavioral couple therapy.

CHAPTER 22

Putting It All Together

Elizabeth's CBT

In this chapter, we review the treatment of Elizabeth, our client with borderline personality and a long history of suicidal ideation and self-injurious behaviors. Figure 22.1 shows the points at which various interventions were introduced into the therapy. Elizabeth was treated with 26 outpatient sessions over 6 months, delivered approximately once per week, although in some weeks she received two sessions. Dark gray shading shows that a strategy was heavily emphasized during that session; light gray shading shows that a strategy was present, but not heavily emphasized.

Therapy Assessment

The therapist first met Elizabeth in the hospital, where she was being kept on a 72-hour involuntary hold after reporting acute suicidal ideation and cutting herself severely enough to require significant medical attention. This was Elizabeth's third psychiatric hospitalization in the past year, and her twelfth overall. Each time, she was hospitalized after an episode of suicidal ideation and nonsuicidal self-injury (NSSI), usually cutting herself with a sharp object but sometimes burning herself with a cigarette. Elizabeth's left forearm was wrapped in bandages at the time of her first meeting with the therapist, and several older scars were visible on her right forearm. Because the therapist held privileges at the hospital, it was possible to meet with Elizabeth prior to her discharge in order to begin discussing a transfer to outpatient care.

Hospital staff had already done a careful diagnostic interview and risk assessment. Elizabeth met DSM-5 criteria for borderline personality disorder, as well as major depressive disorder. The therapist followed up with additional questions about suicidal ideation and behavior. It was determined that Elizabeth was not at imminent risk for suicide. She had chronic suicidal ideation and engaged in repetitive NSSI, but at the time of the discussion she denied an intent to kill herself. This, of course, would need to be reevaluated frequently throughout the treatment.

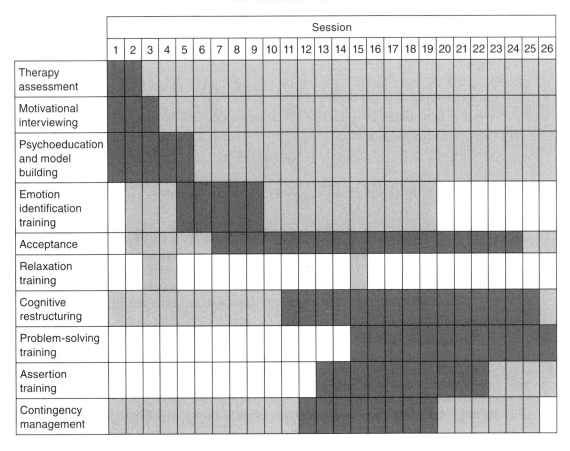

FIGURE 22.1. Session-by-session description of Elizabeth's CBT.

The aim of the initial meeting in the hospital was to discuss the possibility of outpatient treatment and to secure Elizabeth's initial agreement to participate. Here, we join them midway through the conversation, after introductions and basic risk assessment.

T: I know we've been talking about the possibility of having you see me for therapy after you come out of the hospital, but I'd like to get your thoughts on that.

E: I don't know. I mean, I guess I can come see you, but it's not like it's going to help much.

T: I see. So you're pretty doubtful about whether therapy is going to help.

E: Yeah.

T: I'm curious, what do you base that impression on?

E: I guess just the way I feel. I just feel so sad and depressed and I feel like I can't do anything anymore. Everything goes wrong. And nothing ever seems to help, at least not for long. I've had every treatment in the book. And I just get so frustrated that all I want to do is die.

T: OK. So we have two reasons why you would think this way about therapy. First, you feel really depressed, so sad that it's hard to imagine feeling better. And the second is—and tell me if I'm hearing this right—when you've tried things to get better in the past, they haven't been successful.

E: Right.

T: Can I ask for some clarification on that second point? What kinds of things have you tried in order to get better?

E: Well, I've been in the hospital like a dozen times or so.

T: And that hasn't helped.

E: Well, I feel safe while I'm in here, but then as soon as I go home everything goes back to where it was.

T: OK, so these trips to the hospital aren't solving the problem. What else have you tried?

E: I've been on just about every medication there is. I don't think there's a single med out there that I haven't tried.

T: I see. And those didn't help?

E: Maybe a little. I felt a little less depressed with the antidepressants, but not a whole lot. And it didn't stop me from wanting to kill myself or hurt myself.

T: How about therapy?

E: Oh, I've been in therapy forever. Since I was a teenager.

T: I see. And the therapy wasn't helpful, either?

E: Total waste of time. I'd just sit there in someone's office and talk about how my week went, talk about my childhood, and stuff like that, and then I go home and don't feel any better and the therapist collects a check. And it goes like that for years.

T: Wow, sounds like that was a really disappointing experience for you. I can see why you'd feel burned out on the whole therapy thing. What about cognitive-behavioral therapy, or CBT? Have you heard of that?

E: Is that like DBT? I've heard of DBT.

T: Yes, DBT is a kind of CBT. I know, it gets a little confusing with all of the initials. But the basic idea here, whether we call it DBT or CBT, is that the therapy isn't just sitting around and talking about your childhood or how your week went; it's actually learning skills that you can use to make your life better going forward. Is that something you've tried?

E: No, I haven't had anything like that.

T: Ah, so there is something here that you haven't tried yet. Would you be surprised to know that this kind of treatment actually helps a lot of people with the same kind of problems you're experiencing?

E: I didn't know that.

T: It does. Now, of course, that's no guarantee that it will help you, but it would seem like the odds are pretty good. That doesn't mean you'll never have any more problems, but I think that we could help you get things going better than they currently are.

Note that the therapist has already begun some basic CBT procedures in this initial conversation. The therapist uses *empathy*, rather than confrontation, when discussing Elizabeth's attitudes toward treatment; for example, the therapist points out that her pessimism about treatment is understandable based on her prior experiences. This is a tricky balancing act—Elizabeth seems to have a cognitive distortion here, and yet there are some understandable reasons why she might think this way. For all clients, and perhaps particularly for those with borderline personality, both validation and challenging are important—a dichotomy that Linehan (1993) calls a "dialectic." At this stage of the game, and given the therapist's aims for this conversation, it seemed prudent to do more validation than challenging. There is an ever-so-slight challenge, however, when the therapist points out that Elizabeth hasn't tried CBT, which contradicts her statement that she's had "every treatment in the book."

The therapist uses a bit of *psychoeducation* to help raise Elizabeth's awareness of the potential effectiveness of CBT, while at the same time keeping it realistic by pointing out that success can't be guaranteed.

The therapist also begins to use the language of CBT by differentiating thoughts (e.g., her belief that therapy won't help) and feelings (e.g., feeling sad).

Motivational Interviewing

Motivational interviewing strategies were used in the initial inpatient visit in order to get Elizabeth thinking about the possibility of changing. In particular, the therapist was interested in whether Elizabeth would be motivated to end her cycle of NSSI and hospitalization and replace it with a program of skills-based outpatient CBT. Elizabeth appeared to be in the contemplation stage of change (Prochaska & DiClemente, 1982); therefore, the therapist aimed to help her weigh the pros and cons of changing, and to develop discrepancy by helping her see how her behavior was interfering with her happiness (W. R. Miller & Rollnick, 2013).

T: So we have this cycle that you're in. Things go badly, and you feel terrible, and eventually you do something that hurts you, or you have really strong urges to do something that hurts you. And so then you go in the hospital, and you feel safer for a while, but then you come out of the hospital and things are mostly back to where they were, no better. I'm wondering what your thoughts are about changing that pattern.

E: I don't think there's anything I can do besides go to the hospital when I feel unsafe. Are you saying I shouldn't go to the hospital? Because if you are, you can count me out. I need the hospital to be there for me. It's what keeps me alive.

T: No, I'm not saying that at all. You have the right to go to the hospital just like everyone else. What I am saying is that you seem to be stuck in a rut here. And I'm wondering whether getting out of that rut is something that you'd want to do.

E: Well, I do want to feel better.

T: OK, so there's that. There's a bit of a dilemma here, because on one hand you don't want to give up the ability to go to the hospital, and on the other hand you don't feel good now and you'd like to feel better. Am I hearing it right?

E: Yeah.

T: And going to the hospital is giving you a brief feeling of safety, but it's not really making you feel better, at least in the long run. I wonder, in fact, whether the whole pattern is part of what's keeping you stuck.

E: What do you mean?

T: Well, let me ask it this way. Do you have a way of feeling better besides hurting yourself or going to the hospital?

E: No, not really.

T: So there's the problem. You don't know how to really feel better, and the only thing you know how to do is to hurt yourself or go to the hospital, and so you rely on that to get you by. But in the meantime life isn't really getting better, and you still haven't learned how to make yourself feel better.

E: Yeah, I get that.

T: So if we had something that would help you learn how to feel better—I mean actually better, not temporarily better like hurting yourself or going to the hospital— what would be your interest in that?

E: So you're going to get me not to kill myself or hurt myself.

T: Well, not exactly. I mean, I think that's a good goal, but it's just part of the picture. I mean, if all we do is keep you alive and your life continues to stink, that wouldn't be a very satisfactory outcome. I think what would be really helpful would be if you had a life that you felt was worth living. Now, of course, we can't get you there if you're dead, because I'm pretty sure I can't help a dead person. But I wonder whether it would be worth it to you to stay alive for a while to see if this treatment has promise for you. And we can discuss your suicidal thoughts and actions as we go.

E: I guess it would be worth it.

T: So this is an agreement? I do my best as a therapist, and you stay alive so we can do this work?

E: Yeah, I can agree to that.

T: Now, the things you do to hurt yourself. I know that it feels like you don't have a lot of control over that . . .

E: . . . I don't have any control over that.

T: Understood. Would you be willing to make that something we work on together? That is, could we agree that we'd work toward having you get control over that and stop hurting yourself?

E: Sometimes that's the only thing that works.

T: Yes, I get that. And I agree that it does work, in a certain way. So I'm not putting my foot down and saying you can't ever hurt yourself. But could we agree that our work should aim to decrease your need to do that, perhaps by finding better, healthier ways of responding that actually work for you in the long run?

E: I guess I could agree to that.

There are several aspects of this conversation to note, many of which are derived from the stylistic aspects of Linehan and colleagues (Linehan, 1993; Linehan & Dexter-Mazza, 2008). First, the therapist displays a lack of fear of Elizabeth's suicidal ideation and history of NSSI. This is treated as just one aspect of her overall problem and isn't handled with kid gloves. Note as well that the therapist doesn't treat Elizabeth like someone who is so fragile that she can't handle this kind of discussion. The therapist uses language that is frank and honest, and even humorous at times. She's probably not used to having people talk to her like this.

The therapist begins to discuss Elizabeth's hospitalizations and NSSI in behavioral terms, alluding to the likely existence of skill deficits (e.g., "You don't know how to really feel better") and escape/negative reinforcement (e.g., "Going to the hospital is giving you a brief feeling of safety").

The therapist doesn't make the conversation all about suicidality and NSSI. True, those are the most dramatic qualities of Elizabeth's problems, and the therapist makes a point of discussing their unhelpfulness (e.g., "I'm pretty sure I can't help a dead person"). But the therapist points out that these things are happening for a reason and that part of treatment should be to address those reasons (e.g., "I would think that what would be really helpful would be if you had a life that you felt was worth living").

The therapist secures a preliminary agreement from Elizabeth. However, rather than a no-suicide contract, the therapist engages Elizabeth in a commitment to treatment, which, naturally, includes remaining alive (see Rudd, Mandrusiak, & Joiner, 2006, for discussion). The therapist also secures a commitment to work on the NSSIs together. This is different from the therapist's insisting that Elizabeth stop hurting herself before entering therapy (that would be a bit like insisting that a depressed patient stop being depressed before we start depression treatment). But at least we know that Elizabeth is willing to work on this problem.

Initial Treatment Planning

The therapist began by looking for evidence-based treatments for borderline personality disorder and major depressive disorder. Consulting *www.psychologicaltreatments.org*, the therapist saw that for borderline personality disorder, there was strong research support for the use of dialectical behavior therapy (DBT). The therapist found freely available information on DBT and consulted a published treatment manual on that topic. For major depressive disorder, the website indicated that there was strong research support for a number of CBT packages, including behavioral activation, cognitive therapy, and problem-solving therapy. The therapist consulted published treatment manuals on these interventions. As always, the aim of consulting a treatment manual was not to "script" the therapy but rather to get an idea of what kinds of interventions were likely to be successful and should be included in the CBT. The therapist also noted that there was a fair amount of overlap across the various packages (DBT, behavioral activation, cognitive therapy, and problem-solving therapy). Therefore, the therapist recognized that it was not necessary to somehow apply four different treatments; rather, the aim was to distill those packages into the necessary component interventions and create an individualized treatment for Elizabeth.

Based on reviewing the available literature, the therapist hypothesized that the following treatment elements *might* be effective:

- Developing a positive, collaborative working relationship, with careful attention to possible alliance ruptures.
- Emotion regulation strategies, possibly beginning with training in identifying emotions.
- Acceptance for negative emotional states.
- Cognitive restructuring of maladaptive core beliefs.
- Training in effective problem solving.
- Training in assertive interpersonal behavior.

As always, this initial game plan was just a start. It was assumed that the therapist would learn more about Elizabeth along the way and that interventions could be added, subtracted, or modified as needed.

Psychoeducation and Model Building

After Elizabeth was discharged from the hospital, she did as agreed and attended her first outpatient therapy session. The therapist's primary aim was to develop a working model of the problem that would help Elizabeth understand some of the reasons why the problem was persisting.

> T: I'd like to start trying to see if we can understand exactly what's happening and why. Perhaps we could start by talking in some detail about the events that resulted in you going to the hospital this last time. What can you think of that led to the hospitalization?
>
> E: I cut myself.
>
> T: Yes, you did. So why do you think that happened?
>
> E: My boyfriend and I got in a fight and I just did it.
>
> T: OK, so you and your boyfriend had a fight. How did that lead to your cutting yourself?
>
> E: What do you mean?
>
> T: Well, do you always cut yourself whenever you have a fight with someone?
>
> E: No.
>
> T: Let's say I decide to pick a fight with you today. Not that I plan to, but let's just say I do. Would you cut yourself?
>
> E: No.
>
> T: Why not?
>
> E: Well, because I don't even really know you. So if you picked a fight with me it wouldn't matter.
>
> T: It wouldn't, would it? I mean, who am I?
>
> E: Yeah, I'd just think you were some nut job and not come back.
>
> T: But not cut yourself.
>
> E: No.
>
> T: So it seems that there's more to it than just a fight. If it were that simple, then you'd cut yourself every time someone, even me, had a fight with you. So what is it about this particular fight with this particular person?
>
> E: Well, he's important to me.
>
> T: And so you interpreted the fight how?
>
> E: I guess that he didn't really understand me or care about me.
>
> T: So you had something you were trying to communicate to him . . .
>
> E: . . . And all he did was argue and eventually start blaming me for everything.
>
> T: I see. And how were you feeling at that time?
>
> E: I don't know. Just shocked, I guess.

T: Angry?

E: Yeah, I guess.

T: Sad?

E: Yeah.

T: Scared?

E: A little, maybe, yeah.

T: So I'm seeing kind of a progression of events here. Let me show you what I'm thinking of, but you tell me if it sounds accurate. (*Takes out a piece of paper and draws, as
shown in Figure 22.2.*) You have the fight with your boyfriend, up here. Really it's
you trying to express yourself and him not getting it.

E: Right.

T: And it sounds like what really makes this a trigger—what really makes it bothersome for you—is not just that you had a fight, it's that this is someone who's really
important to you, and you think that he's just blaming you, and that he doesn't
understand you, and that he doesn't care. These are thoughts. They're the interpretations that you make.

E: Are you saying I'm wrong about him?

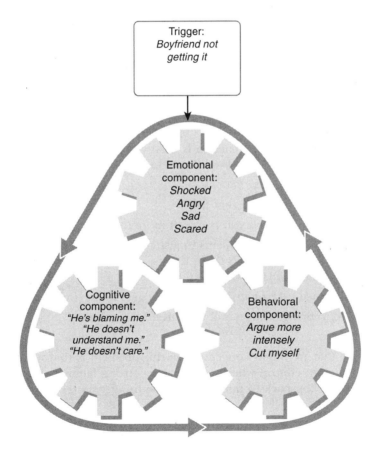

FIGURE 22.2. Initial model developed during Elizabeth's therapy assessment.

T: No, I'm not saying that at all. I've never met him, so how could I know? He might be a great guy who loves you, he might be a rotten guy who doesn't care, he might be somewhere in between. Who knows? The point here is just for us to notice that those thoughts were there, that they were part of how you reacted.

E: OK.

T: And while this is going on, you also notice yourself having some feelings. You felt shocked, you felt angry, sad, scared. These are what's going on in your gut, in your body. They're not words, like the thoughts are; they're more of a sensation. I'll put them here, and can you see how they're connected to the thoughts?

E: I'm not sure I see that.

T: Well, think back to the idea of me picking a fight with you. And that doesn't really matter. Meaning you'd interpret that fight differently from this fight. Would you feel the same amount of anger, fear, sadness, and so on?

E: No. I'd be annoyed, but not like this.

T: Right. So interpretations have an effect on how you feel.

E: Wait, so are you just saying I misinterpret things and that's why I feel bad?

T: Not necessarily. It's true that your thoughts and interpretations can affect your feelings. But your feelings can also affect your thoughts. They kind of go around and around like that. That's what happens to all of us.

E: Because I don't think I'm wrong about him.

T: Are you interpreting what I'm saying as telling you that you're wrong?

E: I guess, yeah.

T: I'm not. You could be spot-on accurate. Right now, I just want us to be aware that thoughts and interpretations are part of your reaction.

E: OK.

T: And the other part of your reaction is what you actually did. I know that cutting yourself was part of it. What else did you do?

E: I guess I just argued more.

T: More, as in more words, different tone?

E: I guess I was just trying to express myself more intensely so he'd get it.

T: So you have this process that seems to just ramp up and up, right? You think this way, you feel this way, you do these things, and you kind of just feel worse and worse as you go along. Does that sound right?

E: Yeah. It's like once I start getting upset it just gets worse.

T: And it's hard to bring it down and feel OK.

E: Exactly.

T: So one way that we might conceptualize this problem is that it's hard for you to feel like you're in control when you're having strong feelings. It's hard for you to get yourself feeling back to normal. And the things you try seem to just add fuel to the fire.

Note that the therapist sidesteps several potential conflicts with Elizabeth during this discussion. In particular, Elizabeth seems to bristle at the idea that her thoughts might be inaccurate. This was a matter of clinical judgment. The therapist could have pressed

Elizabeth, asking her to examine the evidence or other aspects of cognitive restructuring. However, doing so would have risked upsetting the tenuous therapeutic relationship. The therapist is satisfied, at this point, to just point out the fact that thoughts exist and that they are related to emotions and behaviors. The therapist also helps Elizabeth understand that her thoughts are important by constructing a hypothetical scenario (the therapist picking a fight with Elizabeth) and pointing out that she would probably not cut herself under those circumstances—therefore, Elizabeth's interpretations must play a key role in determining her emotional and behavioral response.

The therapist is using psychoeducation to define Elizabeth's problem in terms of emotion regulation, which is central to many theories of borderline personality and NSSI (Linehan, 1993; Nock, 2009). This is a relatively destigmatizing way to begin the process of educating Elizabeth about the nature of her problems.

Note as well that the therapist picks up on an unhealthy CRB: Elizabeth's tendency to quickly assume that others are telling her she is wrong or are otherwise confronting her. The therapist gently points this out in the form of a question ("Are you interpreting what I'm saying as telling you that you're wrong?") and clarifies the issue ("I'm not"). Later, there might be more substantive discussion of CRBs, but for now, given the early aims of the treatment, the therapist opted to tread lightly.

In this session and the next, the therapist and Elizabeth add more detail to her model.

T: Let's keep going with building our understanding of why things happened the way they did. We know that you had a reaction to your boyfriend not getting it, and that your reaction had something to do with your thoughts, something to do with your feelings, and something to do with your actions. What was the effect of your actions here? For example, when you argued more intensely, how did that affect things?

E: I don't think it helped much.

T: What makes you say that?

E: He didn't get it.

T: Hmm. So arguing more intensely doesn't clue him in and make him understand. Any downside to it? Did arguing more intensely make anything worse?

E: I think he just got angrier and angrier.

T: I see. So you're upset, and you argue more intensely, and then he gets more upset . . .

E: . . . and then I get more upset.

T: And around and around it goes. A nasty cycle.

E: Yeah.

T: I'll write that here on our diagram [see Figure 22.3]. There were some negative effects of that particular action. How about the cutting? What were the effects of that?

E: I guess I feel better when I cut.

T: So in this particular instance, what did feeling better mean? I know that you were feeling shocked, angry, sad, and scared. Did something change?

E: After I cut myself I felt less mad, you know? And I wasn't so sad any more. Like I had something else to focus on instead of how bad I was feeling inside.

T: I see. So cutting gave you some relief. And what about the argument you were having at the time? What happened to that?

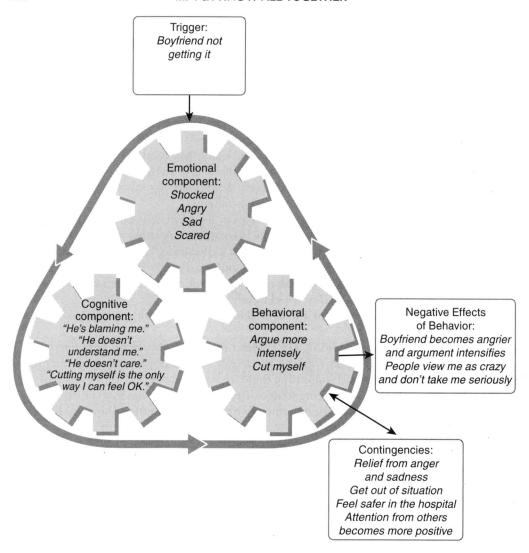

FIGURE 22.3. Expanded model during Elizabeth's therapy assessment.

E: Well, it ended, and my boyfriend had to drive me to the hospital. He was still really pissed, though.

T: But not actively arguing with you?

E: No, just kind of steaming. But also concerned about me.

T: So cutting ended the argument and got you out of that situation, at least temporarily. And maybe your boyfriend softened up a little afterward. Any downside to cutting?

E: Well, I went to the hospital.

T: Was that a downside to you?

E: I don't know . . . maybe not . . . they're nice in the hospital and I feel safer.

T: So it's a nicer environment, feeling safer.

E: Yeah.

T: How about the impact on your relationships outside of the hospital? Good impact? Bad impact?

E: Bad.

T: In what way?

E: I guess people don't take me as seriously because I'm a cutter.

T: Why would cutting make them not take you seriously?

E: I guess I'm just the crazy one, you know? Like, "Oh boy, here she goes again, being her usual crazy self."

T: So it becomes easier for them to dismiss you and harder for them to understand that you actually have something to say.

E: Yeah.

T: But, of course, you do have something to say.

E: I do, yeah.

T: So when you cut yourself there are some positives and negatives that happen as a result. On the positive side, you get some real short-term relief from bad feelings, and it helps you escape from a bad situation and get to an environment where you feel safe and people are nice. And who could blame you for wanting those things? These are pretty temporary, though. And there's a downside, which might be a little more long term, which is that the relationships you have with other people get uglier, and people start thinking that you're crazy and then they don't take you as seriously.

E: Right.

T: And having people you care about not take you seriously is a trigger for you.

E: Yeah, so it gets worse.

T: I think so, yeah.

Elizabeth is beginning to connect the dots. She's articulating at least a preliminary understanding of the long-term, negative consequences of her behaviors, including NSSI. The therapist is also alluding to both positive reinforcement (reinforcement) and negative reinforcement (escape) but is being careful here. Were the therapist to emphasize the reinforcing properties of NSSI too strongly, Elizabeth might jump to the conclusion that the therapist thinks her behaviors are solely "manipulative" in nature. Chances are, Elizabeth's already heard plenty of other people make that argument. Remember that from our perspective, behaviors are the way they are for several reasons, including the person's reinforcement histories. Doing a behavior that has been reinforced is not being manipulative; it's just doing what worked before.

Tracking Elizabeth's Progress

Elizabeth's problems are complex and multidimensional, and therefore the therapist had to make some decisions about what to measure on an ongoing basis. As noted in Chapter 7, threats to safety of self or others should take priority. Therefore, the therapist opted to have Elizabeth track the frequency of NSSI and the severity of suicidal ideation using a daily journal. For the sake of clarity, the therapist reviewed the definition with Elizabeth:

NSSI was defined as any nonaccidental behavior that resulted in damage to bodily tissues, ranging from minor scratches to deep cuts. At each session, the therapist added up the number of NSSI behaviors for the previous week. The therapist explained carefully that the aim of this measurement was not to punish her for self-injury, but rather to get a sense of how well the treatment was or was not working. Suicidal ideation was rated on a 0–10 scale. The therapist made note of her ratings but did not make this an explicit focus of the session unless there was an obvious "jump" in her self-reported suicidal ideation. Rather, it was assumed that suicidal ideation would be rather chronic, and the therapist opted to focus more heavily on the behavioral target of NSSI. The therapist also used the Depression Anxiety Stress Scales (DASS; Lovibond & Lovibond, 1995), with particular attention to her Depression subscale.

Given the hypothesized role of emotion regulation deficits, the therapist also opted to administer the Difficulties in Emotion Regulation Scale (DERS; Gratz & Roemer, 2004) at the beginning of treatment. It didn't seem critical to administer the DERS on a weekly basis; rather, the therapist opted to use it once every few weeks to look for problems and positive changes. Elizabeth scored particularly high at pretreatment on three DERS subscales: Lack of Emotional Awareness (Awareness), Difficulty Engaging in Goal-Directed Behavior (Goals) and Limited Access to Emotion Regulation Strategies (Strategies). These two subscales are shown in Figure 22.4.

Emotion Identification Training

As noted in Chapter 19, for some clients, training in recognizing emotions is the first step in successful emotion regulation. Elizabeth's high score on the DERS-Awareness scale, as well as the therapist's observations of fuzzy descriptions of her emotional states, suggested that this early training would be helpful. Here, the therapist works with Elizabeth to help her with emotion identification, beginning with psychoeducation about the adaptive and maladaptive effects of emotion.

> T: Let's talk more about feelings. As we've discussed, it seems like a big part of the problem is that you have a hard time keeping your feelings from getting the better of you. That doesn't mean that emotions are bad; in fact, they're very important for us. Can you think of how emotions can be important?
>
> E: Um . . . I don't really know.

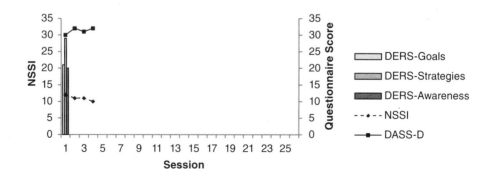

FIGURE 22.4. Elizabeth's measures at Session 4.

T: Well, think of it this way. Have you ever started to step off of a curb, and then there's a car coming that you didn't see, so you quickly jumped back on the curb?

E: Yeah.

T: OK, so what caused you to jump back onto the curb?

E: A feeling?

T: Right. Do you know what that feeling was?

E: Maybe scared?

T: That's exactly right. You felt scared—fear—and that fear made you jump back onto the curb. It's a survival mechanism that we all have.

E: Sometimes I wish I could just walk out into traffic and get run over.

T: Yes, you do have thoughts like that. Those wishes you have, the things you say to yourself, are thoughts. And I definitely want to discuss those thoughts with you as we go along. But for now, I want to stay on the topic of the feelings that you experience. Can you recognize how, from a survival standpoint, the fear was basically a helpful thing?

E: Yeah, I get that.

T: But of course fear can be unhelpful at times as well. Have you ever experienced unhelpful fear?

E: Sure, all the time.

T: Such as?

E: Well, like just the other day when I just started feeling scared for no reason and was feeling like I was having an anxiety attack. Or when I just got so worried that my boyfriend was going to walk out on me, and what was going to become of me, and so on. That was unhelpful.

T: How do you know it was unhelpful?

E: Well, it just felt really bad.

T: It did, and let me suggest an addition to that. In those instances, the fear was unhelpful because it didn't lead you to actually do anything for yourself. See, the fear on the curb was helpful because it motivated you to get back on the curb. And the fear for no reason, or the fear that your boyfriend was going to leave you, was unhelpful because it didn't motivate you to take healthy action. So feelings are helpful when they motivate us to do things that are good for us, and they're unhelpful when they don't.

E: I get it.

T: Let's try another feeling, like anger. When can anger be helpful? Remember, a helpful feeling is one that motivates you to take healthy action.

E: Um . . . maybe if someone does something I don't like and I tell them so?

T: Yes, exactly right! If the feeling of anger motivates you to stand up for yourself in a way that is healthy for you and for everyone else, then that's helpful anger. How about unhelpful anger? Ever have that?

E: Oh yeah, all the time.

T: Can you give me an example?

E: Well, when I just get so mad I cut myself, that's not really helpful.

T: It isn't, is it? Because cutting doesn't actually make anything better. It only hurts you. So you see, any feeling can be helpful or unhelpful.

E: But I shouldn't feel angry.

T: Says who?

E: I don't know; I just shouldn't. It's not nice.

T: Nice people don't get angry?

E: No.

T: You really believe that?

E: Well, they don't cut themselves and scream at people and get into fights.

T: That's a bit different from feeling angry, though, isn't it? Angry is a feeling, and things like cutting, screaming, and fighting are actions.

E: But if I didn't feel angry I wouldn't do those things.

T: That's true. Now, imagine that if we could somehow remove all of the anger from your brain, like if we had some kind of anger-erasing pill, life wouldn't go so well for you that way either. Sure, you might not cut and scream and fight, but you also wouldn't do things like stand up for yourself. You need anger in your life, just like I need anger in my life, just like everyone does. The problem is not so much the fact that you have angry feelings; it's that once you have them, you don't quite know what to do about them, how to use those feelings in ways that are helpful to you.

E: I guess that's true.

T: I think it's helpful for us to look again at what you're doing and why. Previously, you told me about some of the short-term things you're trying to accomplish with your actions, like cutting and going to the hospital. You mentioned that when you do those things, you feel a sense of relief from anger and sadness, and you get out of the stressful situation and go somewhere that you feel safer and get more positive attention. So it seems like all of these actions have something in common; can you see what it is?

E: Um . . . I guess I'm trying to feel better than I do?

T: Yes; that's how I see it as well. So you have a couple of different things going on here. First, you have a feeling. And that's perfectly fine; it's a feeling. But because you really don't like that feeling and don't want it, you try all kinds of things to feel better. And sometimes they work, kind of, for a while, but they don't really offer you any long-term relief.

E: No, I feel worse.

T: Exactly. So from that perspective, what's the bigger problem here? Your feelings, or your efforts to get away from your feelings?

E: I shouldn't get as mad as I do.

T: Well, let's think about it this way. Right now you're passing judgment on yourself for feeling angry. That is, you have some angry feelings, and then you have some ideas about how bad it is to feel that way, right?

E: Yeah.

T: So imagine that your angry feeling is a snowball up at the top of a hill. It's pure and white and clean and natural. Can you imagine that? Now imagine that this snowball, your angry feeling, starts rolling downhill. And as it rolls, it starts picking up stuff, like leaves and sticks. Maybe some dog poop. The leaves and the sticks and the dog poop are what you're adding to the emotion. So when you tell yourself you shouldn't feel mad, there's a stick that just got stuck to the snowball. And then you feel upset with yourself for feeling this way. There's a leaf. And you think "I really have to do something about this feeling." There's some dog poop. And what does your snowball look like by the time it gets to the bottom of the hill?

E: Nasty. Covered in leaves and dirt and dog poop.

T: Right. Your anger started off as a regular old feeling, very natural. It didn't feel good, but it was a clean discomfort. But along the way you put a lot of judgments and rules and self-deprecation and control efforts on it, and now your clean feeling is covered up with a lot of dirty discomfort. So now you have both clean and dirty discomfort going on.

E: I hate it.

T: And by hating it, there's another leaf on the snowball.

E: But this is bullshit. I shouldn't have to suffer like that.

T: I completely agree. That is, I don't want you to have to suffer like that. You've been suffering for too long. Can I point something out? When you said this is bullshit and you shouldn't have to suffer, you threw a little more dirt on the snowball. You see, what happens is that whenever you judge this problem or decide it's bad or that you need to fix it, you're not solving the problem, you're just adding more dirty discomfort onto it.

E: Well, so how the hell am I supposed to feel any better?

T: The trick is to scrape the leaves and dirt and poop off the snowball. All those judgments and rules and control efforts; you need to see that they're doing more harm than good.

E: But then how do I stop feeling mad?

T: Maybe you don't. Maybe that's just it. Maybe it makes sense just to have a clean snowball of anger. And then we can work on some ways to deal with that clean snowball of anger in ways that are healthy and that work for you.

E: I don't want a stupid clean snowball of anger. I want to feel better.

T: And by not wanting it, there's some more dirt. I realize this can be a frustrating way to think about it. And I don't ask you to believe it just now. I just want to put this idea in your head for now. Maybe the snowball, in its pure form, is something you could learn to live with. And maybe by learning to live with it, you wouldn't have all the dirt and poop that's causing you so much suffering.

E: I guess I get that.

T: We could even look a little farther uphill, before the snowball started getting dirty with judgments and rules and self-deprecation. Perhaps we'd find that it didn't even start out as anger.

E: You mean I'm not really angry?

T: No, I don't mean that. You're angry and that's very real and very understandable. But often we find that just before the anger, there was another emotion. Maybe it was fear, or feeling hurt. Have you ever noticed that?

E: Maybe hurt.

T: Like you felt hurt at first and then . . .

E: And then I got mad at the person who hurt me.

T: And maybe yourself, too?

E: Yeah.

T: So maybe we need to pay attention to the hurt feeling in addition to the anger.

A couple of stylistic points to consider here:

• The therapist is stressing to Elizabeth that emotions, in their raw form, are basically helpful. Many clients mistakenly assume that their emotions are bad or unhealthy and that therefore they should try not to experience them. As we know, however, attempts to suppress thoughts or emotions are generally unhelpful and may even intensify the very thoughts and emotions the person is trying to suppress (Hofmann et al., 2009; Wegner et al., 1993; Wegner et al., 1987).

• The therapist is illustrating a model of Elizabeth's problem based on emotion dysregulation. That is, the therapist is suggesting that although emotions (even unpleasant ones) are normal, Elizabeth has a hard time channeling those emotions into healthy action. The therapist notes further that Elizabeth's short-term efforts to control her emotions, rather than the emotions themselves, are a major driving force of the problem.

• The therapist is careful not to reinforce Elizabeth's expression of suicidal ideation. Again, the therapist understood that Elizabeth had chronic suicidal thoughts and that the therapy could easily be derailed if they had to pause therapy and discuss every instance of suicidal ideation. So the therapist noted that Elizabeth's statement had been heard, but "bookmarked" it for later.

• The therapist makes use of metaphor (Mennin & Fresco, 2013) to clarify for Elizabeth the distinction between "clean" (naturally occurring) discomfort and "dirty" (artificially self-inflicted) discomfort (Hayes et al., 2012). Elizabeth clearly finds this discussion confusing and frustrating, which the therapist validates (without backing off from the subject). (A quick side note that the terms *clean* and *dirty* may have excessive connotations [e.g., sexual meanings] for some clients; to avoid having the message get lost among the connotations, the therapist could select an alternative metaphor or language.)

• The therapist begins to discuss with Elizabeth the possibility that her angry feelings could be secondary to more primary ("clean") emotions such as feeling afraid or hurt. The therapist validates the presence of all of Elizabeth's emotions—the aim is not to tell her that she's "wrong" or "neurotic" for feeling angry—but suggests a possible sequence of emotional reactions.

Next, the therapist works with Elizabeth to help her identify her emotions more accurately.

T: So when you're feeling something, like angry or scared or sad, how do you know you're feeling it?

E: I think a lot of the time I don't really know what I'm feeling. I feel bad, but that's about all I know. I just know it's really bad and I have to do something.

T: I think a lot of people have that problem. When we don't pay close attention to what's going on inside us, it can be hard to know what we're feeling—and then it's hard to know what to do. But it's important to be able to identify your feelings, to put some words to them. For example, can you identify what you're feeling right now?

E: No.

T: But you feel something.

E: Yeah.

T: Can I make an observation? I notice that your brow is furrowed. Do you notice that?

E: Now I do, yeah.

T: So maybe that's a clue. Take a minute to pay attention to the rest of your body. What else do you notice?

E: I guess my hands are gripping the armrests.

T: Good. What else?

E: Um . . . not much else. Oh, my jaw is a little tight.

T: OK, so furrowed brow, clenched hands, tight jaw. How about inside you? Like your heart, or your breathing?

E: I guess my breathing is a little shallow. I don't really notice anything with my heart.

T: How about in your thinking? What kind of thoughts are going through your mind?

E: I'm thinking that I don't get this whole snowball thing about my feelings.

T: OK. So let's look at what we have. Your brow is furrowed, and your hands are clenched, and your jaw is tight, and your breathing is shallow, and you're thinking about how you don't get it. Add those up for me. What feeling label might you attach to all of this?

E: Um . . . frustrated, I guess?

T: Yes, frustrated would be a good way to describe it. Angry?

E: Maybe.

T: So let's make a note of this. When you notice these things happening in your body and in your thoughts, maybe that's a signal that you're feeling frustrated or perhaps angry.

Over the next few sessions, the therapist and Elizabeth spent much of their session time identifying her emotions and clarifying the "clean" versus "dirty" aspects of what she was experiencing. Elizabeth seemed to get better at using emotional descriptions for her internal experience, although she continued to make self-judgmental comments (which the therapist pointed out to her as "dirty" discomfort).

The therapist readministered the DERS at Session 6. As shown in Figure 22.5, she was reporting some improvement in emotional awareness, although her difficulty engaging in

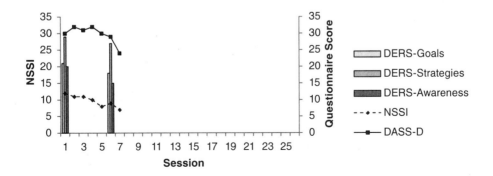

FIGURE 22.5. Elizabeth's measures at Session 7.

goal-directed behavior and limited access to emotion regulation strategies hadn't changed much. There did seem to be a noticeable improvement in her NSSI and level of depression, although clearly she had quite a way to go.

Acceptance

The therapist had been "planting seeds" of acceptance from the beginning of treatment. Starting in Session 7, the therapist increased the focus of sessions on that topic, given Elizabeth's improvement in her ability to identify how she was feeling. Here, the therapist provides psychoeducation about the topic.

T: You really seem to be doing better in terms of your ability to notice what you're feeling.

E: Yeah, but that doesn't stop me from feeling like garbage.

T: No, I wouldn't imagine that it would. Not by itself, anyway. Recognizing how you feel is the first step, and now there are more steps to take. We talked a few weeks back about how your feelings can be kind of like a snowball rolling downhill; do you remember that?

E: Yeah, and it picks up dirt and shit along the way.

T: Right. So let me suggest a way forward here. We need to scrape the shit off your snowball. That is, when you have a feeling, we need to figure out how to help you not add more suffering to it.

E: But I think the problem is just that I get so sad and angry.

T: I have a different take on it. I think that if you just felt sad and angry, you wouldn't be suffering so much. The way I look at it, it seems that the suffering is something you add to it—not on purpose, but because you're trying to feel better. And it has this unintended consequence of adding more suffering to your feelings. So you start with sadness or whatever, and then you try to do things to get less sad, and then you have sadness plus suffering.

E: But even if I scrape the shit off my snowball, I still have the snowball.

T: Yes, you do. If you stop adding suffering to your feeling, you still have the feeling. And what then?

E: Then I feel terrible.

T: I think then you feel normal.

E: But I'm not happy.

T: Uninterrupted happiness isn't normal. Can you imagine someone who always felt happy and never got sad or angry or scared? Wouldn't that strike you as weird?

E: Yeah, I get it, but I feel sad and angry and scared all the time.

T: I suspect that you feel the way you do, as much as you do, because you've invested so much energy in trying not to feel that way. It's understandable why you'd put your energy into that, but it seems like in this case, it's just not a workable strategy. You know those Chinese finger trap things? You put your two fingers inside and then get stuck?

E: Yeah. I hate those things.

T: Well, you're kind of living in one. You get stuck in something, like a feeling, and you can't get out. You pull and you pull to get out, and what happens?

E: I can't get out.

T: Right. The trap gets tighter around your fingers and holds you there. And so you're really stuck. So how do you get out of the trap?

E: You have to push your fingers in.

T: Right. And what happens then?

E: It loosens up and then you can get out.

T: Yes. And so it is with your feelings. You pull against them and you just get stuck in them. So maybe we need to try doing the opposite of that. And the opposite of struggling against your feelings is accepting them.

E: So you're saying I should just accept that I'm depressed and that I feel like shit, and then everything will be fine. That makes no sense.

T: No. Depression is a shit-covered snowball. The snowball is sadness, a regular, normal, even healthy feeling. The shit is all of the judgments and struggle and avoidance and suffering you stuck to it. What I'm suggesting is that you accept the snowball and get rid of the shit. Be sad without suffering.

E: OK, I think I get it.

T: Let's try something. Would you be willing to experiment with some feelings right here with me? Can you think of something that has the potential to make you have some sad feelings?

E: Sure. I had an argument with my case manager on the phone yesterday and she was really rude to me and then she said I was just being irrational and maybe I needed to be in the hospital again. I just felt like she doesn't care about me at all.

T: And you felt sad about that.

E: Yeah.

T: So let's experiment with that. I'm going to write that on a piece of paper. (*Does so.*) "My case manager doesn't care about me." I agree this is a saddening thought. Now, can you look at this piece of paper? What feelings come up?

E: Sad and angry.

T: OK, sad and angry. Keep looking at it. What do you feel like doing?

E: I feel like ripping it up.

T: So that would be you trying to get away from your feelings. Let's try just looking at it instead. Just look at it for a while and tell me what comes up for you.

E: I'm kind of telling myself that maybe I made too big a deal about it and that I shouldn't have gotten so upset.

T: Bah. That's you trying to talk yourself out of how you feel. She was rude to you. Your feelings are perfectly valid.

E: OK.

T: Can I hand this paper to you?

E: OK.

T: (*Hands the paper to Elizabeth.*) Now, don't try to feel better about this. Just notice how you're feeling.

E: I'm sad.

T: Yes.

E: I don't like what's written here.

T: No. But this is what's on your mind, so there it is. So how about we just look at it for a while? Perhaps over time it will just start to look like ink on a piece of paper, rather than something you need to do anything about.

The therapist ended this session by asking Elizabeth to put the piece of paper in her pocket as a tangible example of accepting an unpleasant thought and emotion. Over the next few sessions, the therapist and Elizabeth continued working on accepting emotions, using various strategies. In one session, they experimented with visualizing her thoughts and feelings as if they were clouds passing overhead; in another, they simply sat quietly for much of the session, simply noting any emotions or thoughts that arose. In each instance, the therapist redirected Elizabeth away from attempts to judge or control her inner experiences and toward "peaceful coexistence" with them. Elizabeth was consistently encouraged to redirect her energy toward building a life that was consistent with her longer-term goals and values.

A Wrinkle in the Plan

After the 10th session, the therapist received a phone call from Elizabeth indicating that she was in the hospital again. Reportedly, she had cut herself and taken an overdose of over-the-counter painkillers. The therapist needed to decide how best to handle the situation.

The therapist obtained Elizabeth's consent to coordinate with the inpatient staff in order to maximize continuity of care. The therapist explained to staff what Elizabeth had been working on in outpatient CBT and what her strengths and challenges had been.

Elizabeth asked the therapist to visit her in the hospital and provide additional treatment sessions. The therapist had a dilemma here. On one hand, this was an example of assertive communication (a healthy CRB), which the therapist wanted to reinforce. On the other hand, the therapist remembered that positive attention from others was a potential reinforcer for Elizabeth's NSSI and hospitalizations, and the therapist did not wish to add to the reinforcement for unhealthy behavior. In addition, complying with Elizabeth's request ran the risk of creating an unworkable staff dynamic on the inpatient unit, with unclear definitions of who was responsible for what aspects of her care. The therapist opted to partially honor Elizabeth's request by agreeing to speak to her by telephone for 5 minutes daily to check in.

Importantly, the therapist did not catastrophize the incident. After all, Elizabeth had a long history of NSSI and hospitalization, so it was perhaps not surprising that she would enter the hospital again at some point during treatment. The therapist did not view this as a treatment failure; rather, the NSSI and hospitalization were viewed as working material for upcoming outpatient sessions.

Elizabeth spent 72 hours in the hospital, and the therapist agreed to see her on the day of her discharge. The therapist could have opted to just see Elizabeth at her regularly scheduled time, and there would be some merit to this plan from a reinforcement perspective. However, in this case the therapist determined that a certain degree of flexibility would be more helpful. As shown in Figure 22.6, Elizabeth's depression and NSSI had spiked.

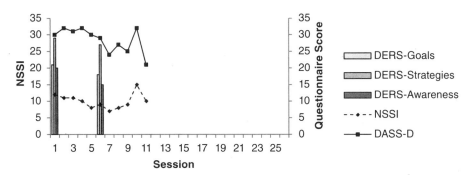

FIGURE 22.6. Elizabeth's measures at Session 11.

The initial discussion afforded a unique opportunity to discuss the therapeutic relationship.

E: I almost didn't call you.

T: I'm glad you did, but I'm curious as to what was holding you back.

E: I thought you'd be mad at me.

T: Why would I be mad at you?

E: For hurting myself and going in the hospital again. I failed and I didn't want to talk about it.

T: So you thought that it was a failure, and that if I knew it was a failure, I'd be mad at you.

E: Yeah.

T: Nothing could be further from the truth, you know. (*long pause*) There's no failure here, and even if there was a failure, I certainly wouldn't be mad about it.

E: I know you don't want me to do that stuff.

T: Well, first of all, what I want isn't really the issue here. More important is getting you to the kind of life that you want. Yeah, I think you'd be better off not hurting yourself, and we've talked about that. But I also understand that this is a pretty long-standing pattern, and it can be hard to change things. Personally I'm glad that you decided to call me and start working on this, rather than just letting it fester.

Because threats to safety of self or others are the highest treatment priority, it made sense to spend most of Elizabeth's session on that topic. The therapist's aims were to understand what happened, assess safety and establish a safety plan, and use the incident as a learning example. Here is an excerpt of the latter part of that discussion.

T: Let's examine this incident some more and see if it can help us understand more about what happens with you. We've been spending some time talking about thoughts, feelings, and actions. Can you tell me what happened, and what your thoughts, feelings, and actions were?

E: I don't know; I was just so mad I wanted to scream or kill someone or kill myself.

T: So you've identified a feeling there, being mad. How did you know you were mad?

E: I was just all tight and tense and clenching my jaw and pacing.

T: Yeah, that sounds pretty mad, all right. Let's back up just a bit. What was going on that had you so mad?

E: Oh, it was just something stupid.

T: Such as?

E: I just had a stupid fight with my boyfriend and he told me he wished he never started dating me because I was crazy and he wished he could just start over with someone else.

T: What made you think that was stupid? That doesn't sound stupid at all. He said something very nasty to you. Why wouldn't you be angry about that?

E: I just got too emotional.

T: What does "too emotional" mean? It sounds like you're judging yourself for what you felt.

E: I guess I am.

T: That judging is some dirty discomfort, but it seems like you had every reason to feel angry. That was pretty natural. Did you notice any feelings before the anger?

E: I guess I felt hurt by what he said.

T: You felt hurt. Understandable. And then that turned into anger? What was that process like?

E: I thought that it was over, and he thinks I'm a nut case, so screw it.

T: Screw it, meaning what?

E: Meaning what's the point? I might as well just be crazy.

T: Like "If he thinks that way, I'll show him how crazy I can be"?

E: Yeah.

T: It seems like you fell into a pattern of yours, a pretty well-worn groove. It started off with a conflict with someone whose opinion matters to you. That set you off, like it often does.

E: Yeah.

T: And then you have some feelings about that, like you felt hurt, and then you felt angry. And it sounds like you also judged yourself for feeling angry, as you often do. So now you were not only angry, but you were angry about being angry. And the feelings just keep ratcheting up and up. And you fell into that same trap of thinking that things were just hopeless, and you might as well act the way he seems to expect you to. So you do the one thing you know will reliably get you some short-term relief from the situation.

E: Yeah, this is what happens over and over again.

T: Right, it's a pattern that once you start, it's hard to stop. We're working on that. So let's think about what you can do next time that might interrupt that pattern before it gets to a crisis point.

By the following session, Elizabeth's depression and NSSI had resumed a downward course. Across the therapy, the therapist paid attention to Elizabeth's reported NSSI behaviors, yet was careful not to let those reports dominate and derail the conversation (which would not only have stalled the CBT but might also have provided reinforcement for the behavior). The therapist treated these behaviors as just one part of the overall problem, responding calmly and directly when they came up. Here's an example:

> T: I see from your diary that you cut yourself twice this week.
>
> E: Yeah, I was just so mad and upset that I couldn't help it.
>
> T: It feels out of control to you. But you're working on it. Anything happening that requires immediate medical attention?
>
> E: No, it wasn't deep and it's not infected.
>
> T: OK. Let's set an agenda for what we're going to talk about this week.

Cognitive Restructuring

As you can see in the description so far, the therapist had been introducing the idea of interpretations from the beginning of treatment. At times, the therapist had challenged Elizabeth's distorted thoughts, although the challenge had been fairly gentle given the precarious therapeutic relationship and the more important aim of validating Elizabeth's internal experience.

Beginning in Session 11, the therapist addressed interpretations more directly, using many of the strategies described in Chapter 14, including examining the evidence, considering alternatives, and scaling. They did not use formal cognitive restructuring sheets (e.g., those shown in Appendix B), although the therapist did discuss the concept of cognitive distortions and helped Elizabeth identify distortions and more adaptive thoughts in session.

From the discussion of interpretations, the therapist moved fairly rapidly to addressing Elizabeth's core beliefs. The therapist thought that a move in this direction would prove fruitful, given the long-standing (some would say "characterological") nature of Elizabeth's problem and the apparent inflexibility of her behaviors over time and across situations. The therapist hypothesized that Elizabeth's interpretations were being driven by deeply held yet unexamined beliefs about herself, about others, and about the world. Here, the therapist combines two strategies, pattern detection and downward arrow, to elicit one of Elizabeth's core beliefs.

> T: You mentioned that part of what really got you feeling upset during the argument with your boyfriend was that his opinion mattered to you, and that as far as you could see, his opinion wasn't a good one.
>
> E: Yeah, it just feels like he blames me for everything.
>
> T: Is that a feeling, or a thought?
>
> E: It's a thought.
>
> T: Yes. And you also think that much of the time he doesn't understand you.
>
> E: He doesn't.
>
> T: Perhaps not. I'm wondering what bothers you about that.
>
> E: Well, he's my boyfriend. Or at least he claims to be. So he should get me.

T: And so here's someone who's supposed to understand you, and instead he doesn't understand you. He blames you. And you've also had the thought that he just flat out doesn't care.

E: I don't think he does care. Whatever. It doesn't matter.

T: You say it doesn't matter, but I wonder about that. I think this really bugs you. And why wouldn't it?

E: Yeah, I mean, that's not how a relationship's supposed to be, right?

T: I don't think I'd be happy in that kind of a situation.

E: Well, I'm not happy.

T: No. What I'd like to understand is what this all means for you. It's supposed to be one way, and instead it's another way. And so what do you make of that?

E: What I make of that is that it sucks.

T: It sucks because . . .

E: It sucks because he's supposed to be there for me.

T: He should support you.

E: Yeah.

T: He should have a connection with you.

E: Yeah, and he doesn't.

T: Do you take that to mean something about relationships? About other people?

E: Well, yeah, it's just like you don't know who you're dealing with. People are supposed to be there for you.

T: And they're not.

E: Right.

T: So it seems like we have an important part of your thought process here. There's this basic idea that you can't count on people for support, for love, for connection. They'll let you down.

E: Yeah, so I'm on my own.

T: Would I be mistaken if I guessed that this issue has come up for you before? Not just with this boyfriend?

E: No, you wouldn't be mistaken.

T: Where do you suppose it started? Where did you first learn that you couldn't count on anyone?

E: My parents. They split up when I was really young. And my mom, I don't know, she just kind of lost it and wasn't there for me. And my dad just split and I hardly ever saw him again.

The therapist and Elizabeth have identified what Young et al. (2003) term an *abandonment/instability* core belief. The therapist opted to flesh out some of the learning history behind this belief; subsequent discussion revealed a good deal of childhood neglect that taught Elizabeth that she could not rely on others for support or connection.

Note that in this case the learning experience was in childhood and had a traumatic aspect to it. We should remember, however, that the development of maladaptive core beliefs requires neither childhood learning nor traumatic experience. Sometimes it's there, sometimes it's not. Endless searching for childhood trauma, at the expense of present-oriented interventions, is not productive.

Later, the therapist used a similar discussion to reveal a *defectiveness/shame* core belief (Young et al., 2003) in which Elizabeth believed herself to be worthless and unimportant (see Figure 22.7). The therapist also noted that Elizabeth had an *attentional bias* toward signs that others were arguing with her or otherwise failing to support her, while simultaneously ignoring signs of support. This, too, was added to the model.

As the maladaptive core beliefs were identified, the therapist helped Elizabeth to understand why they were unhelpful to her by discussing the pros and cons of the belief.

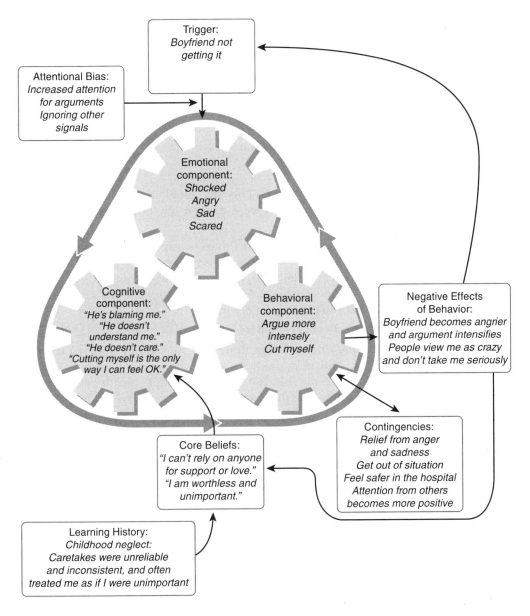

FIGURE 22.7. Expanded model for Elizabeth.

T: This basic idea you have that you can't count on people for support or love. Do you get a sense that you're always carrying this belief around, to some extent?

E: Yeah, I guess it's always there, like in the background.

T: So that's very important. When we have a deep-down belief about how things are, that belief tends to impact how we perceive things, how we react to them. Does that make sense?

E: I'm not sure.

T: Think about it this way. Imagine that the beliefs that you have about yourself, about other people, about the world are like colored lenses in your glasses. So if you have blue-tinted glasses on, how does the world look to you?

E: It looks blue.

T: Right. Is it blue?

E: Well no, it's not really blue.

T: It just looks that way because of the glasses.

E: Right.

T: And if you took those glasses off?

E: Things wouldn't look blue.

T: You'd see the world as it actually was.

E: Yeah, but it's not like I made this all up. This isn't just all in my head. I haven't been able to count on people. My parents were terrible; my boyfriends left; even my therapists have fired me.

T: I understand that. Those are really hard things to experience, and it's not at all surprising that you would come away from those experiences with the belief that you can't count on people. But let's talk for a minute about the pros and cons of continuing to carry that belief around. Let's start with pros. What's good or helpful about believing that you can't count on anyone?

E: Well, it's true. That's what's good about it.

T: Right, so from where you sit, this is how things are, and so why wouldn't you hang on to that belief? If we look at it another way, maybe we could identify what the advantage is to you of believing this. If it's true that people can't be relied on, and you believe that you can't rely on them, then what?

E: Well, then I'm expecting it.

T: So you don't get caught off guard.

E: Right. Like I don't put my faith in someone and then get disappointed.

T: So let's list that as an advantage. (*Draws a line down the center of a piece of paper.*) Over here, on the pro side, let's write that this belief protects you from unexpected disappointment. What else is a pro?

E: Um . . . I guess it forces me to rely on myself?

T: Do you really see that as a pro? That is, has this really turned out to be a good development in your life?

E: I guess not.

T: Seems like we'd at least need to put a big question mark by it. How about cons? What's the downside of believing that you can't rely on anyone for love and support?

E: I don't see a downside. It's how it is.

T: Let's step outside of the belief for a minute and think more about it. Would you say that this belief has overall made you a happier person?

E: No.

T: What has it done?

E: Well, I guess it's depressing.

T: Yeah, so it doesn't feel good to believe this. Right or wrong, it's unpleasant to you. I'll write that down on the con side. If we go back to the idea about your beliefs being a filter on how you view the world—blue glasses make the world look blue—how has your belief colored your view of things? Let's start with relationships with boyfriends, since that's been a really important topic. How has this basic belief affected how you think about your relationships?

E: I guess I kind of go into relationships thinking that when it gets right down to it, this person isn't going to be there for me.

T: Ah. And what's the effect of that?

E: I don't know . . . maybe I'm kind of more edgy in relationships?

T: Seems like that could easily happen. So perhaps this edginess is also a con of the belief. What about when things do start to go wrong in a relationship, like you have a disagreement or something? How does your belief affect you then?

E: I guess I'm like "Here we go again, this is all going to shit because he's not really supporting me."

T: So you assume this is going to turn out the way it's turned out in the past.

E: Yeah, and then I get super depressed.

T: Yes. And it seems like part of what depresses you is not this particular disagreement with this particular boyfriend; it's the fact that you see the episode as part of a never-ending pattern and that it just seems to confirm what you already think about other people.

In considering how (and whether) to challenge Elizabeth's core beliefs, the therapist had to balance several factors. It was clear that Elizabeth believed that others would not adequately support her. One concern, therefore, was that Elizabeth might perceive a direct challenge to her beliefs as evidence that the therapist did not support her. Particularly with clients who have borderline personality characteristics, there is a need to walk a fine line between validating and challenging (Linehan, 1993). At the same time, however, it was clear to the therapist that Elizabeth's core beliefs were having an ongoing negative effect on her mood and interpersonal functioning and needed to be addressed. The therapist opted to try the strategy of *talking to the core belief* (Young et al., 2003). This would allow Elizabeth to explore both sides of the issue in a way that minimized the risk of interpersonal conflict with the therapist.

T: I'd like to try looking at this belief that you can't rely on anyone from a different perspective. I'd like to have you really get behind this belief 100% and say why this belief is totally right. And then I'll ask you to switch perspectives and talk about it from another angle. Would that be OK with you?

E: Sure.

T: OK, so for now, totally believe this 100% and talk about your position on whether or not you can rely on people for love, support, connection, and so on.

E: I can't rely on people. They just let me down.

T: Say more about that. Who can't you rely on?

E: I can't rely on anyone.

T: Good. Tell me more about why you can't.

E: Everyone's just looking out for themselves. And when I really need someone to be there for me, they're going to put their own needs before mine. There's no one that I can just trust and be myself with and know that they're going to support me, no matter what.

T: OK. Now let's try something new. I'd like you to switch chairs with me. (*They do so.*) Now I want you to be the other way of looking at things. Maybe a healthier way, one that doesn't depress you, make you edgy in relationships, and so on. You don't have to believe what you say; let's just see if you can come up with a response. Can you reply to what you just said?

E: Not really; I think she's right. So I guess I would say "Yeah, you're totally right."

T: Yes, you believe that. I understand. Right now, though, try to think of whether there's any other way of looking at it that you can articulate, even if you don't believe it.

E: (*long pause*) This is stupid.

T: Seems like maybe I'm asking you to do something that doesn't make any sense?

E: Yeah.

T: OK, I hear that. I don't want to have you do things that are stupid. Would it help if I explained my thinking more about this?

E: Yeah, it would.

T: OK. What I'm thinking is that you have this particular belief, and it seems that the belief might be doing more harm than good. Now, it might be true or it might not be true, or it might be somewhere in the middle. But it seems like you hang onto this belief so strongly that you end up being more depressed and more reactive than you actually need to be. So I'm interested in having you try thinking about things from a different angle, like voicing two different perspectives. At the end of it, you might conclude that you were right in the first place, or you might not. But either way, you will have considered your beliefs a bit more objectively and decided what you will choose to believe, rather than just letting your beliefs control you without really being aware of them. Does that make sense?

E: Yeah, I get that.

T: I'm glad you gave me the opportunity to explain it a bit more. How would you feel about proceeding?

E: We can do it.

T: OK. So try being that alternative perspective now. You just heard one side saying that you can't rely on anyone, no one's there for you, and people are just looking out for themselves. How could you respond to that?

E: I guess not everyone's like that.

T: Can you say more? Explain that a bit?

E: Well, I like to believe there are some decent people in the world.

T: (*playfully*) That's a little weak, don't you think?

E: (*Smiles.*) Yeah.

T: Can you come up with some examples?

E: I guess I've had therapists that didn't abandon me or drop me. I dropped them.

T: OK, and so you take what from that?

E: I guess not everyone in the world is like that. There are some people who will be there for me.

T: Now let's switch back and have you be the belief side again. Can you respond to that?

E: (*as the belief side*) Well, just because a therapist doesn't drop you, that doesn't mean that they really care about you or support you. They could just want to get paid. You can't look at someone who's being paid to talk to you and say that means that people are nice and caring and so on.

T: Now switch back and be the healthy Elizabeth side again.

E: (*as the healthy side*) OK, maybe I don't really know whether my therapists truly cared about me. But I've had friends who supported me, at least for a while.

T: Now be the belief side again.

E: (*as the belief side*) Yeah, for a while, but they didn't stick around forever. Your whole life has been people coming and going, looking like they're on your side for a while, and then eventually just giving up on you and leaving. That's not support. That's not love.

T: Now be the healthy side again.

E: (*as the healthy side*) Maybe I had something to do with that, though.

T: Can you say more about that?

E: I mean, I can sometimes push people away. And so maybe it's not all about people not loving and supporting me.

The bulk of the next several sessions was spent discussing Elizabeth's maladaptive core beliefs. From time to time, the therapist would use the "empty chair" strategy as shown above; however, as Elizabeth became more comfortable and less defensive over the discussion of core beliefs, the therapist introduced more direct strategies such as examining the evidence, considering alternatives, and scaling (see Chapter 16).

Elizabeth's NSSI and depression continued to decrease, as evidenced by her weekly diary and questionnaire scores (see Figure 22.8). It was also noted on the DERS that

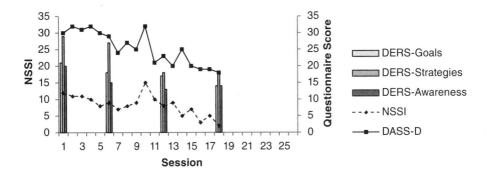

FIGURE 22.8. Elizabeth's measures at Session 18.

Elizabeth was reporting somewhat better ability to engage in goal-directed behavior despite the presence of negative emotions.

A Wrinkle in the Relationship

Beginning around the midway point in treatment, the therapist was beginning to feel annoyed by Elizabeth. Elizabeth was often late for sessions, often would come without having completed all of her homework assignments, and often seemed defensive in sessions. Elizabeth's statement that "this is stupid" during the core belief exercise described above seemed to be part of an overall pattern in which Elizabeth generally seemed dismissive of therapy in general and of the therapist in particular. The therapist was no longer looking forward to Elizabeth's sessions but rather felt a sense of dread and draining of energy as each session approached. Clearly, an *alliance rupture* had occurred (see Chapter 7).

The therapist took these feelings as a prompt to obtain consultation from a trusted colleague. Given the high likelihood of therapist burnout, ongoing consultation is a formal aspect of some forms of CBT for borderline personality, such as DBT (Linehan, 1993). The therapist and colleague openly discussed the therapist's feelings about Elizabeth and worked to identify ways to improve the situation.

The therapist did some self-directed CBT (see Chapter 7) to try to understand the issue more clearly. Specifically, the therapist identified the following:

- The therapist frequently interpreted Elizabeth's behavior as a sign that Elizabeth was deliberately trying to make life difficult for the therapist, or that the therapist was somehow failing. The therapist recognized these thoughts as reflecting the cognitive distortion of *personalizing* and remembered that Elizabeth had a long and powerful learning history that had shaped her behaviors.

- The therapist also noted that as these negative thoughts and feelings became more prominent, the therapist tended to act more aloof toward Elizabeth, taking less time to explore her feelings and making more curt behavioral recommendations. These behaviors, in turn, likely exacerbated Elizabeth's perceptions of not being cared for, resulting in more maladaptive behavior on her part and creating a vicious cycle.

- The therapist realized that the behavioral reaction to Elizabeth might have reflected a skill deficit—the therapist's own discomfort with addressing aversive interpersonal situations directly and assertively. By being aloof and curt, the therapist was using an avoidance strategy that was clearly not working.

The therapist therefore resolved to make two changes. First, the therapist increased the use of overt signals of empathy, genuineness, and unconditional positive regard as a way to reassure Elizabeth that she was being heard and that the therapist had a basic concern and liking for her. Second, the therapist placed a greater emphasis on identifying CRBs in the session, confronting unhealthy CRBs in a respectfully assertive manner, and reinforcing healthy CRBs. Here's an example:

E: This is stupid.

T: I've noticed that you seem to say that a lot.

E: Well, it is.

T: That, to me, feels like you're pushing me away and being dismissive.

E: I'm not trying to be dismissive.

T: Perhaps not. But I'm wondering whether you can see how I would perceive your actions, and how that might make me feel?

E: I guess so.

T: Perhaps more importantly for you, I wonder whether this is a pattern for you? That is, is it possible that you give off that dismissing, pushing away message to other people as well?

E: Maybe.

T: So perhaps that's something you and I should watch for. I'd like to be able to point it out to you when I see it; would that be OK?

E: Yeah, that's OK.

The therapist also took the initiative in eliciting Elizabeth's thoughts and feelings about the therapeutic relationship and used this information as a way of bringing the problem into the room and working on Elizabeth's maladaptive beliefs.

T: How do you think we're doing, working together as a team?

E: What do you mean?

T: Well, whenever two people are working together on something, it can sometimes go really well, and it can sometimes go not so well. I'd be interested to know how you think we're doing.

E: OK, I guess.

T: You sound a little unsure. Can I point something out to you? It seems like sometimes you say things like "this is stupid," or you look away with a frown, when we're talking. Have you noticed that?

E: I guess so, yeah.

T: What do you suppose that's about?

E: I dunno. Sometimes I just get mad. I know I shouldn't.

T: Who says you shouldn't get mad? People get mad all the time.

E: But you're my therapist.

T: So that means no one's allowed to get mad at me?

E: I guess not.

T: Remember that your feelings are perfectly fine. If you're mad, you're mad. I'd be interested to understand what gets you mad, though, when we're talking. Do you have a sense of that?

E: I guess sometimes it seems like you're not really listening to me.

T: Hmm. So I seem not to be listening. I can see why that would make someone mad. How do I give you that impression?

E: I don't know, it's almost more of like a feeling that I get, like you're listening but not really listening, you know? Like you don't really get me.

T: Like I'm not really connecting with you.

E: Exactly, yeah.

T: And I should be connecting with you.

E: Yes.

T: It seems like maybe what's happening is that when you're talking to me, sometimes this just feels like one more example of how someone you're supposed to be able to rely on is letting you down.

E: Yeah.

T: So that just makes that core belief get even stronger. Well, let me tell you that I want to listen to you very carefully, and I want you to be able to feel a good connection, and I want you to feel supported. So I apologize if I haven't conveyed that very well, and I'd like to see if we can fix this.

Problem-Solving Training and Assertion Training

As the discussion about core beliefs was unfolding, the therapist also began introducing training for behavioral skill deficits (see Chapter 12). Specifically, from the ongoing discussion it became evident that Elizabeth had difficulties with problem solving and assertive communication (see Figure 22.9). These skill deficits were thought to contribute to Elizabeth's rather inflexible choice of argumentative, aggressive, and self-injurious behaviors because she lacked the skill to select other, healthier, responses to external stressors.

Assertion training began within the context of the discussion of unhealthy CRBs. As the therapist pointed out maladaptive interpersonal communication (i.e., communication that was passive or aggressive, rather than assertive), they took the opportunity to bring the problem into the room and work on it then and there. Here's an example:

T: How was the homework from last week?

E: I didn't do it.

T: Hmm. What was the reason you didn't do it?

E: It was stupid.

T: I see. Stupid, meaning you didn't think it was a good idea?

E: Yeah.

T: And when we discussed the homework assignment at our last session, did you know then that you didn't think it was a good idea?

E: Yeah, I didn't like it.

T: It's interesting that you didn't mention that. I suggested something to you that didn't sound right to you, and you didn't speak up about it. You just said "OK" and then didn't do it. So would you call that passive, assertive, or aggressive?

E: I guess maybe passive. Or passive -aggressive.

T: Yeah, sounds that way. So what could you have done that would have been assertive?

E: Um . . . I guess tell you that I didn't like the assignment?

T: Yes, you could have told me that you didn't like the idea. What would have been a good way to tell me that? For example, if you thought the idea was stupid, what

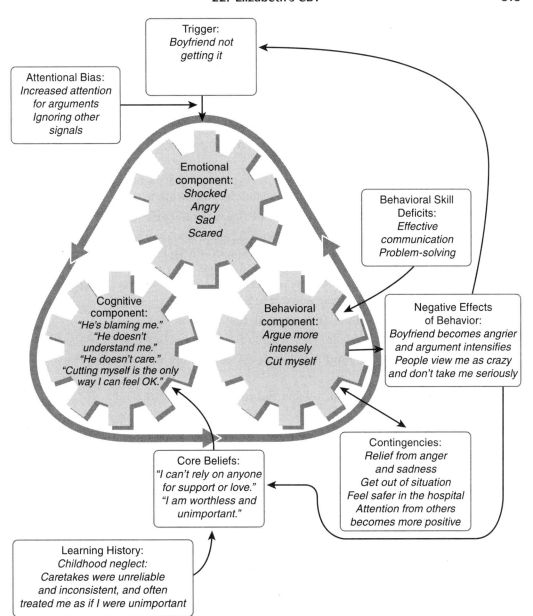

FIGURE 22.9. Expanded model for Elizabeth.

about telling me "This is stupid and you're out of your mind if you think I'm going to do it"?

E: Well no, that wouldn't be nice.

T: No, it wouldn't. That would be aggressive, wouldn't it?

E: Yeah.

T: So what would have been an assertive response?

E: I guess something like "I don't think this is a good idea, and here's why I think that"?

T: Yes, that would have been assertive. Let's practice that right now. I'll be you, and you be me. And you give me just a ridiculous homework assignment.

E: OK. Um. . . . This week I want you to wear your underwear on your head all week.

T: Well, I don't think that's a very good idea for me. I don't see how wearing my underwear on my head will help me. Can you explain why you would want me to do that? So that's how I might say it. Notice that my tone was pretty neutral here; I didn't call you stupid, I just told you my concern about it. Now you try. Elizabeth, I'd like you to wear your underwear on your head this week.

E: (*Laughs nervously.*) Um. . . . I don't think that's a good idea.

T: . . . and tell me why.

E: I don't think that's a good idea because I don't think wearing underwear on my head will help me. At all.

T: Hold up there just a sec. Good, but did you need the "at all?"

E: Maybe not.

T: That was putting kind of an aggressive exclamation point on it. My reaction, as the listener, was that it felt like you were trying to tell me I was an idiot for even suggesting it. Can you see how someone could have that reaction?

E: I guess so.

T: Try saying it again but without the zinger this time.

As Elizabeth's assertive communication skill grew, the therapist (with Elizabeth's explicit approval) encouraged her to practice in everyday life, starting with "safer" people such as store clerks and moving on to more challenging people such as her case worker, her physician, and her boyfriend.

Problem-solving training was initiated as an emotion regulation strategy. Elizabeth's maladaptive behaviors largely reflected efforts to feel better. The therapist redirected her toward actually dealing with the things that were troubling her through teaching and practice of appropriate problem solving (see Chapter 12). During one session, Elizabeth had run out of her medications and was feeling increasingly upset. The therapist used this incident as a way of introducing the topic.

T: Running out of your meds is definitely a problem. What do you think you could do about it?

E: (*tearful*) I don't know. No one ever listens.

T: So there's a problem here that needs to be addressed. But it's hard to know what to do, especially when you're feeling really upset, like you are now. Whenever we're feeling really strong emotions, it can be hard to come up with good solutions to problems. Let me give you something to try. I want you to remember the letters SSTA. They stand for "stop, slow down, think, act." At the end of our meeting today, I'll give you a handout that has this written on it to help you remember. When we say "stop," that means we use our feelings as a signal that there's a problem, and we need to pause for a moment and get ready to solve it. So, for example, how are you feeling right now?

E: Overwhelmed.

T: Yes. What does that feel like in your body?

E: I guess my heart's racing, and my breathing is kind of shallow, and I'm tight all over, and I just feel like crying.

T: Brain going a mile a minute?

E: Yeah.

T: OK. So pay attention to those feelings. This is your signal to stop. In fact, you could even try saying "stop" to yourself. Now, we want to slow down. When your brain's racing like that, and your heart's racing, and you're breathing like that, it's going to be really hard to get into a good problem-solving mode. So how can you slow yourself down?

E: I don't know.

T: Perhaps one thing you could do would be to take a little time-out for yourself. Maybe work on some slow breathing, from the diaphragm, like I showed you a while back.

E: I can do that some of the time, but a lot of the time when I'm trying to deal with a problem I'm in the middle of having a discussion with someone, so it's not like I can just walk out.

T: Hmm, I see what you mean. So maybe we could try doing something a bit more subtle. What if you tried just yawning?

E: Yawning?

T: Yeah, you know, like this. (*Yawns and stretches.*) Even if you don't really have to yawn, just faking it. It would buy you a few seconds.

E: I could try that.

T: Let's try it now. Can you yawn along with me? (*They do so.*)

E: I actually started really yawning in the middle of it.

T: Yeah, that happens. Your body gets tricked into yawning when you go through the motions. And that also helps slow things down for you. Feeling like we can try tackling the problem?

E: I can try.

T: OK, so let's go to the "think" stage. I like to use a worksheet at first, like this one (*pulling out Problem-Solving Worksheet from Appendix B*), until it becomes second nature. I'll give you some blank copies of this at the end of our meeting today.

The therapist and Elizabeth then went through the stages of problem definition/formulation, generation of alternatives, decision making, and solution implementation/verification described in Chapter 12. Formal problem solving became part of Elizabeth's homework, with an assignment to work on solving one minor to moderate problem each day using the worksheet. Over subsequent sessions, the therapist continued problem-solving work with Elizabeth, and she gradually addressed more complex problems.

Elizabeth's NSSI and depression continued to decrease, as shown in Figure 22.10. In addition, her DERS at Session 22 suggested that she was making further progress in her ability to use emotion regulation strategies.

Termination

Termination should be managed carefully for all clients; however, in Elizabeth's case this seemed particularly important. Elizabeth had identified a core belief that she could not rely on others for support, love, and connection. Although she had been working on this belief and was able to spot it and challenge it, the therapist knew that a deeply held belief is never erased. Rather, Elizabeth had learned a new way of thinking that could usually override her core beliefs. But under certain circumstances, it was quite likely that this belief would be reactivated.

The therapist knew that Elizabeth was nearing a logical termination point—her NSSI behaviors (which were the original treatment target) were well controlled, her depression (which was a secondary target) had shown *clinically significant change* and was now closer to the normal than the pathological range, she was displaying fewer unhealthy CRBs and more healthy CRBs in session, and she was reliably using appropriate emotion regulation strategies. At the same time, however, the therapist did not want to reactivate Elizabeth's maladaptive core beliefs and make her feel abandoned.

The best approach was to begin the discussion about termination well in advance, to discuss the issue frankly, and to engage Elizabeth in development of the termination plan. Here is an excerpt of a conversation from Session 22.

> T: Your scores look really good today. I see here that you're still not doing things to hurt yourself, which is really good to see, and your depression seems way down. Does that seem accurate?
>
> E: Yeah. I really do think that I'm doing a lot better.
>
> T: That's good to hear. One thing I find very encouraging is that you seem to be doing

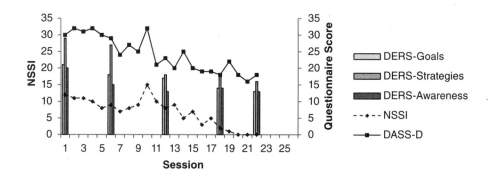

FIGURE 22.10. Elizabeth's measures at Session 22.

a lot better in terms of your ability to use the emotion regulation strategies we've been talking about. I think that's going to continue to be very helpful to you.

E: I think so, too.

T: This seems like a good time for us to review where we are in terms of the goals we had set for ourselves at the start of our treatment. I remember that we wanted to keep you alive and not hurting yourself, and you wanted to feel less depressed, and you wanted to feel like you were living a life that was reasonably satisfying to you. Where do you think we stand on those issues?

E: I think we're doing good. I don't feel very depressed, although I have my ups and downs. And I feel safe these days; I don't feel like I need to go to the hospital. And I'm getting along better with people. I'm not getting into arguments and fights nearly as much.

T: That's really great to hear. I'm happy that you're doing well. You've put in a lot of work and you've earned it. Let me bring you back to a conversation we had right at the start. It wasn't entirely clear at that time how long the treatment was going to be, and I had suggested that we let your progress be our guide and that when it felt like we had accomplished what we set out to accomplish, that would be a good time for us to talk about stopping the treatment. Have we reached that point?

E: I don't know. I mean, I really like talking to you.

T: I like talking to you, too. What would stopping the treatment mean to you?

E: Um . . . (becoming tearful) I guess I would feel like I was on my own again.

T: With no one to support you.

E: Yeah. I don't think I can do that.

T: It's easy to understand why you might have that kind of thought. You have a long history of people bailing on you. And that's what this would feel like? That I'm bailing on you?

E: Yeah. I know you're not, but it feels that way.

T: So you know that this isn't the same thing as what you've experienced before.

E: But even if I'm doing well now, what happens a week from now, or a month from now, if I'm not doing well? What am I going to do?

T: Well, that's a very good question. What would you do? Let's think of it as a problem to be solved. So what are the alternatives?

E: Um . . . I guess I could just go crazy and go to the hospital.

T: Yes, that's one solution. What else?

E: I could try doing the stuff we talked about.

T: You mean like problem solving and acceptance, and that kind of thing.

E: Yeah.

T: Yes, you could. What else?

E: Um . . . could I call you?

T: Yes, you certainly could. Stopping this treatment doesn't mean good-bye forever.

E: That's good to know that I could call you later.

T: What if we tried something out? What if we agreed to meet for, say, four more sessions, but we spaced them out a bit more? For example, instead of coming to see me next week, you could instead see me in 2 weeks. And we'll see how things went. And if things went well, we could have the following visit in 3 weeks, and so on. That way you can test the waters and see how you do with seeing less of me.

E: We could try that.

Over the next four sessions, which were gradually spaced out, Elizabeth did show some increase in depression (see Figure 22.11). This was predictable, as Elizabeth was apprehensive about ending therapy and was having more time between sessions. However, the increase was not particularly severe. Importantly, she did not show an increase in NSSI or problems with emotion regulation. By Session 26, Elizabeth and the therapist agreed that termination was appropriate, although Elizabeth was welcome to recontact the therapist as needed in the future.

Roads Not Taken

I conclude the discussion of Elizabeth's treatment by highlighting some of the critical decisions about what the therapist decided not to do.

Greater Structure and More Rigid Boundaries

Working with clients who have borderline personality characteristics usually involves making constant decisions between structure and flexibility. The therapist could have used more rigid structure, such as not contacting Elizabeth when she was in the hospital, not making an extra appointment for her, adhering to a fixed number of sessions, and not inviting additional contact after termination. The therapist could have also opted to use less self-disclosure in treatment. Such measures, however, would likely have been counterproductive, making it much more difficult to establish a solid therapeutic alliance (which was already a challenge). The therapist, therefore, opted to be flexible when it seemed reasonable to do so. Had Elizabeth been more intrusive (e.g., constantly asking for emergency sessions, calling the therapist at home), the therapist might well have opted to firm up the boundaries and reestablish the mutual expectations for treatment. The therapist did draw a line at certain TIBs, such as failing to do homework, missing sessions, or acting in a hostile manner during sessions. The therapist made it clear that certain things were

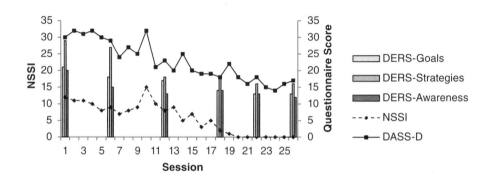

FIGURE 22.11. Elizabeth's measures at Session 26.

expected of Elizabeth during treatment and at the same time used these TIBs as a starting point for therapeutic work.

Requiring a No-Suicide Contract

Many clinicians treating clients with suicidal ideation and behavior opt to use a no-suicide contract, a formal agreement in which the client agrees not to harm him- or herself. Although such contracts may be intuitively appealing, there is no empirical evidence suggesting that they actually reduce the risk of suicide (Rudd et al., 2006). Rather, the therapist opted to obtain a treatment agreement from the client, which includes an implicit requirement that Elizabeth remain alive.

Using a Formal Skills Group in Addition to Individual Therapy

Many clinicians treating borderline personality recommend participation in an ongoing skill-training group in addition to individual CBT (Linehan & Dexter-Mazza, 2008). Separating the skill training from the other elements of CBT has some merit, particularly given the importance of skill training in variations of CBT such as DBT: Use of trained skills strongly predicts improvements in depression, suicidality, and other symptoms (Neacsiu, Rizvi, & Linehan, 2010; Stepp, Epler, Jahng, & Trull, 2008), and some evidence suggests that skill training alone can be an effective intervention for borderline personality disorder (Harley, Baity, Blais, & Jacobo, 2007; Soler et al., 2009; Valentine, Bankoff, Poulin, Reidler, & Pantalone, 2015). However, such skill-training groups are not available in many parts of the country, and Elizabeth did not have ready access to one. (This is one of many instances in which the scientific ideal bumps into the practical reality.) The therapist therefore opted to include skill training as a major component of the individual CBT.

Exposure

Elizabeth did not appear to be suffering from symptoms of posttraumatic stress disorder or another fear-based problem; therefore, exposure was not used in this treatment. It's worth noting, however, that many people with borderline personality do have PTSD symptoms, often stemming from abuse that occurred in childhood. In such cases, exposure therapy can be helpful. Many clinicians would recommend some degree of emotion regulation training—for example, relaxation or breathing training—prior to exposure, given the difficulty clients with borderline personality have in tolerating strong emotions. But it's important to note that we don't skip the exposure when the client needs it.

Hospitalizing Elizabeth

It was not uncommon during treatment for Elizabeth to express thoughts of NSSI and suicide. To be certain, safety must always be the highest priority for any clinician, and roughly 10% of clients with borderline personality do eventually kill themselves (Paris, 2003). In some cases, hospitalization cannot be avoided. However, many experts caution against the reflexive use of hospitalization for clients with borderline personality who have recurrent NSSI and suicidal ideation (e.g., Gunderson, 2011; Linehan, 1993; Paris, 2004). There is no clear evidence that recurrent hospitalization actually prevents suicide in such clients (Paris, 2004), and the safety precautions taken on an inpatient unit risk reinforcing the very behaviors the clinician is trying to decrease (Linehan, 1993). That is, suicidal and self-injurious behaviors are usually reinforced with more attention and clinical care, resulting in a regressive process. The end result may be the "psychiatrization" (a great term from Paris, 2004, p. 243) of the client, in which the client is rewarded for increasing levels of suicidal behavior and uses the hospital to substitute for practicing adaptive coping skills. The therapist in this case opted to continue treating Elizabeth as an outpatient, providing an extra session in the week when needed, while continuing to monitor suicidal risk.

Treating Elizabeth Forever

By definition, personality disorders are chronic. Many clients do not respond well to treatment, and even after successful treatment, most clients with borderline personality disorder continue to experience some degree of clinically significant problems (Kroger, Harbeck, Armbrust, & Kliem, 2013; McMain, Guimond, Streiner, Cardish, & Links, 2012). In Elizabeth's case, after 6 months of treatment she was certainly not depression-free, nor was she a master of emotion regulation. It would be both impractical and counterproductive, however, to provide a never-ending treatment to Elizabeth. There is a point of diminishing returns in any treatment, and it can often be difficult to determine when one has reached that point. In Elizabeth's case, her treatment goals had been met, and she was no longer engaging in NSSI. The decision to terminate treatment was made collaboratively with Elizabeth (and, indeed, the therapist had to correct some maladaptive beliefs about ending therapy), with the understanding that Elizabeth could return to CBT if and when it was needed.

Further Reading

Behavioral Therapies

Barkley, R. A. (1997). *Defiant children: A clinician's manual for assessment and parent training* (2nd ed.). New York: Guilford Press.

Bellack, A. S., & Hersen, M. (1979). *Research and practice in social skill training.* New York: Springer.

Goldstein, A. P., McGinnis, E., Sprafkin, R. P., Gershaw, N. J., & Klein, P. (1997). *Skillstreaming the adolescent: New strategies and perspectives for teaching prosocial skills* (rev. ed.). Champaign, IL: Research Press.

Kazdin, A. E. (1989). *Behavior modification in applied settings* (5th ed.). Pacific Grove, CA: Brooks/Cole.

Kohlenberg, R. J., & Tsai, M. (1991). *Functional analytic psychotherapy: Creating intense and curative therapeutic relationships.* New York: Plenum Press.

Nezu, A. M., Nezu, C. M., & D'Zurilla, T. (2013). *Problem-solving therapy: A treatment manual.* New York: Springer.

CBT Textbooks

Antony, M. M., & Roemer, L. (2011). *Behavior therapy.* Washington, DC: American Psychological Association.

Clark, D. M., & Fairburn, C. G. (1997). *The science and practice of cognitive behaviour therapy.* New York: Oxford University Press.

Hofmann, S. G. (2012). *An introduction to modern CBT: Psychological solutions to mental health problems.* Chichester, UK: Wiley-Blackwell.

Leahy, R. L. (1996). *Cognitive therapy: Basic principles and applications.* Northvale, NJ: Jason Aronson.

Ledley, D. R., Marx, B. P., & Heimberg, R. G. (2010). *Making cognitive-behavioral therapy work: Clinical process for new practitioners* (2nd ed). New York: Guilford Press.

Otto, M. W., Simon, N. M., Olatunji, B. O., Sung, S. C., & Pollack, M. H. (2011). *10-minute CBT: Integrating cognitive-behavioral strategies into your practice.* New York: Oxford University Press.

Wright, J. H., Basco, M. R., & Thase, M. E. (2006). *Learning cognitive-behavior therapy: An illustrated guide.* Arlington, VA: American Psychiatric Publishing.

Cognitive Therapy

Beck, A. T., Emery, G., & Greenberg, R. L. (1985). *Anxiety disorders and phobias: A cognitive perspective.* New York: Basic Books.

Beck, A. T., Freeman, A., & Davis, D. D. (2004). *Cognitive therapy of personality disorders* (2nd ed.). New York: Guilford Press.

Beck, A. T., Rush, A. J., Shaw, B. F., & Emery, G. (1979). *Cognitive therapy of depression.* New York: Guilford Press.

Young, J. E., Klosko, J. S., & Weishaar, M. E. (2003). *Schema therapy: A practitioner's guide.* New York: Guilford Press.

Couples and Families

Datillo, F. M. (2010). *Cognitive-behavioral therapy with couples and families: A comprehensive guide for clinicians.* New York: Guilford Press.

Epstein, N. B., & Baucom, D. H. (2002). *Enhanced cognitive-behavioral therapy for couples: A contextual approach.* Washington, DC: American Psychological Association.

Gottman, J. M. (1999). *The marriage clinic: A scientifically based marital therapy.* New York: Norton.

Jacobson, N. S., & Margolin, G. (1979). *Marital therapy: Strategies based on social learning and behavior exchange principles.* New York: Brunner/Mazel.

Diagnosis-Specific Treatment Manual Series

Advances in psychotherapy–Evidence-based practice. Cambridge, MA: Hogrefe. Series available at *www.hogrefe.com/program/books/book-series/advances-in-psychotherapy-evidence-based-practice.html.*

Treatments that work. New York: Oxford University Press. Series available at *http://global.oup.com/us/companion.websites/umbrella/treatments.*

Emotion Regulation

Kring, A. M., & Sloan, D. M. (Eds.). (2010). *Emotion regulation and psychopathology: A transdiagnostic approach to etiology and treatment.* New York: Guilford Press.

Inpatient CBT

Wright, J. H., Thase, M. E., Beck, A. T., & Ludgate, J. W. (1993). *Cognitive therapy with inpatients: Developing a cognitive milieu.* New York: Guilford Press.

Mindfulness- and Acceptance-Based Therapies

Hayes, S. C., Strosahl, K. D., & Wilson, K. G. (2012). *Acceptance and commitment therapy* (2nd ed.): *The process and practice of mindful change.* New York: Guilford Press.

Linehan, M. M. (1993). *Cognitive-behavioral treatment of borderline personality disorder.* New York: Guilford Press.

Linehan, M. M. (2015). *Skills manual for treating borderline personality disorder.* New York: Guilford Press.

Orsillo, S. M., & Roemer, L. (Eds.). (2005). *Acceptance-and mindfulness-based approaches to anxiety: Conceptualization and treatment.* New York: Springer.

Segal, Z. V., Williams, J. M. G., & Teasdale, J. D. (2013). *Mindfulness-based cognitive therapy for depression* (2nd ed.). New York: Guilford Press.

Wells, A. (2009). *Metacognitive therapy for anxiety and depression.* New York: Guilford Press.

Motivational Interviewing

Miller, W. R., & Rollnick, S. (2013). *Motivational interviewing* (3rd ed.): *Helping people change.* New York: Guilford Press.

The Therapeutic Relationship

Norcross, J. C. (Ed.). (2011). *Psychotherapy relationships that work: Evidence-based responsiveness* (2nd ed.). New York: Oxford University Press.

Safran, J., & Segal, Z. (1996). *Interpersonal process in cognitive therapy.* Northvale, NJ: Jason Aronson.

Treatment Compendia

Antony, M. M., & Barlow, D. H. (Eds.). (2010). *Handbook of assessment and treatment planning for psychological disorders* (2nd ed.). New York: Guilford Press.

Barlow, D. H. (Ed.). (2014). *Clinical handbook of psychological disorders: A step-by-step treatment manual* (5th ed.). New York: Guilford Press.

Tools for the Clinician

Blank Meaty Conceptualization Form

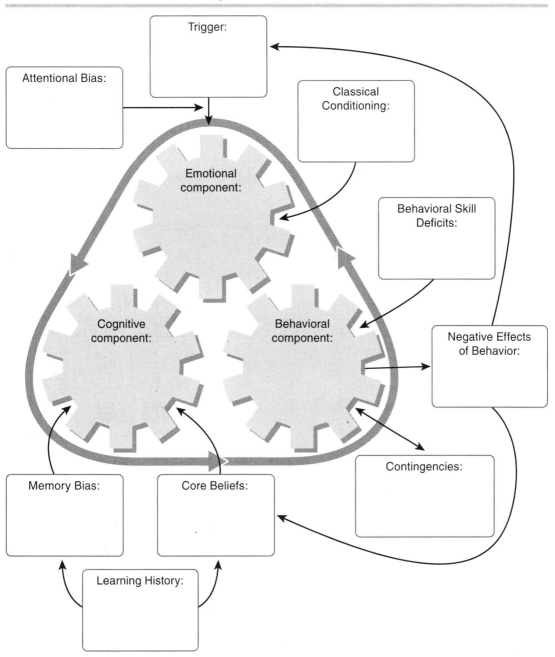

From *Doing CBT* by David F. Tolin. Copyright © 2016 The Guilford Press. Permission to photocopy this form is granted to purchasers of this book for personal use or use with individual clients (see copyright page for details). Purchasers can download enlarged versions of this form (see the box at the end of the table of contents).

Behavior Self-Monitoring Form

The behavior to monitor is: _____

Each time the behavior occurs, complete a row of the form.

Date and time	What was happening right *before* the behavior?	How many times did you do the behavior?	How long did you do the behavior?	What happened right *after* the behavior?

From *Doing CBT* by David F. Tolin. Copyright © 2016 The Guilford Press. Permission to photocopy this form is granted to purchasers of this book for personal use or use with individual clients (see copyright page for details). Purchasers can download enlarged versions of this form (see the box at the end of the table of contents).

Clinician Monitoring Form for Behavior: Frequency and Duration

The behavior to monitor is: _____

Each time the behavior occurs, complete a row of the form.

Date and time	Antecedents: Describe what was happening right *before* the behavior.	How many times did the client do the behavior?	How long did the client do the behavior?	Consequences: Describe what happened right *after* the behavior.

From *Doing CBT* by David F. Tolin. Copyright © 2016 The Guilford Press. Permission to photocopy this form is granted to purchasers of this book for personal use or use with individual clients (see copyright page for details). Purchasers can download enlarged versions of this form (see the box at the end of the table of contents).

Clinician Monitoring Form for Behavior: Check-Ins

The behavior to monitor is: _____

Defined as: _____

_____

Behavior will be monitored at the following intervals: _____

_____

Observation	1	2	3	4	5	6	7	8	9
Behavior present?	Y N	Y N	Y N	Y N	Y N	Y N	Y N	Y N	Y N

Observation	10	11	12	13	14	15	16	17	18
Behavior present?	Y N	Y N	Y N	Y N	Y N	Y N	Y N	Y N	Y′ N

Observation	19	20	21	22	23	24	25	26	27
Behavior present?	Y N	Y N	Y N	Y N	Y N	Y N	Y N	Y N	Y N

Observation	28	29	30	31	32	33	34	35	36
Behavior present?	Y N	Y N	Y N	Y N	Y N	Y N	Y N	Y N	Y N

Observation	37	38	39	40	41	42	43	44	45
Behavior present?	Y N	Y N	Y N	Y N	Y N	Y N	Y N	Y N	Y N

Observation	46	47	48	49	50	51	52	53	54
Behavior present?	Y N	Y N	Y N	Y N	Y N	Y N	Y N	Y N	Y N

Observation	55	56	57	58	59	60	61	62	63
Behavior present?	Y N	Y N	Y N	Y N	Y N	Y N	Y N	Y N	Y N

Observation	64	65	66	67	68	69	70	71	72
Behavior present?	Y N	Y N	Y N	Y N	Y N	Y N	Y N	Y N	Y N

Observation	73	74	75	76	77	78	79	80	81
Behavior present?	Y N	Y N	Y N	Y N	Y N	Y N	Y N	Y N	Y N

A. Total number of "yes" ratings: _____

B. Total number of ratings made: _____

C. Proportion of "yes" ratings (A ÷ B) _____

From *Doing CBT* by David F. Tolin. Copyright © 2016 The Guilford Press. Permission to photocopy this form is granted to purchasers of this book for personal use or use with individual clients (see copyright page for details). Purchasers can download enlarged versions of this form (see the box at the end of the table of contents).

Behavior Star Chart

Identify the desired behavior, and indicate how you will reward that behavior. Put a star on the chart for each day that the desired behavior occurs.

The desired behavior is: _____

Defined as: _____

_____

The reward for the desired behavior is: _____ per _____ stars earned.

	Sun	Mon	Tues	Wed	Thurs	Fri	Sat	Total
Week 1								
Week 2								
Week 3								
Week 4								

From *Doing CBT* by David F. Tolin. Copyright © 2016 The Guilford Press. Permission to photocopy this form is granted to purchasers of this book for personal use or use with individual clients (see copyright page for details). Purchasers can download enlarged versions of this form (see the box at the end of the table of contents).

Token Economy Chart for Institutions

Identify the desired behavior, and indicate how you will reward that behavior. Circle YES or NO for each shift in which the desired behavior occurs.

The desired behavior is: _____

Defined as: _____

_____

The reward for the desired behavior is: _____ per _____ YESes circled

Behavior (_____) present? Y/N			Total
Shift 1	Shift 2	Shift 3	
Monday Y N	Y N	Y N	
Tuesday Y N	Y N	Y N	
Wednesday Y N	Y N	Y N	
Thursday Y N	Y N	Y N	
Friday Y N	Y N	Y N	
Saturday Y N	Y N	Y N	
Sunday Y N	Y N	Y N	

List of items that can be purchased:

Item, activity, or privilege	Token cost

From *Doing CBT* by David F. Tolin. Copyright © 2016 The Guilford Press. Permission to photocopy this form is granted to purchasers of this book for personal use or use with individual clients (see copyright page for details). Purchasers can download enlarged versions of this form (see the box at the end of the table of contents).

Contingency Contract

Use this form to make a contract with yourself. Indicate what changes you intend to make, and how you will reward yourself for making those changes.

Date: _____

I, _____, intend to make the following behavior change(s):

1.

2.

3.

My reward system for making these change(s) will be:

1. When I _____, I will _____.

2. When I _____, I will _____.

3. When I _____, I will _____.

My penalty system (optional) for not making these change(s) will be:

1. When I _____, I will _____.

2. When I _____, I will _____.

3. When I _____, I will _____.

This system will remain in place until _____.

_____   _____

Signature   Co-signature (if applicable)

From *Doing CBT* by David F. Tolin. Copyright © 2016 The Guilford Press. Permission to photocopy this form is granted to purchasers of this book for personal use or use with individual clients (see copyright page for details). Purchasers can download enlarged versions of this form (see the box at the end of the table of contents).

Activity Monitoring Form

For the entire day, write down everything you do, and rate each hour's activity on a scale of 0–10 for mastery (the extent to which you felt a sense of accomplishment) and pleasure (the extent to which you enjoyed yourself), with 0 meaning absolutely no pleasure or sense of accomplishment, and 10 meaning maximum pleasure or sense of accomplishment.

Time	Activity	Mastery (0–10)	Pleasure (0–10)
6–7			
7–8			
8–9			
9–10			
10–11			
11–12			
12–1			
1–2			
2–3			
3–4			
4–5			
5–6			
6–7			
7–8			
8–9			
9–10			
10–11			
11–12			
12–1			
1–2			
2–3			
3–4			
4–5			
5–6			

From *Doing CBT* by David F. Tolin. Copyright © 2016 The Guilford Press. Permission to photocopy this form is granted to purchasers of this book for personal use or use with individual clients (see copyright page for details). Purchasers can download enlarged versions of this form (see the box at the end of the table of contents).

Mastery and Pleasure Checklist

Please look at the activities listed below. For each one, indicate:

1. How much of a *sense of accomplishment* you would experience if you did that activity.
2. How much *pleasure* you would experience if you did that activity.

	Accomplishment			Pleasure		
1. Getting together with friends	None	A little	A lot	None	A little	A lot
2. Getting together with family	None	A little	A lot	None	A little	A lot
3. Going to a party	None	A little	A lot	None	A little	A lot
4. Going to a restaurant	None	A little	A lot	None	A little	A lot
5. Going to a park, the beach, or the woods	None	A little	A lot	None	A little	A lot
6. Going shopping	None	A little	A lot	None	A little	A lot
7. Going to a movie or to the theater	None	A little	A lot	None	A little	A lot
8. Watching TV or listening to the radio	None	A little	A lot	None	A little	A lot
9. Going to a sporting event	None	A little	A lot	None	A little	A lot
10. Going to a concert	None	A little	A lot	None	A little	A lot
11. Individual sport _____	None	A little	A lot	None	A little	A lot
12. Group sport _____	None	A little	A lot	None	A little	A lot
13. Exercise or working out	None	A little	A lot	None	A little	A lot
14. Reading	None	A little	A lot	None	A little	A lot
15. Playing board or card games	None	A little	A lot	None	A little	A lot
16. Playing video or computer games	None	A little	A lot	None	A little	A lot
17. Doing crosswords, Sudoku, or puzzles	None	A little	A lot	None	A little	A lot
18. Writing	None	A little	A lot	None	A little	A lot
19. Taking a class or other educational activity	None	A little	A lot	None	A little	A lot
20. Singing or playing a musical instrument	None	A little	A lot	None	A little	A lot
21. Dancing	None	A little	A lot	None	A little	A lot
22. Doing art work (e.g., painting, sculpture, photography)	None	A little	A lot	None	A little	A lot
23. Doing crafts (e.g., scrapbooking, knitting, sewing)	None	A little	A lot	None	A little	A lot
24. Woodworking	None	A little	A lot	None	A little	A lot
25. Fixing things around the house	None	A little	A lot	None	A little	A lot
26. Cleaning the house	None	A little	A lot	None	A little	A lot
27. Cooking	None	A little	A lot	None	A little	A lot
28. Working in the yard	None	A little	A lot	None	A little	A lot
29. Getting a makeover or haircut	None	A little	A lot	None	A little	A lot
30. Getting a manicure or pedicure	None	A little	A lot	None	A little	A lot
31. Getting a massage	None	A little	A lot	None	A little	A lot
32. Other _____	None	A little	A lot	None	A little	A lot

From *Doing CBT* by David F. Tolin. Copyright © 2016 The Guilford Press. Permission to photocopy this form is granted to purchasers of this book for personal use or use with individual clients (see copyright page for details). Purchasers can download enlarged versions of this form (see the box at the end of the table of contents).

Exposure Hierarchy

The goal of this form is to help you identify *exposure* exercises to face a fear. Think of as many things as you can that would cause you to feel fear and that you would ordinarily avoid. You could expose yourself to certain activities or situations, certain objects, unpleasant thoughts, or unpleasant feelings or body sensations.

For each item, assign a *fear level*, meaning how much fear or discomfort you would experience if you were to do that activity, with 0 meaning absolutely no fear or discomfort, and 100 meaning the worst fear or discomfort you could possibly imagine.

Exposure Hierarchy for My Fear: _____

Activity	Fear Level (0–100)
1.	
2.	
3.	
4.	
5.	
6.	
7.	
8.	
9.	
10.	
11.	
12.	
13.	
14.	
15.	

From *Doing CBT* by David F. Tolin. Copyright © 2016 The Guilford Press. Permission to photocopy this form is granted to purchasers of this book for personal use or use with individual clients (see copyright page for details). Purchasers can download enlarged versions of this form (see the box at the end of the table of contents).

Safety Behavior List

The goal of this form is to help you identify *safety behaviors* that can interfere with successful exposure therapy. Think of as many things as you can that you would normally want to do in order to distract yourself, increase your sense of safety, or relax or feel better; or things or people that you would normally want to bring with you when facing a fear.

During and after exposure, I will not do the following things that distract me:

1.

2.

3.

4.

During and after exposure, I will not do the following things that increase my sense of safety:

1.

2.

3.

4.

During and after exposure, I will not do the following things to relax or feel better:

1.

2.

3.

4.

During and after exposure, I will not bring the following things or people with me:

1.

2.

3.

4.

From *Doing CBT* by David F. Tolin. Copyright © 2016 The Guilford Press. Permission to photocopy this form is granted to purchasers of this book for personal use or use with individual clients (see copyright page for details). Purchasers can download enlarged versions of this form (see the box at the end of the table of contents).

Problem-Solving Worksheet

Step 1. Write down the problem, using objective language. Be as clear as possible. Describe why this is a problem, and what you want to see happen.

My problem is: _____.

This is a problem because: _____.

My goal for this problem is: _____.

Step 2. Write as many possible solutions to the problem as you can think of in column 1. Defer judgment on whether or not they would work or be possible; just be as creative as possible.

Potential Solution	Pros	Cons

Step 3. For each potential solution, write down the likely pros (what would be good about it) and cons (what would be bad about it). Write the pros and cons in columns 2 and 3. Consider whether the solution would work, whether you could actually do it, and what the likely effects would be on you and on others.

Step 4. Write down which solution(s) you want to try first.

I will try: _____.

Step 5. After trying your solution(s), evaluate the outcome.

Overall, how satisfied are you with the results? _____

From *Doing CBT* by David F. Tolin. Copyright © 2016 The Guilford Press. Permission to photocopy this form is granted to purchasers of this book for personal use or use with individual clients (see copyright page for details). Purchasers can download enlarged versions of this form (see the box at the end of the table of contents).

Thought Monitoring Form

The goal of this exercise is to help you record your *interpretations*. That is, the aim is to understand what you think about things.

Carry this form with you throughout the day. Whenever you find yourself experiencing a strong emotion, please write down what was happening (the situation), your interpretation(s), and your emotion(s) or physical sensation(s). Please also rate the strength of your emotional or physical response on a scale from 0 (not at all) to 100 (the strongest it has ever been).

Situation	Interpretation(s)	Emotion(s) (0–100)
Late for work	I'll never succeed in this job	Sadness 65

From *Doing CBT* by David F. Tolin. Copyright © 2016 The Guilford Press. Permission to photocopy this form is granted to purchasers of this book for personal use or use with individual clients (see copyright page for details). Purchasers can download enlarged versions of this form (see the box at the end of the table of contents).

Cognitive Distortions

Cognitive distortions are errors of thinking that everyone makes from time to time. However, when we make the same kind of thinking error repeatedly, it negatively affects our emotions and our actions.

Cognitive Distortion	Examples
Probability Overestimation: Predicting a low-probability event without evidence to support it (or in the face of contradicting evidence).	• If I go to the mall, I'll have a heart attack. • Everyone at the party is going to hate me. • My plane will crash.
"Catastrophizing": Exaggerating the significance of an event; making mountains out of molehills.	• If I faint in a public place, it will be the most humiliating thing ever and I will never be able to show my face in public again. • My husband is late for dinner; he's probably lying dead in a ditch somewhere. • If my partner leaves me, I'll be all alone forever and will never find love again. • If I get anxious, I'll be anxious forever and will never be happy again.
Overgeneralization: Seeing isolated negative events as a global or never-ending pattern.	• I failed a test; therefore, I can't do anything right and I'll never succeed. • I had an argument with my spouse; therefore, I have a lousy marriage. • My friend did not call me this weekend; therefore, no one cares about me.
Personalizing: Blaming yourself for external events, or believing that external events are in some way related to you.	• My boss has a sour look on her face. I must have done something to make her mad. • If I had just been a better parent, my kids would have received better grades in school.
All-or-nothing thinking: Seeing things in black and white categories.	• If I can't do it perfectly, I'm a failure. • If my family doesn't support everything I do, that means they don't love me.
"Should" Statements: Making "rules" about how you or others should or must behave—and getting upset when the "rules" are broken—even if those rules aren't recognized by the rest of the world.	• People should be nice to me all of the time. • I should always put other people first, and I'm rotten if I fail to do so.

(continued)

From *Doing CBT* by David F. Tolin. Copyright © 2016 The Guilford Press. Permission to photocopy this form is granted to purchasers of this book for personal use or use with individual clients (see copyright page for details). Purchasers can download enlarged versions of this form (see the box at the end of the table of contents).

Cognitive Distortion	Examples
Mind Reading: Inferring what someone else is thinking or feeling, without sufficient evidence.	• I'm certain that they don't like me. • My wife thinks I'm a lousy husband, even if she doesn't say so.
Emotional Reasoning: Assuming that your emotions reflect the way things really are: "I feel it; therefore, it must be true."	• This situation must be dangerous; otherwise, why would I feel so anxious? • My husband is a jerk because I'm so angry at him all the time.
Minimizing: Downplaying the significance of events, or making unrealistically "permissive" statements to oneself.	• Just one drink won't hurt. I can keep it under control. • I won't get caught this time. • Everyone's making too big a deal out of this.

Examining the Evidence for Interpretations

The goal of this exercise is to help you examine the evidence for and against a particular *interpretation*—that is, evidence that would support the interpretation, and evidence that would not support the interpretation.

After you have identified the evidence for and against your interpretation, try to write down a new interpretation that is consistent with *all* of the available evidence.

Interpretation: _____

Evidence *for* interpretation	Evidence *against* interpretation

New, balanced interpretation

From *Doing CBT* by David F. Tolin. Copyright © 2016 The Guilford Press. Permission to photocopy this form is granted to purchasers of this book for personal use or use with individual clients (see copyright page for details). Purchasers can download enlarged versions of this form (see the box at the end of the table of contents).

Thought Change Record

When you notice yourself feeling distressed, write down the triggering event, your interpretation of the triggering event, and the emotion(s) you experienced. Then check any cognitive distortions that might be present in your interpretations. Try writing a new, more realistic interpretation, and recheck your emotions to see if rethinking the situation led to a change.

Triggering event	Interpretation	Emotion(s)	Intensity of emotion(s) (0–100)	Cognitive distortions (check all that apply)	New interpretation	Emotion(s)	Intensity of emotion(s) (0–100)
				☐ Probability overestimation ☐ Catastrophizing ☐ Overgeneralization ☐ Personalizing ☐ All-or-nothing thinking ☐ "Should" statements ☐ Mind reading ☐ Emotional reasoning ☐ Minimizing			
				☐ Probability overestimation ☐ Catastrophizing ☐ Overgeneralization ☐ Personalizing ☐ All-or-nothing thinking ☐ "Should" statements ☐ Mind reading ☐ Emotional reasoning ☐ Minimizing			

From *Doing CBT* by David F. Tolin. Copyright © 2016 The Guilford Press. Permission to photocopy this form is granted to purchasers of this book for personal use or use with individual clients (see copyright page for details). Purchasers can download enlarged versions of this form (see the box at the end of the table of contents).

Core Beliefs Checklist

Below is a series of things that people sometimes believe. Please read each one and circle the response indicating how much you usually believe it to be true. There are no right or wrong answers here; the goal is simply to get a better understanding of how you usually think.

Belief	How much you believe it		
1. People can't be trusted.	I don't believe this	I kind of believe this	I totally believe this
2. Other people's needs are more important than my own.	I don't believe this	I kind of believe this	I totally believe this
3. I can't handle upsetting things.	I don't believe this	I kind of believe this	I totally believe this
4. I'm not as competent as other people.	I don't believe this	I kind of believe this	I totally believe this
5. I must always make others happy.	I don't believe this	I kind of believe this	I totally believe this
6. I don't fit in with other people.	I don't believe this	I kind of believe this	I totally believe this
7. My inner feelings are shameful.	I don't believe this	I kind of believe this	I totally believe this
8. I'm not safe.	I don't believe this	I kind of believe this	I totally believe this
9. No one in my life will stick around.	I don't believe this	I kind of believe this	I totally believe this
10. I can't control myself.	I don't believe this	I kind of believe this	I totally believe this
11. I am no good.	I don't believe this	I kind of believe this	I totally believe this
12. What I want and how I feel isn't important.	I don't believe this	I kind of believe this	I totally believe this
13. My life is ruined.	I don't believe this	I kind of believe this	I totally believe this
14. Others won't be there for me.	I don't believe this	I kind of believe this	I totally believe this
15. I must be on guard at all times.	I don't believe this	I kind of believe this	I totally believe this

(continued)

From *Doing CBT* by David F. Tolin. Copyright © 2016 The Guilford Press. Permission to photocopy this form is granted to purchasers of this book for personal use or use with individual clients (see copyright page for details). Purchasers can download enlarged versions of this form (see the box at the end of the table of contents).

Belief	How much you believe it		
16. I am defective or inferior.	I don't believe this	I kind of believe this	I totally believe this
17. The usual rules don't apply to me.	I don't believe this	I kind of believe this	I totally believe this
18. I am dangerous.	I don't believe this	I kind of believe this	I totally believe this
19. I am a failure.	I don't believe this	I kind of believe this	I totally believe this
20. My moods are dangerous.	I don't believe this	I kind of believe this	I totally believe this
21. If I'm not perfect, I'm worthless.	I don't believe this	I kind of believe this	I totally believe this
22. I am inadequate.	I don't believe this	I kind of believe this	I totally believe this
23. No one cares about me.	I don't believe this	I kind of believe this	I totally believe this
24. If something bad happens, I am to blame.	I don't believe this	I kind of believe this	I totally believe this
25. I should never have to be uncomfortable.	I don't believe this	I kind of believe this	I totally believe this
26. I'm only as good as what I can accomplish.	I don't believe this	I kind of believe this	I totally believe this
27. Others will hurt me, manipulate me, or take advantage of me.	I don't believe this	I kind of believe this	I totally believe this
28. I have no future.	I don't believe this	I kind of believe this	I totally believe this
29. The world is against me.	I don't believe this	I kind of believe this	I totally believe this
30. People who do wrong should be punished.	I don't believe this	I kind of believe this	I totally believe this
31. I can't take care of myself.	I don't believe this	I kind of believe this	I totally believe this
32. I must always be the best.	I don't believe this	I kind of believe this	I totally believe this
33. Bad things will always happen to me.	I don't believe this	I kind of believe this	I totally believe this
34. I am helpless.	I don't believe this	I kind of believe this	I totally believe this

(continued)

Belief	How much you believe it		
35. I can do no wrong.	I don't believe this	I kind of believe this	I totally believe this
36. I need to be special.	I don't believe this	I kind of believe this	I totally believe this
37. I have to be admired.	I don't believe this	I kind of believe this	I totally believe this
38. The world is a dangerous place.	I don't believe this	I kind of believe this	I totally believe this
39. Everything that can go wrong, will go wrong.	I don't believe this	I kind of believe this	I totally believe this
40. I deserve to be punished.	I don't believe this	I kind of believe this	I totally believe this
41. I shouldn't get close to anyone.	I don't believe this	I kind of believe this	I totally believe this
42. I'm incompetent.	I don't believe this	I kind of believe this	I totally believe this
43. There is danger everywhere.	I don't believe this	I kind of believe this	I totally believe this
44. I can't control what happens to me.	I don't believe this	I kind of believe this	I totally believe this
45. I should never show weakness.	I don't believe this	I kind of believe this	I totally believe this
46. The bad things that have happened in my life are my fault.	I don't believe this	I kind of believe this	I totally believe this
47. Things need to be perfect.	I don't believe this	I kind of believe this	I totally believe this
48. Mistakes cannot be tolerated.	I don't believe this	I kind of believe this	I totally believe this
49. People will judge me negatively.	I don't believe this	I kind of believe this	I totally believe this
50. I must be in control at all times.	I don't believe this	I kind of believe this	I totally believe this
51. There's a right and wrong way to do everything.	I don't believe this	I kind of believe this	I totally believe this
52. I must succeed in everything I do.	I don't believe this	I kind of believe this	I totally believe this
53. I will fail at whatever I do.	I don't believe this	I kind of believe this	I totally believe this

(continued)

Belief	How much you believe it		
54. I will lose control of myself if I'm not careful.	I don't believe this	I kind of believe this	I totally believe this
55. I can't do anything without help.	I don't believe this	I kind of believe this	I totally believe this
56. I am worthless.	I don't believe this	I kind of believe this	I totally believe this
57. I am responsible for everything.	I don't believe this	I kind of believe this	I totally believe this
58. I can't rely on other people.	I don't believe this	I kind of believe this	I totally believe this
59. I will always get a raw deal.	I don't believe this	I kind of believe this	I totally believe this
60. I am mentally disturbed, weird, or crazy.	I don't believe this	I kind of believe this	I totally believe this
61. Without approval from others, I am worthless.	I don't believe this	I kind of believe this	I totally believe this
62. Disaster will strike at any time.	I don't believe this	I kind of believe this	I totally believe this
63. Uncertainty is intolerable.	I don't believe this	I kind of believe this	I totally believe this
64. No one understands me.	I don't believe this	I kind of believe this	I totally believe this
65. I am damaged.	I don't believe this	I kind of believe this	I totally believe this
66. I'm unlovable.	I don't believe this	I kind of believe this	I totally believe this
67. I can't trust myself.	I don't believe this	I kind of believe this	I totally believe this
68. I am weak.	I don't believe this	I kind of believe this	I totally believe this
69. People need to follow the highest moral or ethical standards.	I don't believe this	I kind of believe this	I totally believe this
70. I am superior or gifted.	I don't believe this	I kind of believe this	I totally believe this
71. I'm stupid.	I don't believe this	I kind of believe this	I totally believe this
72. My needs are more important than those of other people.	I don't believe this	I kind of believe this	I totally believe this

Examining the Evidence for Core Beliefs

The goal of this exercise is to help you examine the evidence for and against a particular *core belief*—that is, evidence that would support the core belief, and evidence that would not support the core belief.

After you have identified the evidence for and against your core belief, try to write down a new belief that is consistent with *all* of the available evidence.

Core belief: _____

Evidence **for** core belief	Evidence **against** core belief

New, balanced core belief

From *Doing CBT* by David F. Tolin. Copyright © 2016 The Guilford Press. Permission to photocopy this form is granted to purchasers of this book for personal use or use with individual clients (see copyright page for details). Purchasers can download enlarged versions of this form (see the box at the end of the table of contents).

References

Abelson, J. L., Weg, J. G., Nesse, R. M., & Curtis, G. C. (2001). Persistent respiratory irregularity in patients with panic disorder. *Biological Psychiatry, 49,* 588–595.

Abramowitz, J. S., Tolin, D. F., & Street, G. P. (2001). Paradoxical effects of thought suppression: A meta-analysis of controlled studies. *Clinical Psychology Review, 21,* 683–703.

Abramson, L. Y., Metalsky, G. I., & Alloy, L. B. (1989). Hopelessness depression: A theory-based subtype of depression. *Psychological Review, 96,* 358–372.

Achenbach, T. M. (1991). *Integrative guide for the 1991 CBCL/4–18, YSR, and TRF profiles.* Burlington: University of Vermont, Department of Psychiatry.

Adams, T. G., Brady, R. E., Lohr, J. M., & Jacobs, W. J. (2015). A meta-analysis of CBT components for anxiety disorders. *Behavior Therapist, 38,* 87–97.

Agras, W. S., Leitenberg, H., Barlow, D. H., Curtis, N. A., Edwards, J., & Wright, D. (1971). Relaxation in systematic desensitization. *Archives of General Psychiatry, 25,* 511–514.

Aite, A., Barrault, S., Cassotti, M., Borst, G., Bonnaire, C., Houde, O., . . . Moutier, S. (2014). The impact of alexithymia on pathological gamblers' decision making: A preliminary study of gamblers recruited in "sportsbook" casinos. *Cognitive and Behavioral Neurology, 27,* 59–67.

Albano, A. M. (2003). Treatment of social anxiety disorder. In M. A. Reinecke, F. M. Dattilio, & A. Freeman (Eds.), *Cognitive therapy with children and adolescents: A casebook for clinical practice* (2nd ed., pp. 128–161). New York: Guilford Press.

Alden, L. E. (1989). Short-term structured treatment for avoidant personality disorder. *Journal of Consulting and Clinical Psychology, 57,* 756–764.

Alden, L. E., & Mellings, T. M. (2004). Generalized social phobia and social judgments: The salience of self- and partner-information. *Journal of Anxiety Disorders, 18,* 143–157.

Alden, L. E., & Wallace, S. T. (1995). Social phobia and social appraisal in successful and unsuccessful social interactions. *Behaviour Research and Therapy, 33,* 497–505.

Allen, L. B., Tsao, J. C. I., Seidman, L. C., & Ehrenreich-May, J. (2012). A unified, transdiagnostic treatment for adolescents with chronic pain and comorbid anxiety and depression. *Cognitive and Behavioral Practice, 19,* 56–67.

Alnaes, R., & Torgersen, S. (1997). Personality and personality disorders predict development and relapses of major depression. *Acta Psychiatrica Scandinavica, 95,* 336–342.

American Psychiatric Association. (2013). *Diagnostic and statistical manual of mental disorders* (5th ed.). Arlington, VA: Author.

American Psychological Association. (2003). Guidelines on multicultural education, training, research, practice, and organizational change for psychologists. *American Psychologist, 58,* 377–402.

Amir, N., Beard, C., Burns, M., & Bomyea, J. (2009). Attention modification program in individuals with generalized anxiety disorder. *Journal of Abnormal Psychology, 118,* 28–33.

Amir, N., Beard, C., Taylor, C. T., Klumpp, H., Elias, J., Burns, M., & Chen, X. (2009). Attention training in individuals with generalized social phobia: A randomized controlled trial. *Journal of Consulting and Clinical Psychology, 77,* 961–973.

Amir, N., Weber, G., Beard, C., Bomyea, J., & Taylor, C. T. (2008). The effect of a single-session attention modification program on response to a public-speaking challenge in socially anxious individuals. *Journal of Abnormal Psychology, 117,* 860–868.

Ansell, E. B., Pinto, A., Edelen, M. O., Markowitz, J. C., Sanislow, C. A., Yen, S., . . . Grilo, C. M. (2011). The association of personality disorders with the prospective 7-year course of anxiety disorders. *Psychological Medicine, 41,* 1019–1028.

Antshel, K. M., & Remer, R. (2003). Social skills training in children with attention deficit hyperactivity disorder: A randomized-controlled clinical trial. *Journal of Clinical Child and Adolescent Psychology, 32,* 153–165.

Arch, J. J., Eifert, G. H., Davies, C., Plumb Vilardaga, J. C., Rose, R. D., & Craske, M. G. (2012). Randomized clinical trial of cognitive behavioral therapy (CBT) versus acceptance and commitment therapy (ACT) for mixed anxiety disorders. *Journal of Consulting and Clinical Psychology, 80,* 750–765.

Areán, P. A., Perri, M. G., Nezu, A. M., Schein, R. L., Christopher, F., & Joseph, T. X. (1993). Comparative effectiveness of social problem-solving therapy and reminiscence therapy as treatments for depression in older adults. *Journal of Consulting and Clinical Psychology, 61,* 1003–1010.

Areán, P. A., Raue, P., Mackin, R. S., Kanellopoulos, D., McCulloch, C., & Alexopoulos, G. S. (2010). Problem-solving therapy and supportive therapy in older adults with major depression and executive dysfunction. *American Journal of Psychiatry, 167,* 1391–1398.

Arntz, A. (2002). Cognitive therapy versus interoceptive exposure as treatment of panic disorder without agoraphobia. *Behaviour Research and Therapy, 40,* 325–341.

Arntz, A., Dreessen, L., Schouten, E., & Weertman, A. (2004). Beliefs in personality disorders: A test with the Personality Disorder Belief Questionnaire. *Behaviour Research and Therapy, 42,* 1215–1225.

Aronson, E., & Mills, J. (1959). The effect of severity of initiation on liking for a group. *Journal of Abnormal and Social Psychology, 59,* 177–181.

Asnaani, A., Sawyer, A. T., Aderka, I. M., & Hofmann, S. G. (2013). Effect of suppression, reappraisal, and acceptance of emotional pictures on acoustic eye-blink startle magnitude. *Journal of Experimental Psychopathology, 4,* 182–193.

Atkinson, R. C., & Shiffrin, R. M. (1968). Human memory: A proposed system and its control processes. In K. W. Spence & J. T. Spence (Eds.), *The psychology of learning and motivation* (Vol. 2, pp. 89–195). New York: Academic Press.

Ayllon, T., & Azrin, N. H. (1968). *The token economy: A motivational system for therapy and rehabilitation.* New York: Appleton-Century-Crofts.

Azrin, N. H., & Nunn, R. G. (1973). Habit-reversal: A method of eliminating nervous habits and tics. *Behaviour Research and Therapy, 11,* 619–628.

Bach, P., & Hayes, S. C. (2002). The use of acceptance and commitment therapy to prevent the rehospitalization of psychotic patients: A randomized controlled trial. *Journal of Consulting and Clinical Psychology, 70,* 1129–1139.

Baer, R. A. (2003). Mindfulness training as a clinical intervention: A conceptual and empirical review. *Clinical Psychology: Science and Practice, 10,* 125–143.

Bailey, J. R., Gross, A. M., & Cotton, C. R. (2011). Challenges associated with establishing a token economy in a residential care facility. *Clinical Case Studies, 10,* 278–290.

Bakal, D. A., Demjen, S., & Kaganov, J. A. (1981). Cognitive behavioral treatment of chronic headache. *Headache, 21,* 81–86.

Baker, S. R., & Edelmann, R. J. (2002). Is social phobia related to lack of social skills? Duration of skill-related behaviours and ratings of behavioural adequacy. *British Journal of Clinical Psychology, 41,* 243–257.

Bandura, A. (1973). *Aggression: A social learning theory analysis.* Englewood Cliffs, NJ: Prentice Hall.

Bandura, A. (1977). Self-efficacy: Toward a unifying theory of behavioral change. *Psychological Review, 84,* 191–215.

Bandura, A. (1982). Self-efficacy mechanism in human agency. *American Psychologist, 37,* 122–147.

Bandura, A., Ross, D., & Ross, S. A. (1963a). Imitation of film-mediated aggressive models. *Journal of Abnormal and Social Psychology, 66,* 3–11.

Bandura, A., Ross, D., & Ross, S. A. (1963b). Vicarious reinforcement and imitative learning. *Journal of Abnormal Psychology, 67,* 601–607.

Barber, J. P., & DeRubeis, R. J. (1989). On second thought: Where the action is in cognitive therapy for depression. *Cognitive Therapy and Research, 13,* 441–457.

Bargh, J. A. (1992). The ecology of automaticity: Toward establishing the conditions needed to produce automatic processing effects. *American Journal of Psychology, 105,* 181–199.

Bargh, J. A., Chaiken, S., Govender, R., & Pratto, F. (1992). The generality of the automatic attitude activation effect. *Journal of Personality and Social Psychology, 62,* 893–912.

Bargh, J. A., & Ferguson, M. J. (2000). Beyond behaviorism: On the automaticity of higher mental processes. *Psychological Bulletin, 126,* 925–945.

Barkley, R. A. (1997). *Defiant children: A clinician's manual for assessment and parent training* (2nd ed.). New York: Guilford Press.

Barlow, D. H. (2002). *Anxiety and its disorders: The nature and treatment of anxiety and panic* (2nd ed.). New York: Guilford Press.

Barlow, D. H., & Allen, L. B. (2004). Scientific basis of psychological treatments for anxiety disorders: Past, present, and future. In J. M. Gorman (Ed.), *Fear and anxiety: The benefits of translational research* (pp. 171–191). Washington, DC: American Psychiatric.

Barlow, D. H., Gorman, J. M., Shear, M. K., & Woods, S. W. (2000). Cognitive-behavioral therapy, imipramine, or their combination for panic disorder: A randomized controlled trial. *Journal of the American Medical Association, 283,* 2529–2536.

Barlow, D. H., O'Brien, G. T., & Last, C. G. (1984). Couples treatment of agoraphobia. *Behavior Therapy, 15,* 41–58.

Barrett, L. F., & Wager, T. D. (2006). The structure of emotion: Evidence from neuroimaging studies. *Current Directions in Psychological Science, 15,* 79–83.

Barrett, P. M., Dadds, M. R., & Rapee, R. M. (1996). Family treatment of childhood anxiety: A controlled trial. *Journal of Consulting and Clinical Psychology, 64,* 333–342.

Baucom, D. H. (1982). A comparison of behavioral contracting and problem-solving/communications training in behavioral marital therapy. *Behavior Therapy, 13,* 162–174.

Baucom, D. H., Shoham, V., Mueser, K. T., Daiuto, A. D., & Stickle, T. R. (1998). Empirically supported couple and family interventions for marital distress and adult mental health problems. *Journal of Consulting and Clinical Psychology, 66,* 53–88.

Bechara, A., & Damasio, A. R. (2007). The somatic marker hypothesis: A neural theory of economic decision. *Games and Economic Behavior, 52,* 336–372.

Bechara, A., Damasio, A. R., Damasio, H., & Anderson, S. W. (1994). Insensitivity to future consequences following damage to human prefrontal cortex. *Cognition, 50,* 7–15.

Beck, A. T. (1976). *Cognitive therapy and the emotional disorders.* New York: International Universities Press.

Beck, A. T., Emery, G., & Greenberg, R. L. (1985). *Anxiety disorders and phobias: A cognitive perspective.* New York: Basic Books.

Beck, A. T., & Freeman, A. (1990). *Cognitive therapy of personality disorders.* New York: Guilford Press.

Beck, A. T., Freeman, A., & Davis, D. D. (2004). *Cognitive therapy of personality disorders* (2nd ed.). New York: Guilford Press.

Beck, A. T., Rush, A. J., Shaw, B. F., & Emery, G. (1979). *Cognitive therapy of depression.* New York: Guilford Press.

Beck, A. T., & Steer, R. A. (1993). *Beck Anxiety Inventory Manual.* San Antonio, TX: Psychological Corp.

Beck, A. T., Steer, R. A., & Brown, G. K. (1996). *Manual for the Beck Depression Inventory* (2nd ed.). San Antonio, TX: Psychological Corp.

Beck, J. G., & Heimberg, R. G. (1983). Self-report assessment of assertive behavior: A critical analysis. *Behavior Modification, 7,* 451–487.

Becker, C. B., Darius, E., & Schaumberg, K. (2007).

An analog study of patient preferences for exposure versus alternative treatments for posttraumatic stress disorder. *Behaviour Research and Therapy, 45,* 2861–2873.

Becker, C. B., Zayfert, C., & Anderson, E. (2004). A survey of psychologists' attitudes towards and utilization of exposure therapy for PTSD. *Behaviour Research and Therapy, 42,* 277–292.

Beidas, R. S., Benjamin, C. L., Puleo, C. M., Edmunds, J. M., & Kendall, P. C. (2010). Flexible applications of the Coping Cat program for anxious youth. *Cognitive and Behavioral Practice, 17,* 142–153.

Beidel, D. C., Turner, S. M., & Morris, T. L. (2000). Behavioral treatment of childhood social phobia. *Journal of Consulting and Clinical Psychology, 68,* 1072–1080.

Beidel, D. C., Turner, S. M., & Young, B. J. (2006). Social effectiveness therapy for children: Five years later. *Behavior Therapy, 37,* 416–425.

Bell, A. C., & D'Zurilla, T. J. (2009). Problem-solving therapy for depression: A meta-analysis. *Clinical Psychology Review, 29,* 348–353.

Bellack, A. S., Morrison, R. L., Wixted, J. T., & Mueser, K. T. (1990). An analysis of social competence in schizophrenia. *British Journal of Psychiatry, 156,* 809–818.

Bellack, A. S., Sayers, M., Mueser, K. T., & Bennett, M. (1994). Evaluation of social problem solving in schizophrenia. *Journal of Abnormal Psychology, 103,* 371–378.

Ben-Porath, Y. S., & Tellegen, A. (2008). *MMPI-2-RF: Manual for administration, scoring and interpretation.* Minneapolis: University of Minnesota Press.

Berenz, E. C., Rowe, L., Schumacher, J. A., Stasiewicz, P. R., & Coffey, S. F. (2012). Prolonged exposure therapy for posttraumatic stress disorder among individuals in a residential substance use treatment program: A case series. *Professional Psychology: Research and Practice, 43,* 154–161.

Berglund, N., Vahlne, J. O., & Edman, A. (2003). Family intervention in schizophrenia: Impact on family burden and attitude. *Social Psychiatry and Psychiatric Epidemiology, 38,* 116–121.

Berking, M., Ebert, D., Cuijpers, P., & Hofmann, S. G. (2013). Emotion regulation skills training enhances the efficacy of inpatient cognitive behavioral therapy for major depressive disorder: A randomized controlled trial. *Psychotherapy and Psychosomatics, 82,* 234–245.

Berking, M., Wupperman, P., Reichardt, A., Pejic, T., Dippel, A., & Znoj, H. (2008). Emotion-regulation skills as a treatment target in psychotherapy. *Behaviour Research and Therapy, 46,* 1230–1237.

Berman, D. E., & Dudai, Y. (2001). Memory extinction, learning anew, and learning the new: Dissociations in the molecular machinery of learning in cortex. *Science, 291,* 2417–2419.

Bernstein, D. A., & Borkovec, T. (1973). *Progressive*

relaxation training: A manual for the helping professions. Champaign, IL: Research Press.

Beutler, L. E., Moleiro, C., & Talebi, H. (2002). Resistance in psychotherapy: What conclusions are supported by research. *Journal of Clinical Psychology, 58,* 207-217.

Bickel, W. K., & Marsch, L. A. (2001). Toward a behavioral economic understanding of drug dependence: Delay discounting processes. *Addiction, 96,* 73-86.

Biener, L., & Abrams, D. B. (1991). The contemplation ladder: Validation of a measure of readiness to consider smoking cessation. *Health Psychology, 10,* 360-365.

Bierman, K. L. (1988). The clinical implications of childrens' conceptions of social relationships. In S. R. Shirk (Ed.), *Cognitive development and child psychotherapy* (pp. 247-269). New York: Plenum Press.

Bilsker, D., & Forster, P. (2003). Problem-solving intervention for suicidal crises in the psychiatric emergency service. *Crisis, 24,* 134-136.

Bloch, L., Moran, E. K., & Kring, A. M. (2010). On the need for conceptual and definitional clarity in emotion regulation research on psychopathology. In A. M. Kring & D. M. Sloan (Eds.), *Emotion regulation and psychopathology: A transdiagnostic approach to etiology and treatment* (pp. 88-104). New York: Guilford Press.

Bloch, S., Lemeignan, M., & Aguilera, N. (1991). Specific respiratory patterns distinguish among human basic emotions. *International Journal of Psychophysiology, 11,* 141-154.

Blondon, K., Klasnja, P., Coleman, K., & Pratt, W. (2014). An exploration of attitudes toward the use of patient incentives to support diabetes self-management. *Psychology and Health, 29,* 552-563.

Bögels, S. M. (2006). Task concentration training versus applied relaxation, in combination with cognitive therapy, for social phobia patients with fear of blushing, trembling, and sweating. *Behaviour Research and Therapy, 44,* 1199-1210.

Bonn, J. A., Readhead, C. P., & Timmons, B. H. (1984). Enhanced adaptive behavioural response in agoraphobic patients pretreated with breathing retraining. *Lancet, 2,* 665-669.

Bootzin, R. R. (1979). Effects of self-control procedures for insomnia. *American Journal of Clinical Biofeedback, 2,* 70-77.

Bordin, E. S. (1979). The generalizability of the psychoanalytic concept of the working alliance. *Psychotherapy: Theory, Research, and Practice, 16,* 252-260.

Bordin, E. S. (1994). Theory and research on the therapeutic working alliance: New directions. In A. O. Horvath & L. S. Greenberg (Eds.), *The working alliance: Theory, research, and practice* (pp. 13-37). New York: Wiley.

Borkovec, T. D. (1994). The nature, functions, and origins of worry. In C. G. L. Davey & F. Tallis (Eds.), *Worrying: Perspectives on theory, assessment, and treatment* (pp. 5-33). New York: Wiley.

Borkovec, T. D., & Costello, E. (1993). Efficacy of applied relaxation and cognitive-behavioral therapy in the treatment of generalized anxiety disorder. *Journal of Consulting and Clinical Psychology, 61,* 611-619.

Borkovec, T. D., Grayson, J. B., & Cooper, K. M. (1978). Treatment of general tension: Subjective and physiological effects of progressive relaxation. *Journal of Consulting and Clinical Psychology, 46,* 518-528.

Borkovec, T. D., & Nau, S. D. (1972). Credibility of analogue therapy rationales. *Journal of Behavior Therapy and Experimental Psychiatry, 3,* 257-260.

Borkovec, T. D., & Roemer, L. (1995). Perceived functions of worry among generalized anxiety disorder subjects: Distraction from more emotionally distressing topics? *Journal of Behavior Therapy and Experimental Psychiatry, 26,* 25-30.

Borkovec, T. D., & Ruscio, A. M. (2001). Psychotherapy for generalized anxiety disorder. *Journal of Clinical Psychiatry, 62* (Suppl. 11), 37-42; discussion 43-45.

Boschen, M. J., & Casey, L. M. (2008). The use of mobile telephones as adjuncts to cognitive behavioral psychotherapy. *Professional Psychology: Research and Practice, 39,* 546-552.

Bothe, D. A., Grignon, J. B., & Olness, K. N. (2014). The effects of a stress management intervention in elementary school children. *Journal of Developmental and Behavioral Pediatrics, 35,* 62-67.

Bouton, M. E. (1993). Context, time, and memory retrieval in the interference paradigms of Pavlovian learning. *Psychological Bulletin, 114,* 80-99.

Bower, G. H. (1981). Mood and memory. *American Psychologist, 36,* 129-148.

Brady, K. T., Dansky, B. S., Back, S. E., Foa, E. B., & Carroll, K. M. (2001). Exposure therapy in the treatment of PTSD among cocaine-dependent individuals: Preliminary findings. *Journal of Substance Abuse Treatment, 21,* 47-54.

Brantley, J. (2003). *Calming your anxious mind: How mindfulness and compassion can free you from anxiety, fear, and panic.* Oakland, CA: New Harbinger.

Brehm, J. W. (1956). Postdecision changes in the desirability of alternatives. *Journal of Abnormal Psychology, 52,* 384-389.

Breuer, J., & Freud, S. (1955). Studies on hysteria. In J. Strachey (Ed., & Trans.), *The standard edition of the complete psychological works of Sigmund Freud* (Vol. 2). London: Hogarth Press. (Original work published 1893-1895)

Brewin, C. R., Christodoulides, J., & Hutchinson, G. (1996). Intrusive thoughts and intrusive memories in a nonclinical sample. *Cognition and Emotion, 10,* 107-112.

Brosschot, J. F., Gerin, W., & Thayer, J. F. (2006).

The perseverative cognition hypothesis: A review of worry, prolonged stress-related physiological activation, and health. *Journal of Psychosomatic Research, 60,* 113–124.

Brown, M. Z., Comtois, K. A., & Linehan, M. M. (2002). Reasons for suicide attempts and nonsuicidal self-injury in women with borderline personality disorder. *Journal of Abnormal Psychology, 111,* 198–202.

Brown, T. A., Chorpita, B. F., Korotitsch, W., & Barlow, D. H. (1997). Psychometric properties of the Depression Anxiety Stress Scales (DASS) in clinical samples. *Behaviour Research and Therapy, 35,* 79–89.

Brown, T. A., DiNardo, P. A., & Barlow, D. H. (1994). *Anxiety Disorders Interview Schedule for DSM-IV.* San Antonio, TX: Psychological Corp.

Bryant, R. A., & Harvey, A. G. (1995). Processing threatening information in posttraumatic stress disorder. *Journal of Abnormal Psychology, 104,* 537–541.

Bryant, R. A., Mastrodomenico, J., Hopwood, S., Kenny, L., Cahill, C., Kandris, E., & Taylor, K. (2013). Augmenting cognitive behaviour therapy for post-traumatic stress disorder with emotion tolerance training: A randomized controlled trial. *Psychological Medicine, 43,* 2153–2160.

Burlingame, G. M., McClendon, D. T., & Alonso, J. (2011). Cohesion in group therapy. In J. C. Norcross (Ed.), *Psychotherapy relationships that work: Evidence-based responsiveness* (2nd ed., pp. 110–131). New York: Oxford University Press.

Bushman, B. J. (2002). Does venting anger feed or extinguish the flame? Catharsis, rumination, distraction, anger, and aggressive responding. *Personality and Social Psychology Bulletin, 28,* 724–731.

Bushman, B. J., Baumeister, R. F., & Stack, A. D. (1999). Catharsis, aggression, and persuasive influence: Self-fulfilling or self-defeating prophecies? *Journal of Personality and Social Psychology, 76,* 367–376.

Butzlaff, R. L., & Hooley, J. M. (1998). Expressed emotion and psychiatric relapse: A meta-analysis. *Archives of General Psychiatry, 55,* 547–552.

Byrne, M., Carr, A., & Clark, M. (2004). The efficacy of couples-based interventions for panic disorder with agoraphobia. *Journal of Family Therapy, 26,* 105–125.

Bywaters, M., Andrade, J., & Turpin, G. (2004). Intrusive and non-intrusive memories in a non-clinical sample: The effects of mood and affect on imagery vividness. *Memory, 12,* 467–478.

Cain, C. K., Blouin, A. M., & Barad, M. (2004). Adrenergic transmission facilitates extinction of conditional fear in mice. *Learning and Memory, 11,* 179–187.

Caldirola, D., Bellodi, L., Caumo, A., Migliarese, G., & Perna, G. (2004). Approximate entropy of respiratory patterns in panic disorder. *American Journal of Psychiatry, 161,* 79–87.

Callaghan, G. M., Summers, C. J., & Weidman, M. (2003). The treatment of histrionic and narcissistic personality disorder behaviors: A single-subject demonstration of clinical improvement using functional analytic psychotherapy. *Journal of Contemporary Psychotherapy, 33,* 321–339.

Campbell-Sills, L., & Barlow, D. H. (2007). Incorporating emotion regulation into conceptualizations and treatments of anxiety and mood disorders. In J. J. Gross (Ed.), *Handbook of emotion regulation* (pp. 542–559). New York: Guilford Press.

Campbell-Sills, L., Barlow, D. H., Brown, T. A., & Hofmann, S. G. (2005). Effects of suppression and acceptance of emotional responses of individuals with anxiety and mood disorders. *Behaviour Research and Therapy, 44,* 1251–1263.

Carlson, C. R., & Hoyle, R. H. (1993). Efficacy of abbreviated progressive muscle relaxation training: A quantitative review of behavioral medicine research. *Journal of Consulting and Clinical Psychology, 61,* 1059–1067.

Carroll, L. J., & Yates, B. T. (1981). Further evidence for the role of stimulus control training in facilitation of weight reduction after behavioral therapy. *Behavior Therapy, 45,* 503.

Carton, J. S., & Schweitzer, J. B. (1996). Use of a token economy to increase compliance during hemodialysis. *Journal of Applied Behavior Analysis, 29,* 111–113.

Castonguay, L. G., & Beutler, L. E. (2006). *Principles of therapeutic change that work.* New York: Oxford University Press.

Chadwick, P., Hughes, S., Russell, D., Russell, I., & Dagnan, D. (2009). Mindfulness groups for distressing voices and paranoia: A replication and randomized feasibility trial. *Behavioural and Cognitive Psychotherapy, 37,* 403–412.

Chambless, D. L., Bryan, A. D., Aiken, L. S., Steketee, G., & Hooley, J. M. (1999). The structure of expressed emotion: A three-construct representation. *Psychological Assessment, 11,* 67–76.

Chambless, D. L., Caputo, G. C., Bright, P., & Gallagher, R. (1984). Assessment of fear of fear in agoraphobics: The Body Sensations Questionnaire and the Agoraphobic Cognitions Questionnaire. *Journal of Consulting and Clinical Psychology, 52,* 1090–1097.

Chaplin, E. W., & Levine, B. A. (1981). The effects of total exposure duration and interrupted versus continuous exposure in flooding therapy. *Behavior Therapy, 12,* 360–368.

Chartrand, T. L., van Baaren, R. B., & Bargh, J. A. (2006). Linking automatic evaluation to mood and information processing style: Consequences for experienced affect, impression formation, and stereotyping. *Journal of Experimental Psychology: General, 135,* 70–77.

Chen, M., & Bargh, J. A. (1999). Consequences of automatic evaluation: Immediate behavioral predispositions to approach and avoid the stimulus. *Personality and Social Psychology Bulletin, 25,* 215–224.

Chiles, J. A., & Strosahl, K. (1995). *The suicidal patient: Principles of assessment, treatment, and case management.* Washington, DC: American Psychiatric Press.

Clark, D. M., Salkovskis, P. M., Hackmann, A., Wells, A., Ludgate, J., & Gelder, M. (1999). Brief cognitive therapy for panic disorder: A randomized controlled trial. *Journal of Consulting and Clinical Psychology, 67,* 583–589.

Clark, L. A., & Watson, D. (1991). Tripartite model of anxiety and depression: Psychometric evidence and taxonomic implications. *Journal of Abnormal Psychology, 100,* 316–336.

Cloitre, M., Courtois, C. A., Charuvastra, A., Carapezza, R., Stolbach, B. C., & Green, B. L. (2011). Treatment of complex PTSD: Results of the ISTSS expert clinician survey on best practices. *Journal of Traumatic Stress, 24,* 615–627.

Cloitre, M., Stovall-McClough, K. C., Nooner, K., Zorbas, P., Cherry, S., Jackson, C. L., . . . Petkova, E. (2010). Treatment for PTSD related to childhood abuse: A randomized controlled trial. *American Journal of Psychiatry, 167,* 915–924.

Coid, J., Yang, M., Tyrer, P., Roberts, A., & Ullrich, S. (2006). Prevalence and correlates of personality disorder in Great Britain. *British Journal of Psychiatry, 188,* 423–431.

Conger, R. D., Ge, X., Elder, G. H., Jr., Lorenz, F. O., & Simons, R. L. (1994). Economic stress, coercive family process, and developmental problems of adolescents. *Child Development, 65,* 541–561.

Conklin, C. Z., Bradley, R., & Westen, D. (2006). Affect regulation in borderline personality disorder. *Journal of Nervous and Mental Disease, 194,* 69–77.

Conrad, A., & Roth, W. T. (2007). Muscle relaxation therapy for anxiety disorders: It works but how? *Journal of Anxiety Disorders, 21,* 243–264.

Cook, R., Brewer, R., Shah, P., & Bird, G. (2013). Alexithymia, not autism, predicts poor recognition of emotional facial expressions. *Psychological Science, 24,* 723–732.

Cooper, M., Cohen-Tovee, E., Todd, G., Wells, A., & Tovee, M. (1997). The Eating Disorder Belief Questionnaire: Preliminary development. *Behaviour Research and Therapy, 35,* 381–388.

Costin, J., & Chambers, S. M. (2007). Parent management training as a treatment for children with oppositional defiant disorder referred to a mental health clinic. *Clinical Child Psychology and Psychiatry, 12,* 511–524.

Cox, B. J., Endler, N. S., Lee, P. S., & Swinson, R. P. (1992). A meta-analysis of treatments for panic disorder with agoraphobia: Imipramine, alprazolam, and in vivo exposure. *Journal of Behavior Therapy and Experimental Psychiatry, 23,* 175–182.

Coyne, J. C. (1976). Toward an interactional description of depression. *Psychiatry, 39,* 28–40.

Craske, M. G., & Barlow, D. H. (2001). Panic disorder and agoraphobia. In D. H. Barlow (Ed.), *Clinical handbook of psychological disorders* (3rd ed., pp. 1–59). New York: Guilford Press.

Craske, M. G., Kircanski, K., Zelikowsky, M., Mystkowski, J., Chowdhury, N., & Baker, A. (2008). Optimizing inhibitory learning during exposure therapy. *Behaviour Research and Therapy, 46,* 5–27.

Craske, M. G., Niles, A. N., Burklund, L. J., Wolitzky-Taylor, K. B., Vilardaga, J. C., Arch, J. J., . . . Lieberman, M. D. (2014). Randomized controlled trial of cognitive behavioral therapy and acceptance and commitment therapy for social phobia: Outcomes and moderators. *Journal of Consulting and Clinical Psychology, 82,* 1034–1048.

Creed, A. T., & Funder, D. C. (1998). Social anxiety: From the inside and outside. *Personality and Individual Differences, 25,* 19–33.

Crowe, L. M., Beauchamp, M. H., Catroppa, C., & Anderson, V. (2011). Social function assessment tools for children and adolescents: A systematic review from 1988 to 2010. *Clinical Psychology Review, 31,* 767–785.

Cuijpers, P., van Straten, A., & Warmerdam, L. (2007a). Behavioral activation treatments of depression: A meta-analysis. *Clinical Psychology Review, 27,* 318–326.

Cuijpers, P., van Straten, A., & Warmerdam, L. (2007b). Problem solving therapies for depression: A meta-analysis. *European Psychiatry, 22,* 9–15.

Curtis, R. C., & Miller, K. (1986). Believing another likes or dislikes you: Behaviors making the beliefs come true. *Journal of Personality and Social Psychology, 51,* 284–290.

D'Cruz, A. M., Ragozzino, M. E., Mosconi, M. W., Shrestha, S., Cook, E. H., & Sweeney, J. A. (2013). Reduced behavioral flexibility in autism spectrum disorders. *Neuropsychology, 27,* 152–160.

D'Zurilla, T. J., Chang, E. C., Nottingham, E. J., & Faccini, L. (1998). Social problem-solving deficits and hopelessness, depression, and suicidal risk in college students and psychiatric inpatients. *Journal of Clinical Psychology, 54,* 1091–1107.

D'Zurilla, T. J., & Goldfried, M. R. (1971). Problem solving and behavior modification. *Journal of Abnormal Psychology, 78,* 107–126.

D'Zurilla, T. J., & Nezu, A. M. (1982). Social problem solving in adults. In P. C. Kendall (Ed.), *Advances in cognitive-behavioral research and therapy* (pp. 201–274). New York: Academic Press.

D'Zurilla, T. J., & Nezu, A. M. (1999). *Problem-solving therapy: A social competence approach to clinical intervention.* New York: Springer.

da Costa, I. G., Rapoff, M. A., Lemanek, K., &

Goldstein, G. L. (1997). Improving adherence to medication regimens for children with asthma and its effect on clinical outcome. *Journal of Applied Behavior Analysis, 30,* 687–691.

Dagnan, D., Chadwick, P., & Proudlove, J. (2000). Toward assessment of suitability of people with mental retardation for cognitive therapy. *Cognitive Therapy and Research, 24,* 627–636.

Daiuto, A. D., Baucom, D. H., Epstein, N., & Dutton, S. S. (1998). The application of behavioral couples therapy to the assessment and treatment of agoraphobia: Implications of empirical research. *Clinical Psychology Review, 18,* 663–687.

Darcy, K., Davila, J., & Beck, J. G. (2005). Is social anxiety associated with both interpersonal avoidance and interpersonal dependence? *Cognitive Therapy and Research, 29,* 171–186.

Datillo, F. M. (2010). *Cognitive-behavioral therapy with couples and families: A comprehensive guide for clinicians.* New York: Guilford Press.

Davey, G. C. L., Tallis, F., & Capuzzo, N. (1996). Beliefs about the consequences of worrying. *Cognitive Therapy and Research, 20,* 499–520.

Davila, J., Hammen, C., Burge, D., Daley, S. E., & Paley, B. (1996). Cognitive/interpersonal correlates of adult interpersonal problem-solving strategies. *Cognitive Therapy and Research, 20,* 465–480.

Davis, P. K., & Rehfeldt, R. A. (2007). Functional skills training for people with intellectual and developmental disabilities. In J. W. Jacobson, J. A. Mulick, & J. Rojahn (Eds.), *Handbook of intellectual and developmental disabilities* (pp. 581–599). New York: Springer.

Dawes, R. M., Faust, D., & Meehl, P. E. (1989). Clinical versus actuarial judgment. *Science, 243,* 1668–1674.

de Berardis, D., Campanella, D., Gambi, F., Sepede, G., Salini, G., Carano, A., . . . Ferro, F. M. (2005). Insight and alexithymia in adult outpatients with obsessive–compulsive disorder. *European Archives of Psychiatry and Clinical Neuroscience, 255,* 350–358.

de Berardis, D., Campanella, D., Nicola, S., Gianna, S., Alessanro, C., Chiara, C., . . . Ferro, F. M. (2008). The impact of alexithymia on anxiety disorders: A review of the literature. *Current Psychiatry Reviews, 4,* 80–86.

De Gucht, V., & Heiser, W. (2003). Alexithymia and somatisation: Quantitative review of the literature. *Journal of Psychosomatic Research, 54,* 425–434.

de Panfilis, C., Ossola, P., Tonna, M., Catania, L., & Marchesi, C. (2015). Finding words for feelings: The relationship between personality disorders and alexithymia. *Personality and Individual Differences, 74,* 285–291.

de Shazer, S. (1988). *Clues: Investigating solutions in brief therapy.* New York: Norton.

Deacon, B. J., Fawzy, T. I., Lickel, J. J., & Wolitzky-Taylor, K. B. (2011). Cognitive defusion versus cognitive restructuring in the treatment of negative self-referential thoughts: An investigation of process and outcome. *Journal of Cognitive Psychotherapy, 25,* 218–232.

Deacon, B. J., & Maack, D. J. (2008). The effects of safety behaviors on the fear of contamination: An experimental investigation. *Behaviour Research and Therapy, 46,* 537–547.

Deacon, B. J., Sy, J. T., Lickel, J. J., & Nelson, E. A. (2010). Does the judicious use of safety behaviors improve the efficacy and acceptability of exposure therapy for claustrophobic fear? *Journal of Behavior Therapy and Experimental Psychiatry, 41,* 71–80.

Deci, E. L., Koestner, R., & Ryan, R. M. (1999). A meta-analytic review of experiments examining the effects of extrinsic rewards on intrinsic motivation. *Psychological Bulletin, 125,* 627–668; discussion 692–700.

Deckersbach, T., Holzel, B. K., Eisner, L. R., Stange, J. P., Peckham, A. D., Dougherty, D. D., . . . Nierenberg, A. A. (2012). Mindfulness-based cognitive therapy for nonremitted patients with bipolar disorder. *CNS Neuroscience and Therapeutics, 18,* 133–141.

Deffenbacher, J. L. (2011). Cognitive-behavioral conceptualization and treatment of anger. *Cognitive and Behavioral Practice, 18,* 212–221.

Deffenbacher, J. L., Filetti, L. B., Lynch, R. S., Dahlen, E. R., & Oetting, E. R. (2002). Cognitive-behavioral treatment of high anger drivers. *Behaviour Research and Therapy, 40,* 895–910.

Deffenbacher, J. L., Lynch, R. S., Oetting, E. R., & Kemper, C. C. (1996). Anger reduction in early adolescents. *Journal of Counseling Psychology, 43,* 149–157.

Deffenbacher, J. L., & Stark, R. S. (1992). Relaxation and cognitive-relaxation treatments of general anger. *Journal of Counseling Psychology, 39,* 158–167.

Delgado, M. R., Nearing, K. I., Ledoux, J. E., & Phelps, E. A. (2008). Neural circuitry underlying the regulation of conditioned fear and its relation to extinction. *Neuron, 59,* 829–838.

Dempsey, J. A., Forster, H. V., Gledhill, N., & doPico, G. A. (1975). Effects of moderate hypoxemia and hypocapnia on CSF [H+] and ventilation in man. *Journal of Applied Physiology, 38,* 665–674.

Derogatis, L. R. (1992). *The Symptom Checklist–90 Revised.* Minneapolis, MN: NCS Assessments.

DeRubeis, R. J., Evans, M. D., Hollon, S. D., Garvey, M. J., Grove, W. M., & Tuason, V. B. (1990). How does cognitive therapy work? Cognitive change and symptom change in cognitive therapy and pharmacotherapy for depression. *Journal of Consulting and Clinical Psychology, 58,* 862–869.

DiClemente, R. J., & Wingood, G. M. (1995). A randomized controlled trial of an HIV sexual risk-reduction intervention for young African-American women. *Journal of the American Medical Association, 274,* 1271–1276.

Diekhof, E. K., Geier, K., Falkai, P., & Gruber, O. (2011). Fear is only as deep as the mind allows: A coordinate-based meta-analysis of neuroimaging studies on the regulation of negative affect. *Neuro-Image, 58,* 275–285.

Diener, E., Emmons, R. A., Larsen, R. J., & Griffin, S. (1985). The Satisfaction with Life Scale. *Journal of Personality Assessment, 49,* 71–75.

Dimidjian, S., Hollon, S. D., Dobson, K. S., Schmaling, K. B., Kohlenberg, R. J., Addis, M. E., . . . Jacobson, N. S. (2006). Randomized trial of behavioral activation, cognitive therapy, and antidepressant medication in the acute treatment of adults with major depression. *Journal of Consulting and Clinical Psychology, 74,* 658–670.

Dobson, K. S. (1989). A meta-analysis of the efficacy of cognitive therapy for depression. *Journal of Consulting and Clinical Psychology, 57,* 414–419.

Doty, D. W. (1975). Role playing and incentives in the modification of the social interaction of chronic psychiatric patients. *Journal of Consulting and Clinical Psychology, 43,* 676–682.

Duckworth, M. P. (2003). Assertiveness skills and the management of related factors. In W. O'Donohue, J. E. Fisher, & S. C. Hayes (Eds.), *Cognitive behavior therapy: Applying empirically supported techniques in your practice* (pp. 16–22). Hoboken, NJ: Wiley.

Dugas, M. J., Freeston, M. H., & Ladouceur, R. (1997). Intolerance of uncertainty and problem orientation in worry. *Cognitive Therapy and Research, 21,* 593–606.

Dworkin, R. H., Turk, D. C., Revicki, D. A., Harding, G., Coyne, K. S., Peirce-Sandner, S., . . . Melzack, R. (2009). Development and initial validation of an expanded and revised version of the Short-Form McGill Pain Questionnaire (SF-MPQ-2). *Pain, 144,* 35–42.

Dykman, B. M., Horowitz, L. M., Abramson, L. Y., & Usher, M. (1991). Schematic and situational determinants of depressed and nondepressed students' interpretation of feedback. *Journal of Abnormal Psychology, 100,* 45–55.

Edinger, J. D., Wohlgemuth, W. K., Radtke, R. A., Marsh, G. R., & Quillian, R. E. (2001). Cognitive behavioral therapy for treatment of chronic primary insomnia: A randomized controlled trial. *Journal of the American Medical Association, 285,* 1856–1864.

Ehlers, A., & Breuer, P. (1992). Increased cardiac awareness in panic disorder. *Journal of Abnormal Psychology, 101,* 371–382.

Ehlers, A., Mayou, R. A., & Bryant, B. (1998). Psychological predictors of chronic posttraumatic stress disorder after motor vehicle accidents. *Journal of Abnormal Psychology, 107,* 508–519.

Ehring, T., Welboren, R., Morina, N., Wicherts, J. M., Freitag, J., & Emmelkamp, P. M. G. (2014). Meta-analysis of psychological treatments for posttraumatic stress disorder in adult survivors of childhood abuse. *Clinical Psychology Review, 34,* 645–657.

Eich, E. (1995). Searching for mood dependent memory. *Psychological Science, 6,* 67–75.

Eisler, R. M., Frederiksen, L. W., & Peterson, G. L. (1978). The relationship of cognitive variables to the expression of assertiveness. *Behavior Therapy, 9,* 419–427.

Eisler, R. M., Miller, P. M., & Hersen, M. (1973). Components of assertive behavior. *Journal of Clinical Psychology, 29,* 295–299.

Ekers, D., Carman, S., & Schlich, T. (2004). Successful outcome of exposure and response prevention in the treatment of obsessive compulsive disorder in a patient with schizophrenia. *Behavioural and Cognitive Psychotherapy, 32,* 375–378.

Ekman, P. (1992a). An argument for basic emotions. *Cognition and Emotion, 6,* 169–200.

Ekman, P. (1992b). Facial expressions of emotion: An old controversy and new findings. *Philosophical Transactions of the Royal Society of London. Series B: Biological Sciences, 335,* 63–69.

Eldar, S., & Bar-Haim, Y. (2010). Neural plasticity in response to attention training in anxiety. *Psychological Medicine, 40,* 667–677.

Elder, G. H., Caspi, A., & Downey, D. (1983). Problem behavior in family relationships: A multigenerational analysis. In A. Sorensen, F. Weinert, & L. Sherrod (Eds.), *Human development: Interdisciplinary perspective* (pp. 93–118). Hillsdale, NJ: Erlbaum.

Ellard, K. K., Fairholme, C. P., Boisseau, C. L., Farchione, T. J., & Barlow, D. H. (2010). Unified protocol for the transdiagnostic treatment of emotional disorders: Protocol development and initial outcome data. *Cognitive and Behavioral Practice, 17,* 88–101.

Elliott, R. (2003). Executive functions and their disorders. *British Medical Bulletin, 65,* 49–59.

Elliott, S. N., & Gresham, F. M. (1993). Social skills interventions for children. *Behavior Modification, 17,* 287–313.

Ellis, A. (1977). The basic clinical theory of rational-emotive therapy. In A. Ellis & R. Grieger (Eds.), *Handbook of rational-emotive therapy* (pp. 3–34). New York: Springer.

Ellis, A. (2001). *Overcoming destructive beliefs, feelings, and behaviors: New directions for rational emotive behavior therapy.* Amherst, NY: Prometheus Books.

Endicott, J., Nee, J., Harrison, W., & Blumenthal, R. (1993). Quality of Life Enjoyment and Satisfaction Questionnaire: A new measure. *Psychopharmacology Bulletin, 29,* 321–326.

Engle-Friedman, M. (1994). Primary insomnia. In C. G. Last & M. Hersen (Eds.), *Adult behavior therapy casebook* (pp. 279–294). New York: Plenum Press.

Epstein, L. H., Masek, B. J., & Marshall, W. R. (1978). A nutritionally based school program for control of eating in obese children. *Behavior Therapy, 9,* 766–778.

Epstein, N. B., & Baucom, D. H. (2002). *Enhanced cognitive-behavioral therapy for couples: A contextual approach.* Washington, DC: American Psychological Association.

Epstein, N. B., Baucom, D. H., & Rankin, L. A. (1993). Treatment of marital conflict: A cognitive-behavioral approach. *Clinical Psychology Review, 13,* 45–57.

Eskin, M., Ertekin, K., & Demir, H. (2008). Efficacy of a problem-solving therapy for depression and suicide potential in adolescents and young adults. *Cognitive Therapy and Research, 32,* 227–245.

Esteves, F., Parra, C., Dimberg, U., & Ohman, A. (1994). Nonconscious associative learning: Pavlovian conditioning of skin conductance responses to masked fear-relevant facial stimuli. *Psychophysiology, 31,* 375–385.

Fairburn, C., & Beglin, S. (2008). Eating Disorder Examination. In C. Fairburn (Ed.), *Cognitive behavior therapy and eating disorders* (pp. 265–308). New York: Guilford Press.

Farb, N. A., Anderson, A. K., Mayberg, H., Bean, J., McKeon, D., & Segal, Z. V. (2010). Minding one's emotions: Mindfulness training alters the neural expression of sadness. *Emotion, 10,* 25–33.

Farb, N. A., Segal, Z. V., Mayberg, H., Bean, J., McKeon, D., Fatima, Z., & Anderson, A. K. (2007). Attending to the present: Mindfulness meditation reveals distinct neural modes of self-reference. *Social Cognitive and Affective Neuroscience, 2,* 313–322.

Feeny, N. C., Hembree, E. A., & Zoellner, L. A. (2003). Myths regarding exposure therapy for PTSD. *Cognitive and Behavioral Practice, 10,* 85–90.

Ferster, C. B. (1972). Clinical reinforcement. *Seminars in Psychiatry, 4,* 101–111.

Ferster, C. B. (1973). A functional analysis of depression. *American Psychologist, 28,* 857–870.

Festinger, L. (1962). Cognitive dissonance. *Scientific American, 207,* 93–102.

First, M. B., Spitzer, R. L., Gibbon, M., & Williams, J. B. W. (1995). *Structured Clinical Interview for DSM-IV Axis I Disorders–Patient Edition (SCID I/P, version 2.0).* New York: Biometrics Research Department.

Flor, H., & Turk, D. C. (2011). *Chronic pain: An integrated biobehavioral approach.* Seattle, WA: IASP Press.

Flynn, L., & Healy, O. (2012). A review of treatments for deficits in social skills and self-help skills in autism spectrum disorders. *Research in Autism Spectrum Disorders, 6,* 431–441.

Foa, E. B., Ehlers, A., Clark, D. M., Tolin, D. F., & Orsillo, S. M. (1999). The Post-Traumatic Cognitions Inventory (PTCI): Development and validation. *Psychological Assessment, 11,* 303–314.

Foa, E. B., & Kozak, M. J. (1986). Emotional processing of fear: Exposure to corrective information. *Psychological Bulletin, 99,* 20–35.

Foa, E. B., Kozak, M. J., Goodman, W. K., Hollander, E., Jenike, M. A., & Rasmussen, S. A. (1995). DSM-IV field trial: Obsessive–compulsive disorder. *American Journal of Psychiatry, 152,* 90–96.

Foa, E. B., Liebowitz, M. R., Kozak, M. J., Davies, S., Campeas, R., Franklin, M. E., . . . Tu, X. (2005). Randomized, placebo-controlled trial of exposure and ritual prevention, clomipramine, and their combination in the treatment of obsessive-compulsive disorder. *American Journal of Psychiatry, 162,* 151–161.

Foa, E. B., Riggs, D. S., Dancu, C. V., & Rothbaum, B. O. (1993). Reliability and validity of a brief instrument for assessing post-traumatic stress disorder. *Journal of Traumatic Stress, 6,* 459–473.

Foa, E. B., & Rothbaum, B. O. (1998). *Treating the trauma of rape: Cognitive-behavioral therapy for PTSD.* New York: Guilford Press.

Foa, E. B., Zoellner, L. A., Feeny, N. C., Hembree, E. A., & Alvarez-Conrad, J. (2002). Does imaginal exposure exacerbate PTSD symptoms? *Journal of Consulting and Clinical Psychology, 70,* 1022–1028.

Folstein, M. F., Folstein, S. E., & McHugh, P. R. (1975). Mini-mental state: A practical method for grading the cognitive state of patients for clinicians. *Journal of Psychiatric Research, 12,* 189–198.

Forman, E. M., Herbert, J. D., Moitra, E., Yeomans, P. D., & Geller, P. A. (2007). A randomized controlled effectiveness trial of acceptance and commitment therapy and cognitive therapy for anxiety and depression. *Behavior Modification, 31,* 772–799.

Fox, L. (1962). Effecting the use of efficient study habits. *Journal of Mathematics, 1,* 75–86.

Frank, E., & Levenson, J. (2010). *Interpersonal psychotherapy.* Washington, DC: American Psychological Association.

Frank, J. D. (1974). *Persuasion and healing* (rev. ed.). New York: Schocken Books.

Franklin, M. E., & Tolin, D. F. (2007). *Treating trichotillomania: Cognitive behavior therapy for hair pulling and related problems.* New York: Springer.

Frederick, B. P., & Olmi, D. J. (1994). Children with attention-deficit/hyperactivity disorder: A review of the literature on social skills deficits. *Psychology in the Schools, 31,* 288–296.

Freedman, J. L., & Fraser, S. C. (1966). Compliance without pressure: The foot-in-the-door technique. *Journal of Personality and Social Psychology, 4,* 195–202.

Freeman, D., Garety, P. A., Kuipers, E., Fowler, D., Bebbington, P. E., & Dunn, G. (2007). Acting on persecutory delusions: The importance of safety seeking. *Behaviour Research and Therapy, 45,* 89–99.

Freeston, M. H., Gagnon, F., Ladouceur, R., Thibodeau, N., Letarte, H., & Rheaume, J. (1994).

Health-related intrusive thoughts. *Journal of Psychosomatic Research, 38,* 203–215.

Freud, S. (1958). The dynamics of transference. In J. Strachey (Ed., & Trans.), *The standard edition of the complete psychological works of Sigmund Freud* (Vol. 12, pp. 99–108). London: Hogarth Press. (Original work published 1912)

Freud, S. (1965). *New introductory lectures on psychoanalysis.* New York: Norton. (Original work published 1933)

Frewen, P. A., Dozois, D. J., Neufeld, R. W., & Lanius, R. A. (2008). Meta-analysis of alexithymia in post-traumatic stress disorder. *Journal of Traumatic Stress, 21,* 243–246.

Fried, R. (1993). The role of respiration in stress and stress control: Toward a theory of stress as a hypoxic phenomenon. In P. M. Lehrer & R. L. Woolfolk (Eds.), *Principles and practice of stress management* (pp. 301–331). New York: Guilford Press.

Friedberg, R. D. (2006). A cognitive-behavioral approach to family therapy. *Journal of Contemporary Psychotherapy, 36,* 159–165.

Frijda, N. H. (1987). Emotion, cognitive structure, and action tendency. *Cognition and Emotion, 1,* 115–143.

Frisch, M. B., Cornell, J., Villanueva, M., & Retzlaff, P. J. (1992). Clinical validation of the Quality of Life Inventory: A measure of life satisfaction for use in treatment planning and outcome assessment. *Psychological Assessment: A Journal of Consulting and Clinical Psychology, 4,* 92–101.

Frueh, B. C., Grubaugh, A. L., Cusack, K. J., Kimble, M. O., Elhai, J. D., & Knapp, R. G. (2009). Exposure-based cognitive-behavioral treatment of PTSD in adults with schizophrenia or schizoaffective disorder: A pilot study. *Journal of Anxiety Disorders, 23,* 665–675.

Frye-Cox, N. E., & Hesse, C. R. (2013). Alexithymia and marital quality: The mediating roles of loneliness and intimate communication. *Journal of Family Psychology, 27,* 203–211.

Fydrich, T., Chambless, D. L., Perry, K. J., Buergener, F., & Beazley, M. B. (1998). Behavioral assessment of social performance: A rating system for social phobia. *Behaviour Research and Therapy, 36,* 995–1010.

Gabbard, G. O. (2014). *Psychodynamic psychiatry in clinical practice: DSM-5 edition* (5th ed.). Washington, DC: American Psychiatric Press.

Gallagher-Thompson, D., Arean, P., Rivera, P., & Thompson, L. W. (2001). A psychoeducational intervention to reduce distress in Hispanic family caregivers: Results of a pilot study. *Clinical Gerontologist, 23,* 17–32.

Garb, H. N. (2005). Clinical judgment and decision making. *Annual Review of Clinical Psychology, 1,* 67–89.

Garland, E. L., Manusov, E. G., Froeliger, B., Kelly, A., Williams, J. M., & Howard, M. O. (2014). Mindfulness-oriented recovery enhancement for chronic pain and prescription opioid misuse: Results from an early-stage randomized controlled trial. *Journal of Consulting and Clinical Psychology, 82,* 448–459.

Gaudiano, B. A., & Herbert, J. D. (2006). Acute treatment of inpatients with psychotic symptoms using acceptance and commitment therapy: Pilot results. *Behaviour Research and Therapy, 44,* 415–437.

Geen, R. G., Stonner, D., & Shope, G. L. (1975). The facilitation of aggression by aggression: Evidence against the catharsis hypothesis. *Journal of Personality and Social Psychology, 31,* 721–726.

Gerard, H. B., & Mathewson, G. C. (1966). The effects of severity of initiation on liking for a group: A replication. *Journal of Experimental Social Psychology, 2,* 278–287.

Gilbert, C. (1999). Hyperventilation and the body. *Accident and Emergency Nursing, 7,* 130–140.

Gilboa-Schechtman, E., Foa, E. B., Shafran, N., Aderka, I. M., Powers, M. B., Rachamim, L., . . . Apter, A. (2010). Prolonged exposure versus dynamic therapy for adolescent PTSD: A pilot randomized controlled trial. *Journal of the American Academy of Child and Adolescent Psychiatry, 49,* 1034–1042.

Glass, C. R., & Arnkoff, D. B. (1989). Behavioral assessment of social anxiety and social phobia. *Clinical Psychology Review, 9,* 75–90.

Glombiewski, J. A., Sawyer, A. T., Gutermann, J., Koenig, K., Rief, W., & Hofmann, S. G. (2010). Psychological treatments for fibromyalgia: A meta-analysis. *Pain, 151,* 280–295.

Goldfried, M. R. (1982). Resistance and clinical behavior therapy. In P. L. Wachtel (Ed.), *Resistance: Psychodynamic and behavioral approaches* (pp. 95–113). New York: Plenum Press.

Goldfried, M. R., & Davison, G. C. (1994). *Clinical behavior therapy.* New York: Wiley.

Goldstein, A. P., & Kanfer, F. H. (1979). *Maximizing treatment gains: Transfer enhancement in psychotherapy.* New York: Academic Press.

Goodman, W. K., Price, L. H., Rasmussen, S. A., Mazure, C., Fleischmann, R. L., Hill, C. L., . . . Charney, D. S. (1989). The Yale–Brown Obsessive-Compulsive Scale: I. Development, use, and reliability. *Archives of General Psychiatry, 46,* 1006–1011.

Gotlib, I. H. (1983). Perception and recall of interpersonal feedback: Negative bias in depression. *Cognitive Therapy and Research, 7,* 399–412.

Gotlib, I. H., & Robinson, L. A. (1982). Responses to depressed individuals: Discrepancies between self-report and observer-rated behavior. *Journal of Abnormal Psychology, 91,* 231–240.

Gottman, J. M. (1999). *The marriage clinic: A scientifically based marital therapy.* New York: Norton.

Gottman, J. M., Markman, H., & Notarius, C. (1977). The topography of marital conflict: A sequential analysis of verbal and nonverbal behavior. *Journal of Marriage and the Family, 39,* 461–477.

Gottman, J. M., Notarius, C., Markman, H., Bank, S., Yoppi, B., & Rubin, M. E. (1976). Behavior exchange theory and marital decision making. *Journal of Personality and Social Psychology, 34,* 14–23.

Granholm, E., Holden, J., Link, P. C., & McQuaid, J. R. (2014). Randomized clinical trial of cognitive behavioral social skills training for schizophrenia: Improvement in functioning and experiential negative symptoms. *Journal of Consulting and Clinical Psychology, 82,* 1173–1185.

Gratz, K. L., & Gunderson, J. G. (2006). Preliminary data on an acceptance-based emotion regulation group intervention for deliberate self-harm among women with borderline personality disorder. *Behavior Therapy, 37,* 25–35.

Gratz, K. L., & Roemer, L. (2004). Multidimensional assessment of emotion regulation and dysregulation: Development, factor structure, and initial validation of the Difficulties in Emotion Regulation Scale. *Journal of Psychopathology and Behavioral Assessment, 26,* 41–54.

Gratz, K. L., Tull, M. T., & Levy, R. (2013). Randomized controlled trial and uncontrolled 9-month follow-up of an adjunctive emotion regulation group therapy for deliberate self-harm among women with borderline personality disorder. *Psychological Medicine, 44,* 2099–2112.

Grave, J., & Blissett, J. (2004). Is cognitive behavior therapy developmentally appropriate for young children? A critical review of the evidence. *Clinical Psychology Review, 24,* 399–420.

Grayson, J. B., Foa, E. B., & Steketee, G. (1982). Habituation during exposure treatment: Distraction vs. attention-focusing. *Behaviour Research and Therapy, 20,* 323–328.

Grecucci, A., Pappaianni, E., Siugzdaite, R., Theunnick, A., & Job, R. (2015). Mindful emotion regulation: Exploring the neurocognitive mechanisms behind mindfulness. *BioMed Research International, 2015,* Article ID670724, 9 pp.

Green, C. E., Freeman, D., Kuipers, E., Bebbington, P., Fowler, D., Dunn, G., & Garety, P. A. (2008). Measuring ideas of persecution and social reference: The Green et al. Paranoid Thought Scales (GPTS). *Psychological Medicine, 38,* 101–111.

Greenberg, L. S. (2004). Emotion-focused therapy. *Clinical Psychology and Psychotherapy, 11,* 3–16.

Greenberg, L. S., & Safran, J. D. (1987). *Emotion in psychotherapy: Affect, cognition, and the process of change.* New York: Guilford Press.

Greenberger, D., & Padesky, C. A. (2016). *Mind over mood* (2nd ed.): *Change how you feel by changing the way you think.* New York: Guilford Press.

Greenstein, D. K., Franklin, M. E., & McGuffin, P.

(1999). Measuring motivation to change: An examination of the University of Rhode Island Change Assessment Questionnaire (URICA) in an adolescent sample. *Psychotherapy and Psychosomatics, 36,* 47–55.

Grilo, C. M., Stout, R. L., Markowitz, J. C., Sanislow, C. A., Ansell, E. B., Skodol, A. E., . . . McGlashan, T. H. (2010). Personality disorders predict relapse after remission from an episode of major depressive disorder: A 6-year prospective study. *Journal of Clinical Psychiatry, 71,* 1629–1635.

Gross, J. J. (1998). The emerging field of emotion regulation: An integrative review. *Review of General Psychology, 2,* 271–299.

Gross, J. J., & Thompson, R. A. (2007). Emotion regulation: Conceptual foundations. In J. J. Gross (Ed.), *Handbook of emotion regulation* (pp. 3–24). New York: Guilford Press.

Gross, P. R., & Eifert, G. H. (1990). Components of generalized anxiety: The role of intrusive thoughts vs. worry. *Behaviour Research and Therapy, 28,* 421–428.

Groves, P. M., & Thompson, R. F. (1970). Habituation: A dual-process theory. *Psychological Review, 77,* 419–450.

Grynberg, D., Chang, B., Corneille, O., Maurage, P., Vermeulen, N., Berthoz, S., & Luminet, O. (2012). Alexithymia and the processing of emotional facial expressions (EFEs): Systematic review, unanswered questions and further perspectives. *PLoS ONE, 7,* e42429.

Gulpek, D., Kelemence Kaplan, F., Kesebir, S., & Bora, O. (2014). Alexithymia in patients with conversion disorder. *Nordic Journal of Psychiatry, 68,* 300–305.

Gunderson, J. G. (2011). Clinical practice: Borderline personality disorder. *New England Journal of Medicine, 364,* 2037–2042.

Gutierrez, O., Luciano, C., Rodriguez, M., & Fink, B. C. (2004). Comparison between an acceptance-based and a cognitive-control-based protocol for coping with pain. *Behavior Therapy, 35,* 767–783.

Hagenaars, M. A., van Minnen, A., & Hoogduin, K. A. L. (2010). The impact of dissociation and depression on the efficacy of prolonged exposure treatment for PTSD. *Behaviour Research and Therapy, 48,* 19–27.

Hahlweg, K., & Markman, H. J. (1988). Effectiveness of behavioral marital therapy: Empirical status of behavioral techniques in preventing and alleviating marital distress. *Journal of Consulting and Clinical Psychology, 56,* 440–447.

Hall, S. M., & Hall, R. G. (1982). Clinical series in the behavioral treatment of obesity. *Health Psychology, 1,* 359–372.

Hallion, L. S., & Ruscio, A. M. (2011). A meta-analysis of the effect of cognitive bias modification on anxiety and depression. *Psychological Bulletin, 137,* 940–958.

Hallion, L. S., Ruscio, A. M., & Jha, A. P. (2014). Fractionating the role of executive control in control over worry: A preliminary investigation. *Behaviour Research and Therapy, 54*, 1–6.

Halvorsen, J. O., Stenmark, H., Neuner, F., & Nordahl, H. M. (2014). Does dissociation moderate treatment outcomes of narrative exposure therapy for PTSD?: A secondary analysis from a randomized controlled clinical trial. *Behaviour Research and Therapy, 57*, 21–28.

Harley, R. M., Baity, M. R., Blais, M. A., & Jacobo, M. C. (2007). Use of dialectical behavior therapy skills training for borderline personality disorder in a naturalistic setting. *Psychotherapy Research, 17*, 351–358.

Harley, R. M., Sprich, S., Safren, S., Jacobo, M. C., & Fava, M. (2008). Adaptation of dialectical behavior therapy skills training group for treatment-resistant depression. *Journal of Nervous and Mental Disease, 196*, 136–143.

Harned, M. S., Korslund, K. E., & Linehan, M. M. (2014). A pilot randomized controlled trial of dialectical behavior therapy with and without the dialectical behavior therapy prolonged exposure protocol for suicidal and self-injuring women with borderline personality disorder and PTSD. *Behaviour Research and Therapy, 55*, 7–17.

Harrell, A. W., Mercer, S. H., & DeRosier, M. E. (2009). Improving the social-behavioral adjustment of adolescents: The effectiveness of a social skills group intervention. *Journal of Child and Family Studies, 18*, 378–387.

Hartmann, A. S., Thomas, J. J., Greenberg, J. L., Rosenfield, E. H., & Wilhelm, S. (2015). Accept, distract, or reframe? An exploratory experimental comparison of strategies for coping with intrusive body image thoughts in anorexia nervosa and body dysmorphic disorder. *Psychiatry Research, 225*(3), 643–650.

Hatcher, S., Sharon, C., Parag, V., & Collins, N. (2011). Problem-solving therapy for people who present to hospital with self-harm: Zelen randomised controlled trial. *British Journal of Psychiatry, 199*, 310–316.

Hawton, K., & Kirk, J. (1989). Problem-solving. In K. Hawton, P. M. Salkovskis, J. Kirk, & D. M. Clark (Eds.), *Cognitive behaviour therapy for psychiatric problems: A practical guide* (pp. 406–426). New York: Oxford University Press.

Hayes, S. C. (Ed.). (1989). *Rule-governed behavior: Cognition, contingencies, and instructional control.* New York: Plenum Press.

Hayes, S. C., & Pankey, J. (2003). Acceptance. In W. O'Donohue, J. E. Fisher, & S. C. Hayes (Eds.), *Cognitive behavior therapy: Applying empirically supported techniques in your practice* (pp. 4–9). Hoboken, NJ: Wiley.

Hayes, S. C., Strosahl, K. D., & Wilson, K. G. (1999). *Acceptance and commitment therapy: An experiential approach to behavior change.* New York: Guilford Press.

Hayes, S. C., Strosahl, K. D., & Wilson, K. G. (2012). *Acceptance and commitment therapy* (2nd ed.): *The process and practice of mindful change.* New York: Guilford Press.

Hayes-Skelton, S. A., Roemer, L., & Orsillo, S. M. (2013). A randomized clinical trial comparing an acceptance-based behavior therapy to applied relaxation for generalized anxiety disorder. *Journal of Consulting and Clinical Psychology, 81*, 761–773.

Hayes-Skelton, S. A., Usmani, A., Lee, J. K., Roemer, L., & Orsillo, S. M. (2012). A fresh look at potential mechanisms of change in applied relaxation for generalized anxiety disorder: A case series. *Cognitive and Behavioral Practice, 19*, 451–462.

Hedtke, K. A., Kendall, P. C., & Tiwari, S. (2009). Safety-seeking and coping behavior during exposure tasks with anxious youth. *Journal of Clinical Child and Adolescent Psychology, 38*, 1–15.

Heimberg, R. G., & Becker, R. E. (2002). *Cognitive-behavioral group therapy for social phobia: Basic mechanisms and clinical strategies.* New York: Guilford Press.

Heimberg, R. G., Horner, K. J., Juster, H. R., Safren, S. A., Brown, E. J., Schneier, F. R., & Liebowitz, M. R. (1999). Psychometric properties of the Liebowitz Social Anxiety Scale. *Psychological Medicine, 29*, 199–212.

Heimberg, R. G., Liebowitz, M. R., Hope, D. A., Schneier, F. R., Holt, C. S., Welkowitz, L. A., . . . Klein, D. F. (1998). Cognitive behavioral group therapy versus phenelzine therapy for social phobia: 12-week outcome. *Archives of General Psychiatry, 55*, 1133–1141.

Heimberg, R. G., Montgomery, D., Madsen, C. H., & Heimberg, J. S. (1977). Assertion training: A review of the literature. *Behavior Therapy, 8*, 953–971.

Hembree, E. A., Foa, E. B., Dorfan, N. M., Street, G. P., Kowalski, J., & Tu, X. (2003). Do patients drop out prematurely from exposure therapy for PTSD? *Journal of Traumatic Stress, 16*, 555–562.

Herbert, J. D., Gaudiano, B. A., Rheingold, A. A., Myers, V. H., Dalrymple, K., & Nolan, E. M. (2005). Social skills training augments the effectiveness of cognitive behavioral group therapy for social anxiety disorder. *Behavior Therapy, 36*, 125–138.

Herrnstein, R. J. (1970). On the law of effect. *Journal of the Experimental Analysis of Behavior, 13*, 243–266.

Hersen, M. (1976). Token economies in institutional settings: Historical, political, deprivation, ethical, and generalization issues. *Journal of Nervous and Mental Disease, 162*, 206–211.

Hester, R., Dixon, V., & Garavan, H. (2006). A consistent attentional bias for drug-related material in active cocaine users across word and picture versions of the emotional Stroop task. *Drug and Alcohol Dependence, 81,* 251–257.

Hinton, D. E., Chhean, D., Pich, V., Safren, S. A., Hofmann, S. G., & Pollack, M. H. (2005). A randomized controlled trial of cognitive-behavior therapy for Cambodian refugees with treatment-resistant PTSD and panic attacks: A cross-over design. *Journal of Traumatic Stress, 18,* 617–629.

Hofmann, S. G. (2008). Common misconceptions about cognitive mediation of treatment change: A commentary to Longmore and Worrell (2007). *Clinical Psychology Review, 28,* 67–70.

Hofmann, S. G., & Asmundson, G. J. (2008). Acceptance and mindfulness-based therapy: New wave or old hat? *Clinical Psychology Review, 28,* 1–16.

Hofmann, S. G., Heering, S., Sawyer, A. T., & Asnaani, A. (2009). How to handle anxiety: The effects of reappraisal, acceptance, and suppression strategies on anxious arousal. *Behaviour Research and Therapy, 47,* 389–394.

Hoge, E. A., Bui, E., Marques, L., Metcalf, C. A., Morris, L. K., Robinaugh, D. J., . . . Simon, N. M. (2013). Randomized controlled trial of mindfulness meditation for generalized anxiety disorder: Effects on anxiety and stress reactivity. *Journal of Clinical Psychiatry, 74,* 786–792.

Hollon, S. D., & Kendall, P. C. (1980). Cognitive self-statements in depression: Development of an automatic thoughts questionnaire. *Cognitive Therapy and Research, 4,* 383–395.

Hölzel, B. K., Lazar, S. W., Gard, T., Schuman-Olivier, Z., Vago, D. R., & Ott, U. (2011). How does mindfulness meditation work? Proposing mechanisms of action from a conceptual and neural perspective. *Perspectives on Psychological Science, 6,* 537–559.

Hong, R. Y. (2007). Worry and rumination: Differential associations with anxious and depressive symptoms and coping behavior. *Behaviour Research and Therapy, 45,* 277–290.

Hood, H. K., Antony, M. M., Koerner, N., & Monson, C. M. (2010). Effects of safety behaviors on fear reduction during exposure. *Behaviour Research and Therapy, 48,* 1161–1169.

Hooley, J. M. (1985). Expressed emotion: A review of the critical literature. *Clinical Psychology Review, 5,* 119–139.

Horley, K., Williams, L. M., Gonsalvez, C., & Gordon, E. (2003). Social phobics do not see eye to eye: A visual scanpath study of emotional expression processing. *Journal of Anxiety Disorders, 17,* 33–44.

Horney, K. (1950). *Neurosis and human growth: The struggle toward self-realization.* New York: Norton.

Houck, P. R., Spiegel, D. A., Shear, M. K., & Rucci, P. (2002). Reliability of the self-report version of the Panic Disorder Severity Scale. *Depression and Anxiety, 15,* 183–185.

Hunt, M. G. (1998). The only way out is through: Emotional processing and recovery after a depressing life event. *Behaviour Research and Therapy, 36,* 361–384.

Huppert, J. D., Bufka, L. F., Barlow, D. H., Gorman, J. M., Shear, M. K., & Woods, S. W. (2001). Therapists, therapist variables, and cognitive-behavioral therapy outcome in a multicenter trial for panic disorder. *Journal of Consulting and Clinical Psychology, 69,* 747–755.

Husain, N., Afsar, S., Ara, J., Fayyaz, H., Rahman, R. U., Tomenson, B., . . . Chaudhry, I. B. (2014). Brief psychological intervention after self-harm: Randomised controlled trial from Pakistan. *British Journal of Psychiatry, 204,* 462–470.

Ilardi, S. S., Craighead, W. E., & Evans, D. D. (1997). Modeling relapse in unipolar depression: The effects of dysfunctional cognitions and personality disorders. *Journal of Consulting and Clinical Psychology, 65,* 381–391.

Institute of Medicine. (2008). *Treatment of posttraumatic stress disorder: An assessment of the evidence.* Washington, DC: National Academies Press.

Ison, M. S. (2001). Training in social skills: An alternative technique for handling disruptive child behavior. *Psychological Reports, 88,* 903–911.

Izard, C. E. (1977). *Human emotions.* New York: Plenum Press.

Izard, C. E., & Ackerman, B. P. (2000). Motivational, organizational, and regulatory functions of discrete emotions. In M. Lewis & J. M. Haviland-Jones (Eds.), *Handbook of emotions* (2nd ed., pp. 253–264). New York: Guilford Press.

Izci, F., Gultekin, B. K., Saglam, S., Koc, M. I., Zincir, S. B., & Atmaca, M. (2014). Temperament, character traits, and alexithymia in patients with panic disorder. *Journal of Neuropsychiatric Disease and Treatment, 10,* 879–885.

Jackson, D. A., & Wallace, R. F. (1974). The modification and generalization of voice loudness in a fifteen-year-old retarded girl. *Journal of Applied Behavior Analysis, 7,* 461–471.

Jacobs, G. D., Rosenberg, P. A., Friedman, R., Matheson, J., Peavy, G. M., Domar, A. D., & Benson, H. (1993). Multifactor behavioral treatment of chronic sleep-onset insomnia using stimulus control and the relaxation response: A preliminary study. *Behavior Modification, 17,* 498–509.

Jacobson, E. (1929). *Progressive relaxation.* Chicago: University of Chicago Press.

Jacobson, N. S., Dobson, K. S., Truax, P. A., Addis, M. E., Koerner, K., Gollan, J. K., . . . Prince, S. E. (1996). A component analysis of cognitive-behavioral treatment for depression. *Journal of Consulting and Clinical Psychology, 64,* 295–304.

Jacobson, N. S., Follette, W. C., & Revenstorf, D. (1984). Toward a standard definition of clinically significant change. *Behavior Therapy, 17,* 308–311.

Jacobson, N. S., Holtzworth-Munroe, A., &

Schmaling, K. B. (1989). Marital therapy and spouse involvement in the treatment of depression, agoraphobia, and alcoholism. *Journal of Consulting and Clinical Psychology, 57,* 5–10.

Jacobson, N. S., & Margolin, G. (1979). *Marital therapy: Strategies based on social learning and behavior exchange principles.* New York: Brunner/Mazel.

Jain, S., Shapiro, S. L., Swanick, S., Roesch, S. C., Mills, P. J., Bell, I., & Schwartz, G. E. (2007). A randomized controlled trial of mindfulness meditation versus relaxation training: Effects on distress, positive states of mind, rumination, and distraction. *Annals of Behavioral Medicine, 33,* 11–21.

Jayawickreme, N., Cahill, S. P., Riggs, D. S., Rauch, S. A., Resick, P. A., Rothbaum, B. O., & Foa, E. B. (2014). *Primum non nocere* (first do no harm): Symptom worsening and improvement in female assault victims after prolonged exposure for PTSD. *Depression and Anxiety, 31,* 412–419.

Johnson-Laird, P. N., Mancini, F., & Gangemi, A. (2006). A hyper-emotion theory of psychological illnesses. *Psychological Review, 113,* 822–841.

Joiner, T. E., Jr., Voelz, Z. R., & Rudd, M. D. (2001). For suicidal young adults with comorbid depressive and anxiety disorders, problem-solving treatment may be better than treatment as usual. *Professional Psychology: Research and Practice, 32,* 278–282.

Jonas, D. E., Cusack, K., Forneris, C. A., Wilkins, T. M., Sonis, J., Middleton, J. C., . . . Gaynes, B. N. (2013). *Psychological and pharmacological treatments for adults with posttraumatic stress disorder (PTSD): Comparative effectiveness review No. 92.* Rockville, MD: Agency for Healthcare Research and Quality.

Jonsson, H., & Hougaard, E. (2009). Group cognitive behavioural therapy for obsessive-compulsive disorder: A systematic review and meta-analysis. *Acta Psychiatrica Scandinavica, 119,* 98–106.

Kabat-Zinn, J. (1982). An outpatient program in behavioral medicine for chronic pain patients based on the practice of mindfulness meditation: Theoretical considerations and preliminary results. *General Hospital Psychiatry, 4,* 33–47.

Kabat-Zinn, J. (1994). *Wherever you go, there you are: Mindfulness meditation in everyday life.* New York: Hyperion.

Kalisch, R. (2009). The functional neuroanatomy of reappraisal: Time matters. *Neuroscience and Biobehavioral Reviews, 33,* 1215–1226.

Kamphuis, J. H., & Telch, M. J. (2000). Effects of distraction and guided threat reappraisal on fear reduction during exposure-based treatments for specific fears. *Behaviour Research and Therapy, 38,* 1163–1181.

Kanfer, F. H. (1971). The maintenance of behavior by self-generated stimuli and reinforcement. In A. Jacobs & L. Sachs (Eds.), *The psychology of private events* (pp. 39–59). New York: Academic Press.

Kano, M., Ito, M., & Fukudo, S. (2011). Neural substrates of decision making as measured with the Iowa Gambling Task in men with alexithymia. *Psychosomatic Medicine, 73,* 588–597.

Kanter, J. W., Manos, R. C., Bowe, W. M., Baruch, D. E., Busch, A. M., & Rusch, L. C. (2010). What is behavioral activation? A review of the empirical literature. *Clinical Psychology Review, 30,* 608–620.

Kanter, J. W., Weeks, C. E., Bonow, J. T., Landes, S. J., Callaghan, G. M., & Follette, W. C. (2009). Assessment and case conceptualization. In M. Tsai, R. J. Kohlenberg, J. W. Kanter, B. Kohlenberg, W. C. Follette, & G. M. Callaghan (Eds.), *A guide to functional analytic psychotherapy: Awareness, courage, love, and behaviorism* (pp. 37–59). New York: Springer.

Kashdan, T. B., & Roberts, J. E. (2007). Social anxiety, depressive symptoms, and post-event rumination: Affective consequences and social contextual influences. *Journal of Anxiety Disorders, 21,* 284–301.

Kassinove, H. (1986). Self-reported affect and core irrational thinking: A preliminary analysis. *Journal of Rational-Emotive Therapy, 4,* 119–130.

Kassinove, H., & Tafrate, R. C. (2002). *Anger management: The complete treatment guidebook for practitioners.* Atascadero, CA: Impact.

Kaufman, J., Birmaher, B., Brent, D., Rao, U., Flynn, C., Moreci, P., . . . Ryan, N. (1997). Schedule for Affective Disorders and Schizophrenia for School-Age Children—Present and Lifetime Version (K-SADS-PL): Initial reliability and validity data. *Journal of the American Academy of Child and Adolescent Psychiatry, 36,* 980–988.

Kazdin, A. E. (1989). *Behavior modification in applied settings* (5th ed.). Pacific Grove, CA: Brooks/Cole.

Kazdin, A. E. (1997). Parent management training: Evidence, outcomes, and issues. *Journal of the American Academy of Child and Adolescent Psychiatry, 36,* 1349–1356.

Kazdin, A. E. (2008). *The Kazdin method for parenting the defiant child.* New York: Houghton Mifflin Harcourt.

Kazdin, A. E., Esveldt-Dawson, K., French, N. H., & Unis, A. S. (1987). Effects of parent management training and problem-solving skills training combined in the treatment of antisocial child behavior. *Journal of the American Academy of Child and Adolescent Psychiatry, 26,* 416–424.

Kazdin, A. E., Siegel, T. C., & Bass, D. (1992). Cognitive problem-solving skills training and parent management training in the treatment of antisocial behavior in children. *Journal of Consulting and Clinical Psychology, 60,* 733–747.

Keating, C. F., Pomerantz, J., Pommer, S. D., Ritt, S. J., Miller, L. M., & McCormick, J. (2005). Going to college and unpacking hazing: A functional approach to decrypting initiation practices among undergraduates. *Group Dynamics: Theory, Research, and Practice, 9,* 104–126.

Kehle-Forbes, S. M., Polusny, M. A., MacDonald, R., Murdoch, M., Meis, L. A., & Wilt, T. J. (2013). A systematic review of the efficacy of adding nonexposure components to exposure therapy for posttraumatic stress disorder. *Psychological Trauma: Theory, Research, Practice, and Policy, 5,* 317–322.

Keinan, G. (1987). Decision making under stress: Scanning of alternatives under controllable and uncontrollable threats. *Journal of Personality and Social Psychology, 52,* 639–644.

Keltner, D., & Gross, J. J. (1999). Functional accounts of emotions. *Cognition and Emotion, 13,* 467–480.

Kemeny, M. E., Foltz, C., Cavanagh, J. F., Cullen, M., Giese-Davis, J., Jennings, P., . . . Ekman, P. (2012). Contemplative/emotion training reduces negative emotional behavior and promotes prosocial responses. *Emotion, 12,* 338–350.

Kendall, P. C., & Hedtke, K. (2006). *Cognitive-behavioral therapy for anxious children: Therapist manual.* Ardmore, PA: Workbook.

Kendall, P. C., & Hollon, S. D. (1989). Anxious self-talk: Development of the Anxious Self-Statements Questionnaire (ASSQ). *Cognitive Therapy and Research, 13,* 81–93.

Kendall, P. C., Robin, J. A., Hedtke, K. A., Suveg, C., Flannery-Schroeder, E., & Gosch, E. (2006). Considering CBT with anxious youth? Think exposures. *Cognitive and Behavioral Practice, 12,* 136–148.

Key, F., Craske, M. G., & Reno, R. M. (2003). Anxiety-based cognitive-behavioral therapy for paranoid beliefs. *Behavior Therapy, 34,* 97–115.

Kim, E. J. (2005). The effect of the decreased safety behaviors on anxiety and negative thoughts in social phobics. *Journal of Anxiety Disorders, 19,* 69–86.

Kingdon, D. G., & Turkington, D. (1991). The use of cognitive behavior therapy with a normalizing rationale in schizophrenia: Preliminary report. *Journal of Nervous and Mental Disease, 179,* 207–211.

Kingdon, D. G., & Turkington, D. (2006). The ABCs of cognitive-behavioral therapy for schizophrenia. *Psychiatric Times, 23,* 49–50.

Kirby, K. C., Benishek, L. A., Dugosh, K. L., & Kerwin, M. E. (2006). Substance abuse treatment providers' beliefs and objections regarding contingency management: Implications for dissemination. *Drug and Alcohol Dependence, 85,* 19–27.

Kircanski, K., Craske, M. G., & Bjork, R. A. (2008). Thought suppression enhances memory bias for threat material. *Behaviour Research and Therapy, 46,* 462–476.

Klein, D. F. (1993). False suffocation alarms, spontaneous panics, and related conditions: An integrative hypothesis. *Archives of General Psychiatry, 50,* 306–317.

Kliem, S., Kroger, C., & Kosfelder, J. (2010). Dialectical behavior therapy for borderline personality disorder: A meta-analysis using mixed-effects

modeling. *Journal of Consulting and Clinical Psychology, 78,* 936–951.

Klonsky, E. D. (2007). The functions of deliberate self-injury: A review of the evidence. *Clinical Psychology Review, 27,* 226–239.

Klumpp, H., & Amir, N. (2010). Preliminary study of attention training to threat and neutral faces on anxious reactivity to social stressor in social anxiety. *Cognitive Therapy and Research, 34,* 263–271.

Kohlenberg, R. J., & Tsai, M. (1991). *Functional analytic psychotherapy: Creating intense and curative therapeutic relationships.* New York: Plenum Press.

Kohlenberg, R. J., & Tsai, M. (1994). Functional analytic psychotherapy: A radical behavioral approach to treatment and integration. *Journal of Psychotherapy Integration, 4,* 175–201.

Kohn, L. P., Oden, T., Muñoz, R. F., Robinson, A., & Leavitt, D. (2002). Adapted cognitive behavioral group therapy for depressed low-income African American women. *Community Mental Health Journal, 38,* 497–504.

Kohn, M. A., Kwan, E., Gupta, M., & Tabas, J. A. (2005). Prevalence of acute myocardial infarction and other serious diagnoses in patients presenting to an urban emergency department with chest pain. *Journal of Emergency Medicine, 29,* 383–390.

Kozak, M. J., & Foa, E. B. (1997). *Mastery of obsessive-compulsive disorder: A cognitive-behavioral approach.* New York: Oxford University Press.

Kozak, M. J., Foa, E. B., & Steketee, G. (1998). Process and outcome of exposure treatment with obsessive-compulsives: Psychophysiological indicators of emotional processing. *Behavior Therapy, 19,* 157–169.

Krampe, H., Wagner, T., Stawicki, S., Bartels, C., Aust, C., Kroener-Herwig, B., . . . Ehrenreich, H. (2006). Personality disorder and chronicity of addiction as independent outcome predictors in alcoholism treatment. *Psychiatric Services, 57,* 708–712.

Kroger, C., Harbeck, S., Armbrust, M., & Kliem, S. (2013). Effectiveness, response, and dropout of dialectical behavior therapy for borderline personality disorder in an inpatient setting. *Behaviour Research and Therapy, 51,* 411–416.

Krüger, A., Kleindienst, N., Priebe, K., Dyer, A. S., Steil, R., Schmal, C., & Bohus, M. (2014). Nonsuicidal self-injury during an exposure-based treatment in patients with posttraumatic stress disorder and borderline features. *Behaviour Research and Therapy, 61,* 136–141.

Kuehlwein, K. T. (2000). Enhancing creativity in cognitive therapy. *Journal of Cognitive Psychotherapy, 14,* 175–187.

Kurtz, M. M., & Mueser, K. T. (2008). A meta-analysis of controlled research on social skills training for schizophrenia. *Journal of Consulting and Clinical Psychology, 76,* 491–504.

Ladouceur, R., Dugas, M. J., Freeston, M. H., Leger,

E., Gagnon, F., & Thibodeau, N. (2000). Efficacy of a cognitive-behavioral treatment for generalized anxiety disorder: Evaluation in a controlled clinical trial. *Journal of Consulting and Clinical Psychology, 68,* 957–964.

Lambert, M. J., Hansen, N. B., Umphress, V., Lunnen, K. M., Okiishi, J., Burlingame, G. M., . . . Reisinger, C. R. (1996). *Administration and scoring manual for the Outcome Questionnaire (OQ-45.2).* Wilmington, DE: American Professional Credentialing Services.

Lang, P. J. (1971). The application of psychophysiological methods to the study of psychotherapy and behavior modification. In A. Bergin & S. Garfield (Eds.), *Handbook of psychotherapy and behavior change* (pp. 75–125). New York: Wiley.

Lazarus, A. A. (1967). In support of technical eclecticism. *Psychological Reports, 21,* 415–416.

Lazarus, A. A., & Beutler, L. E. (1993). On technical eclectisism. *Journal of Counseling and Development, 71,* 381–385.

Lazarus, A. A., Beutler, L. E., & Norcross, J. C. (1992). The future of technical eclecticism. *Psychotherapy, 29,* 11–20.

Lazarus, R. S. (1984). On the primacy of cognition. *American Psychologist, 39,* 124–129.

Leahy, R. L. (1998). Cognitive therapy of childhood depression. In S. R. Shirk (Ed.), *Cognitive development and child psychotherapy* (pp. 187–206). New York: Plenum Press.

Ledgerwood, D. M., Arfken, C. L., Petry, N. M., & Alessi, S. M. (2014). Prize contingency management for smoking cessation: A randomized trial. *Drug and Alcohol Dependence, 140,* 208–212.

LeDoux, J. E., & Phelps, E. A. (2000). Emotional networks in the brain. In M. Lewis & J. M. Haviland-Jones (Eds.), *Handbook of emotions* (2nd ed., pp. 157–172). New York: Guilford Press.

Lee, J. (1993). *Facing the fire: Experiencing and expressing anger appropriately.* New York: Bantam.

Leff, J. P., & Vaughn, C. (1985). *Expressed emotion in families: Its significance for mental illness.* New York: Guilford Press.

Leichsenring, F., & Rabung, S. (2008). Effectiveness of long-term psychodynamic psychotherapy: A meta-analysis. *Journal of the American Medical Association, 300,* 1551–1565.

Lejuez, C. W., Hopko, D. R., & Hopko, S. D. (2001). A brief behavioral activation treatment for depression: Treatment manual. *Behavior Modification, 25,* 255–286.

Leon, A. C., Solomon, D. A., Mueller, T. I., Turvey, C. L., Endicott, J., & Keller, M. B. (1999). The Range of Impaired Functioning Tool (LIFE-RIFT): A brief measure of functional impairment. *Psychological Medicine, 29,* 869–878.

LePage, J. P. (1999). The impact of a token economy on injuries and negative events on an acute psychiatric unit. *Psychiatric Services, 50,* 941–944.

LePage, J. P., DelBen, K., Pollard, S., McGhee, M., VanHorn, L., Murphy, J., . . . Mogge, N. (2003). Reducing assaults on an acute psychiatric unit using a token economy: A 2-year follow-up. *Behavioral Interventions, 18,* 179–190.

Lerner, J. S., Gonzalez, R. M., Small, D. A., & Fischhoff, B. (2003). Effects of fear and anger on perceived risks of terrorism: A national field experiment. *Psychological Science, 14,* 144–150.

Lester, G. W., Beckham, E., & Baucom, D. H. (1980). Implementation of behavioral marital therapy. *Journal of Marital and Family Therapy, 6,* 189–199.

Levenson, R. W. (1992). Autonomic nervous system differences among emotions. *Psychological Science, 3,* 23–27.

Levenson, R. W. (1999). The intrapersonal functions of emotion. *Cognition and Emotion, 13,* 481–504.

Levenson, R. W., Ekman, P., & Friesen, W. V. (1990). Voluntary facial action generates emotion-specific autonomic nervous system activity. *Psychophysiology, 27,* 363–384.

Levitt, J. T., & Cloitre, M. (2006). A clinician's guide to STAIR/MPE: Treatment for PTSD related to childhood abuse. *Cognitive and Behavioral Practice, 12,* 40–52.

Levy, H. C., & Radomsky, A. S. (2014). Safety behaviour enhances the acceptability of exposure. *Cognitive Behaviour Therapy, 43,* 83–92.

Leweke, F., Leichsenring, F., Kruse, J., & Hermes, S. (2012). Is alexithymia associated with specific mental disorders? *Psychopathology, 45,* 22–28.

Lewin, A. B., Park, J. M., Jones, A. M., Crawford, E. A., De Nadai, A. S., Menzel, J., . . . Storch, E. A. (2014). Family-based exposure and response prevention therapy for preschool-aged children with obsessive–compulsive disorder: A pilot randomized controlled trial. *Behaviour Research and Therapy, 56,* 30–38.

Lewinsohn, P. M. (1974). A behavioural approach to depression. In M. M. Katz (Ed.), *The psychology of depression: Contemporary theory and research* (pp. 157–185). New York: Wiley.

Lewinsohn, P. M., Biglan, A., & Zeiss, A. M. (1976). Behavioral treatment for depression. In P. O. Davidson (Ed.), *Behavioral management of anxiety, depression, and pain* (pp. 91–146). New York: Brunner/Mazel.

Lewinsohn, P. M., Mischel, W., Chaplin, W., & Barton, R. (1980). Social competence and depression: The role of illusory self-perceptions. *Journal of Abnormal Psychology, 89,* 203–212.

Lewis, M. (2000). The emergence of human emotions. In M. Lewis & J. M. Haviland-Jones (Eds.), *Handbook of emotions* (2nd ed., pp. 265–280). New York: Guilford Press.

Lewis, S., Tarrier, N., Haddock, G., Bentall, R., Kinderman, P., Kingdon, D., . . . Dunn, G. (2002). Randomised controlled trial of cognitive-behavioural therapy in early schizophrenia: Acute-phase outcomes. *British Journal of Psychiatry Supplement, 43*, s91–s97.

Ley, R. (1985). Blood, breath, and fears: A hyperventilation theory of panic attacks and agoraphobia. *Clinical Psychology Review, 5*, 271–285.

Leyro, T. M., Zvolensky, M. J., & Bernstein, A. (2010). Distress tolerance and psychopathological symptoms and disorders: A review of the empirical literature among adults. *Psychological Bulletin, 136*, 576–600.

Liberman, R. P. (1982). Assessment of social skills. *Schizophrenia Bulletin, 8*, 62–83.

Liberman, R. P., Wallace, C. J., Falloon, I. R., & Vaughn, C. E. (1981). Interpersonal problem-solving therapy for schizophrenics and their families. *Comprehensive Psychiatry, 22*, 627–630.

Lichstein, K. L., & Schreibman, L. (1976). Employing electric shock with autistic children: A review of the side effects. *Journal of Autism and Childhood Schizophrenia, 6*, 163–173.

Linehan, M. M. (1993). *Cognitive-behavioral treatment of borderline personality disorder*. New York: Guilford Press.

Linehan, M. M. (2015). *DBT siskills training manual*. New York: Guilford Press.

Linehan, M. M., Armstrong, H. E., Suarez, A., Allmon, D., & Heard, H. L. (1993). Dialectical behavior therapy for borderline personality disorder. In D. H. Barlow (Ed.), *Clinical handbook of psychological disorders: A step-by-step treatment manual* (3rd ed., pp. 470–522). New York: Guilford Press.

Linehan, M. M., Camper, P., Chiles, J. A., Strosahl, K., & Shearin, E. (1987). Interpersonal problem solving and parasuicide. *Cognitive Therapy and Research, 11*, 1–12.

Linehan, M. M., Comtois, K. A., Murray, A. M., Brown, M. Z., Gallop, R. J., Heard, H. L., . . . Lindenboim, N. (2006). Two-year randomized controlled trial and follow-up of dialectical behavior therapy vs. therapy by experts for suicidal behaviors and borderline personality disorder. *Archives of General Psychiatry, 63*, 757–766.

Linehan, M. M., & Dexter-Mazza, E. T. (2008). Dialectical behavior therapy for borderline personality disorder. In D. H. Barlow (Ed.), *Clinical handbook of psychological disorders: A step-by-step treatment manual* (4th ed., pp. 365–420). New York: Guilford Press.

Linehan, M. M., & Egan, K. J. (1979). Modification of social skill deficits in children. In A. S. Bellack & M. Hersen (Eds.), *Research and practice in social skills training* (pp. 237–271). New York: Springer.

Linehan, M. M., Schmidt, H., III, Dimeff, L. A., Craft, J. C., Kanter, J., & Comtois, K. A. (1999). Dialectical behavior therapy for patients with borderline personality disorder and drug-dependence. *American Journal on Addictions, 8*, 279–292.

Linscheid, T. R., Iwata, B. A., Ricketts, R. W., Williams, D. E., & Griffin, J. C. (1990). Clinical evaluation of the self-injurious behavior inhibiting system (SIBIS). *Journal of Applied Behavior Analysis, 23*, 53–78.

Llera, S. J., & Newman, M. G. (2010). Effects of worry on physiological and subjective reactivity to emotional stimuli in generalized anxiety disorder and nonanxious control participants. *Emotion, 10*, 640–650.

Loftus, E. F., Loftus, G. R., & Messo, J. (1987). Some facts about "weapon focus." *Law and Human Behavior, 11*, 55–62.

Lohr, J. M., Olatunji, B. O., & Sawchuk, C. N. (2007). A functional analysis of danger and safety signals in anxiety disorders. *Clinical Psychology Review, 27*, 114–126.

Long, P., Forehand, R., Wierson, M., & Morgan, A. (1994). Does parent training with young noncompliant children have long-term effects? *Behaviour Research and Therapy, 32*, 101–107.

Longmore, R. J., & Worrell, M. (2007). Do we need to challenge thoughts in cognitive behavior therapy? *Clinical Psychology Review, 27*, 173–187.

Lopata, C., Thomeer, M. L., Volker, M. A., Toomey, J. A., Nida, R. E., Lee, G. K., . . . Rodgers, J. D. (2010). RCT of a manualized social treatment for high-functioning autism spectrum disorders. *Journal of Autism and Developmental Disorders, 40*, 1297–1310.

Lopez, E. L. (1981). Increasing intrinsic motivation with performance-contingent reward. *Journal of Psychology, 108*, 59–65.

Lovibond, S. H., & Lovibond, P. F. (1995). *Manual for the Depression Anxiety Stress Scales*. Sydney: Psychology Foundation of Australia.

Lowe, R., & Ziemke, T. (2011). The feeling of action tendencies: On the emotional regulation of goal-directed behavior. *Frontiers in Psychology, 2*, 346.

Ludgate, J. W., Wright, J. H., Bowers, W., & Camp, G. F. (1993). Individual cognitive therapy with inpatients. In J. H. Wright, M. E. Thase, A. T. Beck, & J. W. Ludgate (Eds.), *Cognitive therapy with inpatients: Developing a cognitive milieu* (pp. 91–120). New York: Guilford Press.

Luoma, J. B., & Hayes, S. C. (2003). Cognitive defusion. In W. O'Donohue, J. E. Fisher, & S. C. Hayes (Eds.), *Cognitive behavior therapy: Applying empirically supported techniques in your practice* (pp. 71–78). Hoboken, NJ: Wiley.

Lyubomirsky, S., Caldwell, N. D., & Nolen-Hoeksema, S. (1998). Effects of ruminative and distracting responses to depressed mood on retrieval of autobiographical memories. *Journal of Personality and Social Psychology, 75*, 166–177.

Lyubomirsky, S., & Nolen-Hoeksema, S. (1995). Effects of self-focused rumination on negative thinking and interpersonal problem solving. *Journal of Personality and Social Psychology, 69*, 176–190.

Macaskill, N. D. (1996). Improving clinical outcomes in REBT/CBT: The therapeutic uses of tape-recording. *Journal of Rational-Emotive and Cognitive-Behavior Therapy, 14,* 199–207.

Mahoney, M. J. (1977). Cognitive therapy and research: A question of questions. *Cognitive Therapy and Research, 1,* 1–3.

Maley, R. F., Feldman, G. L., & Ruskin, R. S. (1973). Evaluation of patient improvement in a token economy treatment program. *Journal of Abnormal Psychology, 82,* 141–144.

Mandelberg, J., Laugeson, E. A., Cunningham, T. D., Ellingsen, R., Bates, S., & Frankel, F. (2014). Long-term treatment outcomes for parent-assisted social skills training for adolescents with autism spectrum disorders: The UCLA PEERS program. *Journal of Mental Health Research in Intellectual Disabilities, 7,* 45–73.

Mansell, W., & Jones, S. H. (2006). The Brief-HAPPI: A questionnaire to assess cognitions that distinguish between individuals with a diagnosis of bipolar disorder and non-clinical controls. *Journal of Affective Disorders, 93,* 29–34.

Manzoni, G. M., Pagnini, F., Castelnuovo, G., & Molinari, E. (2008). Relaxation training for anxiety: A ten-years systematic review with meta-analysis. *BMC Psychiatry, 8,* 41.

March, J. S., & Mulle, K. (1998). *OCD in children and adolescents: A cognitive-behavioral treatment manual.* New York: Guilford Press.

Marcks, B. A., & Woods, D. W. (2005). A comparison of thought suppression to an acceptance-based technique in the management of personal intrusive thoughts: A controlled evaluation. *Behaviour Research and Therapy, 43,* 433–445.

Marcks, B. A., & Woods, D. W. (2007). Role of thought-related beliefs and coping strategies in the escalation of intrusive thoughts: An analog to obsessive–compulsive disorder. *Behaviour Research and Therapy, 45,* 2640–2651.

Marlatt, G. A., & Gordon, J. R. (1985). *Relapse prevention: Maintenance strategies in the treatment of addictive behaviors.* New York: Guilford Press.

Martell, C. R., Addis, M. E., & Jacobson, N. S. (2001). *Depression in context: Strategies for guided action.* New York: Norton.

Martinez, C. R., & Eddy, J. M. (2005). Effects of culturally adapted parent management training on Latino youth behavioral health outcomes. *Journal of Consulting and Clinical Psychology, 73,* 841–851.

Martinez, J. M., Kent, J. M., Coplan, J. D., Browne, S. T., Papp, L. A., Sullivan, G. M., . . . Gorman, J. M. (2001). Respiratory variability in panic disorder. *Depression and Anxiety, 14,* 232–237.

Masters, J. C., Burish, T. G., Hollon, S. D., & Rimm, D. C. (1987). *Behavior therapy: Techniques and empirical findings* (3rd ed.). New York: Harcourt Brace Jovanovich.

Matson, J. L., & Boisjoli, J. A. (2009). The token economy for children with intellectual disability and/ or autism: A review. *Research in Developmental Disabilities, 30,* 240–248.

Matson, J. L., & Kazdin, A. E. (1981). Punishment in behavior modification: Pragmatic, ethical, and legal issues. *Clinical Psychology Review, 1,* 197–210.

Matson, J. L., & Wilkins, J. (2009). Psychometric testing methods for children's social skills. *Research in Developmental Disabilities, 30,* 249–274.

Maxmen, J. S., & Ward, N. G. (1995). *Essential psychopathology and its treatment* (2nd ed.). New York: Norton.

Maydeu-Olivares, A., & D'Zurilla, T. J. (1996). A factor-analytic study of the Social Problem-Solving Inventory: An integration of theory and data. *Cognitive Therapy and Research, 20,* 115–133.

Mayer, J. A., & Frederiksen, L. W. (1986). Encouraging long-term compliance with breast self-examination: The evaluation of prompting strategies. *Journal of Behavioral Medicine, 9,* 179–189.

Mazzeo, S. E., & Espelage, D. L. (2002). Association between childhood physical and emotional abuse and disordered eating behaviors in female undergraduates: An investigation of the mediating role of alexithymia and depression. *Journal of Counseling Psychology, 49,* 86–100.

McCullough, L., Kuhn, N., Andrews, S., Kaplan, A., Wolf, J. E., & Hurley, C. L. (2003). *Treating affect phobia: A manual for short-term dynamic psychotherapy.* New York: Guilford Press.

McDonagh, A., Friedman, M., McHugo, G., Ford, J., Sengupta, A., Mueser, K., . . . Descamps, M. (2005). Randomized trial of cognitive-behavioral therapy for chronic posttraumatic stress disorder in adult female survivors of childhood sexual abuse. *Journal of Consulting and Clinical Psychology, 73,* 515–524.

McDowell, J. J. (1982). The importance of Herrnstein's mathematical statement of the law of effect for behavior therapy. *American Psychologist, 37,* 771–779.

McFall, R. M. (1982). A review and reformulation of the concept of social skills. *Behavioral Assessment, 4,* 1–33.

McGinnis, J. C., Friman, P. C., & Carlyon, W. D. (1999). The effect of token rewards on "intrinsic" motivation for doing math. *Journal of Applied Behavior Analysis, 32,* 375–379.

McKay, D., Gavigan, C. A., & Kulchycky, S. (2004). Social skills and sex-role functioning in borderline personality disorder: Relationship to self-mutilating behavior. *Cognitive Behaviour Therapy, 33,* 27–35.

McMahon, R. J., & Forehand, R. L. (2003). *Helping the noncompliant child* (2nd ed.): *Family-based treatment for oppositional behavior.* New York: Guilford Press.

McMain, S. F., Guimond, T., Streiner, D. L., Cardish, R. J., & Links, P. S. (2012). Dialectical behavior therapy compared with general psychiatric management for borderline personality disorder: Clinical outcomes and functioning over a 2-year follow-up. *American Journal of Psychiatry, 169,* 650–661.

McNeil, C. B., Eyberg, S., Eisenstadt, T. H., Newcomb, K., & Funderburk, B. (1991). Parent–child interaction therapy with behavior problem children: Generalization of treatment effects to the school setting. *Journal of Clinical Child Psychology, 20,* 140–151.

Meichenbaum, D. (1977). *Cognitive-behavior modification: An integrative approach.* New York: Plenum Press.

Mennin, D. S. (2006). Emotion regulation therapy: An integrative approach to treatment-resistant anxiety disorders. *Journal of Contemporary Psychotherapy, 36,* 95–105.

Mennin, D. S., & Fresco, D. M. (2013). Emotion regulation therapy. In J. J. Gross (Ed.), *Handbook of emotion regulation* (2nd ed., pp. 469–490). New York: Guilford Press.

Mennin, D. S., Heimberg, R. G., Turk, C. L., & Fresco, D. M. (2002). Applying an emotion regulation framework to integrative approaches to generalized anxiety disorder. *Clinical Psychology: Science and Practice, 9,* 85–90.

Mennin, D. S., Heimberg, R. G., Turk, C. L., & Fresco, D. M. (2005). Preliminary evidence for an emotion dysregulation model of generalized anxiety disorder. *Behaviour Research and Therapy, 43,* 1281–1310.

Meuret, A. E., Rosenfield, D., Hofmann, S. G., Suvak, M. K., & Roth, W. T. (2009). Changes in respiration mediate changes in fear of bodily sensations in panic disorder. *Journal of Psychiatric Research, 43,* 634–641.

Meuret, A. E., Rosenfield, D., Wilhelm, F. H., Zhou, E., Conrad, A., Ritz, T., & Roth, W. T. (2011). Do unexpected panic attacks occur spontaneously? *Biological Psychiatry, 70,* 985–991.

Meuret, A. E., Wilhelm, F. H., Ritz, T., & Roth, W. T. (2008). Feedback of end-tidal pCO_2 as a therapeutic approach for panic disorder. *Journal of Psychiatric Research, 42,* 560–568.

Meuret, A. E., Wolitzky-Taylor, K. B., Twohig, M. P., & Craske, M. G. (2012). Coping skills and exposure therapy in panic disorder and agoraphobia: Latest advances and future directions. *Behavior Therapy, 43,* 271–284.

Meyer, T. J., Miller, M. L., Metzger, R. L., & Borkovec, T. D. (1990). Development and validity of the Penn State Worry Questionnaire. *Behaviour Research and Therapy, 28,* 487–495.

Meyerbroker, K., & Emmelkamp, P. M. (2010). Virtual reality exposure therapy in anxiety disorders: A systematic review of process-and-outcome studies. *Depression and Anxiety, 27,* 933–944.

Meyers, A. W., Thackwray, D. E., Johnson, D. B., & Schleser, R. (1983). A comparison of prompting strategies for improving appointment compliance of hypertensive individuals. *Behavior Therapy, 14,* 267–274.

Michaliszyn, D., Marchand, A., Bouchard, S., Martel, M. O., & Poirier-Bisson, J. (2010). A randomized, controlled clinical trial of in virtuo and in vivo exposure for spider phobia. *Cyberpsychology, Behavior, and Social Networking, 13,* 689–695.

Miller, P. M. (1972). The use of behavioral contracting in the treatment of alcoholism: A case report. *Behavior Therapy, 3,* 593–596.

Miller, S. D., Duncan, B. L., Sorrell, R., & Brown, G. S. (2005). The partners for change outcome management system. *Journal of Clinical Psychology, 61,* 199–208.

Miller, W. R., & Rollnick, S. (2002). *Motivational interviewing: Preparing people for change* (2nd ed.). New York: Guilford Press.

Miller, W. R., & Rollnick, S. (2013). *Motivational interviewing: Helping people change* (3rd ed.). New York: Guilford Press.

Miller, W. R., Wilbourne, P. L., & Hettema, J. E. (2003). What works? A summary of alcohol treatment outcome research. In R. K. Hester & W. R. Miller (Eds.), *Handbook of alcoholism treatment approaches: Effective alternatives* (3rd ed., pp. 13–63). Boston: Allyn & Bacon.

Millon, T., Millon, C., Davis, R. D., & Grossman, S. (2009). *MCMI-III: Millon Clinical Multiaxial Inventory-III (MCMI-III): Manual.* Minneapolis: Pearson/PsychCorp.

Mills, K. L., Teesson, M., Back, S. E., Brady, K. T., Baker, A. L., Hopwood, S., . . . Ewer, P. L. (2012). Integrated exposure-based therapy for co-occurring posttraumatic stress disorder and substance dependence: A randomized controlled trial. *Journal of the American Medical Association, 308,* 690–699.

Milosevic, I., & Radomsky, A. S. (2008). Safety behaviour does not necessarily interfere with exposure therapy. *Behaviour Research and Therapy, 46,* 1111–1118.

Mineka, S., & Oehlberg, K. (2008). The relevance of recent developments in classical conditioning to understanding the etiology and maintenance of anxiety disorders. *Acta Psychologica, 127,* 567–580.

Miranda, J., Azocar, F., Organista, K. C., Dwyer, E., & Areane, P. (2003). Treatment of depression among impoverished primary care patients from ethnic minority groups. *Psychiatric Services, 54,* 219–225.

Miranda, J., Bernal, G., Lau, A., Kohn, L., Hwang, W. C., & LaFromboise, T. (2005). State of the science on psychosocial interventions for ethnic minorities. *Annual Review of Clinical Psychology, 1,* 113–142.

Moberly, N. J., & Watkins, E. R. (2008). Ruminative self-focus and negative affect: An experience sampling study. *Journal of Abnormal Psychology, 117,* 314–323.

Mogg, K., Bradley, B. P., Hyare, H., & Lee, S. (1998). Selective attention to food-related stimuli in hunger: Are attentional biases specific to emotional and psychopathological states, or are they also found in normal drive states? *Behaviour Research and Therapy, 36,* 227–237.

Monti, P. M., Kadden, R. M., Rohsenow, D. J., Cooney, N. L., & Abrams, D. B. (2002). *Treating alcohol dependence: A coping skills training guide* (2nd ed.). New York: Guilford Press.

Moore, R. G., Watts, F. N., & Williams, J. M. (1988). The specificity of personal memories in depression. *British Journal of Clinical Psychology, 27*(Pt. 3), 275–276.

Moors, A. (2010). Automatic constructive appraisal as a candidate cause of emotion. *Emotion Review, 2,* 139–156.

Moors, A., & De Houwer, J. (2006). Automaticity: A theoretical and conceptual analysis. *Psychological Bulletin, 132,* 297–326.

Morey, L. C. (1991). *The Personality Assessment Inventory professional manual.* Odessa, FL: Psychological Assessment Resources.

Morgan, H., & Raffle, C. (1999). Does reducing safety behaviours improve treatment response in patients with social phobia? *Australian and New Zealand Journal of Psychiatry, 33,* 503–510.

Morillo, C., Belloch, A., & Garcia-Soriano, G. (2007). Clinical obsessions in obsessive–compulsive patients and obsession-relevant intrusive thoughts in non-clinical, depressed and anxious subjects: Where are the differences? *Behaviour Research and Therapy, 45,* 1319–1333.

Morin, C. M., & Espie, C. A. (2003). *Insomia: A clinical guide to assessment and treatment.* New York: Kluwer Academic/Plenum Press.

Moritz, S., & Laudan, A. (2007). Attention bias for paranoia-relevant visual stimuli in schizophrenia. *Cognitive Neuropsychiatry, 12,* 381–390.

Morone, N. E., Greco, C. M., & Weiner, D. K. (2008). Mindfulness meditation for the treatment of chronic low back pain in older adults: A randomized controlled pilot study. *Pain, 134,* 310–319.

Morrison, A. P., Turkington, D., Pyle, M., Spencer, H., Brabban, A., Dunn, G., . . . Hutton, P. (2014). Cognitive therapy for people with schizophrenia spectrum disorders not taking antipsychotic drugs: A single-blind randomised controlled trial. *Lancet, 383,* 1395–1403.

Mott, J. M., Sutherland, R. J., Williams, W., Lanier, S. H., Ready, D. J., & Teng, E. J. (2013). Patient perspectives on the effectiveness and tolerability of group-based exposure therapy for posttraumatic stress disorder: Preliminary self-report findings from 20 veterans. *Psychological Trauma: Theory, Research, Practice, and Policy, 5,* 453–461.

Moulds, M. L., & Nixon, R. D. (2006). In vivo flooding for anxiety disorders: Proposing its utility in the treatment posttraumatic stress disorder. *Journal of Anxiety Disorders, 20,* 498–509.

Mueser, K. T., Bellack, A. S., Morrison, R. L., & Wixted, J. T. (1990). Social competence in schizophrenia: Premorbid adjustment, social skill, and domains of functioning. *Journal of Psychiatric Research, 24,* 51–63.

Muller, K. L., & Schultz, L. T. (2012). "Selling" exposure therapy. *Pragmatic Case Studies in Psychotherapy, 8,* 288–295.

Mundt, J. C., Marks, I. M., Shear, M. K., & Greist, J. H. (2002). The Work and Social Adjustment Scale: A simple measure of impairment in functioning. *British Journal of Psychiatry, 180,* 461–464.

Muralidharan, A., Sheets, E. S., Madsen, J., Craighead, L. W., & Craighead, W. E. (2011). Interpersonal competence across domains: Relevance to personality pathology. *Journal of Personality Disorders, 25,* 16–27.

Muran, J. C., Safran, J. D., Gorman, B. S., Samstag, L. W., Eubanks-Carter, C., & Winston, A. (2009). The relationship of early alliance ruptures and their resolution to process and outcome in three time-limited psychotherapies for personality disorders. *Psychotherapy (Chic), 46,* 233–248.

Nacasch, N., Huppert, J. D., Su, Y. J., Kivity, Y., Dinshtein, Y., Yeh, R., & Foa, E. B. (2015). Are 60-minute prolonged exposure sessions with 20-minute imaginal exposure to traumatic memories sufficient to successfully treat PTSD? A randomized noninferiority clinical trial. *Behavior Therapy, 46,* 328–341.

Najmi, S., & Amir, N. (2010). The effect of attention training on a behavioral test of contamination fears in individuals with subclinical obsessive–compulsive symptoms. *Journal of Abnormal Psychology, 119,* 136–142.

Napolitano, L. A., & McKay, D. (2007). Dichotomous thinking in borderline personality disorder. *Cognitive Therapy and Research, 31,* 717–726.

Nasreddine, Z. S., Phillips, N. A., Bedirian, V., Charbonneau, S., Whitehead, V., Collin, I., . . . Chertkow, H. (2005). The Montreal Cognitive Assessment, MoCA: A brief screening tool for mild cognitive impairment. *Journal of the American Geriatrics Society, 53,* 695–699.

Neacsiu, A. D., Eberle, J. W., Kramer, R., Wiesmann, T., & Linehan, M. M. (2014). Dialectical behavior therapy skills for transdiagnostic emotion dysregulation: A pilot randomized controlled trial. *Behaviour Research and Therapy, 59,* 40–51.

Neacsiu, A. D., Rizvi, S. L., & Linehan, M. M. (2010). Dialectical behavior therapy skills use as a mediator and outcome of treatment for borderline personality disorder. *Behaviour Research and Therapy, 48,* 832–839.

Nelson, D. R., Hammen, C., Brennan, P. A., & Ullman, J. B. (2003). The impact of maternal depression on adolescent adjustment: The role of expressed emotion. *Journal of Consulting and Clinical Psychology, 71,* 935–944.

Nevin, J. A. (1992). An integrative model for the

study of behavioral momentum. *Journal of the Experimental Analysis of Behavior, 57,* 301–316.

Newby, J. M., & Moulds, M. L. (2010). Negative intrusive memories in depression: The role of maladaptive appraisals and safety behaviours. *Journal of Affective Disorders, 126,* 147–154.

Newby, J. M., & Moulds, M. L. (2011). Characteristics of intrusive memories in a community sample of depressed, recovered depressed and never-depressed individuals. *Behaviour Research and Therapy, 49,* 234–243.

Newman, C. F. (2002). A cognitive perspective on resistance in psychotherapy. *Journal of Clinical Psychology, 58,* 165–174.

Newman, M. G., & Llera, S. J. (2011). A novel theory of experiential avoidance in generalized anxiety disorder: A review and synthesis of research supporting a contrast avoidance model of worry. *Clinical Psychology Review, 31,* 371–382.

Nezu, A. M., Nezu, C. M., & D'Zurilla, T. J. (2013). *Problem-solving therapy: A treatment manual.* New York: Springer.

Nezu, A. M., Nezu, C. M., Sarayadarian, L., Kalmar, K., & Ronan, G. F. (1986). Social problem solving as a moderator variable between negative life stress and depressive symptoms. *Cognitive Therapy and Research, 10,* 489–498.

Nezu, A. M., & Ronan, G. F. (1985). Life stress, current problems, problem solving, and depressive symptoms: An integrative model. *Journal of Consulting and Clinical Psychology, 53,* 693–697.

Niles, A. N., Burklund, L. J., Arch, J. J., Lieberman, M. D., Saxbe, D., & Craske, M. G. (2014). Cognitive mediators of treatment for social anxiety disorder: Comparing acceptance and commitment therapy and cognitive-behavioral therapy. *Behavior Therapy, 45,* 664–677.

Nock, M. K. (2009). Why do people hurt themselves? New insights into the nature and functions of self-injury. *Current Directions in Psychological Science, 18,* 78–83.

Nock, M. K., & Mendes, W. B. (2008). Physiological arousal, distress tolerance, and social problem-solving deficits among adolescent self-injurers. *Journal of Consulting and Clinical Psychology, 76,* 28–38.

Nolen-Hoeksema, S. (1991). Responses to depression and their effects on the duration of depressive episodes. *Journal of Abnormal Psychology, 100,* 569–582.

Nolen-Hoeksema, S., & Morrow, J. (1993). Effects of rumination and distraction on naturally occurring depressed mood. *Cognition and Emotion, 7,* 561–570.

Norcross, J. C. (Ed.). (1986). *Handbook of eclectic psychotherapy.* New York: Brunner/Mazel.

Norcross, J. C., & Wampold, B. E. (2011). Evidence-based therapy relationships: Research conclusions and clinical practices. In J. C. Norcross (Ed.), *Psychotherapy relationships that work: Evidence-based*

responsiveness (2nd ed., pp. 423–430). New York: Oxford University Press.

Norton, G. R., Allen, G. E., & Hilton, J. (1983). The social validity of treatments for agoraphobia. *Behaviour Research and Therapy, 21,* 393–399.

Norton, P. J., & Hope, D. A. (2001). Analogue observational methods in the assessment of social functioning in adults. *Psychological Assessment, 13,* 59–72.

Norton, P. J., & Price, E. C. (2007). A meta-analytic review of adult cognitive-behavioral treatment outcome across the anxiety disorders. *Journal of Nervous and Mental Disease, 195,* 521–531.

Obsessive Compulsive Cognitions Working Group. (2005). Psychometric validation of the Obsessive Beliefs Questionnaire and the Interpretation of Intrusions Inventory: Part 2. Factor analyses and testing of a brief version. *Behaviour Research and Therapy, 43,* 1527–1542.

Ochsner, K. N., Silvers, J. A., & Buhle, J. T. (2012). Functional imaging studies of emotion regulation: A synthetic review and evolving model of the cognitive control of emotion. *Annals of the New York Academy of Sciences, 1251,* E1–E24.

O'Connor, K., Stip, E., Pelissier, M. C., Aardema, F., Guay, S., Gaudette, G., . . . Leblanc, V. (2007). Treating delusional disorder: A comparison of cognitive-behavioural therapy and attention placebo control. *Canadian Journal of Psychiatry, 52,* 182–190.

O'Driscoll, C., Laing, J., & Mason, O. (2014). Cognitive emotion regulation strategies, alexithymia and dissociation in schizophrenia: A review and meta-analysis. *Clinical Psychology Review, 34,* 482–495.

Ogden, T., & Hagen, K. A. (2008). Treatment effectiveness of Parent Management Training in Norway: A randomized controlled trial of children with conduct problems. *Journal of Consulting and Clinical Psychology, 76,* 607–621.

Ogrodniczuk, J. S., Joyce, A. S., & Abbass, A. A. (2014). Childhood maltreatment and somatic complaints among adult psychiatric outpatients: Exploring the mediating role of alexithymia. *Psychotherapy and Psychosomatics, 83,* 322–324.

Ohayon, M. M. (2000). Prevalence of hallucinations and their pathological associations in the general population. *Psychiatry Research, 97,* 153–164.

Olatunji, B. O., Etzel, E. N., Tomarken, A. J., Ciesielski, B. G., & Deacon, B. (2011). The effects of safety behaviors on health anxiety: An experimental investigation. *Behaviour Research and Therapy, 49,* 719–728.

Olatunji, B. O., Tolin, D. F., & Lohr, J. M. (2004). Irritable bowel syndrome: Associated features and the efficacy of psychosocial treatments. *Applied and Preventive Psychology, 11,* 125–140.

Ollendick, T. H., Ost, L. G., Reuterskiold, L., Costa, N., Cederlund, R., Sirbu, C., . . . Jarrett, M. A. (2009). One-session treatment of specific phobias in youth: A randomized clinical trial in the United States and Sweden. *Journal of Consulting and Clinical Psychology, 77*, 504–516.

Öst, L. G. (1989). One-session treatment for specific phobias. *Behaviour Research and Therapy, 27*, 1–7.

Öst, L. G. (2014). The efficacy of acceptance and commitment therapy: An updated systematic review and meta-analysis. *Behaviour Research and Therapy, 61*, 105–121.

Öst, L. G., Alm, T., Brandberg, M., & Breitholtz, E. (2001). One vs. five sessions of exposure and five sessions of cognitive therapy in the treatment of claustrophobia. *Behaviour Research and Therapy, 39*, 167–183.

Öst, L. G., Thulin, U., & Ramnero, J. (2004). Cognitive behavior therapy vs. exposure in vivo in the treatment of panic disorder with agoraphobia. *Behaviour Research and Therapy, 42*, 1105–1127.

Öst, L. G., & Westling, B. E. (1995). Applied relaxation vs. cognitive behavior therapy in the treatment of panic disorder. *Behaviour Research and Therapy, 33*, 145–158.

Otto, M. W. (2000). Stories and metaphors in cognitive-behavior therapy. *Cognitive and Behavioral Practice, 7*, 166–172.

Otto, M. W., & Hinton, D. E. (2006). Modifying exposure-based CBT for Cambodian refugees with posttraumatic stress disorder. *Cognitive and Behavioral Practice, 13*, 261–270.

Otto, M. W., Simon, N. M., Olatunji, B. O., Sung, S. C., & Pollack, M. H. (2011). *10-minute CBT: Integrating cognitive-behavioral strategies into your practice*. New York: Oxford University Press.

Padesky, C. A. (1993, September). *Socratic questioning: Changing minds or guiding discovery?* Paper presented at the annual meeting of the European Congress of Behavioural and Cognitive Therapies, London.

Padesky, C. A. (1994). Schema change processes in cognitive therapy. *Clinical Psychology and Psychotherapy, 1*, 267–278.

Papp, L. A., Martinez, J. M., Klein, D. F., Coplan, J. D., Norman, R. G., Cole, R., . . . Gorman, J. M. (1997). Respiratory psychophysiology of panic disorder: Three respiratory challenges in 98 subjects. *American Journal of Psychiatry, 154*, 1557–1565.

Paris, J. (2003). *Personality disorders over time*. Washington, DC: American Psychiatric Press.

Paris, J. (2004). Is hospitalization useful for suicidal patients with borderline personality disorder? *Journal of Personality Disorders, 18*, 240–247.

Park, K. M., Ku, J., Choi, S. H., Jang, H. J., Park, J. Y., Kim, S. I., & Kim, J. J. (2011). A virtual reality application in role-plays of social skills training for schizophrenia: A randomized, controlled trial. *Psychiatry Research, 189*, 166–172.

Patterson, G. R. (1982). *A social learning approach: 3. Coercive family process*. Eugene, OR: Castalia.

Patterson, G. R., DeBaryshe, B. D., & Ramsey, E.

(1989). A developmental perspective on antisocial behavior. *American Psychologist, 44*, 329–335.

Paulhus, D. L., & Morgan, K. L. (1997). Perceptions of intelligence in leaderless groups: The dynamic effects of shyness and acquaintance. *Journal of Personality and Social Psychology, 72*, 581–591.

Pavlov, I. P. (1960). *Conditioned reflexes*. New York: Dover. (Original work published 1927)

Penn, D., Roberts, D. L., Munt, E. D., Silverstein, E., Jones, N., & Sheitman, B. (2005). A pilot study of social cognition and interaction training (SCIT) for schizophrenia. *Schizophrenia Research, 80*, 357–359.

Perls, F. P. (1973). *The Gestalt approach and eyewitness to therapy*. Palo Alto, CA: Science and Behavior Books.

Perowne, S., & Mansell, W. (2002). Social anxiety, self-focused attention, and the discrimination of negative, neutral and positive audience members by their non-verbal behaviours. *Behavioural and Cognitive Psychotherapy, 30*, 11–23.

Perry, Y., Henry, J. D., Nangle, M. R., & Grisham, J. R. (2012). Regulation of negative affect in schizophrenia: The effectiveness of acceptance versus reappraisal and suppression. *Journal of Clinical and Experimental Neuropsychology, 34*, 497–508.

Persons, J. B. (1989). *Cognitive therapy in practice: A case formulation approach*. New York: Norton.

Persons, J. B., & Tompkins, M. A. (2007). Cognitive-behavioral case formulation. In T. D. Eells (Ed.), *Handbook of psychotherapy case formulation* (pp. 290–316). New York: Guilford Press.

Peters, E., Joseph, S., Day, S., & Garety, P. (2004). Measuring delusional ideation: The 21-item Peters et al. Delusions Inventory (PDI). *Schizophrenia Bulletin, 30*, 1005–1022.

Petry, N. M., Alessi, S. M., & Hanson, T. (2007). Contingency management improves abstinence and quality of life in cocaine abusers. *Journal of Consulting and Clinical Psychology, 75*, 307–315.

Petry, N. M., Alessi, S. M., & Rash, C. J. (2013). Contingency management treatments decrease psychiatric symptoms. *Journal of Consulting and Clinical Psychology, 81*, 926–931.

Petry, N. M., & Carroll, K. M. (2013). Contingency management is efficacious in opioid-dependent outpatients not maintained on agonist pharmacotherapy. *Psychology of Addictive Behaviors, 27*, 1036–1043.

Petry, N. M., DePhilippis, D., Rash, C. J., Drapkin, M., & McKay, J. R. (2014). Nationwide dissemination of contingency management: The Veterans Administration initiative. *American Journal on Addictions, 23*, 205–210.

Petry, N. M., Peirce, J. M., Stitzer, M. L., Blaine, J., Roll, J. M., Cohen, A., . . . Li, R. (2005). Effect of prize-based incentives on outcomes in stimulant abusers in outpatient psychosocial treatment programs: A National Drug Abuse Treatment

Clinical Trials Network Study. *Archives of General Psychiatry, 62,* 1148–1156.

Pham, M. T. (2007). Emotion and rationality: A critical review and interpretation of empirical evidence. *Review of General Psychology, 11,* 155–178.

Piacentini, J., Bergman, R. L., Chang, S., Langley, A., Peris, T., Wood, J. J., & McCracken, J. (2011). Controlled comparison of family cognitive behavioral therapy and psychoeducation/relaxation training for child obsessive–compulsive disorder. *Journal of the American Academy of Child and Adolescent Psychiatry, 50,* 1149–1161.

Pieper, S., Brosschot, J. F., van der Leeden, R., & Thayer, J. F. (2010). Prolonged cardiac effects of momentary assessed stressful events and worry episodes. *Psychosomatic Medicine, 72,* 570–577.

Pierce, K. A., & Kirkpatrick, D. R. (1992). Do men lie on fear surveys? *Behaviour Research and Therapy, 30,* 415–418.

Pincus, D. B., May, J. E., Whitton, S. W., Mattis, S. G., & Barlow, D. H. (2010). Cognitive-behavioral treatment of panic disorder in adolescence. *Journal of Clinical Child and Adolescent Psychology, 39,* 638–649.

Platt, J. J., & Hermalin, J. (1989). Social skill deficit interventions for substance abusers. *Psychology of Addictive Behaviors, 3,* 114–133.

Platt, J. J., & Metzger, G. (1978). Cognitive interpersonal problem-solving skills and the maintenance of treatment success in heroin addicts. *Psychology of Addictive Behaviors, 1,* 5–13.

Plaud, J. J., & Gaither, G. A. (1996). Behavioral momentum: Implications and development from reinforcement theories. *Behavior Modification, 20,* 183–201.

Polischuk, D., & Collins, D. (1991). Sharks, mice and bears: A group-counseling experience with adolescents. *Journal of Child and Youth Care, 6,* 41–47.

Ponniah, K., & Hollon, S. D. (2008). Empirically supported psychological interventions for social phobia in adults: A qualitative review of randomized controlled trials. *Psychological Medicine, 38,* 3–14.

Poppen, R. (1998). *Behavioral relaxation training and assessment* (2nd ed.). Thousand Oaks, CA: Sage.

Powers, M. B., Halpern, J. M., Ferenschak, M. P., Gillihan, S. J., & Foa, E. B. (2010). A meta-analytic review of prolonged exposure for posttraumatic stress disorder. *Clinical Psychology Review, 30,* 635–641.

Powers, M. B., Smits, J. A., & Telch, M. J. (2004). Disentangling the effects of safety-behavior utilization and safety-behavior availability during exposure-based treatment: A placebo-controlled trial. *Journal of Consulting and Clinical Psychology, 72,* 448–454.

Powers, M. B., Smits, J. A., Whitley, D., Bystritsky, A., & Telch, M. J. (2008). The effect of attributional processes concerning medication taking on return of fear. *Journal of Consulting and Clinical Psychology, 76,* 478–490.

Prasko, J., Diveky, T., Grambal, A., Kamaradova, D., Mozny, P., Sigmundova, Z., . . . Vyskocilova, J. (2010). Transference and countertransference in cognitive behavioral therapy. *Biomedical Papers of the Medical Faculty of the University Palacky, Olomouc, Czechoslovakia, 154,* 189–197.

Premack, D. (1962). Reversibility of the reinforcement relation. *Science, 136,* 255–257.

Prochaska, J. O., & DiClemente, C. C. (1982). Transtheoretical therapy: Toward a more integrated model of change. *Psychotherapy: Theory, Research, and Practice, 19,* 276–288.

Purdon, C., Rowa, K., & Antony, M. M. (2005). Thought suppression and its effects on thought frequency, appraisal and mood state in individuals with obsessive–compulsive disorder. *Behaviour Research and Therapy, 43,* 93–108.

Rabavilas, A. D., Boulougouris, J. C., & Stefanis, C. (1976). Duration of flooding sessions in the treatment of obsessive–compulsive patients. *Behaviour Research and Therapy, 14,* 349–355.

Rachman, S. J. (1984). Agoraphobia—a safety-signal perspective. *Behaviour Research and Therapy, 22,* 59–70.

Rachman, S. J. (1993). Obsessions, responsibility, and guilt. *Behaviour Research and Therapy, 31,* 149–154.

Rachman, S. J., & de Silva, P. (1978). Abnormal and normal obsessions. *Behaviour Research and Therapy, 16,* 233–248.

Rachman, S. J., Radomsky, A. S., & Shafran, R. (2008). Safety behaviour: A reconsideration. *Behaviour Research and Therapy, 46,* 163–173.

Rachman, S. J., Shafran, R., Radomsky, A. S., & Zysk, E. (2011). Reducing contamination by exposure plus safety behaviour. *Journal of Behavior Therapy and Experimental Psychiatry, 42,* 397–404.

Rapee, R. M., Spence, S. H., Cobham, V., & Wignall, A. (2000). *Helping your anxious child: A step-by-step guide for parents.* Oakland, CA: New Harbinger.

Ray, R. D., & Zald, D. H. (2012). Anatomical insights into the interaction of emotion and cognition in the prefrontal cortex. *Neuroscience and Biobehavioral Reviews, 36,* 479–501.

Reiss, S., Peterson, R. A., Gursky, D. M., & McNally, R. J. (1986). Anxiety sensitivity, anxiety frequency and the prediction of fearfulness. *Behaviour Research and Therapy, 24,* 1–8.

Resick, P. A., Nishith, P., & Griffin, M. G. (2003). How well does cognitive-behavioral therapy treat symptoms of complex PTSD? An examination of child sexual abuse survivors within a clinical trial. *CNS Spectrums, 8,* 340–355.

Riener, C., Stefanucci, J. K., Proffitt, D., & Clore, G. L. (2011). An effect of mood on the perception of geographical slant. *Cognition and Emotion, 25,* 174–182.

Rimes, K. A., & Watkins, E. (2005). The effects of

self-focused rumination on global negative self-judgements in depression. *Behaviour Research and Therapy, 43,* 1673–1681.

Rinn, R. C., & Markle, A. (1979). Modification of social skill deficits in children. In A. S. Bellack & M. Hersen (Eds.), *Research and practice in social skills training* (pp. 107–129). New York: Springer.

Riskind, J. H. (1997). Looming vulnerability to threat: A cognitive paradigm for anxiety. *Behaviour Research and Therapy, 35,* 685–702.

Roberts, D. L., Combs, D. R., Willoughby, M., Mintz, J., Gibson, C., Rupp, B., & Penn, D. L. (2014). A randomized, controlled trial of social cognition and interaction training (SCIT) for outpatients with schizophrenia spectrum disorders. *British Journal of Clinical Psychology, 53,* 281–298.

Roberts, N. P., Kitchiner, N. J., Kenardy, J., & Bisson, J. I. (2009). Systematic review and meta-analysis of multiple-session early interventions following traumatic events. *American Journal of Psychiatry, 166,* 293–301.

Roemer, L., & Orsillo, S. M. (2003). Mindfulness: A promising intervention strategy in need of further study. *Clinical Psychology: Science and Practice, 10,* 172–178.

Roemer, L., Orsillo, S. M., & Salters-Pedneault, K. (2008). Efficacy of an acceptance-based behavior therapy for generalized anxiety disorder: Evaluation in a randomized controlled trial. *Journal of Consulting and Clinical Psychology, 76,* 1083–1089.

Rogers, C. R. (1957). The necessary and sufficient conditions of therapeutic personality change. *Journal of Consulting Psychology, 21,* 95–103.

Rogers, C. R., & Skinner, B. F. (1956). Some issues concerning the control of human behavior: A symposium. *Science, 124,* 1057–1066.

Ronen, T. (1992). Cognitive therapy with young children. *Child Psychiatry and Human Development, 23,* 19–30.

Rood, L., Roelofs, J., Bogels, S. M., & Arntz, A. (2012). The effects of experimentally induced rumination, positive reappraisal, acceptance, and distancing when thinking about a stressful event on affect states in adolescents. *Journal of Abnormal Child Psychology, 40,* 73–84.

Rosenfield, D., Zhou, E., Wilhelm, F. H., Conrad, A., Roth, W. T., & Meuret, A. E. (2010). Change point analysis for longitudinal physiological data: Detection of cardio-respiratory changes preceding panic attacks. *Biological Psychology, 84,* 112–120.

Ross, J. A. (1974). The use of contingency contracting in controlling adult nailbiting. *Journal of Behavior Therapy and Experimental Psychiatry, 5,* 105–106.

Rossello, J., & Bernal, G. (1999). The efficacy of cognitive-behavioral and interpersonal treatments for depression in Puerto Rican adolescents. *Journal of Consulting and Clinical Psychology, 67,* 734–745.

Rottenberg, J., Gross, J. J., & Gotlib, I. H. (2005). Emotion context insensitivity in major depressive disorder. *Journal of Abnormal Psychology, 114,* 627–639.

Rotter, J. B. (1966). Generalized expectancies for internal versus external control of reinforcement. *Psychological Monographs, 80,* 1–28.

Rowa, K., Paulitzki, J. R., Ierullo, M. D., Chiang, B., Antony, M. M., McCabe, R. E., & Moscovitch, D. A. (2015). A false sense of security: Safety behaviors erode objective speech performance in individuals with social anxiety disorder. *Behavior Therapy, 46,* 304–314.

Rowa, K., & Purdon, C. (2003). Why are certain intrusive thoughts more upsetting than others? *Behavioural and Cognitive Psychotherapy, 31,* 1–11.

Rudd, M. D., Mandrusiak, M., & Joiner, T. E. (2006). The case against no-suicide contracts: The commitment to treatment statement as a practice alternative. *Journal of Clinical Psychology, 62,* 243–251.

Saavedra, L. M., Silverman, W. K., Morgan-Lopez, A. A., & Kurtines, W. M. (2010). Cognitive behavioral treatment for childhood anxiety disorders: Long-term effects on anxiety and secondary disorders in young adulthood. *Journal of Child Psychology and Psychiatry and Allied Disciplines, 51,* 924–934.

Safran, J. D., & Muran, J. C. (2000). *Negotiating the therapeutic alliance: A relational treatment guide.* New York: Guilford Press.

Safran, J. D., Muran, J. C., & Eubanks-Carter, C. (2011). Repairing alliance ruptures. In J. C. Norcross (Ed.), *Psychotherapy relationships that work: Evidence-based responsiveness* (2nd ed., pp. 224–238). New York: Oxford University Press.

Safran, J. D., & Segal, Z. V. (1996). *Interpersonal process in cognitive therapy.* Northvale, NJ: Aronson.

Salkovskis, P. M. (1985). Obsessional–compulsive problems: A cognitive-behavioural analysis. *Behaviour Research and Therapy, 23,* 571–583.

Salkovskis, P. M. (1999). An experimental investigation of the role of safety-seeking behaviours in the maintenance of panic disorder with agoraphobia. *Behaviour Research and Therapy, 37,* 559–574.

Salkovskis, P. M., Atha, C., & Storer, D. (1990). Cognitive-behavioural problem solving in the treatment of patients who repeatedly attempt suicide: A controlled trial. *British Journal of Psychiatry, 157,* 871–876.

Salkovskis, P. M., Jones, D. R., & Clark, D. M. (1986). Respiratory control in the treatment of panic attacks: Replication and extension with concurrent measurement of behaviour and pCO_2. *British Journal of Psychiatry, 148,* 526–532.

Saltzman, A., & Goldin, P. (2008). Mindfulness-based stress reduction for school-age children. In L. A. Greco & S. C. Hayes (Eds.), *Acceptance and mindfulness treatments for children and adolescents: A practitioner's guide* (pp. 139–161). Oakland, CA: New Harbinger.

Saunders, J. B., Aasland, O. G., Babor, T. F., de la Fuente, J. R., & Grant, M. (1993). Development of the Alcohol Use Disorders Identification Test (AUDIT): WHO Collaborative Project on Early Detection of Persons with Harmful Alcohol Consumption—II. *Addiction, 88*, 791–804.

Schare, M. L., & Wyatt, K. P. (2013). On the evolving nature of exposure therapy. *Behavior Modification, 37*, 243–256.

Schmaling, K. B., Fruzzetti, A. E., & Jacobson, N. S. (1989). Marital problems. In K. Hawton, P. M. Salkovskis, J. Kirk, & D. M. Clark (Eds.), *Cognitive behaviour therapy for psychiatric problems: A practical guide* (pp. 339–369). New York: Oxford University Press.

Schmidt, N. B., Richey, J. A., Buckner, J. D., & Timpano, K. R. (2009). Attention training for generalized social anxiety disorder. *Journal of Abnormal Psychology, 118*, 5–14.

Schmidt, N. B., Richey, J. A., Cromer, K. R., & Buckner, J. D. (2007). Discomfort intolerance: Evaluation of a potential risk factor for anxiety psychopathology. *Behavior Therapy, 38*, 247–255.

Schmidt, N. B., Woolaway-Bickel, K., Trakowski, J., Santiago, H., Storey, J., Koselka, M., & Cook, J. (2000). Dismantling cognitive-behavioral treatment for panic disorder: Questioning the utility of breathing retraining. *Journal of Consulting and Clinical Psychology, 68*, 417–424.

Schneier, F. R., Heckelman, L. R., Garfinkel, R., Campeas, R., Fallon, B. A., Gitow, A., . . . Liebowitz, M. R. (1994). Functional impairment in social phobia. *Journal of Clinical Psychiatry, 55*, 322–331.

Schniering, C. A., & Rapee, R. M. (2002). Development and validation of a measure of children's automatic thoughts: The Children's Automatic Thoughts Scale. *Behaviour Research and Therapy, 40*, 1091–1109.

Schotte, D. E., & Clum, G. A. (1987). Problem-solving skills in suicidal psychiatric patients. *Journal of Consulting and Clinical Psychology, 55*, 49–54.

Schuppert, H. M., Timmerman, M. E., Bloo, J., van Gemert, T. G., Wiersema, H. M., Minderaa, R. B., . . . Nauta, M. H. (2012). Emotion regulation training for adolescents with borderline personality disorder traits: A randomized controlled trial. *Journal of the American Academy of Child and Adolescent Psychiatry, 51*, 1314–1323.e2.

Schwartz, J., & Bellack, A. S. (1975). A comparison of a token economy with standard inpatient treatment. *Journal of Consulting and Clinical Psychology, 43*, 107–108.

Segal, Z. V., Williams, J. M. G., & Teasdale, J. D. (2013). *Mindfulness-based cognitive therapy for depression* (2nd ed.). New York: Guilford Press.

Segrin, C. (1990). A meta-analytic review of social skill deficits in depression. *Communication Monographs, 57*, 292–308.

Segrin, C. (2000). Social skills deficits associated with depression. *Clinical Psychology Review, 20*, 379–403.

Segrin, C. (2008). Social skills training. In W. O'Donohue, J. E. Fisher, & S. C. Hayes (Eds.), *Cognitive behavior therapy: Applying empirically supported techniques in your practice* (pp. 502–509). Hoboken, NJ: Wiley.

Sehlmeyer, C., Schoning, S., Zwitserlood, P., Pfleiderer, B., Kircher, T., Arolt, V., & Konrad, C. (2009). Human fear conditioning and extinction in neuroimaging: A systematic review. *PLoS ONE, 4*, e5865.

Seid, E. L., & Yalom, V. (2009). Instructor's manual. In A. Freeman, *Depression: A cognitive therapy approach* [DVD]. Available at *www.psychotherapy. net/video/depression-cognitive-therapy*.

Seim, R. W., & Spates, R. (2008, May). *The efficacy of dosed exposure therapy in the treatment of small animal phobias.* Paper presented at the annual meeting of the Association for Psychological Science, Chicago, IL.

Seligman, M. E., Abramson, L. Y., Semmel, A., & von Baeyer, C. (1979). Depressive attributional style. *Journal of Abnormal Psychology, 88*, 242–247.

Sensky, T., Turkington, D., Kingdon, D., Scott, J. L., Scott, J., Siddle, R., . . . Barnes, T. R. (2000). A randomized controlled trial of cognitive-behavioral therapy for persistent symptoms in schizophrenia resistant to medication. *Archives of General Psychiatry, 57*, 165–172.

Shadish, W. R., & Baldwin, S. A. (2005). Effects of behavioral marital therapy: A meta-analysis of randomized controlled trials. *Journal of Consulting and Clinical Psychology, 73*, 6–14.

Shadish, W. R., Montgomery, L. M., Wilson, P., Wilson, M. R., Bright, I., & Okwumabua, T. (1993). Effects of family and marital psychotherapies: A meta-analysis. *Journal of Consulting and Clinical Psychology, 61*, 992–1002.

Shafran, R., Cooper, Z., & Fairburn, C. G. (2002). Clinical perfectionism: A cognitive-behavioural analysis. *Behaviour Research and Therapy, 40*, 773–791.

Shafran, R., Lee, M., Cooper, Z., Palmer, R. L., & Fairburn, C. G. (2007). Attentional bias in eating disorders. *International Journal of Eating Disorders, 40*, 369–380.

Shapiro, D. (1989). *Psychotherapy of neurotic character.* New York: Basic Books.

Shawyer, F., Farhall, J., Mackinnon, A., Trauer, T., Sims, E., Ratcliff, K., . . . Copolov, D. (2012). A randomised controlled trial of acceptance-based cognitive behavioural therapy for command hallucinations in psychotic disorders. *Behaviour Research and Therapy, 50*, 110–121.

Shear, M. K., Brown, T. A., Barlow, D. H., Money, R., Sholomskas, D. E., Woods, S. W., . . . Papp, L. A. (1997). Multicenter Collaborative Panic Disorder Severity Scale. *American Journal of Psychiatry, 154*, 1571–1575.

Sheehan, D. V. (2008). Sheehan Disability Scale. In A. Rush, M. First, & D. Blacker (Eds.), *Handbook of psychiatric measures* (2nd ed., pp. 100–102). Washington, DC: American Psychiatric Publishing.

Sheehan, D. V., Lecrubier, Y., Sheehan, K. H., Amorim, P., Janavs, J., Weiller, E., . . . Dunbar, G. C. (1998). The Mini-International Neuropsychiatric Interview (M.I.N.I.): The development and validation of a structured diagnostic psychiatric interview for DSM-IV and ICD-10. *Journal of Clinical Psychiatry, 59*(Suppl. 20), 22–33; quiz, 34–57.

Shipherd, J. C., & Beck, J. G. (1999). The effects of suppressing trauma-related thoughts on women with rape-related posttraumatic stress disorder. *Behaviour Research and Therapy, 37,* 99–112.

Shishido, H., Gaher, R. M., & Simons, J. S. (2013). I don't know how I feel, therefore I act: Alexithymia, urgency, and alcohol problems. *Addictive Behaviors, 38,* 2014–2017.

Siev, J., & Chambless, D. L. (2007). Specificity of treatment effects: Cognitive therapy and relaxation for generalized anxiety and panic disorders. *Journal of Consulting and Clinical Psychology, 75,* 513–522.

Sifneos, P. E. (1973). The prevalence of "alexithymic" characteristics in psychosomatic patients. *Psychotherapy and Psychosomatics, 22,* 255–262.

Sifneos, P. E. (1996). Alexithymia: Past and present. *American Journal of Psychiatry, 153,* 137–142.

Simons, J., & Gaher, R. (2005). The Distress Tolerance Scale: Development and validation of a self-report measure. *Motivation and Emotion, 29,* 83–102.

Skinner, B. F. (1938). *The behavior of organisms: An experimental analysis.* New York: Appleton-Century-Crofts.

Skinner, B. F. (1974). *About behaviorism.* New York: Knopf.

Skinner, H. A. (1982). The drug abuse screening test. *Addictive Behaviors, 7,* 363–371.

Sloan, T., & Telch, M. J. (2002). The effects of safety-seeking behavior and guided threat reappraisal on fear reduction during exposure: An experimental investigation. *Behaviour Research and Therapy, 40,* 235–251.

Slocum, S. K., & Tiger, J. H. (2011). An assessment of the efficiency of and child preference for forward and backward chaining. *Journal of Applied Behavior Analysis, 44,* 793–805.

Smith, T. E., Bellack, A. S., & Liberman, R. P. (1996). Social skills training for schizophrenia: Review and future directions. *Clinical Psychology Review, 16,* 599–617.

Smits, J. A., Powers, M. B., Cho, Y., & Telch, M. J. (2004). Mechanism of change in cognitive-behavioral treatment of panic disorder: Evidence for the fear of fear mediational hypothesis. *Journal of Consulting and Clinical Psychology, 72,* 646–652.

Soler, J., Pascual, J. C., Tiana, T., Cebria, A., Barrachina, J., Campins, M. J., . . . Perez, V. (2009). Dialectical behaviour therapy skills training compared to standard group therapy in borderline personality disorder: A 3-month randomised controlled clinical trial. *Behaviour Research and Therapy, 47,* 353–358.

Solomon, R. L., Kamin, L. J., & Wynne, L. C. (1953). Traumatic avoidance learning: The outcomes of several extinction procedures with dogs. *Journal of Abnormal Psychology, 48,* 291–302.

Sotres-Bayon, F., Cain, C. K., & LeDoux, J. E. (2006). Brain mechanisms of fear extinction: Historical perspectives on the contribution of prefrontal cortex. *Biological Psychiatry, 60,* 329–336.

Sotsky, S. M., Glass, D. R., Shea, M. T., Pilkonis, P. A., Collins, J. F., Elkin, I., . . . Moyer, J. (1991). Patient predictors of response to psychotherapy and pharmacotherapy: Findings in the NIMH Treatment of Depression Collaborative Research Program. *American Journal of Psychiatry, 148,* 997–1008.

Speckens, A. E., & Hawton, K. (2005). Social problem solving in adolescents with suicidal behavior: A systematic review. *Suicide and Life-Threatening Behavior, 35,* 365–387.

Spence, S. H. (1994). Cognitive therapy with children and adolescents: From theory to practice. *Journal of Child Psychology and Psychiatry and Allied Disciplines, 35,* 1191–1228.

Spence, S. H., Donovan, C., & Brechman-Toussaint, M. (2000). The treatment of childhood social phobia: The effectiveness of a social skills training-based, cognitive-behavioural intervention, with and without parental involvement. *Journal of Child Psychology and Psychiatry and Allied Disciplines, 41,* 713–726.

Spencer, T. J., Adler, L. A., Meihua, Q., Saylor, K. E., Brown, T. E., Holdnack, J. A., . . . Kelsey, D. K. (2010). Validation of the Adult ADHD Investigator Symptom Rating Scale (AISRS). *Journal of Attention Disorders, 14,* 57–68.

Spurr, J. M., & Stopa, L. (2002). The observer perspective: Effects on social anxiety and performance. *Behaviour Research and Therapy, 22,* 947–975.

Stallard, P. (2002). Cognitive behaviour therapy with children and young people: A selective review of key issues. *Behavioural and Cognitive Psychotherapy, 30,* 297–309.

Stapinski, L. A., Abbott, M. J., & Rapee, R. M. (2010). Evaluating the cognitive avoidance model of generalised anxiety disorder: Impact of worry on threat appraisal, perceived control and anxious arousal. *Behaviour Research and Therapy, 48,* 1032–1040.

Starr, S., & Moulds, M. L. (2006). The role of negative interpretations of intrusive memories in depression. *Journal of Affective Disorders, 93,* 125–132.

Stasiewicz, P. R., Bradizza, C. M., Schlauch, R. C.,

Coffey, S. F., Gulliver, S. B., Gudleski, G. D., & Bole, C. W. (2013). Affect regulation training (ART) for alcohol use disorders: Development of a novel intervention for negative affect drinkers. *Journal of Substance Abuse Treatment, 45,* 433–443.

Staub, E., Tursky, B., & Schwartz, G. E. (1971). Self-control and predictability: Their effects on reactions to aversive stimulation. *Journal of Personality and Social Psychology, 18,* 157–162.

Stefanopoulou, E., Hirsch, C. R., Hayes, S., Adlam, A., & Coker, S. (2014). Are attentional control resources reduced by worry in generalized anxiety disorder? *Journal of Abnormal Psychology, 123,* 330–335.

Stepp, S. D., Epler, A. J., Jahng, S., & Trull, T. J. (2008). The effect of dialectical behavior therapy skills use on borderline personality disorder features. *Journal of Personality Disorders, 22,* 549–563.

Stern, J. B., & Fodor, I. G. (1989). Anger control in children: A review of social skills and cognitive behavioral approaches to dealing with aggressive children. *Child and Family Behavior Therapy, 11,* 1–20.

Stern, R., & Marks, I. (1973). Brief and prolonged flooding: A comparison in agoraphobic patients. *Archives of General Psychiatry, 28,* 270–276.

Stokes, T. F., & Baer, D. M. (1977). An implicit technology of generalization. *Journal of Applied Behavior Analysis, 10,* 349–367.

Stone, M., & Borkovec, T. D. (1975). The paradoxical effect of brief CS exposure on analogue phobic subjects. *Behaviour Research and Therapy, 13,* 51–54.

Storebo, O. J., Gluud, C., Winkel, P., & Simonsen, E. (2012). Social-skills and parental training plus standard treatment versus standard treatment for children with ADHD—the randomised SOSTRA trial. *PLoS ONE, 7,* e37280.

Stotts, A. L., Green, C., Masuda, A., Grabowski, J., Wilson, K., Northrup, T. F., . . . Schmitz, J. M. (2012). A stage I pilot study of acceptance and commitment therapy for methadone detoxification. *Drug and Alcohol Dependence, 125,* 215–222.

Strand, P. S. (2000). A modern behavioral perspective on child conduct disorder: Integrating behavioral momentum and matching theory. *Clinical Psychology Review, 20,* 593–615.

Strupp, H. H., & Binder, J. L. (1984). *Psychotherapy in a new key.* New York: Basic Books.

Stuart, R. B. (1971). A three-dimensional program for the treatment of obesity. *Behaviour Research and Therapy, 9,* 177–186.

Sturmey, P. (2004). Cognitive therapy with people with intellectual disabilities: A selective review and critique. *Clinical Psychology and Psychotherapy, 11,* 222–232.

Sue, D. W. (2001). Multidimensional facets of cultural competence. *Counseling Psychologist, 29,* 790–821.

Sue, D. W., Ivey, A. E., & Pedersen, P. B. (1996). *A theory of multicultural counseling and therapy.* San Francisco: Brooks/Cole.

Sue, S. (1998). In search of cultural competence in psychotherapy and counseling. *American Psychologist, 53,* 440–448.

Sue, S., Zane, N., Nagayama Hall, G. C., & Berger, L. K. (2009). The case for cultural competency in psychotherapeutic interventions. *Annual Review of Psychology, 60,* 525–548.

Suinn, R. M., & Richardson, F. (1971). Anxiety management training: A nonspecific behavior therapy program for anxiety control. *Behavior Therapy, 2,* 498–510.

Sukhodolsky, D. G., Gorman, B. S., Scahill, L., Findley, D., & McGuire, J. (2013). Exposure and response prevention with or without parent management training for children with obsessive-compulsive disorder complicated by disruptive behavior: A multiple-baseline across-responses design study. *Journal of Anxiety Disorders, 27,* 298–305.

Sy, J. T., Dixon, L. J., Lickel, J. J., Nelson, E. A., & Deacon, B. J. (2011). Failure to replicate the deleterious effects of safety behaviors in exposure therapy. *Behaviour Research and Therapy, 49,* 305–314.

Taylor, C. T., & Amir, N. (2010). Attention and emotion regulation. In A. M. Kring & D. M. Sloan (Eds.), *Emotion regulation and psychopathology: A transdiagnostic approach to treatment* (pp. 380–404). New York: Guilford Press.

Taylor, G. J. (1984). Alexithymia: Concept, measurement, and implications for treatment. *American Journal of Psychiatry, 141,* 725–732.

Taylor, G. J., & Bagby, R. M. (2013). Psychoanalysis and empirical research: The example of alexithymia. *Journal of the American Psychoanalytic Association, 61,* 99–133.

Teasdale, J. D., Scott, J., Moore, R. G., Hayhurst, H., Pope, M., & Paykel, E. S. (2001). How does cognitive therapy prevent relapse in residual depression?: Evidence from a controlled trial. *Journal of Consulting and Clinical Psychology, 69,* 347–357.

Teasdale, J. D., Segal, Z. V., Williams, J. M. G., Ridgeway, V. A., Soulsby, J. M., & Lau, M. A. (2000). Prevention of relapse/recurrence in major depression by mindfulness-based cognitive therapy. *Journal of Consulting and Clinical Psychology, 68,* 615–623.

Telch, C. F., Agras, W. S., & Linehan, M. M. (2001). Dialectical behavior therapy for binge eating disorder. *Journal of Consulting and Clinical Psychology, 69,* 1061–1065.

Telch, M. J., Valentiner, D. P., Ilai, D., Young, P. R., Powers, M. B., & Smits, J. A. (2004). Fear activation and distraction during the emotional processing of claustrophobic fear. *Journal of Behavior Therapy and Experimental Psychiatry, 35,* 219–232.

Thoma, P., Friedmann, C., & Suchan, B. (2013). Empathy and social problem solving in alcohol dependence, mood disorders and selected personality disorders. *Neuroscience and Biobehavioral Reviews, 37,* 448–470.

Thompson, R. A. (1994). Emotion regulation: A theme in search of definition. *Monographs of the Society for Research in Child Development, 59,* 25–52.

Thompson, S., & Rapee, R. M. (2002). The effect of situational structure on the social performance of socially anxious and non-anxious participants. *Journal of Behavior Therapy and Experimental Psychiatry, 33,* 91–102.

Thorberg, F. A., Young, R. M., Sullivan, K. A., & Lyvers, M. (2009). Alexithymia and alcohol use disorders: A critical review. *Addictive Behaviors, 34,* 237–245.

Thorndike, E. L. (1901). Animal intelligence: An experimental study of the associative processes in animals. *Psychological Review Monograph Supplement, 2,* 1–109.

Thorsell, J., Finnes, A., Dahl, J., Lundgren, T., Gybrant, M., Gordh, T., & Buhrman, M. (2011). A comparative study of 2 manual-based self-help interventions, acceptance and commitment therapy and applied relaxation, for persons with chronic pain. *Clinical Journal of Pain, 27,* 716–723.

Tisdelle, D. A., & St. Lawrence, J. S. (1986). Interpersonal problem-solving competency: Review and critique of the literature. *Clinical Psychology Review, 6,* 337–356.

Tolin, D. F. (2010). Is cognitive-behavioral therapy more effective than other therapies? A meta-analytic review. *Clinical Psychology Review, 30,* 710–720.

Tolin, D. F. (2012). *Face your fears: A proven plan to beat anxiety, panic, phobias, and obsessions.* Hoboken, NJ: Wiley.

Tolin, D. F., Abramowitz, J. S., Hamlin, C., Foa, E. B., & Synodi, D. S. (2002). Attributions for thought suppression failure in obsessive–compulsive disorder. *Cognitive Therapy and Research, 26,* 505–517.

Tolin, D. F., Abramowitz, J. S., Przeworski, A., & Foa, E. B. (2002). Thought suppression in obsessive–compulsive disorder. *Behaviour Research and Therapy, 40,* 1255–1274.

Tolin, D. F., & Franklin, M. E. (2002). Prospects for the use of cognitive-behavioral therapy in childhood obsessive–compulsive disorder. *Expert Review of Neurotherapeutics, 2,* 89–98.

Tolin, D. F., Gilliam, C. M., Wootton, B. M., Bowe, W., Bragdon, L. B., Davis, E., . . . Hallion, L. S. (in press). Reliability and validity of a structured diagnostic interview for DSM-5 anxiety, mood, and obsessive–compulsive and related disorders. *Assessment.*

Tolin, D. F., Woods, C. M., & Abramowitz, J. S. (2003). Relationship between obsessive beliefs and obsessive–compulsive symptoms. *Cognitive Therapy and Research, 27,* 657–669.

Treadwell, K. R. H., & Tolin, D. F. (2007). Clinical challenges in the treatment of pediatric OCD.

In E. A. Storch, T. K. Murphy, & G. R. Geffken (Eds.), *A comprehensive handbook of child and adolescent obsessive–compulsive disorder* (pp. 273–294). Mahwah, NJ: Erlbaum.

Truax, C. B. (1966). Reinforcement and nonreinforcement in Rogerian psychotherapy. *Journal of Abnormal Psychology, 71,* 1–9.

Tsai, M., Kohlenberg, R. J., Kanter, J. W., & Waltz, J. (2009). Therapeutic technique: The five rules. In M. Tsai, R. J. Kohlenberg, J. W. Kanter, B. Kohlenberg, W. C. Follette, & G. M. Callaghan (Eds.), *A guide to functional analytic psychotherapy: Awareness, courage, love, and behaviorism* (pp. 61–102). New York: Springer.

Tse, W. S., & Bond, A. J. (2004). The impact of depression on social skills. *Journal of Nervous and Mental Disease, 192,* 260–268.

Turk, D. C., Meichenbaum, D., & Genest, M. (1983). *Pain and behavioral medicine: A cognitive-behavioral perspective.* New York: Guilford Press.

Turner, S. M., Beidel, D. C., Dancu, C. V., & Keys, D. J. (1986). Psychopathology of social phobia and comparison to avoidant personality disorder. *Journal of Abnormal Psychology, 95,* 389–394.

Twohig, M. P., Hayes, S. C., Plumb, J. C., Pruitt, L. D., Collins, A. B., Hazlett-Stevens, H., & Woidneck, M. R. (2010). A randomized clinical trial of acceptance and commitment therapy versus progressive relaxation training for obsessive–compulsive disorder. *Journal of Consulting and Clinical Psychology, 78,* 705–716.

Twohig, M. P., & Woods, D. W. (2001). Evaluating the duration of the competing response in habit reversal: A parametric analysis. *Journal of Applied Behavior Analysis, 34,* 517–520.

Valentine, S. E., Bankoff, S. M., Poulin, R. M., Reidler, E. B., & Pantalone, D. W. (2015). The use of dialectical behavior therapy skills training as stand-alone treatment: A systematic review of the treatment outcome literature. *Journal of Clinical Psychology, 71,* 1–20.

Valentiner, D. P., & Smith, S. A. (2008). Believing that intrusive thoughts can be immoral moderates the relationship between obsessions and compulsions for shame-prone individuals. *Cognitive Therapy and Research, 32,* 714–720.

van Aalderen, J. R., Donders, A. R., Giommi, F., Spinhoven, P., Barendregt, H. P., & Speckens, A. E. (2012). The efficacy of mindfulness-based cognitive therapy in recurrent depressed patients with and without a current depressive episode: A randomized controlled trial. *Psychological Medicine, 42,* 989–1001.

van der Heiden, C., Muris, P., & van der Molen, H. T. (2012). Randomized controlled trial on the effectiveness of metacognitive therapy and intolerance-of-uncertainty therapy for generalized anxiety disorder. *Behaviour Research and Therapy, 50,* 100–109.

van Manen, T. G., Prins, P. J., & Emmelkamp, P. M. (2004). Reducing aggressive behavior in boys with a social cognitive group treatment: Results of a randomized, controlled trial. *Journal of the American Academy of Child and Adolescent Psychiatry, 43,* 1478–1487.

van Minnen, A., & Foa, E. B. (2006). The effect of imaginal exposure length on outcome of treatment for PTSD. *Journal of Traumatic Stress, 19,* 427–438.

van Minnen, A., Hendriks, L., & Olff, M. (2010). When do trauma experts choose exposure therapy for PTSD patients? A controlled study of therapist and patient factors. *Behaviour Research and Therapy, 48,* 312–320.

Verheul, R., van den Brink, W., & Hartgers, C. (1998). Personality disorders predict relapse in alcoholic patients. *Addictive Behaviors, 23,* 869–882.

Viane, I., Crombez, G., Eccleston, C., Poppe, C., Devulder, J., Van Houdenhove, B., & De Corte, W. (2003). Acceptance of pain is an independent predictor of mental well-being in patients with chronic pain: Empirical evidence and reappraisal. *Pain, 106,* 65–72.

Visser, S., & Bouman, T. K. (2001). The treatment of hypochondriasis: Exposure plus response prevention vs. cognitive therapy. *Behaviour Research and Therapy, 39,* 423–442.

Vowles, K. E., McNeil, D. W., Gross, R. T., McDaniel, M. L., Mouse, A., Bates, M., . . . McCall, C. (2007). Effects of pain acceptance and pain control strategies on physical impairment in individuals with chronic low back pain. *Behavior Therapy, 38,* 412–425.

Vowles, K. E., Wetherell, J. L., & Sorrell, J. M. (2009). Targeting acceptance, mindfulness, and values-based action in chronic pain: Findings of two preliminary trials of an outpatient group-based intervention. *Cognitive and Behavioral Practice, 16,* 49–58.

Wachtel, P. L. (1982). *Resistance: Psychodynamic and behavioral approaches.* New York: Plenum Press.

Wadsworth, B. J. (1996). *Piaget's theory of cognitive and affective development: Foundations of constructivism.* New York: Longman.

Wahler, R. G., Williams, A. J., & Cerezo, A. (1990). The compliance and predictability hypotheses: Some sequential and correlational analyses of coercive mother–child interactions. *Behavioral Assessment, 12,* 391–407.

Waldeck, T. L., & Miller, L. S. (2000). Social skills deficits in schizotypal personality disorder. *Psychiatry Research, 93,* 237–246.

Wallace, C. J., & Liberman, R. P. (1985). Social skills training for patients with schizophrenia: A controlled clinical trial. *Psychiatry Research, 15,* 239–247.

Walton, K. M., & Ingersoll, B. R. (2013). Improving social skills in adolescents and adults with autism and severe to profound intellectual disability: A review of the literature. *Journal of Autism and Developmental Disorders, 43,* 594–615.

Ware, J. E. (1993). *SF-36 Health Survey Manual and Interpretation Guide.* Boston: Health Institute, New England Medical Center.

Ware, J. E., Kosinski, M., & Keller, S. D. (1996). A 12-item short form health survey: Construction of scales and preliminary tests of reliability and validity. *Medical Care, 34,* 220–233.

Watkins, E., & Brown, R. G. (2002). Rumination and executive function in depression: An experimental study. *Journal of Neurology, Neurosurgery and Psychiatry, 72,* 400–402.

Watson, J. B., & Rayner, R. (1920). Conditioned emotional reactions. *Journal of Experimental Psychology, 3,* 1–14.

Watts, F. N., McKenna, F. P., Sharrock, R., & Trezise, L. (1986). Colour naming of phobia-related words. *British Journal of Psychology, 77*(Pt. 1), 97–108.

Weber, F., & Exner, C. (2013). Metacognitive beliefs and rumination: A longitudinal study. *Cognitive Therapy and Research, 37,* 1257–1261.

Webster-Stratton, C., & Hammond, M. (1997). Treating children with early-onset conduct problems: A comparison of child and parent training interventions. *Journal of Consulting and Clinical Psychology, 65,* 93–109.

Wedig, M. M., & Nock, M. K. (2007). Parental expressed emotion and adolescent self-injury. *Journal of the American Academy of Child and Adolescent Psychiatry, 46,* 1171–1178.

Wegner, D. M., Erber, R., & Zanakos, S. (1993). Ironic processes in the mental control of mood and mood-related thought. *Journal of Personality and Social Psychology, 65,* 1093–1104.

Wegner, D. M., Schneider, D. J., Carter, S. R., & White, T. L. (1987). Paradoxical effects of thought suppression. *Journal of Personality and Social Psychology, 53,* 5–13.

Wells, A. (2009). *Metacognitive therapy for anxiety and depression.* New York: Guilford Press.

Wells, A., Clark, D. M., Salkovskis, P. M., Ludgate, J., Hackmann, A., & Gelder, M. (1995). Social phobia: The role of in-situation safety behaviors in maintaining anxiety and negative beliefs. *Behavior Therapy, 26,* 153–161.

Wells, A., Welford, M., King, P., Papageorgiou, C., Wisely, J., & Mendel, E. (2010). A pilot randomized trial of metacognitive therapy vs. applied relaxation in the treatment of adults with generalized anxiety disorder. *Behaviour Research and Therapy, 48,* 429–434.

Wenzel, A., Graff-Dolezal, J., Macho, M., & Brendle, J. R. (2005). Communication and social skills in socially anxious and nonanxious individuals in the context of romantic relationships. *Behaviour Research and Therapy, 43,* 505–519.

Wenzlaff, R. M., & Wegner, D. M. (2000). Thought

suppression. *Annual Review of Psychology, 51,* 59–91.

Werner, K., & Gross, J. J. (2010). Emotion regulation and psychopathology: A conceptual framework. In A. M. Kring & D. M. Sloan (Eds.), *Emotion regulation and psychopathology: A transdiagnostic approach to etiology and treatment* (pp. 13–37). New York: Guilford Press.

Westen, D. (1994). Toward an integrative model of affect regulation: Applications to social-psychological research. *Journal of Personality, 62,* 641–667.

Westen, D., Novotny, C. M., & Thompson-Brenner, H. (2004). The empirical status of empirically supported psychotherapies: Assumptions, findings, and reporting in controlled clinical trials. *Psychological Bulletin, 130,* 631–663.

Westra, H. A., Stewart, S. H., & Conrad, B. E. (2002). Naturalistic manner of benzodiazepine use and cognitive behavioral therapy outcome in panic disorder with agoraphobia. *Journal of Anxiety Disorders, 16,* 233–246.

Whaley, A. L., & Davis, K. E. (2007). Cultural competence and evidence-based practice in mental health services: A complementary perspective. *American Psychologist, 62,* 563–574.

Wicksell, R. K., Dahl, J., Magnusson, B., & Olsson, G. L. (2005). Using acceptance and commitment therapy in the rehabilitation of an adolescent female with chronic pain: A case example. *Cognitive and Behavioral Practice, 12,* 415–423.

Wilhelm, F. H., Trabert, W., & Roth, W. T. (2001). Characteristics of sighing in panic disorder. *Biological Psychiatry, 49,* 606–614.

Williams, J. M. G., Alatiq, Y., Crane, C., Barnhofer, T., Fennell, M. J., Duggan, D. S., . . . Goodwin, G. M. (2008). Mindfulness-based cognitive therapy (MBCT) in bipolar disorder: Preliminary evaluation of immediate effects on between-episode functioning. *Journal of Affective Disorders, 107,* 275–279.

Williams, J. M. G., Watts, F. N., MacLeod, C., & Mathews, A. (1997). *Cognitive psychology and emotional disorders* (2nd ed.). New York: Wiley.

Williams, M., Teasdale, J., Segal, Z., & Kabat-Zinn, J. (2007). *The mindful way through depression: Freeing yourself from chronic unhappiness.* New York: Guilford Press.

Williams, W. L., & Burkholder, E. (2003). Behavioral chaining. In W. O'Donohue, J. E. Fisher, & S. C. Hayes (Eds.), *Cognitive behavior therapy: Applying empirically supported techniques in your practice* (pp. 33–39). Hoboken, NJ: Wiley.

Wimperis, B. R., & Farr, J. L. (1979). The effects of task content and reward contingency upon task performance and satisfaction. *Journal of Applied Social Psychology, 9,* 229–249.

Wolgast, M., Lundh, L. G., & Viborg, G. (2011). Cognitive reappraisal and acceptance: An experimental comparison of two emotion regulation strategies. *Behaviour Research and Therapy, 49,* 858–866.

Wolpe, J. (1961). The systematic desensitization treatment of neuroses. *Journal of Nervous and Mental Disease, 132,* 189–203.

Wolpe, J. (1990). *The practice of behavior therapy* (4th ed.). New York: Pergamon Press.

Wood, V., Wylie, M. L., & Sheafor, B. (1969). An analysis of a short self-report measure of life satisfaction: Correlation with rater judgments. *Journal of Gerontology, 24,* 465–469.

Wright, J. H., Basco, M. R., & Thase, M. E. (2006). *Learning cognitive-behavior therapy: An illustrated guide.* Arlington, VA: American Psychiatric Association.

Yalom, I. D. (1995). *The theory and practice of group psychotherapy* (4th ed.). New York: Basic Books.

Yerkes, R. M., & Dodson, J. D. (1908). The relation of strength of stimulus to rapidity of habit-formation. *Journal of Comparative Neurology and Psychology, 18,* 459–482.

Yoshizumi, T., & Murase, S. (2007). The effect of avoidant tendencies on the intensity of intrusive memories in a community sample of college students. *Personality and Individual Differences, 43,* 1819–1828.

Young, J. E. (1999). *Cognitive therapy for personality disorders: A schema-focused approach.* Sarasota, FL: Professional Resource Press.

Young, J. E., Klosko, J. S., & Weishaar, M. E. (2003). *Schema therapy: A practitioner's guide.* New York: Guilford Press.

Zajonc, R. B. (1984). On the primacy of affect. *American Psychologist, 39,* 117–123.

Zoellner, L. A., Feeny, N. C., Cochran, B., & Pruitt, L. (2003). Treatment choice for PTSD. *Behaviour Research and Therapy, 41,* 879–886.

Index